HANDBUCH DER UROLOGIE

ENCYCLOPEDIA OF UROLOGY

ENCYCLOPÉDIE D'UROLOGIE

HERAUSGEGEBEN VON · EDITED BY
PUBLIÉE SOUS LA DIRECTION DE

C. E. ALKEN **V. W. DIX** **H. M. WEYRAUCH**
HOMBURG (SAAR) LONDON SAN FRANCISCO

E. WILDBOLZ
BERN

XV

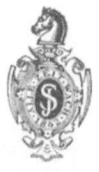

Springer-Verlag Berlin Heidelberg GmbH 1958

UROLOGY IN CHILDHOOD

BY

D. INNES WILLIAMS

M. D., M. CHIR. (CANTAB), F. R. C. S. (ENG.)
SURGEON, ST. PETER'S AND ST. PAUL'S HOSPITALS
GENITO-URINARY SURGEON, THE HOSPITAL FOR SICK CHILDREN
GREAT ORMOND STREET AND WHIPPS CROSS HOSPITAL, LONDON

WITH 162 FIGURES

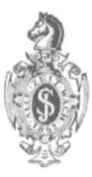

Springer-Verlag Berlin Heidelberg GmbH 1958

© by Springer-Verlag Berlin Heidelberg 1958

Ursprünglich erschienen bei Springer Verlag OHG Berlin Gottigen Heidelberg 1958.

Softcover reprint of the hardcover 1st edition 1958

ISBN 978-3-662-37353-8   ISBN 978-3-662-38095-6 (eBook)
DOI 10.1007/978-3-662-38095-6

Foreword

This volume is concerned with the clinical aspects of urology in childhood; the anatomy, physiology and pathology are discussed only where they have a direct bearing upon the clinical problem, and for a detailed description of these aspects, and of operative technique, the reader is referred to other volumes of this series. Emphasis is laid upon the disorders peculiar to infants and children, so that diseases such as tuberculosis, the manifestations of which in the child differ little from those in the adult, receive less attention. Childhood is deemed to cease with the completion of puberty, though illustrations have sometimes been taken from adolescent cases.

The personal views expressed in this work are based upon experience at The Hospital for Sick Children, Great Ormond Street, at St. Peter's and St. Paul's Hospitals, and at the Institute of Urology, University of London. I am deeply indebted to all my colleagues and assistants at these institutions for their help and co-operation both in the treatment of cases and in the preparation of this volume. I would particularly wish to thank Mr. T. T. TWISTINGTON HIGGINS for introducing me to the urology of childhood, Drs. M. BODIAN, R. C. B. PUGH and L. L. R. WHITE for their assistance in matters of pathology, and for preparing specimens for illustration, Dr. W. W. PAYNE for his advice on biochemistry, Dr. I. A. B. CATHIE for notes on nuclear sexing, Dr. BERNARD SCHLESINGER and Dr. P. R. EVANS for correcting the chapters concerned with renal disease, and Dr. SNAITH for guidance in endocrinology. I must further acknowledge the indispensable assistance which I have received from the Departments of Medical Illustration at The Hospital for Sick Children, and at The Institute of Urology in the preparation of illustrations. For permission to reproduce figures first published in their journals, I am indebted to the Editors of The British Journal of Urology (Figs. 28, 133, 134), The British Medical Journal (Fig. 59), The British Journal of Radiology (Figs. 54, 55, 62) and to Butterworths Medical Publications (Fig. 42).

London, 31st August, 1957   D. Innes Williams

Contents

A. Introduction

I. The basic requirements for paediatric urology

The systematic study of the urological diseases of childhood, which is the theme of this volume, is a comparatively recent development, for although many of the pioneers of urology such as MARION and H. H. YOUNG made important contributions on particular disorders, it is only in the last quarter of a century that the subject as a whole has received the attention which it deserves, and the disorders have been seen in their proper context as problems in the management of infants and children as well as variations on familiar problems in urology.

Recent advances in paediatric urology have come from two distinct groups; on the one hand a number of leading urologists, amongst whom MEREDITH CAMPBELL of New York must be accorded first place, have devoted increasing attention to the special problems of childhood; they have adapted well established methods and instruments to the particular circumstances and shown that the basic principles that have served adult urology well have also an application to children. On the other hand the newly emerged specialists, the paediatric surgeons, have included urology within their scope and have demonstrated how successfully surgical procedures can be undertaken in early infancy when the whole organisation of the unit is geared to the management of children. Both these groups have an important contribution to make, and provided there is a free interchange of ideas, paediatric urology will continue to thrive, not as an independent speciality but as a special interest of a few surgeons whose other work keeps them fully in touch with the broad advances of surgery.

The basic requirement of children's urology therefore is not simply a small cystoscope, it is the whole apparatus of a children's surgical unit. It is true that the special needs of the boy of 8 or 9 years are not numerous, but with the steady advance of paediatrics disorders are increasingly recognised at an early stage, and the most rewarding work is done on children in the first five years of life, when both the physical and psychological needs are entirely different from those of adult patients. Nurses and sisters with a training in children's work are of course indispensable, the resident medical personnel must be accustomed to the postoperative care of infants, and able to perform such special procedures as intravenous infusions into the scalp veins, and it is desirable that all ancilliary workers should have some experience of handling children; the radiographers must be prepared for the child's reluctance to keep still, the laboratory staff must be able to perform chemical estimations on blood obtained by finger or heel prick so that numerous venepunctures can be avoided. In this imperfect world it is unlikely that any surgeon will obtain for his patients all the facilities he desires, and children's urology like any other surgical activity must usually be carried out under conditions which fall a long way short of the ideal, but there can be no doubt that it will yield better results when it is undertaken in a children's unit rather than in a side ward of a urological unit.

The co-operation of the paediatrician is a sine qua non, and many of the cases will only be discovered after investigation in the medical ward, but the surgeon himself must understand sufficient of the management of children to retain full control of the pre- and post-operative care.

II. The nature of genito-urinary disease in children

With the general advance of paediatrics and preventive medicine, acquired disease is becoming less frequent and less severe, and as a consequence the congenital abnormalities provide a steadily increasing proportion of the cases requiring treatment. This general observation is well exemplified in the urological field: whereas in many countries of the Near and Far East where dietary deficiencies are common, vesical calculus is the most important surgical disorder, in Western Europe and America it is now rare. Similarly renal tuberculosis seldom affects young children in England, although it is still reported to be common in parts of Eastern Europe where nutritional and hygienic standards are low.

The external congenital deformities of the genitalia and lower urinary tract constitute a large group of genito-urinary disorders: they range from gross and invariably fatal malformations such as ectopia cloacae to the most minor degrees of hypospadias. Amongst primitive peoples these cases are seldom brought for treatment, perhaps the afflicted children fail to survive, but in countries with a high standard of medical care they pose some of the most perplexing problems, and while a satisfactory solution is often possible, at times the surgeon is pressed to operate upon the hopeless cases with multiple abnormalities, or at the other extreme upon minor and insignificant deformities which involve no handicap if left untreated. The diagnosis is made by simple inspection, and cases therefore reach the surgeon direct from the general practitioner or obstetrician.

By contrast, the "internal" deformities are not immediately apparent: they cause obstruction or predispose to infection or stone formation and produce symptoms simulating acquired disease, yet in childhood a basis in a malformation should always be sought as an explanation. Even the neoplasms of childhood are commonly embryonic tumours, and there is a very real sense in which these too may be considered to be congenital abnormalities. Occasionally a hereditary defect is known and the risks of malformation can be calculated, as in polycystic disease and some forms of intersex; at other times there is a familial tendency but some other factor is required to bring out the malformation, as in hypospadias. Rarely the deviation from normal development can be traced to a definite event during pregnancy, a virus infection, for instance, or exposure to irradiation.

The symptoms of many forms of urinary tract disease are such that their origin is not immediately recognized, and for this reason cases are first seen by the paediatrician rather than the surgeon. Many infants suffering from chronic urinary infection or obstruction are brought up with such complaints as vomiting, loss of weight, or a vague failure to thrive. The causes of such complaints are manifold and involve many systems of the body: it is only by careful abdominal palpation and routine urine tests that the urological cases will be sorted out, and only by further special investigations that an exact diagnosis will be reached. The early diagnosis of urological disease is therefore dependent upon the vigilance of the paediatrician, with whom the surgeon must maintain a close liaison.

The disorders of micturition which are the common symptoms of urinary tract disorders in childhood are discussed later in this volume: retention in Section E; incontinence in Section F; anuria, polyuria and haematuria in Section M. Renal swellings are discussed under the differential diagnosis of nephroblastoma. Frequency has much the same significance as incontinence, for any disorder causing frequency is likely also to cause bed-wetting. A purely diurnal frequency of late onset is sometimes seen in girls with sterile urine and normal bladders: it is likely to have a purely emotional basis and should be treated upon the same lines as diurnal enuresis.

Pain is sometimes a presenting symptom: the hydronephrosis due to congenital pelvi-ureteric obstruction characteristically gives rise to severe attacks of loin pain, while the simple mega-ureters cause a much less acute pain in the abdomen. True ureteric colic due to small calculi is comparatively uncommon, though in older children it does not differ from that seen in adults. Pain accompanies pyelonephritis in older children, but does not appear to be serious in infancy: it may be felt in the loin but is often poorly localized, and may be confused with pain of intestinal origin. The dysplastic kidney is frequently a source of discomfort, but other congenital abnormalities such as horse-shoe kidney or ureteric duplication are unlikely to cause pain unless infected or obstructed. Vague abdominal pains for which no cause can be found are a common complaint in childhood, and if exhaustive investigations are undertaken in all such cases, a few examples of renal anomalies will undoubtedly be discovered, though a relationship between the symptoms and the finding is hard to establish.

III. Urological investigations

1. Collection of urine specimens

A mid-stream specimen of urine taken after retraction of the prepuce should be used in the male child; in the male infant the penis must be carefully cleansed and placed in a test-tube which is strapped in position until the specimen appears. Twenty-four hour samples of urine, usually required for chemical estimations, should be collected from a length of Paul's tubing fixed over the penis.

In the female, only a catheter specimen should be sent for bacteriological investigation, though for routine testing it is reasonable first to examine an ordinary specimen for pus cells. Catheterization is often terrifying to the child and is better performed by a familiar nurse than a strange doctor. Sterility is best maintained by the use of a metal or glass catheter. In infancy, twenty-four hour samples may be collected by sitting the child on a moulded plastic cup which is strapped in position, but this is often less satisfactory and more traumatic than an indwelling catheter.

2. Radiological investigations

As in adult urology, the intravenous pyelogram is the key investigation in most disorders of the upper urinary tract and is the basis upon which suspected urological cases are first sorted out into diagnostic categories.

The normal pyelogram in the infant presents certain minor variations on the adult pattern. The kidney is more "rolled-up" so that the two poles approach one another on the medial aspect; the renal pelvis is therefore relatively small and the first part of the ureter runs directly medially before turning downwards (Fig. 1). During the first months of life the kidney is lobulated and the consequent irregularity of the renal outline at this stage does not indicate scarring. The lumbar ureter is relatively wide in the neonate as in the foetus, and a few small kinks which involve the mucosa and muscularis but not the adventitia, causing transverse linear filling defects, are seen immediately below the pelvis (c.f. Fig. 24).

Time and care spent on obtaining good intravenous pyelograms is well repaid in the avoidance of other investigations, and certain special points applicable to children may be noted here. The investigation carries some risk in uraemia and should not be undertaken with a blood urea exceeding 100 mgm/100 ml: it is in any case unlikely that in these circumstances there will be sufficient concentration of contrast medium to give useful films. The same drugs are used as in adults

1*

(e.g. Hypaque, Bayer) and the dosage may be calculated on the basis of 10 ml plus 1 ml for every year of age, so that a child of ten years receives the full adult dosage of 20 ml. Intravenous administration gives the most satisfactory results and with a skilled operator should be possible in the great majority of children. The opaque medium may be given intramuscularly or subcutaneously together with hyalase (a half dose together with 3 mgm hyalase- in 1 ml of water into each buttock) where suitable veins cannot be found and though good pictures may be obtained, the intravenous method is more reliable.

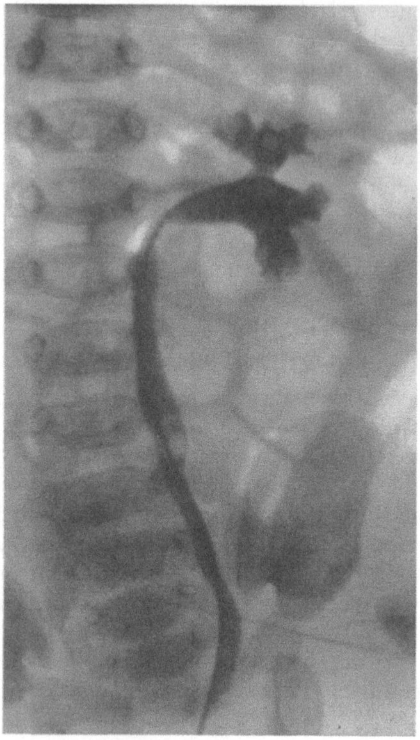

Fig. 1. Normal retrograde pyelogram in a young infant. The film shows the horizontally placed renal pelvis, the "rolled up" form of the kidney, the small kinks at the pelvi-ureteric junction and the relative widening of the lumbar spindle

In children a twelve hour period of dehydration may be possible but it is not practicable in infants and films should be taken 4—5 hours after the last feed. Bowel preparation is only required when there is definite constipation, and then a mild aperient only should be used. In the infant gas shadows in the abdomen are often troublesome, but the renal areas can be cleared by the administration of a fizzy drink which distends the stomach with gas (Fig. 2). Alternatively, tomograms may be used to isolate the pyelographic shadow (BROCKHAUS, FAINSINGER). Compression may be employed in older children, but it is too frightening to the very young. The need for these manoeuvres, and for other modifications of technique such as later films in cases of hydronephrosis or mega-ureter demands the close supervision of the radiologist, and intravenous pyelography should not be regarded as a simple routine procedure. In the male the genital area should be shielded in the films showing the upper tract in order to minimize the irradiation of the testicles.

Retrograde pyelograms present no special difficulties provided the urethra is large enough to admit a cystoscope. Since in infants a single catheterizing instrument must normally be employed, it is preferable that the films should be taken on the cystoscopic table, while the cystoscope is still in situ, and one ureter catheterized after the other. Small ureteric catheters (4F) are essential and must be introduced with the utmost gentleness since it is easy to perforate the renal parenchyma with the tip; this is not usually harmful but the injection of the dye under the capsule produces a confusing picture. Only 2—3 ml of fluid should be injected into the normal renal pelvis of the infant for larger quantities often cause pyelovenous backflow. It is always wise to use an organic compound such as diodone or iodoxyl rather than sodium iodide. Retrograde pyelograms carry a definite risk in cases of hydronephrosis due to pelvi-ureteric obstruction and it is preferable to proceed at once to operation if this condition is present (p. 30).

Simple cystograms may be useful in the diagnosis of vesical diverticula and in doubtful cases the pelvimetry view is valuable in showing small sacs arising immediately behind the ureteric orifices. Usually, however, micturating cysto-grams are employed (see BRODNY and ROBINS, HACKWORTH, STEPHENS) both for the purpose of outlining the urethra (Figs. 3 and 4) and for detecting the presence of vesico-ureteric reflux. Films exposed 2 hours after cystography not infre-

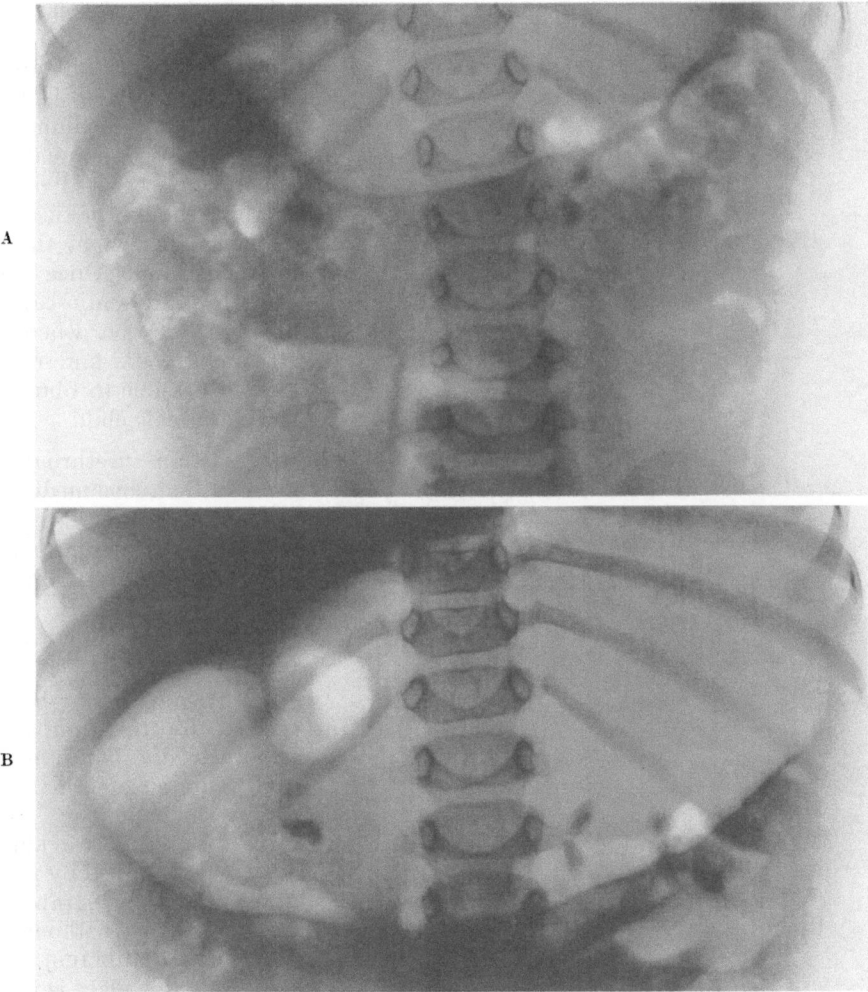

Fig. 2. Renal calculi in a girl aged 1 year: films demonstrating the value of distending the stomach to obtain better definition of the renal area. A before; B after administration of fizzy lemonade

quently outline by reflux dilated ureters which are not shown on intravenous pyelography (Fig. 132). When no serious obstruction is suspected a fine suspension of barium sulphate (25%) is the best contrast medium but is apt to give trouble if there is considerable residual urine. Sodium iodide can cause serious reaction when there is free reflux and it is safer to employ one of the organic iodides (e.g. diodone, at about 15%). The bladder is filled by catheter until it is tense and there is a definite desire to micturate: the catheter is then withdrawn and oblique or AP films are exposed during micturition. It is important that the stream should be flowing freely at the time of the exposure, for half filling or temporary con-

traction of the external sphincter can give very confusing pictures. Cine radiology
with the image intensifier eliminates these difficulties if it is available.

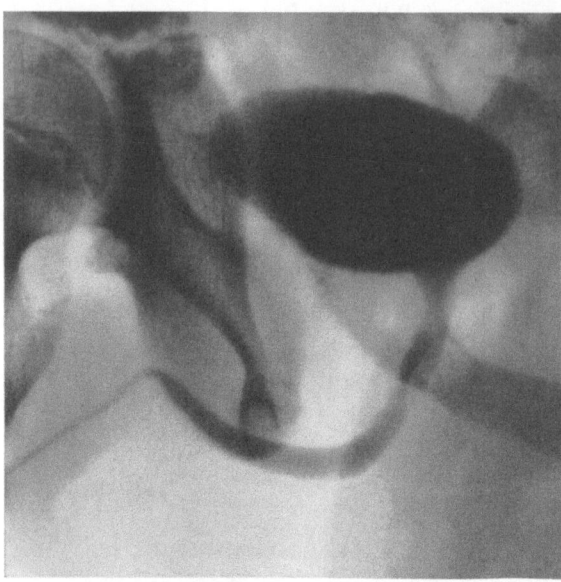

Fig. 3. Normal micturating cysto-urethrogram in the male. A boy
aged 11 years

In chronic retention, and in young infants when active micturition cannot be obtained, an expression cysto-urethrogram may be substituted. Under full anaesthesia the bladder is filled with contrast medium and then expressed manually: a narrow cone centred on the urethra should be used to avoid irradiation of the expressing hand. Once again the films are only capable of interpretation when the stream is good, and this is seldom possible to obtain in the older male child.

Injection urethrograms, even with viscous media, are not often needed except to show the distal limits of a stricture, for even anterior urethral diverticula show better on the micturating films.

Aortography may be performed by the lumbar or femoral route, but it is seldom required for renal conditions in childhood. Adequate information can almost always be obtained by pyelography and aortography is by no mean without its dangers (LANDELIUS). Its most valuable place is in the investigation of hypertension, when anomalies of the renal arteries may be found or pheochromocytomata may be localized.

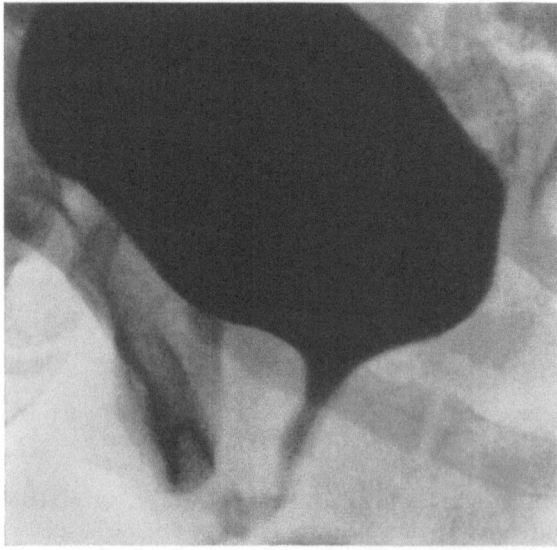

Fig. 4. Normal micturating cysto-urethrogram in a girl aged 7 years

Retroperitoneal air insufflation is helpful in some cases of adrenal tumour. It is conveniently performed by the presacral route, 300—500 ml of air being injected on either side, but anaesthesia is essential for young children and may need to be prolonged as it often takes 1 or 2 hours for the air to reach the right level.

3. Endoscopy

A considerable variety of endoscopic instruments of a size suitable for children is now available (see Volume VI); two models in current use at The Hospital for Sick Children are shown in Fig. 5. Metal bougies and catheters with a suitable curve for children are also essential (McCREA, CAMPBELL).

The female urethra even at birth will normally take an instrument of 11—12F and cystoscopy with ureteric catheterization should always be possible. The male urethra is of extraordinarily variable calibre, and attempts to lay down standards for the various ages are entirely misleading. In many cases the 11F cystoscope

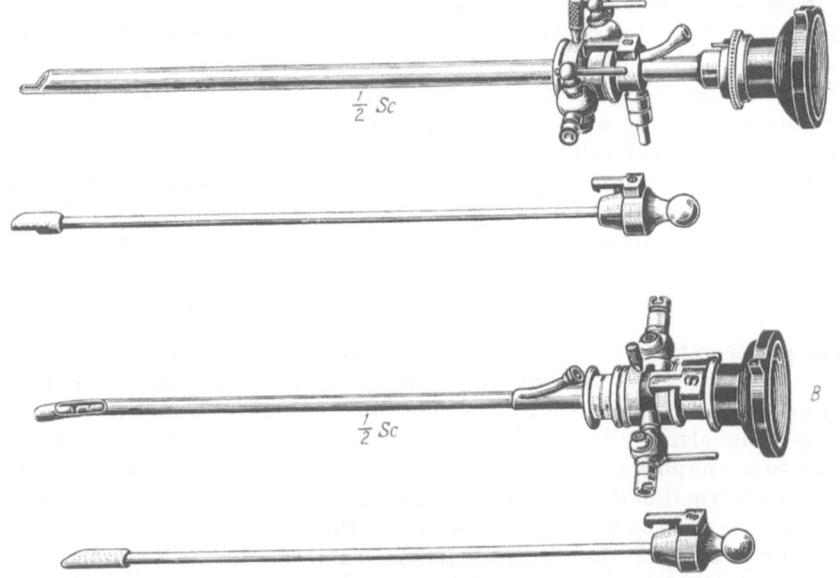

Fig. 5. Endoscopic instruments for children, manufactured by the Genito-Urinary Mfg. Co. Ltd,, London. *A* Urethroscope (MORISON-NASH), made with two sheaths, 11 F and 14 F. Telescope gives an almost direct view, and the bulb is fitted to a separate light carrier. *B* Cysto-Urethroscope (WILLIAMS), approximately 12 F. The sheath is slightly beaked, and the light carried on the convex side. Forsoblique telescope

can be introduced from the age of 1 month onwards, but the urethra in other apparently normal children of a year or eighteen months will not admit the same instrument. The narrowest points are at the external meatus and in the anterior urethra at about the level of the penoscrotal junction: the former may be overcome by meatotomy, but the latter can only be dilated by bougies to a limited extent, and may need to be by-passed by the use of a perineal urethrostomy. This manouevre will enable all males to be cystoscoped, and gives little postoperative trouble provided drainage is ensured for a day or two after operation. General anaesthesia should be employed as a routine in all children.

Many child's cystoscopes have a fixed telescope and no irrigation, so that the bladder must first be washed out and filled with a catheter. Simple inspection of the bladder is not often sufficient, however, and the information usually required concerns the ureters, for which a catheterizing instrument is necessary, or the urethra which demands an irrigating device and a foroblique lens. The cysto-urethroscope illustrated in Fig. 5 attempts to meet both these needs, although in difficult cases the urethroscope with the direct view is preferable.

The normal child's bladder requires no special comment, but the importance of urethroscopy may be emphasized here: no endoscopy is complete unless the whole length of the urethra has been inspected, for important anomalies occur in both anterior and posterior portions.

Resectoscopes suitable for children are also available: my own preference is for the diathermy loop type rather than the cold punch, but the choice must depend largely upon the previous experience of the operator. All such instruments must be used with great caution as there is a danger of producing incontinence in boys and vesicovaginal fistula in girls.

4. Cystometry

This investigation has been employed in a number of diseases, particularly in enuresis and in the neurogenic bladder. While a useful research tool, the method has not been of great practical assistance in either of these conditions, but has a place in the differential diagnosis of the mega-ureters (p. 59). It is seldom possible to obtain a satisfactory record from a child under three years of age, and co-operation is not always easy to obtain later on. Continuous records on a rotating drum are preferable to intermittent observations, and the filling should proceed slowly, at not more than 150—200 drops a minute. The maximum volume is perhaps the most useful figure, but the terminal pressure before active evacuation and the frequency of contractions should also be noted.

IV. Management of surgical cases

The pre-operative treatment of urological cases is discussed under the various diagnostic headings throughout this volume. In general terms the most likely requirements are the sterilization of the urine, and correction of dehydration or electrolyte imbalance. When there is an acute urinary obstruction it may be difficult to accomplish either of these desiderata until drainage is established, but in chronic obstruction it is usually possible and is always helpful. Chemotherapy is discussed on p. 142 and fluid balance on p. 10.

The skin of the genitalia and lower abdomen not infrequently requires treatment in babies and in incontinent children, because of ammonia dermatitis. In hospital, exposure to warm air is the most reliable method of securing an improvement; boracic powder and barrier creams may also be employed (p. 244).

In many chronic urological disorders, there is an accompanying constipation, and some pre-operative bowel preparation is essential: the current medical distaste for the use of aperients is doubtless of value for the healthy child and in many surgical disorders, but it must be impressed on the nursing staff that a mass of faeces in the rectum pre-operatively makes cystoscopy difficult and impedes many operations on the urinary tract, while post-operatively severe constipation interferes with the resumption of normal micturition. In mild cases aperients such as paraffin emulsion are useful, but more severe cases will certainly require a pre-operative enema.

Pre-operative blood transfusion is sometimes necessary when the haemoglobin is low: it will be recalled that if 13 gm/100 ml is taken as 100%, the normal haemoglobin of a new born infant is about 140%; this drops sharply to 75% at the age of 3 months and then rises gradually to 80—90% at six months, where it remains for the rest of the first year. Haemoglobin levels will also vary considerably with the state of hydration, and an accurate calculation of the needs of an infant is therefore difficult. Blood transfusions should always be small, particularly where the blood urea is raised, but may be repeated. In any major operation on an infant, the blood loss should be measured accurately by weighing the swabs and completely replaced by transfusion.

Anaesthetics and pre-operative sedation are now very much in the hands of the specialist anaesthetists, and a full discussion would be out of place here. Infants and very young children normally do best on a barbiturate premedication, nembutal or seconal; older children on omnopon or on a pethidine-largactil mixture. Rectal pentothal is an excellent premedication for operation, but should be avoided before cystoscopy as the fluid is apt to be returned during the procedure.

Open ethyl chloride and ether is undoubtedly the safest anaesthetic for general use, but if an anaesthetist accustomed to children's work is available, a pentothal induction, followed by gas and oxygen, a relaxant and pethidine, provides better conditions for the surgeon, and enables him to make use of the diathermy. In some operations, such as reconstruction of the ectopic bladder where bleeding is profuse, hypotension is valuable: arfonad has been used with success (ANDERSON) in my cases.

A bulky dressing is seldom necessary or desirable, wetting and soiling occur easily, and the exposed wound is always easier to keep clean. Where no drainage is required the wound may be sealed with "Nobecutane" or covered with a single strip of transparent nylon which is stuck to the skin with adhesive. A cradle is necessary to prevent contact with the bedclothes after operations on the external genitalia, and in the very young it may be necessary to restrain the hands. Post-operative vomiting is occasionally troublesome, and in the early stages only small drinks of sweetened water should be given. Ileus and acute dilatation of the stomach are rare complications of urological procedures which require gastric suction.

Neonates, particularly when premature, require special measures which are fully discussed by GROSS and by RICKHAM. They are best nursed in an incubator where a constant temperature can be maintained (85° F for the full term, 90—95° F for the premature baby) with an atmosphere of 50% oxygen, and a relative humidity of 100%. Heat loss is rapid unless these precautions are taken and premature infants are liable to a peculiar hardening of the subcutaneous tissues, sclerema, which is almost always fatal. Massive collapse of the lungs and broncho-pneumonia are also serious hazards: the throat must be kept free from mucus, and the infant's position must be changed frequently. Broad spectrum antibiotics must be avoided if possible, because of the danger of monilia infection. Where operation is required for breast fed infants, the mother should be admitted to hospital as well, so that feeding can be continued without interruption: she may also undertake part of the nursing care and so minimise the risk of cross-infection.

The psychological effects of hospitalization and of operation have been largely disregarded by surgeons in the past, and are not readily appreciated at the ordinary follow-up examination when the chief concern is the healing of the wound or the control of micturition. Yet there is no doubt that the experience of hospitalization is terrifying to the child, and is not infrequently the starting point of serious emotional disorder. The risk is greatest between the ages of 6 months and five years, unfortunately the period at which the most useful urological surgery is undertaken. It is at this stage that the child is most dependent upon his mother, and admission to hospital should be confined to cases in which it is strictly necessary; many procedures such as cystoscopy under anaesthesia, or minor operations such as ligation of a hydrocele sac, can be safely undertaken in out-patients provided facilities for the immediate pre- and post-operative care are available. When admission is essential, the mother should bring the child to the ward, and leave him only when he is comfortably settled in: thereafter daily visiting is important even though it means a minor disturbance at the end of each visit. Some sort of explanation of hospital routine should be given to the child before he comes in, and emphasis should be placed upon the need to "put things right", rather than on the actual operation.

V. Fluid and electrolyte balance in infants

A careful control of fluid and electrolyte balances is of vital importance in all forms of infant surgery, and although urological cases seldom present such difficult problems as the intestinal obstructions, yet renal failure brings with it special hazards.

Renal secretion of urine starts early in foetal life, certainly by $3^1/_2$ months (CAMERON and CHAMBERS). The foetal urine is extremely dilute and contains little urea but much sodium chloride (McCANCE and WIDDOWSON), for probably the kidney is not under hormonal control at this period. The formation of urine contributes to the amniotic fluid, but is in no way essential to the normal development of the foetus; if however there is an obstruction to the urine flow the urinary tract will show all the changes commonly associated with obstruction in post-natal life. The urine changes its composition rapidly after birth, and perhaps even before if there is a failure of the maternal kidneys, but the output of urine during the first two or three days of life is very small, being no more than 30 ml per day. The kidney does not reach full maturity during the first weeks of life and it is often believed to be a relatively inefficient organ at this stage; there is no doubt that if clearance values are related to body surface area as has been customary in the past the kidney of the neonate compares very poorly indeed with the mature organ. McCANCE and WIDDOWSON point out, however, that if these values are correlated with the volume of body water, the factor with which the kidney is directly concerned, then the differences between infant and adults are not nearly so great. The infant cannot produce a very concentrated urine, and though the maximum dilution is as great as in adults, yet simple over-hydration due to a large increase in the water intake cannot be corrected so rapidly. The glomerular filtration rate is a little below normal by any standard, a fact probably correlated with the cap of high columnar cells which is seen on the tips of the glomerular tufts during the first weeks of life (GRUENWALD and POPPER). Tubular reabsorptive functions are fully developed at birth. Urea clearance is relatively poor, and the maintenance of a normal blood urea in an infant depends upon active anabolism, most of the protein ingested being built up into body tissue, and if this process is reversed following trauma or infection the blood urea will rise rapidly despite normal renal function.

Serum phosphate levels are higher in infants than in adults (5.0—8.0 mgm/ 100 ml) as opposed to 2.5—4.5; bicarbonate levels are lower, 20 m Eq/L instead of 27 m Eq/L, and infants are very easily pushed into acidosis.

In the infant as in the adult, 70% of the body weight is water but the extra-cellular compartment is very much larger in the infant, representing 50% of the body weight as opposed to 20%. Moreover, the daily exchange of fluid in the infants represents about half the volume of the extracellular fluid, as against one seventh of that volume in adults (BLAND). It is evident therefore that serious imbalance can occur much more rapidly in infancy, particularly in cases of renal failure where the normal homeostatic function of the kidney is deficient.

The ordinary fluid requirements of a healthy infant may be calculated on the basis of 150 ml/kilo/day ($2^1/_2$ oz. per lb) but very much less is needed in the neonatal period and in post-operative management if a drip is being employed there is a danger of overhydration, so that GROSS calculates the fluid needs at approximately half the normal scale suggested above. The urological disorders which are most often complicated by serious water and electrolyte imbalance are acute infections with septicemia, renal failure, and adrenal deficiency in congenital adrenocortical hyperplasia. Dehydration is a feature of all these states and there is almost always a concomitant loss of electrolytes with a metabolic acidosis. If regular weight charts have been kept, the acute loss of weight accompanying dehydration gives a measure of the amount of water lost (1 pint of water weighs $1^1/_4$ lbs) but in most cases of dehydration must be recognized and estimated clinically from the irritability, thirst, fever, loss of elasticity in the skin and tension in the fontanelles. Haematocrit values in infancy are always high and give little assistance. The serum electrolyte levels should be estimated before starting treatment so that correct repair solutions may be chosen.

Fluids should always be administered by mouth if possible, even though this demands frequent small feeds which may be partially returned as vomit. In these circumstances, it is impossible to estimate with accuracy the fluid intake, and the difficulties of urine collection likewise complicate the measurement of output: the standard fluid requirements give only a general guide therefore and the precise volume of the feeds must be judged from the infant's progress by the ward sister or resident who is seeing the case several times a day. The administration of fluid or feed through a small polyvinyl tube passed through the nose down into the stomach (gavage) is sometimes of value but normal feeding keeps the mouth and throat in a much healthier condition, and is less likely to allow the accumulation of mucus in the pharynx. Parenteral fluid may be given slowly by subcutaneous drip, but absorption is variable, and hyalase has not really proved helpful. Intravenous infusion is the most certain method, though it must always be used with caution because of the dangers of overhydration. In infants the scalp veins are usually employed, but if a drip is required to continue for some time, a vein in the arm or leg should be cut down upon, and a short length of polyethylene tubing inserted.

For the infant who is dehydrated, or in the immediate post-operative periods, a $1/_2$ normal saline solution containing 5% of dextrose may be used, or if the chlorides are raised a simple dextrose solution. When acidosis is present, Hartmann's solution should be given (Sodium lactate 2.26 gms., Sodium chloride 6.0 gms., Potassium chloride 0.4 gms., Calcium chloride 0.2 gms. in water 1000 ml). In acute dehydration fluid may be given at the rate of 6—8 ml/hour/lb body weight; this rate should be halved as the condition improves and later fluid intake should be based on the normal fluid requirements noted above. Milk feeds, diluted at first, should be gradually introduced. Hartmann's solution does not contain sufficient potassium for maintenance if no other feed is taken and 1 gm of potassium chloride should be added to each litre of fluid if parenteral therapy is continued for some days. Plasma infusions are of value when the infant is starving and the plasma proteins are low, it may be given at the rate of 20 ml/kilo/day.

RICKHAM has made a careful study of the metabolic response to surgery in infants, and finds that during the first three weeks of life there are some important differences in post-operative reactions. Neonates exhibit a remarkable resistance to trauma and probably withstand major surgical procedures better than infants of 4 or 5 weeks, but for proper management certain facts must be recognised. The body temperature is rarely raised even with severe infections, it is more likely to be subnormal. Weight loss of 5—10% occurs in most new born children, and those subjected to operation lose little more. The normal urine output during the first two days is not much more than 30 ml/day and post-operative water retention is not easy to estimate, but fluid requirements at this stage are minimal. An increase of nitrogen excretion occurs but is no greater than that found in starvation and as already noted the blood urea may rise considerably because of endogenous protein breakdown. Post-operative retention of sodium and chloride is common but none of the neonates investigated by RICKHAM showed the potassium loss characteristic of the adult post-operative response: this feature only appeared after three weeks of age.

B. Congenital abnormalities of the upper urinary tract

I. Renal agenesis

Unilateral renal agenesis is not a very uncommon condition, though its exact frequency is hard to determine. CAMPBELL found 88 cases in a series of post-mortems on 47,409 children (1 in 528) but since it is apt to accompany other fatal malformations this is probably too high an incidence for the general population. In clinical studies it is very difficult to distinguish from extreme degrees of hypoplasia. The ureter is absent in agenesis of the kidney and commonly the trigone of the bladder has an asymmetrical appearance, undeveloped on the side of the abnormality. Associated malformations of the genital tract, particularly double uterus, are common in the female, and occasionally in the male only a portion of the vas deferens is present. The adrenal of the affected side may be absent, but when present assumes a disc shape because of the absence of local pressure from the kidney.

From the clinical viewpoint, however, interest clearly centres on the solitary kidney and as has been emphasized by many authors (e.g. GUTIERREZ) it is very liable to pathological complications. Such a kidney is naturally hypertrophied and is therefore often easily palpable; in some cases it is also excessively mobile and has given rise to the suspicion of a tumour. Other malformations are not uncommon, the solitary pelvic kidney being a characteristic form. Even with the normally placed organ there may be complications, and the present author has encountered gross mega-ureter in the solitary kidney on 4 occasions in childhood. The exact diagnosis in clinical cases is often difficult although the absence of a functioning kidney will be appreciated from the pyelograms. The asymmetry of the trigone and the absence of the ureteric orifice will lead to the suspicion of renal agenesis, but these features may also be observed in cases of renal "aplasia", and in ectopic ureter.

Bilateral renal agenesis is naturally incompatible with survival, but affected infants not infrequently live some hours or even days after birth. POTTER has drawn attention to this group, having found no less than 20 cases in the course of 5000 autopsies performed in cases of pre-natal or early post-natal death. All cases had hypoplastic lungs and a characteristic facies. There was observed to be an increased width between the eyes, and an unusually prominent fold arising from the inner canthus which swept downwards and outwards to form a wide semi-circle under the orbital space. Flattening and broadening of the nose and large low set ears were characteristic. A somewhat similar but not identical appearance is to be found in cases of extreme hypoplasia and polycystic disease.

II. Renal hypoplasia

Renal hypoplasia, a failure of full development in the kidney is a common accompaniment of other malformations of the urinary tract: when it occurs alone, it may be difficult or impossible to distinguish from atrophic pyelonephritis. The frequency of the true congenital abnormality is therefore hard to assess, there are no reliable estimates of the incidence, and the fact that almost all authors report that girls are much more often affected than boys probably simply reflects the greater liability of the female to acquired infection.

The interest of the hypoplastic kidney lies not simply in its failure to achieve normal size, but in the presence of abnormal tissues within the renal substance. BAGEN-STOSS has, in fact, proposed the use of the term dysplasia as a substitute for hypoplasia in order to indicate the inclusion of primitive renal elements and of tissues normally foreign to the kidney such as cartilage and striated muscle. A kidney which contains "dysplastic" elements may be of any size, from a minute nodule of fibrous tissue to almost normal dimensions, and from the pathologists standpoint, a continuous series can be traced from one extreme to the other. The following classification attempts to reconcile the needs of the clinician with those of the pathologist.

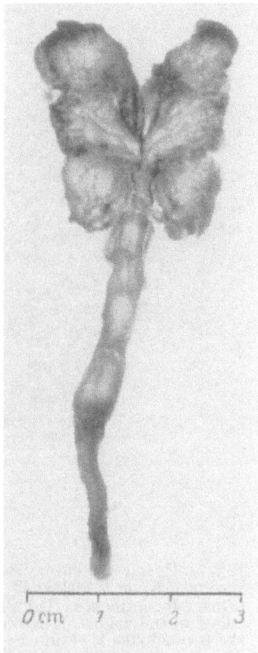

1. Dysplastic kidney with obliterated ureter

This type is often referred to as "aplasia" of the kidney, although in structure it differs only in degree from less severe forms of dysplasia. The kidney is represented by a small fibrous body in which no true nephrons can be found, though some straight and primitive renal tubules may be seen. The ureter is usually atrophic and narrows down at some point to a slender and impermeable thread.

Fig. 6. Dysplastic kidney with obliterated ureter. Nephrectomy specimen from a girl aged 13 years suffering from recurrent urinary infection and hypertension. Contralateral kidney showed pyelonephritic changes

In unilateral cases, symptoms are seldom attributable to the dysplastic kidney, which is functionless and excluded from the urinary tract. As in renal agenesis, however, the contralateral kidney is not only hypertrophied, but is unusually liable to pathological complications. Fig. 6 illustrates a case of a girl with hypertension, an extremely hypoplastic kidney on the left side, and a chronic pyelonephritis in the contralateral organ. The diagnosis is reached by exploration of the loin, though the absence of renal function and the obliteration of the ureter may give a clue. Although the minute kidney is often removed the treatment must naturally be directed chiefly towards the contralateral organ. In bilateral cases, the infant is born dead or dies within a few days of birth.

2. Dysplastic kidney with patent ureter

This type is commoner than the previously described, and includes the majority of so-called hypoplastic kidneys. The size is extremely variable, but the parenchyma is usually distorted by masses of fibrous tissue and cysts, and complicating pyelonephritis is almost always present (Fig. 7). The dysplastic elements may be recognized microscopically: straight radiating tubules reaching the surface of the kidney, proglomeruli without separation of tuft from capsule, masses of cartilage and angiomatous areas (Fig. 8). Other abnormalities of the urinary tract are frequently present, particularly double or ectopic ureters, and only one half of a double kidney may be affected by dysplasia. Sometimes it appears that other malformations are the cause of hypoplasia, and not simply an accompaniment; in lower urinary obstructions which have been present from early foetal life, there is apparently an interference with the maturation of the nephrons, and the kidneys are often hypoplastic rather than hydronephrotic.

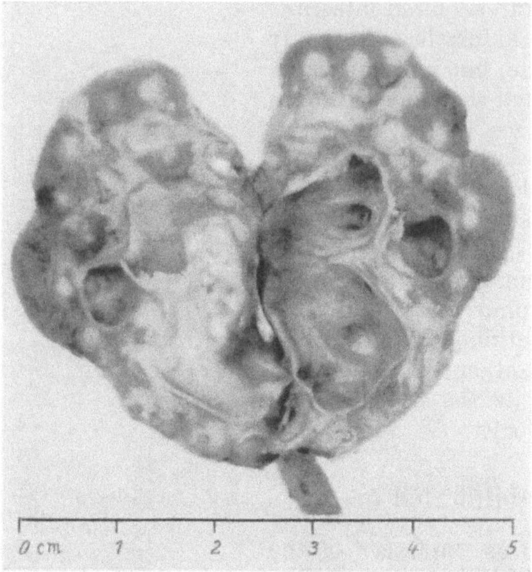

The symptoms may be those of the ureteric abnormality as in the case of the ectopic ureter (Fig. 7), in other instances it is the complicating infection which brings the child to hospital. Recurrent pyuria with pain in the loin on the affected side is the characteristic story. Hypertension is a well recognized complication; it is discussed on p. 211. Bilateral cases (Fig. 9) inevitably progress to a state of chronic renal failure, and many of the cases of renal osteodystrophy (p. 224) are the result of this type of hypoplasia. The course is very prolonged and death may be postponed until adolescence or early adult life, but the downward trend cannot be deflected.

Fig. 7. Dysplastic kidney with patent ureter. Nephrectomy specimen from a girl aged 4 years suffering from dribbling urinary incontinence. The single ureter draining this kidney ended in the vagina. The renal pelvis is hydronephrotic and the parenchyma is studded with islands of fibrosis and hyaline cartilage

Pyelographically these dysplastic kidneys are indistinguishable from the contracted kidneys of chronic pyleonephritis, and the radiological appearances are discussed under that heading. In many unilateral examples there is sufficient function to give an adequate shadow on intravenous pyelography, but in bilateral cases retrograde filling is almost always required for diagnosis. Strictly unilateral cases may be treated by nephrectomy for the control of recurrent infection or hypertension: in bilateral disease, all functioning tissue must be preserved.

3. The miniature kidney

This term conveniently describes the small kidney which is normal in function and architecture; it is unlikely to be the cause of symptoms, provided the abnormality is unilateral. The diagnosis is usually clear from the pyelogram, as in the case illustrated in Fig. 10, the calyces being perfectly formed although perhaps fewer in number than in the normal kidney. It is important to realize that despite the apparently good function, such an organ would be incapable of maintaining life unaided by its fellow and if the disorder is bilateral signs of renal failure will appear some time during childhood or adolescence. Even if the two kidneys, though small, are structurally normal at birth it is inevitable that the

renal insufficiency will lead to gross tubular dilatation and hypertrophy; complicating pyelonephritis practically always occurs with scarring and distortion of

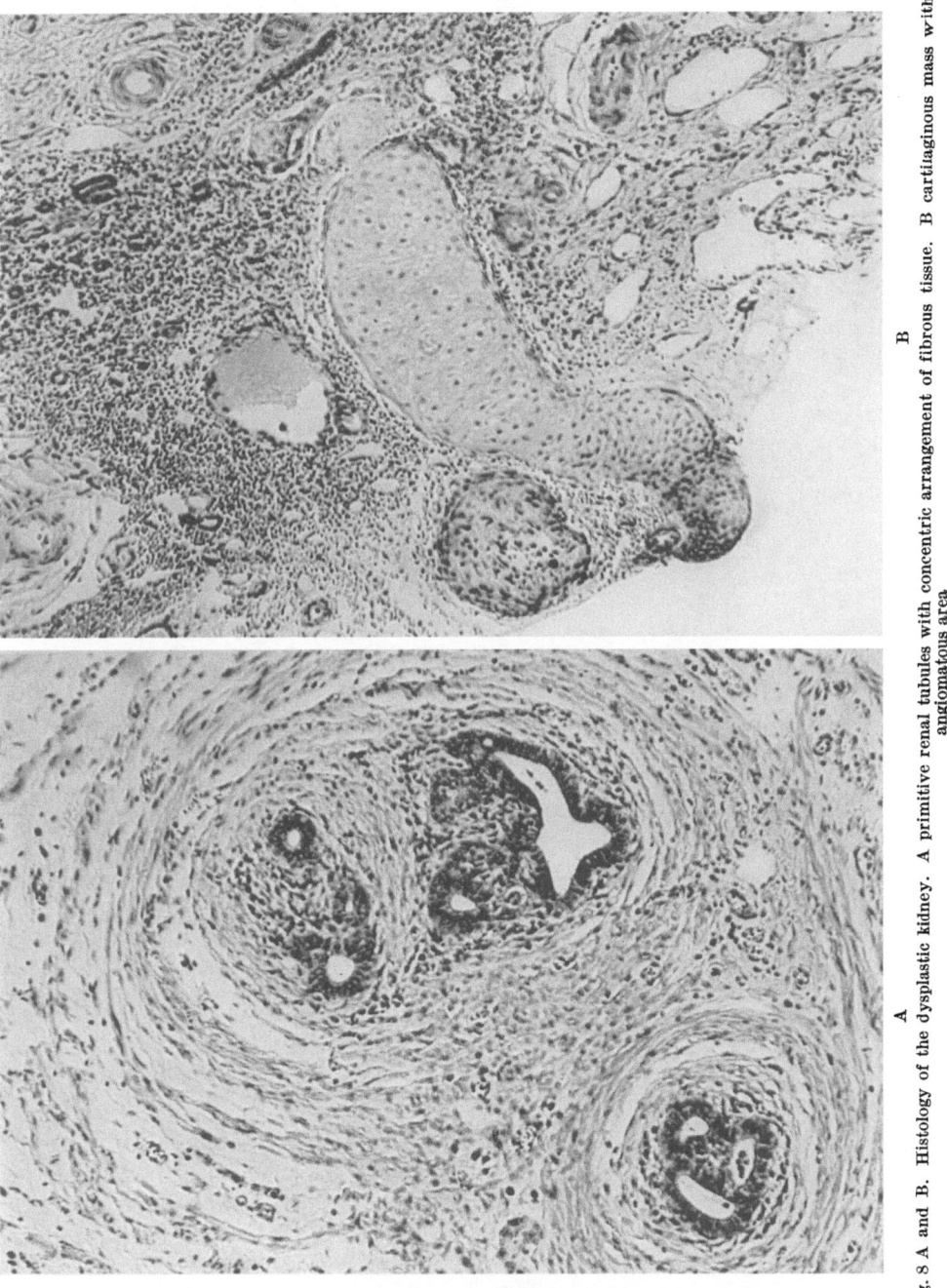

Fig. 8 A and B. Histology of the dysplastic kidney. A primitive renal tubules with concentric arrangement of fibrous tissue. B cartilaginous mass with angiomatous area

the parenchyma. There is often hypertension causing vascular changes, and at
autopsy therefore bilateral hypoplastic kidneys always present a complex appearance which may be avoided in the unilateral.

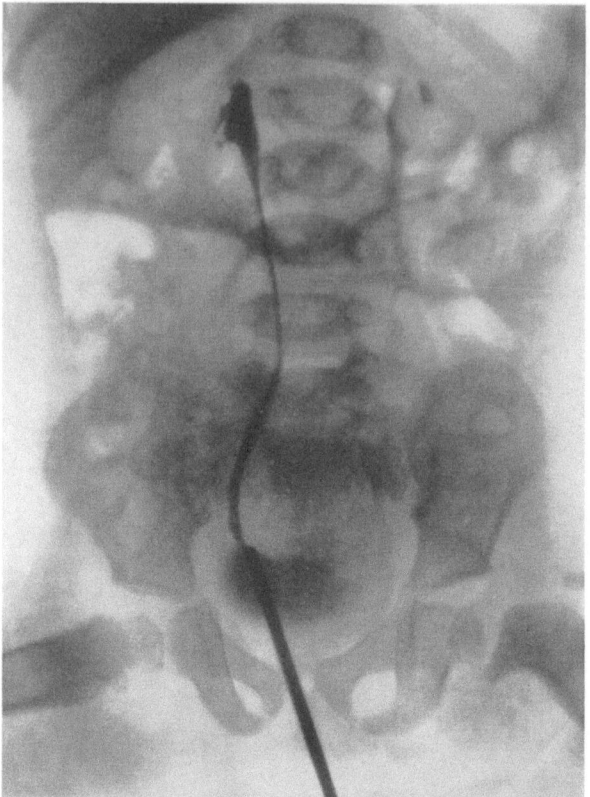

Fig. 9. Bilateral renal hypoplasia. Retrograde pyelogram in a boy aged 3 years with renal osteodystrophy and hypertension. Blood urea 178 mgm/100 ml. Sterile urine and no history of infection

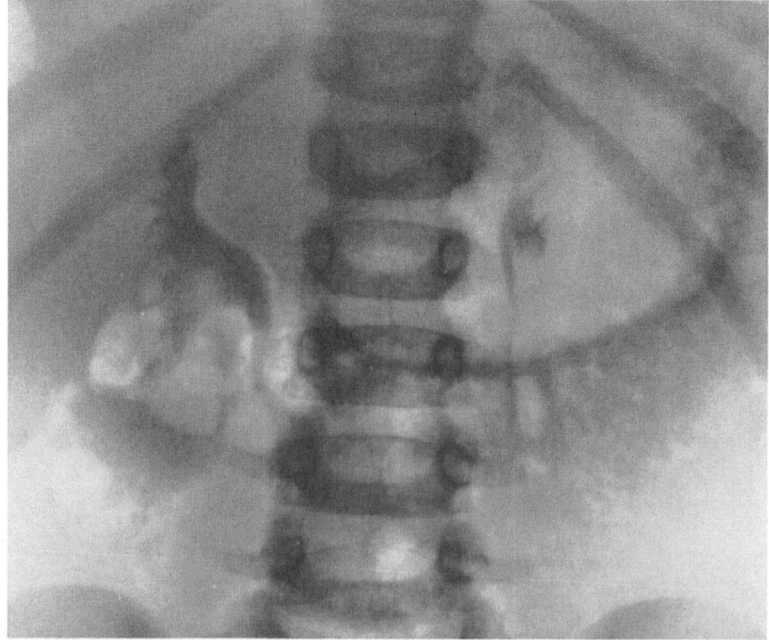

Fig. 10. "Miniature" kidney. Intravenous pyelogram in a boy aged 2 years complaining of painful micturition. Urine sterile. The left kidney is small, but the calyces are regular and show the normal cupping

It is uncertain whether the miniature kidney can be responsible for hypertension; a case reported by HUTCHISON and MONCRIEFF suggests that it can be, but as mentioned on p. 212 it is only during recent years that the importance of minor anomalies of the renal arteries has been recognized, and such lesions may well have been overlooked.

Surgery is scarcely ever required for the miniature kidney, but its presence may contra-indicate surgery for the opposite organ.

III. Cystic disease of the kidneys

Cystic disease of the kidney, although by no means a common affliction, presents in children the most bewildering variety of forms. Unfortunately the term infantile polycystic disease has been used to include a great many of these forms, and the statistics which are usually given relate to the whole group although it is a heterogenous one. Some idea of the relative frequency of cystic disease in children and adults may be gained from the figures of RALL and ODELL who found only six children under the age of ten years in the series of 207 clinical cases, but nine examples, all in infancy, in a post-mortem series of 44 cases. CAMPBELL found 70 cases among a post-mortem series of 15,919 children and states that many of these showed other congenital abnormalities. BELL has given a useful general survey of the problem and POTTER has discussed the neonatal pathology. In this chapter an attempt will be made to survey the various clinico-pathological types.

1. Congenital polycystic disease. Infantile form

The great majority of afflicted infants are stillborn or die within the first few hours of birth: some survive a few months but die of renal failure before their first birthday. Both kidneys are grossly enlarged, but their only divergence from the normal shape is some foetal lobulation. The cut surface presents a honeycomb appearance with thousands of minute oval or elongated cysts arranged in a radial fashion throughout the parenchyma (Fig. 11). They commonly occupy the entire substance of the kidney though in some examples the medullary region and the immediate subcapsular zones are spared. Careful microscopic studies with reconstruction have been carried out by several workers: NORRIS and HERMAN found that the cystic spaces were irregularly dilated tubules lined with a single layer of flattened or cubical epithelium; distended Bowman's capsules were sometimes found and the tubules often anastomosed. In the pyramids blind ending collecting tubules were found. LAMBERT found some glomerular cysts and other tubular cysts which were blind at both ends; he contrasted this state of affairs with adult polycystic disease in which the cysts appear to be dilatations in the course of functioning nephrons. Roos on the other hand, in a kidney which conformed to the usual appearance of polycystic disease found only glomerular cysts. POTTER reported 5 instances of the tubular form and one of the glomerular pattern. It appears from these studies that a degenerative process must have taken place after the formation of the nephrons which resulted in the isolation of segments which later became dilated to form cysts. In this group other urogenital malformations are rare, but it is usual to find cystic changes in the liver and occasionally also in the lungs, pancreas and ovaries.

Infantile polycystic disease occurs in sibs but not in different generations within the family. It does not occur in families affected by adult forms of the disease (FERGUSSON). The renal swellings are considerable and easily palpable, on occasions they have caused dystocia (GONNET et al., BOURLAND). In infants who survive the first days of extra-uterine life the presenting signs are commonly vomiting and failure to thrive; the blood urea is found to be raised, perhaps 60 or 80 mgm-%, and deterioration with other biochemical disturbances is to be expected. Hypertension may occur (PARNELL and KESSEL, PARROT et al.) and death may be due to cardiac rather than renal failure. Spontaneous peri-renal haematoma with hyperthermia has been recorded (CADERAS and BERT). The

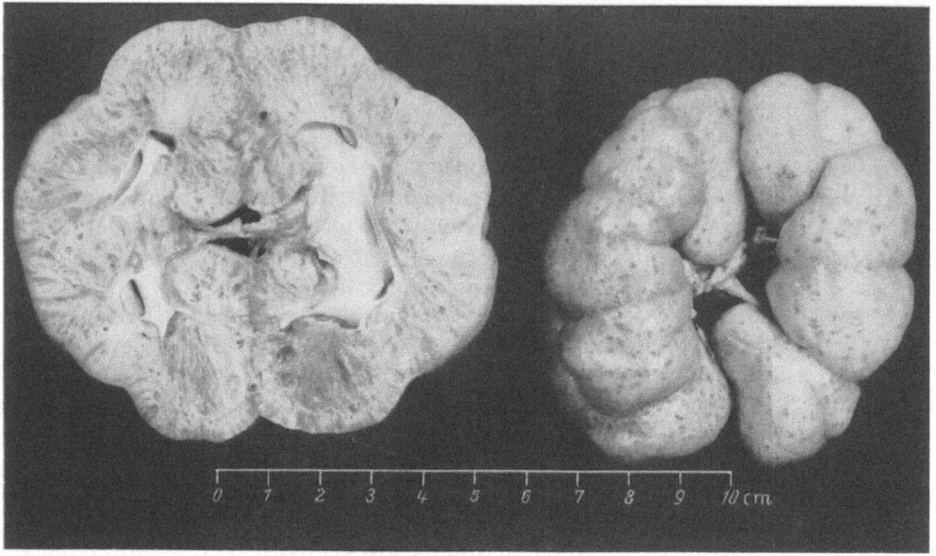

Fig. 11. Infantile polycystic kidneys. Post-mortem specimen from a child dying at 3 months of renal failure. There were also cystic changes in the liver

diagnosis may usually be confirmed by retrograde pyelography, the pelvi-calycine system being enlarged and stretched out in the "spider" fashion seen in adult cases; HINKEL and SANTINI point out however that the pyelograms may be indistinguishable from normal. No treatment can usefully be given.

2. Congenital polycystic disease. Adult form

This is a familial disorder passed from one generation to another which usually causes no symptoms until middle life, but occassionally shows itself during childhood. A detailed description would be out of place in this volume, but briefly it may be stated that the kidney instead of having the uniform honey-comb appearance of the infantile form is distorted by cysts of varying size which are irregularly arranged throughout the parenchyma; in between the cysts there are areas of normal renal tissue. There is some evidence that these cysts are part of functioning nephrons; they gradually enlarge throughout the life span of the individual so that pyelograms which may be virtually normal at first become more and more distorted with the passage of years and the intervening functional tissue is progressively destroyed by the pressure of the growing cysts. It sometimes happens that the cysts in one kidney grow much more rapidly than in the other, giving for a time the appearance of unilateral disease. It is wise, however, to assume that all cases in this group are potentially bilateral so that nephrectomy is only justifiable if there are severe unilateral complications.

Presenting signs during childhood may be haematuria, palpable tumour, or chronic renal failure with rachitic changes (KRETSCHMER). The diagnosis is usually apparent from a consideration of the clinical findings and family history, and it may be confirmed by pyelography, though it must be remembered that where the cysts are small, the deformity will be slight (Fig. 12). Treatment is chiefly concerned with the management of the failing kidney and surgery is seldom required.

Certain reported cases of bilateral polycystic disease present variants on one or other of the two forms described. Thus SMITH and GRAHAM describe a

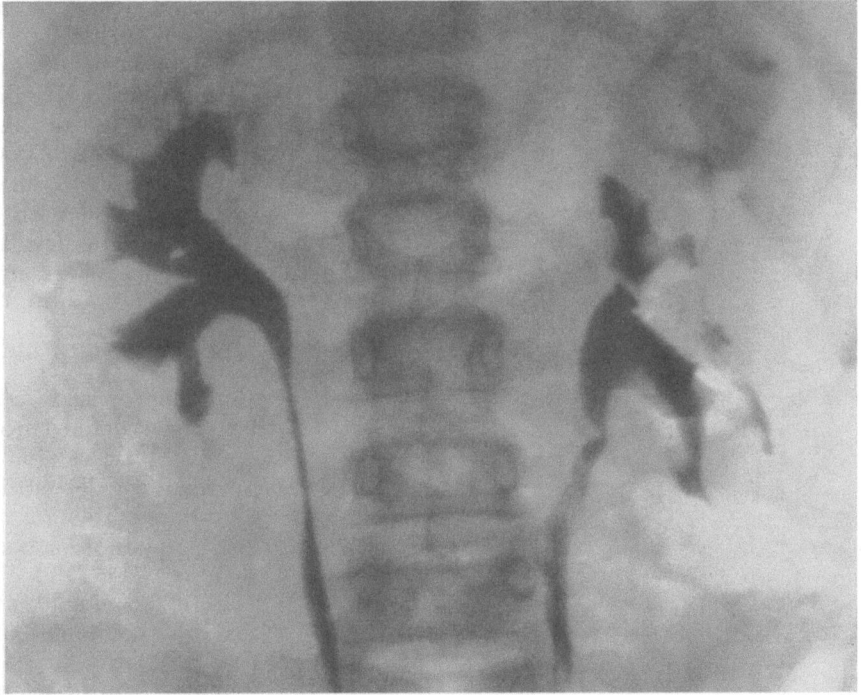

Fig. 12. Polycystic kidneys. Retrograde pyelograms in a girl aged 11 years suffering from haematemesis with portal obstruction. Blood urea 140. Exploration of the kidneys, and biopsy proved the presence of bilateral polycystic disease

girl of 8 years with profound anaemia who died of renal failure and was found to have the medullary region of both kidneys riddled with minute cysts while the cortex was unaffected. LIGHTWOOD and LOOTS report a family of 3 children suffering from cystic disease of the kidneys and liver but two of these children continued to survive into later childhood with symptoms largely attributable to their hepatic condition. The case illustrated in Fig. 12 was investigated on account of the symptoms of portal obstruction.

3. Cystic changes in hypoplastic kidneys and accompanying lower urinary obstruction

Congenital hypoplastic kidneys not infrequently contain cysts, particularly those in which there are many dysplastic elements present in the parenchyma. In bilateral hypoplasia functional deficiency may lead to such extreme tubular dilatation that the kidney has a cystic appearance (GREEN). Bilateral cystic changes are quite commonly found in infants dying within the first few days of life with bladder neck obstruction or urethral valves; some of these cysts communicate with the renal pelvis but others do not, and it appears that the presence of a lower urinary obstruction can interfere with the maturation of the later generations of nephrons. An excellent illustration of this type is given by VAIL and STONE, and the results of micro-dissection have been described by BIALESTOCK.

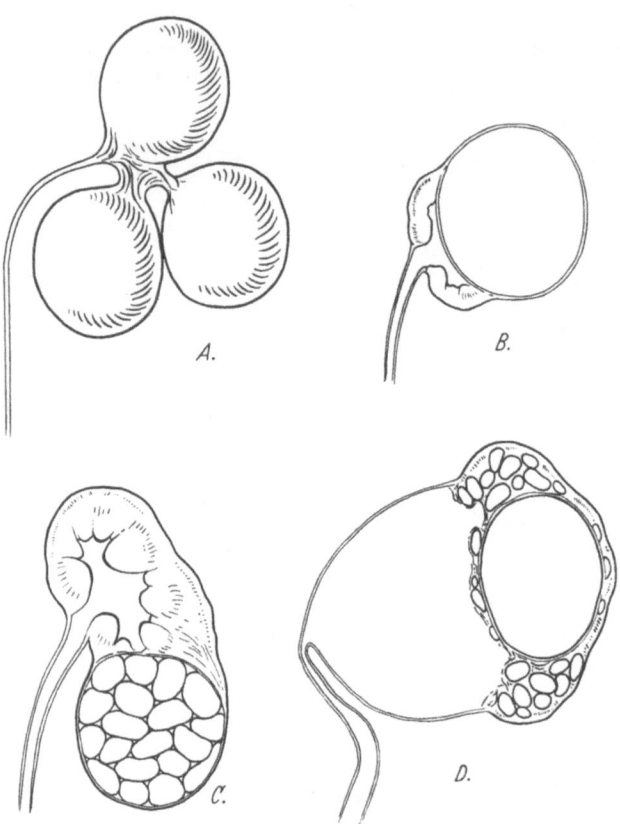

It is doubtless the inclusion of these two types under the heading of bilateral polycystic disease that has led to the impression that in infants this disorder is likely to be associated with other congenital malformations of the urinary tract.

Fig. 13 A—D. Diagrams to show various types of cystic kidneys. *A* The multi-cystic kidney. *B* Large serous cyst. *C* Multilocular cyst. *D* Cystic disease with hydronephrosis

4. Multicystic kidneys

This term is applied to a well defined group of unilateral cases in which a loose conglomeration of cysts resembling a bunch of grapes replaces the kidney (Fig. 13 A). The ureter is commonly atretic at some point in its length, it may be reduced to a minute thread or be altogether absent. The renal arteries are also poorly developed. The cysts are composed of fibrous tissue which is occasionally calcified and are lined by a single layer of flattened epithelium, but they are bound together by tissue which may contain primitive renal elements. The atretic nature of the ureter or renal pelvis and calyces seems to be the essential feature of this type of disease, and in one of my cases a partial atresia of the opposite ureter had caused severe hydronephrosis. Many excellent descriptions of these cases can be found in the literature, particularly those of SCHWARTZ, RAVITCH and SANDFORD, and SPENCE. Clinically most cases have presented with a renal swelling during infancy or have been discovered because of a disease in the contralateral organ. The diagnosis is usually made at laparotomy for suspected tumour, but the characteristic form of the swelling and the atresia of the ureter (with at times absence of the ureteric orifice) may be an indication of the nature of the disorder. Nephrectomy has been the treatment in all suitable cases and since the opposite kidney is usually normal this treatment is successful, though it is perhaps not always necessary.

5. Simple serous cysts (solitary cysts)

This type, though very common in adults and often regarded as an acquired disease, is rare in children. Cases have been presented by CHALKLEY and SUTTON and by CHRISTESON. The literature is reviewed by WEERD and SIMON. One or two large cysts may arise in the periphery of an otherwise normal kidney, and grow to such a size that they distort or displace their parent organ (Fig. 13 B). The disease has usually presented with renal swelling or urinary infection and in most reported cases in children the destruction of the parenchyma was such that a nephrectomy was performed, though uncapping of the cyst is the preferable operation.

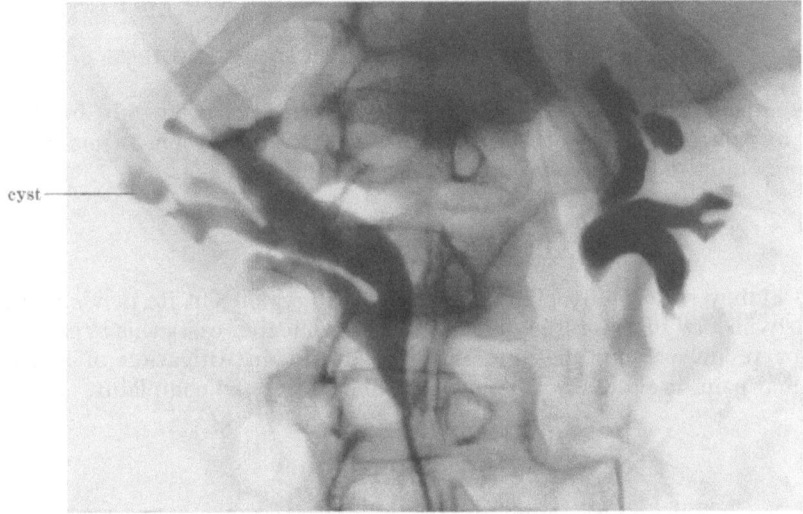

cyst

Fig. 14. Pyelogenic cysts. Retrograde pyelograms: oblique views in a boy aged 11 years suffering from inter-mittent haematuria

6. Multi-locular cysts (cyst-adenoma)

In several publications this type has been confused with the multicystic kidney described above, though it has much more in common with the serous cyst. Within a firm capsule on the periphery of the kidney is a mass of enlarging cysts lined by flattened epithelium and containing within them no renal elements (Fig. 13 C). Although more common in adults, cases have been reported in children, by BURRELL, CHAUVIN, TOULSON and WAGNER. The enlarging mass calls attention to the condition, and together with the distortion of the renal pelvis, gives rise to the suspicion of Wilm's tumour. The diagnosis can only be made with assurance from the histology of the specimen, and nephrectomy must therefore be the treatment. In one case there was also hypertension.

7. Cystic disease with hydronephrosis and pelvi-ureteric obstruction

This rare form has been reported by WAKELEY, HIGGINS et al., and MOORE. In addition to a large pelvic hydronephrosis the parenchyma is entirely replaced by cysts of various sizes (Fig. 13 D). MOORE has used the term spongy kidney to describe his case, but there is no relationship between this type and the disease found in young adults described in the literature as Rein-en-éponge.

8. Pyelogenic cysts

Small cystic spaces (Fig. 14) communicating with the calyceal system may be seen in otherwise normal pyelograms or in association with the hypoplastic kidney. They are usually regarded as calyceal diverticula or pyelogenic cysts and are seldom responsible for symptoms, though occasionally a stone may form in one and be accompanied by recurrent urinary infection. Such cysts when enlarged are difficult to distinguish from "hydrocalycosis" in which there is a dilatation of the entire calyx. WEYRAUCH and FLEMMING, and HART et al. have both reported cases of infants with a single large cyst of the kidney, necessitating nephrectomy, which proved on examination to be a hydrocalycosis.

IV. Malrotated, fused and ectopic kidneys

The anomalies of form and position of the kidneys need only be discussed briefly in this volume, since the disorders which affect them in childhood are less common but otherwise similar to those seen in adult life.

1. Simple malrotation

The kidney is normally placed in the lumbar region but its pelvis is directed anteriorly instead of antero-medially. In uncomplicated cases this type of kidney does not produce symptoms and if found during investigation of enuresis or abdominal pain, it should not be held responsible for the complaint.

2. Horse-shoe kidney

The lower poles of the kidneys are joined to one another by an isthmus of renal tissue which crosses in front of the aorta immediately below the level of the inferior mesenteric arteries. The two pelves are directed forwards, and the ureters run downwards in front of the isthmus: pyelograms show a malrotation and a characteristic medially directed lower calyx (Fig. 15). Other anomalies of the ureters such as a duplication are not uncommon, and there is a liability to the development of hydronephrosis.

GUTIERREZ has described a syndrome in which a simple and uncomplicated horse-shoe kidney is associated with abdominal pain, nausea and constipation, and claims that division of the isthmus combined with nephropexy will relieve these symptoms. Mild abdominal pains are often seen in childhood, and it is difficult to be sure that the renal malformation is responsible: in cases seen by the writer the symptoms have cleared up without surgical interference. Similar considerations apply to the observation of unexplained haematuria associated with the horse-shoe kidney. CHAUVIN and CHAUVIN believe that the anomaly alone can be responsible for bleeding, but as will be seen in Section M, V, unexplained and benign haematuria is relatively common in the pyelographically normal child.

In general, treatment is only required for complications and may follow the same lines as in the normal kidney. Excision of one half of the horse-shoe can be performed: the division of the isthmus presents no special difficulty provided the exposure is good and the possibility of anomalous blood supply is born in mind. The problem of hydronephrosis is discussed on p. 26.

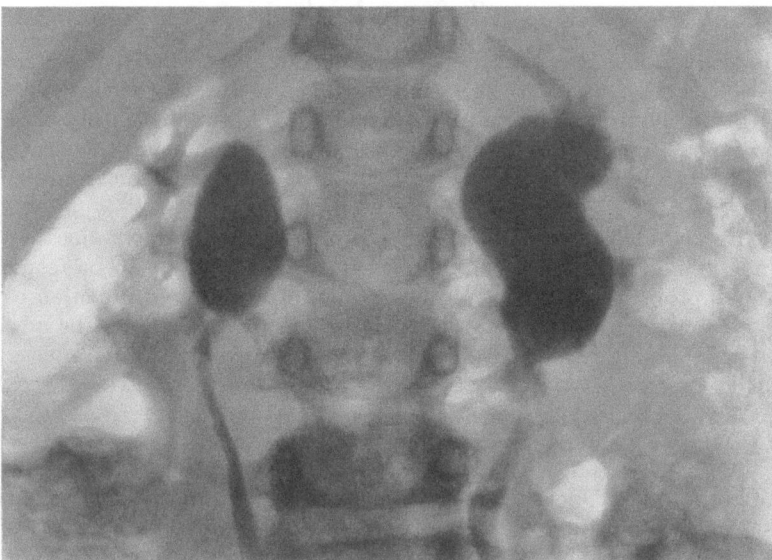

Fig. 15. Horse-shoe kidney. Intravenous pyelogram in a boy with a mild lower urinary obstruction; the renal anomaly is an incidental finding

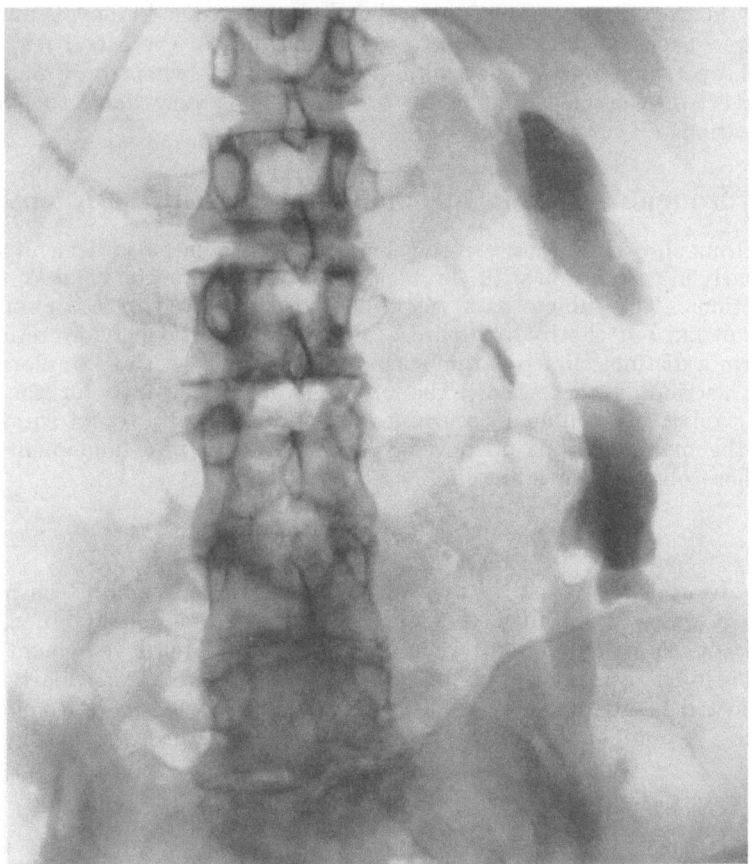

Fig. 16. Crossed ectopia with fusion. Intravenous pyelogram in a girl of 4 years with complex cloacal deformity. Both renal pelves are on the same side of the body, and both are a little dilated

3. Crossed ectopia

The two kidneys are placed on the same side of the body, the crossed organ lying below and medial to the other and usually fused with it (KEUSENHOFF, CARLETON). The ureters enter the bladder in the normal situation on either side of the trigone. Accompanying malformations are common; in the case illustrated in Fig. 16, the child also suffered from a minute bladder which emptied directly into the vagina.

The renal mass is usually palpable on simple abdominal examination and may be a little tender. In the uncomplicated form it is unlikely to be responsible for serious symptoms, but hydronephrosis, stone formation and infection may occur. Surgical operations in the fused cases are difficult, and should be advised only on unassailable indications. BOISSONNAT has, however, recorded a case in which the renal elements were separated at the age of fourteen days.

4. Pelvic ectopia

Unilateral pelvic ectopia is a comparatively common malformation: one kidney is placed at the level of the promontory of the sacrum or actually in the pelvic cavity. Such a kidney usually possesses an anterior pelvis and a blood supply from the lower aorta or iliac artery (THOMPSON and PACE). The mass may be palpable on abdominal or pelvic examination, and may indent the bladder shadow on a cystogram. The fused pelvic kidney, or disc-kidney, is another well recognized type in which the whole renal mass lies in the sacral region, and is drained by two ureters. The solitary pelvic kidney where only one ureter is present is an even more anomalous form, which is very liable to pathological complications (HANLEY).

V. Hydronephrosis due to congenital pelvi-ureteric obstruction

Hydronephrosis is found during childhood in a large variety of disorders, particuarly in association with chronic dilatation of the ureters and lower urinary obstructions. The subject as a whole has been reviewed by CAMPBELL and by KRETSCHMER, but the hydronephroses due to congenital pelvi-ureteric obstruction form a distinct clinico-pathological group and it is with these alone that the present section is concerned. The group gains importance for the urologist from its relatively common occurrence and from the efficacy of surgical treatment: the manifestations do not, however, differ in any fundamental respect from those observed in adult life.

1. Incidence

The disorder may occur at any age, though it is most often seen in children who have passed their fifth year; girls and boys are equally affected. The majority of cases are unilateral when first seen, but a later development of hydronephrosis in the contralateral kidney may be encountered, particularly when the first affected has been removed. The left side is involved more frequently than the right. A familial incidence is rare, but has been recorded (RAFFLE).

2. Pathology

In this type of hydronephrosis the dilatation affects particularly the extra-renal portion of the pelvis and ballooning of the calyces appears later. It seems, in fact, that the disorder occurs only in those kidneys in which there is a well developed pelvis outside the hilum, and it is not seen in the ordinary upper pelvis of the double kidney where there is no clearly defined pelvi-ureteric junction. Hydronephrosis is particularly common in the malrotated kidney. The obstruction is evidently sited at the pelvi-ureteric junction, but the exact findings at operation differ from case to case, and there is a considerable divergence of opinion among observers as to the true causative lesion.

a) Obstruction due to aberrant renal vessels

Many authorities regard vascular obstruction as the commonest form, particularly in children (WHITE and WYATT, CAMPBELL). NIXON in a review of cases at the Hospital for Sick Children found vessels as a contributory cause in 25 out of 78 cases. There remains, however, some doubt as to whether the presence of the vessel alone can obstruct the outflow of urine, or whether it merely exacerbates, by producing a kink, the obstruction due to an intrinsic lesion. The vessels concerned may be arteries or veins or both; they are found in front of the ureter more often than behind and usually run to the lowermost point of the hilum but may be truly aberrant, being derived directly from the aorta or running direct to the lower pole of the kidney. At operation it is sometimes found that the vessel crosses immediately over the pelvi-ureteric junction, and that when these two structures are separated the distended pelvis empties itself; more often the vessel crosses the ureter 1—2 cm distal to the junction and binds it down to the surface of the hydronephrotic sac (Fig. 17). In this event the urine flow is seldom restored by simple freeing of the vessel.

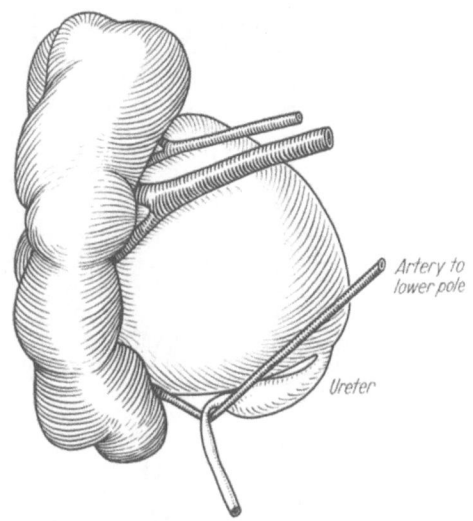

Fig. 17. Hydronephrosis with vascular obstruction of the ureter. Diagrammatic view showing the ureter kinked and bound down to the surface of the hydronephrotic sac by a vessel running to the lower pole of the kidney

b) Kinks and adhesions

Even in the absence of a vessel it is common to find the ureter bound down by dense adhesions to the surface of the distended pelvis so that it is acutely kinked at the pelvi-ureteric junction and at the point where it becomes free. The adhesions cannot be due to inflammation since they are found in sterile cases in the new born. ÖSTLING has emphasized the frequency with which these kinks are found in the hydronephroses of children: he has also demonstrated that a series of kinks involving the muscularis and the mucosa, but not the adventitia, are a normal feature of the upper third of the ureter in the foetus and he postulates that a persistence of one of these could lead to obstruction. The normal foetal kinks are not found precisely at the pelvi-ureteric junction, but they do suggest that at this stage the adventitia forms a loose sleeve around the ureter which, as it condenses, may fix pathological contortions of the ureter. Division of the adhesions alone does not usually allow complete emptying of the pelvis, and it is difficult therefore to regard them as the primary cause of the obstruction.

c) High insertion of the ureter

It is sometimes claimed that an abnormally high position of the pelvi-ureteric junction may be responsible for obstruction: high insertion may be found in the malrotated kidney, but is otherwise rare and probably results simply from asymmetrical distension of the pelvis. In the malrotated, fused or ectopic kidneys the renal pelvis arises from a broad area on the anterior surface of the kidney,

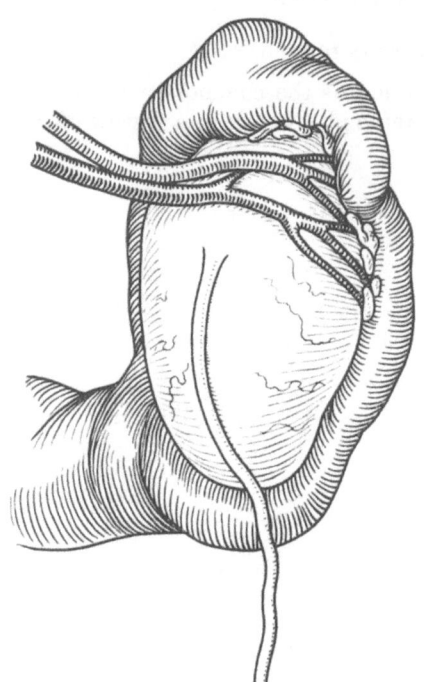

and the ureter therefore springs from the centre of a dome, rather than from a narrow triangular cavity as in the normal kidney (Fig. 18). This type of pelvis which is clearly at a mechanical disadvantage in propelling the urine into the ureter, and a high insertion may increase the difficulties. In the case of the horse-shoe kidney the ureter passes down over the isthmus and it has been suggested that this crossing is responsible for obstruction: in my cases, however, the obstruction has clearly been at a higher level, and often the distension of the hydronephrotic sac has lifted the ureter away from the isthmus.

d) Stenosis

Many authors (e.g. DAVIS) believe that a narrowing of the ureter immediately below the pelvi-ureteric junction is the primary cause of the hydronephrosis, and that other findings such as kinks and involvement with vessels are secondary developments. In the congenital type of stenosis there is seldom any suggestion of a fibrotic stricture, the muscular wall is in fact thinner than normal at the site

Fig. 18. Hydronephrosis in the horse-shoe kidney. Diagrammatic view showing the dome-like pelvis, the high insertion of the ureter, and the isthmus of the kidney

of the narrowing, and at times muscular fibres are completely absent. MURNAG-HAN has claimed that an interruption of the circular element of the musculature is a constant finding, and is the primary lesion. Instrumental dilatation of the narrowed segment is usually possible, and some writers have suggested a spasm as the cause of the narrowing.

e) "Unrolled" kidney

The kidney itself in hydronephrosis is often elongated and rather straight: JEWETT has suggested that this unrolling of the kidney is responsible for entangling the ureter with the renal vessels and therefore for causing the hydronephrosis. GRAUHAN on the other hand believes that the presence of hydronephrosis causes the kidney to grow in this shape.

f) Functional disorders

In spite of all these observations, in a proportion of cases operative findings do not suggest any obvious cause of obstruction, and it must be emphasized that the pathology of hydronephrosis cannot be discussed solely in terms of anatomy.

Disorders of function must be taken into account, although our present knowledge of normal physiology is sadly deficient. Intravenous pyelograms show that in normal conditions the upper 2—3 cm of the ureter as well as the renal pelvis forms a reservoir for the urine between the contraction waves, and both these segments are continuously filled throughout the phase of diastole. In hydronephrosis on the other hand the upper ureter is seldom filled at all in the earlier films of the pyelographic series, and in the later, there is often a filling defect immediately below the pelvis. At operation it can be demonstrated that contraction waves occur in the distended pelvis, but are not propagated down to the ureter: some failure of conduction at this point has therefore been suggested. However, the failure of ureteric contractions is probably due to the fact that no urine passes the pelvi-ureteric junction for the ureter can easily be provoked to contraction by distension (ANDERSON). In mild cases, it can sometimes be seen that while the pelvis is lax the upper ureter lies straight, and the contraction waves will be conducted from pelvis to ureter; if the pelvis is then tightly distended with fluid a curious writhing occurs, the junction becomes contorted and waves of contraction no longer reach the ureter. MURNAGHAN has demonstrated this effect in excised specimens and attributes it to the deficiency of circular muscle at the pelvi-ureteric junction in these cases. The adventitial sheath may fix these contortions but does not cause them. It would thus appear that any kidney with a large extra-renal pelvis, an abrupt transition from pelvis to ureter and a deficiency of circular muscle at this point, is liable to hydronephrosis which may be precipitated by a temporary polyuria, producing a load beyond the capacity of an inefficient segment. The formation of kinks and entanglement with vessels accentuates the obstruction, and any operation which restores a straight conical outlet from the pelvis will lead to an improvement.

The consequences of pelvi-ureteric obstruction are well known and need be mentioned only in brief. The muscle of the pelvis becomes hypertrophied, though continual distension may ultimately lead to thinning. The calyces dilate, and there is a progressive destruction of the renal parenchyma as a result of direct pressure, and of vascular obstruction. Urinary stasis may lead to the formation of secondary calculi, and urinary infection with consequent pyelonephritic changes is a common complication.

3. Clinical features

Congenital pelvi-ureteric lesions may be responsible for intermittent acute obstructions or for a slowly progressive distension of the pelvis and calyces. The acute form is the more common and is seen chiefly in children over the age of 5 years. During the attack there is a severe loin pain which does not radiate; it lasts for some hours and is accompanied by vomiting and pallor, but after its cessation the child is well and symptom-free. In the younger children the pain is less well localized and may be referred to the central abdomen, leading perhaps to the diagnosis of appendicitis. In the pelvic ectopic kidney, hydronephrosis may cause lower abdominal pain. At times vomiting is the predominant feature, and such cases are often regarded as examples of the "periodic syndrome" or acidosis. Most children lie down during the attack, but a few find that the adoption of some posture (e.g. the knee-elbow position) leads to relief. No disorder of micturition is to be expected, but in a few cases the pain is accompanied by oliguria and followed by a diuresis. This must clearly be a reflex phenomenon since the volume of the hydronephrotic kidney could not account for the discrepancy in the urine output. During the attack the kidney may be palpable and tender; in the intervals there are usually no abnormal physical signs.

Where the obstruction is less acute, a much more advanced stage of hydronephrosis may be reached with few symptoms. Sometimes there is aching pain in the loin, but often a large abdominal mass is found during routine examination. The latter observation is particularly common in infants in whom the renal enlargement is easily palpable and gives rise to the suspicion of tumour or polycystic disease. Differentiation can be made from the consistency of the swelling, from its variation in size from day to day, and from the pyelographic appearances.

Recurrent urinary infection with some pain in the loin is a third type of presentation. Haematuria may occur with or without infection, in the latter case it is presumed to stem from a pelvic vein ruptured by pressure. Secondary calculi seldom give any clinical indication of their presence, and may be found in symptom-free cases. Hydronephrosis may be discovered during the routine investigation of enuresis and though the renal condition may require treatment it is very unlikely to have any bearing on the complaint. Hypertension occurs on rare occasions in uncomplicated hydronephrosis.

4. Radiological diagnosis

An intravenous pyelogram is the most important part of the investigation, and treatment should not be undertaken without it; even if the hydronephrosis is discovered during laparotomy it is wiser to postpone any operative measures until this examination has been performed as it is often difficult to judge the state of the opposite kidney and ureter from palpation alone.

The common pyelographic appearance is a bulging renal pelvis with no filling of the ureter (Fig. 19A). The size of the pelvis is not of such diagnostic value as its shape: the small tense pelvis shown in Fig. 20 indicates pelvi-ureteric obstruction as much as the larger but slacker form shown in Fig. 21A. Save in the earliest cases the calyces have lost their normal cupped appearance and are clubbed; in advanced disease large round shadows in the dilated calyces are all that can be demonstrated. The upper ureter is not often filled in the earlier films of the series, and in the later it may show the small filling defect illustrated in Fig. 20, immediately distal to the pelvis. Sometimes there is a blob of dye in the kinked up portion of the ureter, where vessels or adhesions bind it down to the dilated renal pelvis. Below the kidney the ureter is normal, or shows a slight atonic dilatation in the lumbar region.

A large renal pelvis with continuous filling of the upper ureter and normal calyces should not be classified as a hydronephrosis (Fig. 22): there is no obstruction and no treatment is required. Such a pelvis is perhaps predisposed to the later development of hydronephrosis, however, and if there are any symptoms at all, periodic X-ray examination may be advisable.

In intermittent hydronephrosis there are characteristic attacks of loin pain, but in the intervals the pyelogram might pass for normal. In the case illustrated in Fig. 23 there was a vessel running from the aorta to the lower pole of the left kidney and the ureteric shadow ceases abruptly at this level. At operation this vessel was found but it could be demonstrated that on distension of the pelvis a kink formed at the pelvi-ureteric junction, and it appeared that obstruction occured at this point, well above the vessel. The decision to explore this type of case is made from a consideration of the type of pain and from the sharp cessation of the ureteric shadow: this appearance contrasts with that shown in Fig. 24; in which there is a transverse linear filling defect in the upper ureter without any deviation of the course of the ureter or any dilatation above. The latter picture may result from a kink of the muscularis within the adventitial

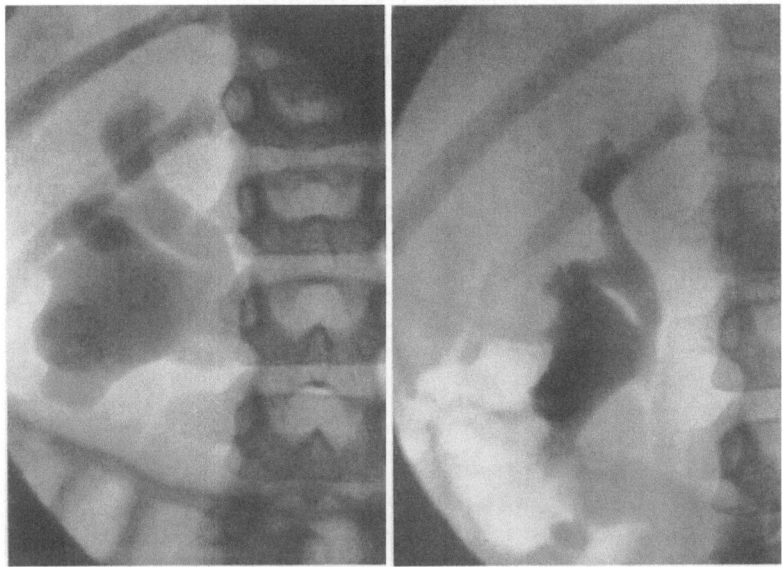

A   B

Fig. 19 A and B. Hydronephrosis. Intravenous pyelograms. A before: B after pyeloplasty. Girl aged 6 years with recurrent loin pain. The pelvis is partially bifurcated as well as being hydronephrotic

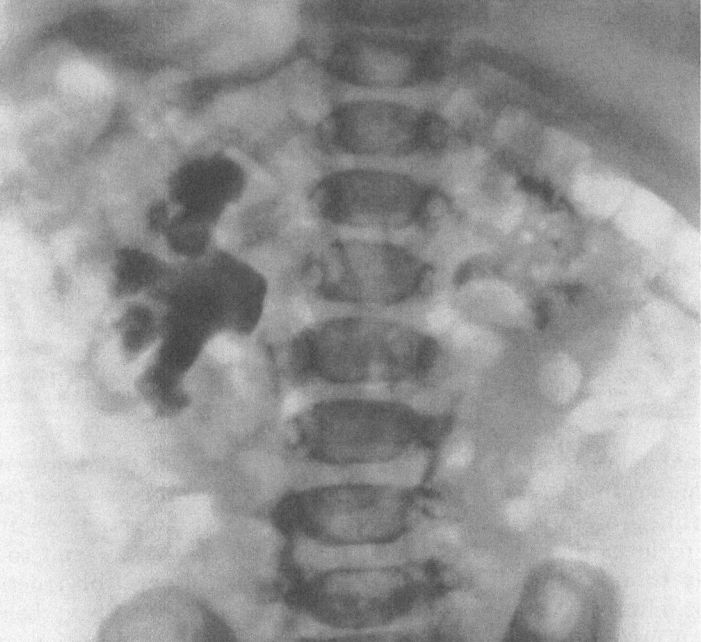

Fig. 20. Right hydronephrosis. Intravenous pyelogram in a girl of 12 months suffering from recurrent urinary infection

layer, of the type normally found in the foetus, and is not associated with obstruction; exploration is not required.

In malrotated kidneys, the pelvis normally appears large in the antero-posterior view: dilatation seen also in the lateral view and dilatation of the calyces indicate true hydronephrosis (Figs. 25 and 26).

The intravenous pyelogram may show no secretion in the affected kidney: this may be due to acute exacerbation of obstruction in a kidney of good function

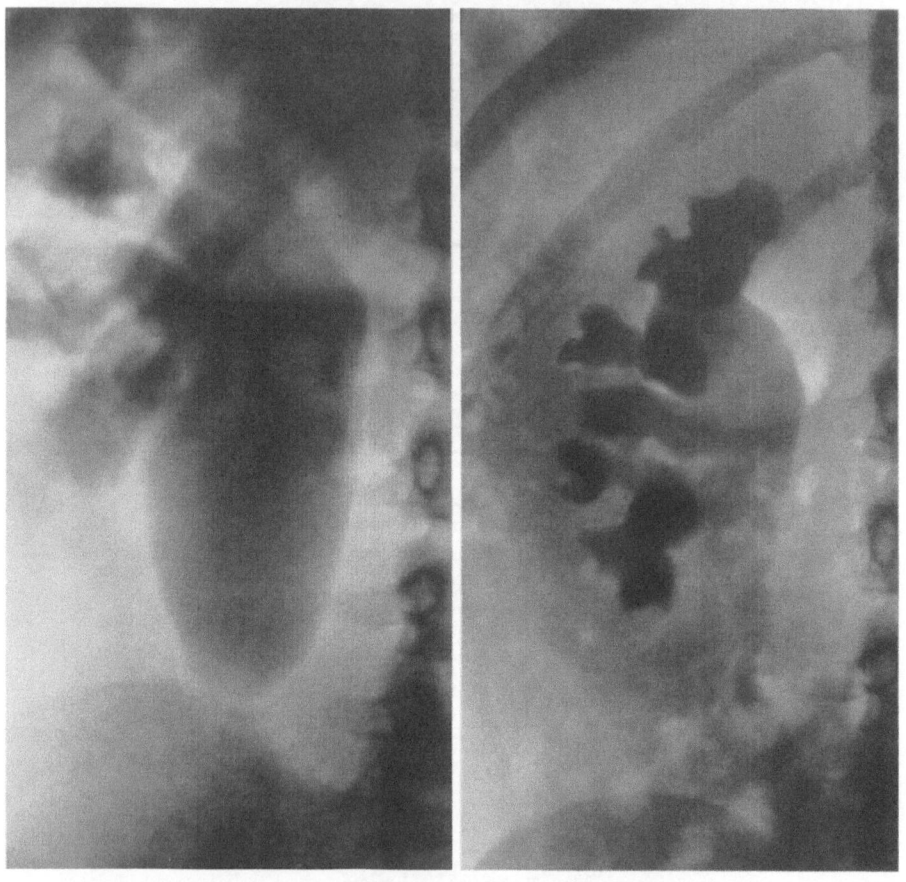

A   B

Fig. 21 A and B. Hydronephrosis. Intravenous pyelograms: A before and B after pyeloplasty. Boy aged 10 years whose opposite kidney had been removed in infancy during laparotomy for abdominal pain

(as in renal colic, a nephrogram is occasionally seen) or to advanced destruction of the parenchyma. A retrograde pyelogram is desirable in these circumstances, though this procedure is not without risks due to infection or trauma; it is wise to perform the examination in the operating theatre and to proceed immediately to operation if the diagnosis of pelvi-ureteric obstruction is made. It is not always possible to fill the obstructed pelvis from below, but the kinked up ureter is usually outlined and gives a clear indication of the nature of the disorder.

It is sometimes claimed that aortography is of value in indicating the type of operation to be undertaken, but in the child it is a difficult procedure and not without risks. In my opinion it is not a justifiable investigation in these cases.

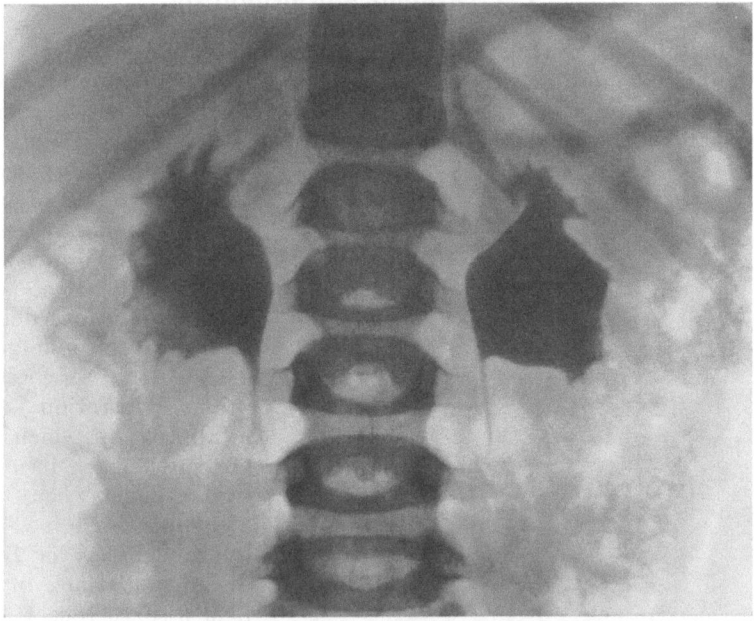

Fig. 22. Large renal pelves without pelvi-ureteric obstruction. Intravenous pyelogram in a girl aged 5 years without renal symptoms. Condition unchanged in 3 year follow-up

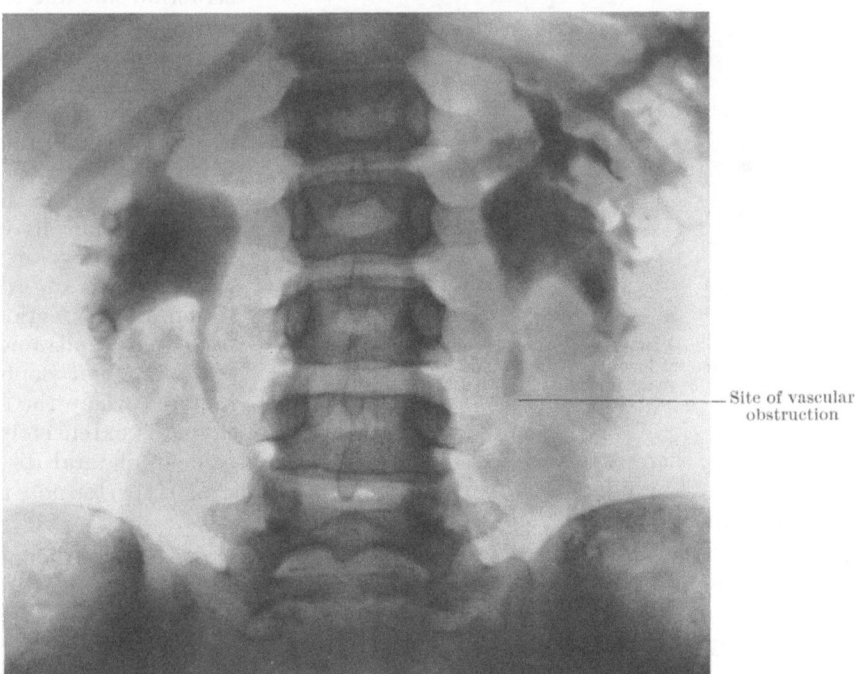

Site of vascular obstruction

Fig. 23. Intermittent hydronephrosis. Intravenous pyelogram in a boy aged 10 years with repeated attacks of severe left loin pain. At operation an aberrant vessel was found to cross the ureter 3 cm below the pelvi-ureteric junction: there was also a kink and potential obstruction at the junction itself (see text).

5. Treatment and prognosis

The aim of treatment is not only to relieve the pain and prevent the recurrences of infection, but also to preserve and improve the functioning renal tissue. During recent years the great value of conservative operations has been recognized and there is now no doubt that they are applicable to the majority of cases (four-fifths of my series). Untreated, the rate of increase of the dilatation may be extremely slow in those cases with intermittent attacks of pain, while in the chronic form deterioration is apt to continue relentlessly despite the absence of symptoms. Operation is desirable in all cases in which a definite obstruction can be demonstrated, though when as in the case illustrated in Fig. 20, the hydronephrosis is first found during an attack of infection, it is wise to repeat the pyelogram some weeks after sterilization of the urine to exclude the possibility that the obstruction was due to temporary spasm.

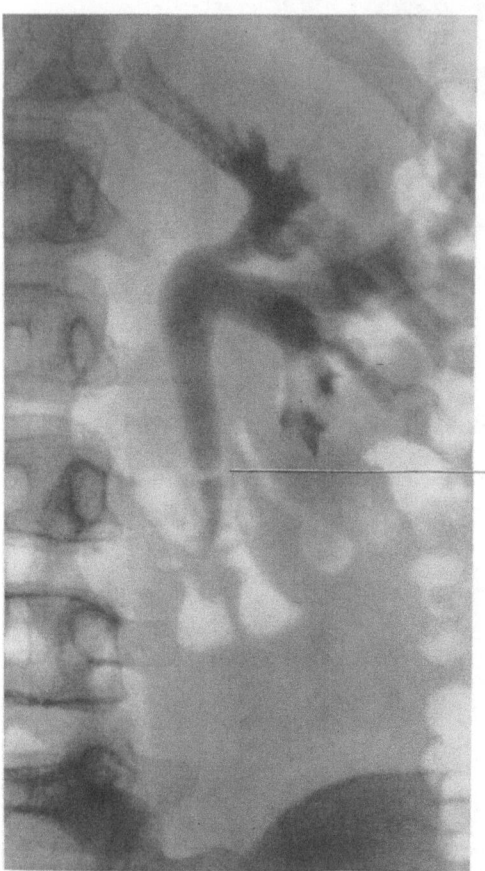

mucosal kink

Fig. 24. Normal kidney with non-obstructive kink below the pelvi-ureteric junction. Intravenous pyelogram in a boy aged 8 years investigated because of enuresis (see text)

Conservative operation is almost obligatory in cases of bilateral hydronephrosis and in the primarily unilateral case when the contralateral kidney has a large, square pelvis which suggests that hydronephrosis may later develop there too. The presence of calyceal dilatation, mild infection or calculi need not contraindicate conservatism, but nephrectomy is required where the renal parenchyma is extensively destroyed or where there is severe pyelonephritis complicating unilateral disease, for in such cases the infection is very difficult to eliminate. Hypertension unquestionably indicates nephrectomy in the unilateral case.

The techniques of conservative surgery are discussed in another volume, but certain expressions of opinion may not be out of place here. Ligature of vessels alone is only justifiable where that procedure results in the immediate collapse of the hydronephrotic sac: in other cases a plastic operation is required, and its use may obviate the need for a ligature which deprives an important area of the kidney of its blood supply. Division of adhesions alone is not an adequate measure, and simple dilatation of the junctional region has given disappointing results. The author has obtained better results with the operation described by

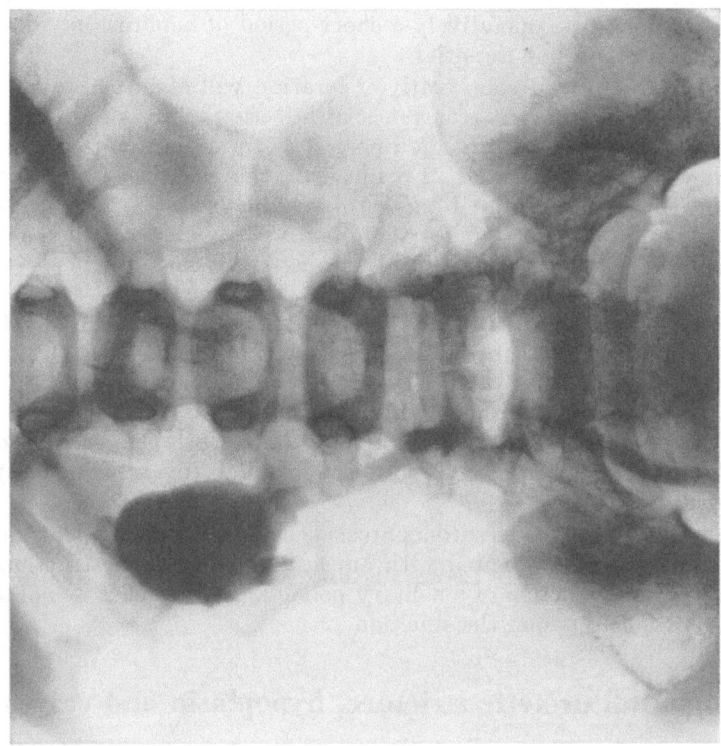

Fig. 26. Bilateral hydronephrosis in the horse-shoe kidney. Intravenous pyelogram in a boy aged 7 years complaining of severe attacks of left loin pain. There is no concentration of dye in the left kidney; on the right side there is a moderate hydronephrosis in a mal-rotated renal pelvis with a medially directed lower calyx. Exploration confirmed [the suspected diagnosis of horse-shoe kidney, the left ureter being kinked and obstructed by a vessel running to the lower pole

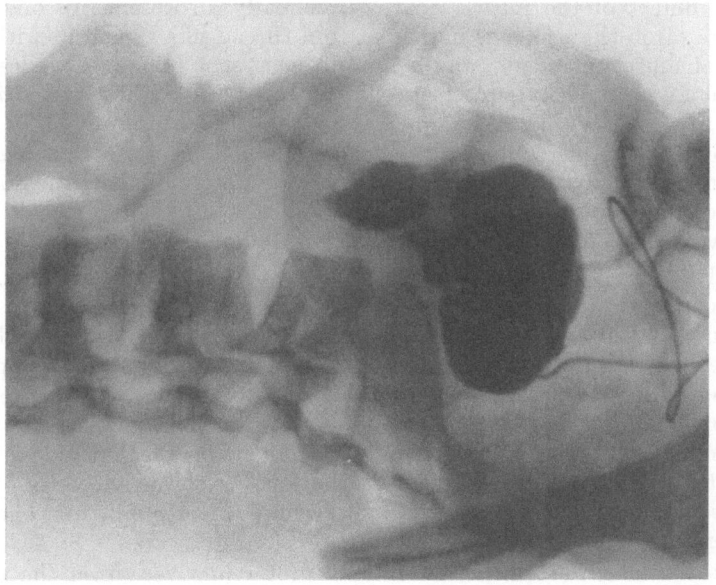

Fig. 25. Hydronephrosis in the pelvic ectopic kidney. Retrograde pyelogram in a girl aged 8 years, suffering from recurrent severe abdominal pains. Treated by nephrectomy

ANDERSON, which is applicable to all types, than with the Foley Y-V-plasty, or with any other procedure. In infected cases it is desirable to sterilize the urine before operation; post-operatively a short period of nephrostomy drainage may be desirable, though not essential.

A satisfactorily performed conservative operation will almost always relieve the attacks of pain, and prevent recurrence of infection: some improvement in renal function is to be expected, though a perfect restoration of normal anatomy is seldom achieved. Figs. 19 B and 21 B illustrate the recovery which may be possible. By contrast, in malrotated and ectopic kidneys the response to plastic operations is seldom satisfactory unless there is a well defined vascular obstruction. In the painful unilateral anomalous hydronephrosis therefore nephrectomy should be the treatment of choice, and in the symptom-free cases operative intervention is scarcely ever justified. Conservative operation for the relief of hydronephrosis in the horse-shoe kidney is sometimes successful: CULP and WINTERRINGER indicate that pyeloplasty should be supplemented by division of the isthmus and nephropexy, though I am not entirely convinced of the value of the latter procedures. With very low kidneys, HESS has performed a direct anastomosis between the renal pelvis and the bladder (pyelocystomosis) and claims good results.

At times a purely intrarenal hydronephrosis is seen in the anomalous kidney: in one of my cases a child presented with anuria due to acute obstruction at a strictured reno-ureteral junction of a solitary pelvic kidney. Relief was obtained by a plastic operation to widen the junction.

VI. Congenital ureteric stricture, hypoplasia and valves

Congenital narrowing of the ureter affects chiefly the pelvi-ureteric junction causing hydronephrosis as already described. Congenital uretero-vesical stricture produces a condition akin to mega-ureter and is discussed in Section C. Between these two points, a congenital narrowing is rare and is usually associated with a defect of the muscle coat, occasionally an absence of one layer only, but more often the ureter is narrowed to a thread-like structure with thin walls devoid of muscle elements, and a minute or absent lumen. This lesion is here described as ureteric hypoplasia though it has received little attention in the literature.

Where there is complete obliteration of the lumen, ureteric hypoplasia is associated with severe dysplasia of the kidney, or with the multicystic kidney. These conditions have already been described, and it will be noted that in them the obliterative process extends up into the pelvis and calyces.

Where only a short segment of ureter is affected, and obliteration of the lumen is not complete, the hypoplastic area will present an obstruction to urine flow and cause partial hydro-ureter or hydronephrosis. This type might be included under the heading of "stricture" but the latter term is usually applied to a narrowing with a thickened wall, and the distinction is worth making because severe and mild forms of hypoplasia may occur in the same patient. Thus in one case under my care, a long hypoplastic segment on the left side led up to a multicystic kidney, a short segment at the level of the pelvic brim on the right caused severe hydronephrosis. Hypoplasia may affect more than one segment of the ureter causing multiple "strictures".

Hypoplasia of the lower end of an ectopic ureter (derived from the upper pelvis of a double kidney) is illustrated in Fig. 27. The lumen was sufficient to allow dribbling incontinence, but had caused considerable dilatation of the proximal segment, and of a blind bifurcation or diverticulum.

The treatment of hypoplasia is by excision and re-anastomosis, or by nephrectomy.

The term ureteric valve should not be applied to a kink which involves the whole ureter: such kinks are an inevitable concomitant of ureteric dilatation, and where this ceases above the bladder as in the simple mega-ureter with supravesical narrow segment, the terminal kink has always a valve-like appearance. True valves consist of mucosal folds within the lumen, and do not involve the muscularis; they are very rare but they have been described in children by ROBERTS and by SIMON et al.

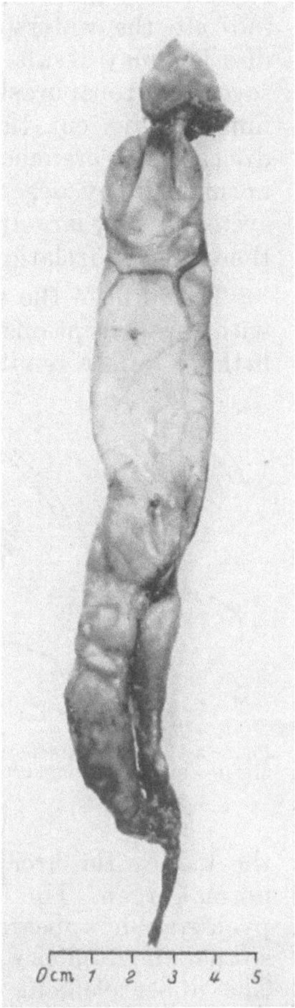

VII. Duplications of the ureter

1. General

Duplication of the ureter in various forms is one of the commonest malformations of the genito-urinary tract, and complications much more frequently give rise to symptoms during childhood than during adult life. The possibility of a duplication must always be borne in mind whenever pyelograms are reviewed, particularly in children with pyuria, renal pain or incontinence, and it must be emphasized that renal function may be so depressed in the affected elements that only one pelvis and ureter is outlined pyelographically. The anatomy of the malformation is therefore described in some detail in this volume, though for embryological details and full references Volume VII should be consulted.

a) Incidence

NATION has reviewed the malformation at all ages, and found 109 cases in the 16000 autopsies: it was more common in females, and in that sex very much more often showed pathological complications. GOYANNA and GREENE found the right side to be affected twice as often as the left, but it must be emphasized that some form of the malformation is very often bilateral, perhaps showing a bifid ureter on one side and a complete duplication on the other. CAMPBELL has reviewed the complications in children.

Fig. 27. Ureteric hypoplasia, with a blind duplication in an ectopic ureter. Operative specimen from a girl aged 7 years with dribbling incontinence due to an ectopic ureter derived from the upper pelvis of a right double kidney. Hemi-nephrectomy with ureterectomy performed. The lower end of the ectopic ureter is narrow and thread-like, the upper end is dilated and there is a distended blind pouch opening in it

b) Anatomy

The malformation arises from the development of an accessory ureteric bud either upon the side of the normal ureter (resulting in an incomplete duplication) or upon the parent Wolffian duct (giving a complete duplication). All derivatives of the ureteric bud are therefore duplicated and differentiation of the nephrons takes place in relation to the two systems, but the mass of meta-nephric tissue into which the ureters grow remains undivided save in the rare instances of supernumerary kidneys. Apart from some increase in length the kidney has a superficially normal appearance and there is no more than a shallow sulcus to indicate the watershed between the two systems of drainage. A more definite division may result from changes in only one renal element as when there is severe hydronephrosis or pyelo-nephritis, but an incision severing the two halves must always cut through renal tissue. The renal artery exhibits a premature division into branches which usually follow, however, the general pattern for the normal kidney described by GRAVES: it sometimes happens that one calyceal system is very largely served by one or two arterial branches, but more frequently there is no correlation between blood supply and urinary drainage.

The form of the pelvi-calyceal systems is similar in all types of duplication: with rare exceptions the upper element is the smaller, its ureter expands very little to form a renal pelvis and there is no true pelvi-ureteric junction. Within

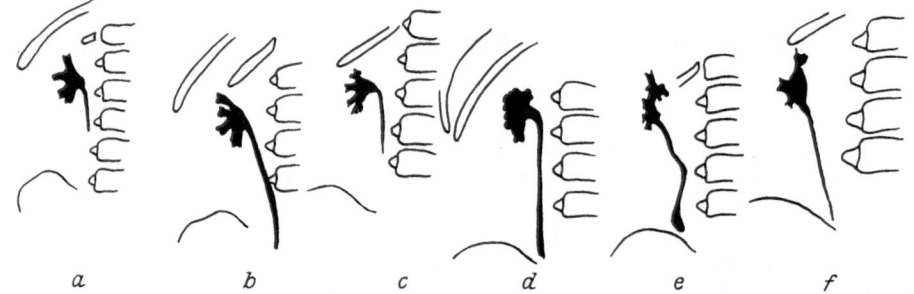

a   b   c   d   e   f

Fig. 28 a—f. Outline tracings of pyelograms, show the lower pelves of double kidneys. In *a* and *b* the upper ureter connected with an ectopic ureterocele. In *c* the ureter was bifid and in *d, e* and *f* the ureter from the upper pelvis terminated in the vagina

the kidney the area of drainage corresponds to the upper major calyx of the normal organ. The lower element is larger and a definite pelvis is formed. The pyelographic appearances of the separate elements should be studied with care so that the duplicity can be readily recognized even if only one pelvis is outlined. The upper element can be identified without difficulty; when only the lower is filled, it can be recognized as part of a double kidney from one or more of the following features (Figs. 28 and 29, 38 and 40).

α) The calyces are fewer in number than in the normal kidney, and the uppermost does not approach the upper limit of the renal shadow.

β) The upper pole of the kidney appears to be rotated outwards and downwards giving the pelvis something of the appearance of a drooping flower. This distortion may be mimicked by a tumour.

γ) The upper calyx is short, and though the cups of the calyces may be directed upwards or medially they are very close to the renal pelvis and there is no elongated infundibulum. Occasionally there is a suggestion of malrotation.

δ) The pelvis is displaced laterally away from the vertebral column, and the ureter instead of being directed at first towards the mid-line and then running down vertically gradually approaches the paravertebral region at the level of the 5th lumbar vertebra.

In cases where the ureter from the upper pelvis ends ectopically the upper element is unusually small and the outline of the lower pelvis less typical. Where the duplication is incomplete the two elements are occasionally of almost equal size, or very rarely the upper may be the larger.

The point of bifurcation of the ureter in incomplete duplication may be placed at any point between the renal pelvis and the bladder, though it is more common in the upper and in the lower third than in the middle. The branches normally run parallel to one another and join at an acute angle, but occasionally one spirals around the other before joining it.

Because of the manner in which the terminal segment of the Wolffian duct is absorbed into the trigone, in the complete duplications the upper pelvis ureter

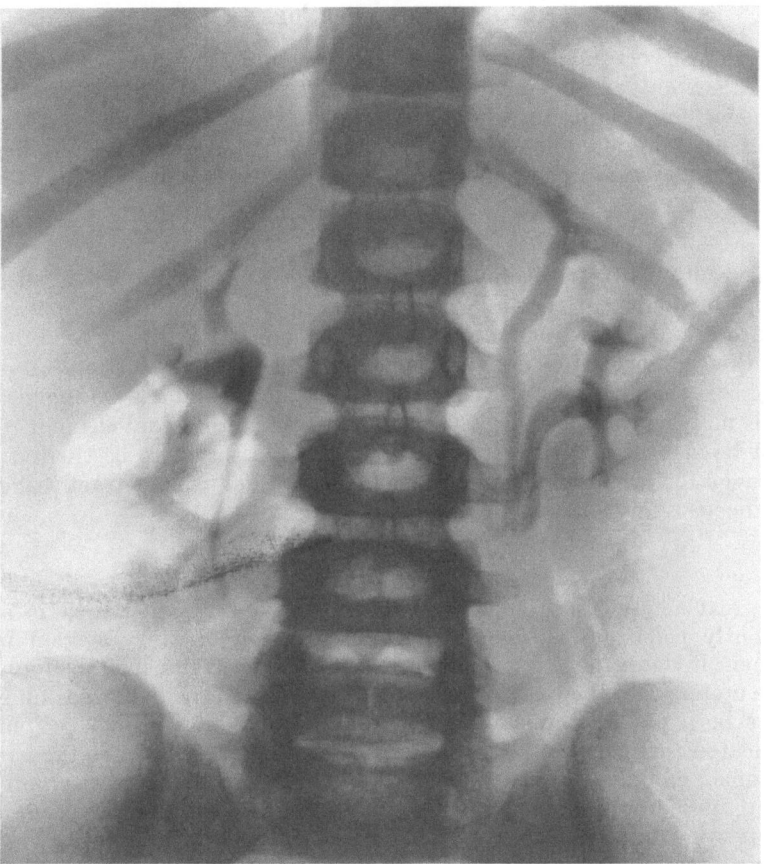

Fig. 29. Left bifid ureter. Intravenous pyelogram in a boy aged 7 years complaining of recurrent loin pain. The pyelogram shows no evident complication and the attacks of pain ceased spontaneously after 3 months

enters the bladder at some point caudal and medial to the ureter from the lower element. Commonly the latter has an orifice at the angle of the trigone which has cystoscopically the normal crescentic appearance, while the former (upper renal element) has a slit-like opening placed on the inferior aspect of the inter-ureteric bar where it is very easily overlooked. At times the opening of the ureter from the upper pelvis becomes even further removed from its normal position, and may be placed at the bladder neck, in the urethra or in other organs; these complications (ectopic endings) and the formation of ureteroceles are discussed in a later section. At other times the orifice of the upper pelvis ureter lies immediately medial, or very rarely medial and superior, to the orifice of the lower pelvis ureter. The common arrangement of the ureteric orifices in complete duplication is often taken to indicate a crossing of the ureters, though in fact the upper pelvis ureter often lies medial to its fellow throughout its length, and it is merely prolonged beyond it at both upper and lower end; the frontal crossing which is shown in pyelograms taken in the antero-posterior view very seldom indicates a true spiralling. In the lumbar region the two ureters are loosely bound together, but as they approach the bladder they become more closely united within Waldeyer's sheath and often share a common adventitial layer.

c) Complications

There are very many cases in which a complete or incomplete duplication never causes any derangement of function, and the malformation is only directly responsible for symptoms where there is an ectopic opening or a ureterocele. Nevertheless, double ureters unquestionably carry an increased liability to complications and certain characteristic ones merit discussion.

α) Recurrent urinary infection

The routine investigation of pyuria in girls not infrequently discloses the presence of double ureters in which there are no additional complications such as hydro-ureter or hydronephrosis, and although it is difficult to prove statistically, this malformation does appear to predispose to infection. It should be emphasized that when the pyelograms reveal no secondary pathological process there is no indication for surgical interference since the renal element responsible cannot be identified with certainty. Cases should therefore be treated along the lines suggested for recurrent infections in the normal urinary tract (page 143) and spontaneous remission is ultimately to be expected.

β) Pain

A great many children suffer vague abdominal pain which is sometimes sufficiently persistent to demand an investigation of every system within the abdomen: it is not therefore surprising that some such cases will be found to have double ureters, and the knowledge of the existence of this malformation frequently worries both parent and child. Where the duplication is pyelographically uncomplicated there should be great hesitation in identifying it as the cause of the symptoms, and unless the pain is very clearly renal in origin, it is wiser not to inform the parents of the findings. There are, however, in children as in adults certain subjects with bifid ureter who suffer colicky pain in the loin, and it has been suggested that in these few there is an interference in the transmission of the peristaltic wave at the point of bifurcation. In these cases an upper pole heminephrectomy has been advised (GUTIERREZ, CAMPBELL), but I have always been reluctant to undertake such a procedure unless an abnormality can be demonstrated radiologically, and in some of my cases the pains have ultimately ceased spontaneously.

γ) Hydronephrosis

The lower pelvis has a definite pelvi-ureteric junction, and is as liable as a normal kidney to congenital obstruction and hydronephrosis. In the author's cases (Fig. 30) and those reported in the literature (e.g. FEYDER and DEMING) the hydronephrosis has been of such a size as to require nephrectomy, but less severe cases will probably be seen and can treated on conservative lines. In the upper element there is very rarely any extra-renal pelvis and congenital pelvi-ureteric obstruction can scarcely occur.

δ) Hydro-ureter

The most marked examples of hydro-ureter with duplications are seen in the ureters with ectopic endings or ureteroceles and affect therefore the upper pole ureter. Chronic dilatation affecting both branches is quite commonly encountered in low bifurcation of the ureter, often with chronic urinary infection. In three of the author's cases this type was associated with dilatation of the contralateral single ureter and the exact importance of the duplication was hard to assess.

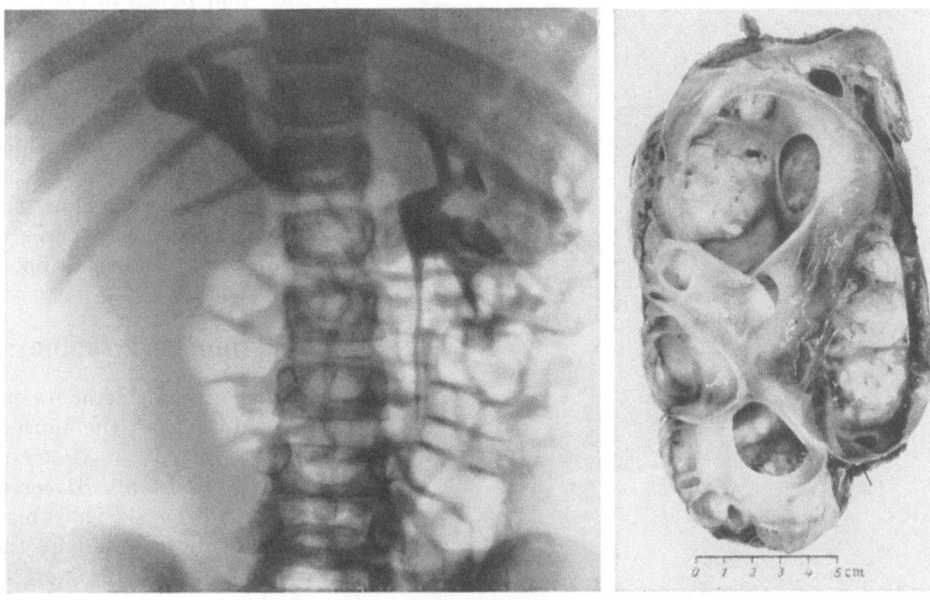

A   B

Fig. 30 A and B. Hydronephrosis due to pelvi-ureteric obstruction in the lower pelvis of a double kidney (bifid ureter). A Intravenous pyelogram showing the displacement of the upper pelvis and distortion suggesting renal tumour. B Nephrectomy specimen

Such cases must be treated in the same way as mega-ureters without this complication; conservative operations on the ureters are seldom successful but nephrectomy must only be performed in the strictly unilateral case. In the complete duplications where both ureters open close together on the trigone, a moderate dilatation of the ureter from the lower pelvis may be seen, usually with pyelonephritis and hypoplasia of the corresponding element. Ten such cases have been treated by the author; they presented with recurrent pyuria and the diagnosis was easily established from pyelograms (Fig. 31). Satisfactory relief was obtained by lower pole heminephrectomy. Other variations are encountered from time to time and many offer the possibility of cure by resection of the affected renal element.

ε) Hypoplasia

Complete or partial hypoplasia is a complication of many types of ureteric duplication and the renal element associated with an ectopic ureter is very often affected in this way.

2. Blind ending duplications

At times one ureter, arising either as a branch of the main duct or independently from the bladder, ends blindly at its upper extremity and makes no contact with renal tissue. Perhaps the commonest site for such malformations is near the lower end (e.g. KRETSCHMER'S case) and where the blind pouch opens immediately adjacent to the ureteric orifice in the bladder it may be difficult to decide whether it should be regarded as a vesical diverticulum or as a ureter. Often there are no symptoms directly attributable to the malformation; the author has thus encountered one in an enuretic child and another during nephro-ureterectomy for ectopic ureter (Fig. 27). In some reports, however, the blind pouch has become distended and has obstructed the normal ureter (HARRIS, CAMP-BELL). Such blind duplications are hardly distinguishable from the true ureteric diverticula which are reported on very rare occasions: CULP in reviewing the literature found eleven cases of which two presented in childhood.

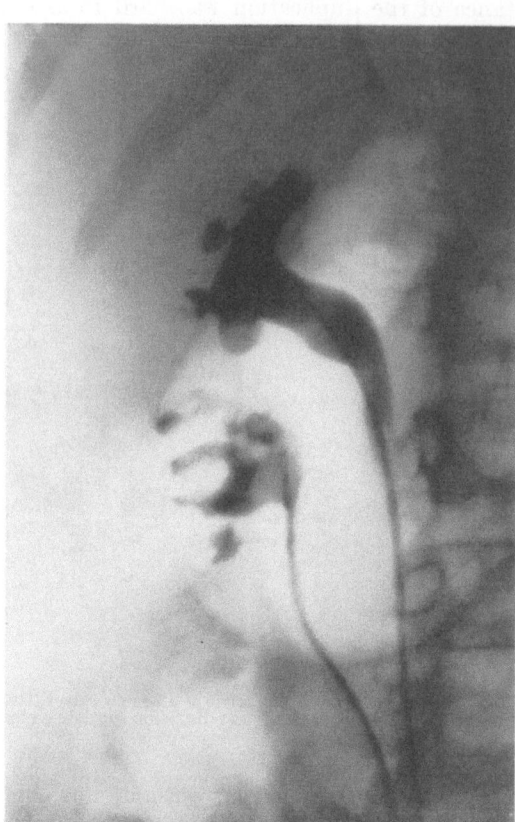

Fig. 31. Complete ureteric duplication with hypoplasia of the lower renal element. Retrograde pyelogram in a girl aged 8 years suffering from recurrent urinary infection. Satisfactory relief obtained from heminephrectomy

3. Supernumerary kidneys

Accessory renal elements entirely separate from the normal kidney are very rare: CARLSON was able to find only 51 cases, recorded at all ages. They may present in childhood as in the case of GLEIZE-RAMBAL et al. The supernumerary organ has almost always an additional malformation such as hydronephrosis or hypoplasia; it is most often found in the iliac fossa or pelvis and its ureter joins that from the normal kidney above the bladder. The hydronephrotic sac may present as a mass in the abdomen causing partial obstruction to the normal kidney. A supernumerary kidney lying above the normal organ and drained by an ectopic ureter is on record (RUBIN).

4. Caudal bifurcation

On rare occasions a ureter which is single above, branches at its lower end: PHOKITIS found 11 cases reported. Where both branches enter the bladder no serious complications are to be expected, but it is recorded that in some, one branch ended in the vagina and caused dribbling incontinence. The diagnosis in these cases is open to some question as the patients had had previous extensive gynaecological operations, and an epithelialized fistula might have formed, but VON RIHMER describes a girl of 17 years whom he investigated for vaginal incontinence and found that the left ureter had a triangular dilatation at its caudal extremity; one angle of the triangle was represented by a small orifice in the region of the bladder neck while the other was formed by an opening into the vagina.

5. Triplications of the ureter

Three or more ureters may drain a single kidney: they may unite or enter the bladder separately. The kidney itself is likely to be anomalous, and is extremely liable to all the complications described for the "double kidney". A case in a child has been reported by SMITH, who also reviews the literature.

VIII. Ectopic ureters

1. General

An ectopic ureter is one which has its termination in the urinary tract at a point distal to the normal site or in some part of the genital tract. The ureter may be single and drain the whole of the corresponding kidney, in which case some associated renal anomaly is common e.g. hypoplasia, malrotation or ectopia. More often the ureteric ectopia is associated with duplication, and the ureter from the upper pelvis, which always opens in the more caudal position, terminates ectopically. There may be bilateral ectopic ureters of either type, or both ureters from the one kidney may end ectopically, though that from the lower pelvis will be nearer the normal situation than that from the upper pelvis. The ureter itself is almost always dilated, sometimes exhibiting a saccular dilatation; the orifice may be wide or strictured. The related renal element is usually small, and complicating pyelonephritis is not uncommon.

The symptoms caused by the presence of an ectopic ureter depend less upon its origin than upon its termination. If it reaches the vesico-urethral canal, it must open somewhere between the site of the normal ureteric orifice, and the final position of the Wolffian duct opening, i.e. the verumontanum in the male, or the region of the external urinary meatus in the female. On the other hand, if the bud originates high up on the Wolffian duct, it will fail to reach the urethra, and will retain its connection with the derivatives of that duct (i.e. the ejaculatory ducts, seminal vesicles or vasa deferentia in the male) or with atrophy of its parent, break through into the Müllerian duct system (vagina or uterus in the female). Openings further afield, into the rectum for instance, are also on record.

For general reviews and full lists of the relevant literature, the reader should consult the works of DEUTICKE, BURFORD et al., CAMPBELL, HEPLER, T. D. MOORE, POLITZER, and VAZQUEZ and VARELA. In the following paragraphs, the various anatomical types of ectopic ureter will be considered separately.

2. Urethral ectopia in the female

A ureter which opens at the bladder neck or into the upper urethra of the female often causes very little disturbance of function and may be symptomless. As with other forms it may be derived from a single or a double kidney, but it should be noted that in the latter case it may drain the lower pelvis, while the ureter from the upper pelvis is more widely ectopic, opening into the vestibule or vagina. The orifice is wide, and clearly visible on urethroscopy but dilatation of the ureter is the rule and may be extreme at the lower end, simulating a urethral diverticulum (WILLMARTH). In this situation the ectopic ureter does not cause incontinence in the child, though it is possible that in adult life, with the relaxation of the external urethral supporting muscles, it may do so (IDBOHRM and SJOSTEDT). Most of the cases present with recurrent or persistent pyuria, and with the symptoms characteristic of infection. The diagnosis will be suspected from the intravenous pyelogram; the corresponding renal element will seldom concentrate the dye sufficiently to cast a clear shadow, but its presence will be indicated by the shape and position of the lower pelvis (see p. 36). Confirmation may be obtained by urethroscopy and catheterization of the ectopic orifice: treatment, when

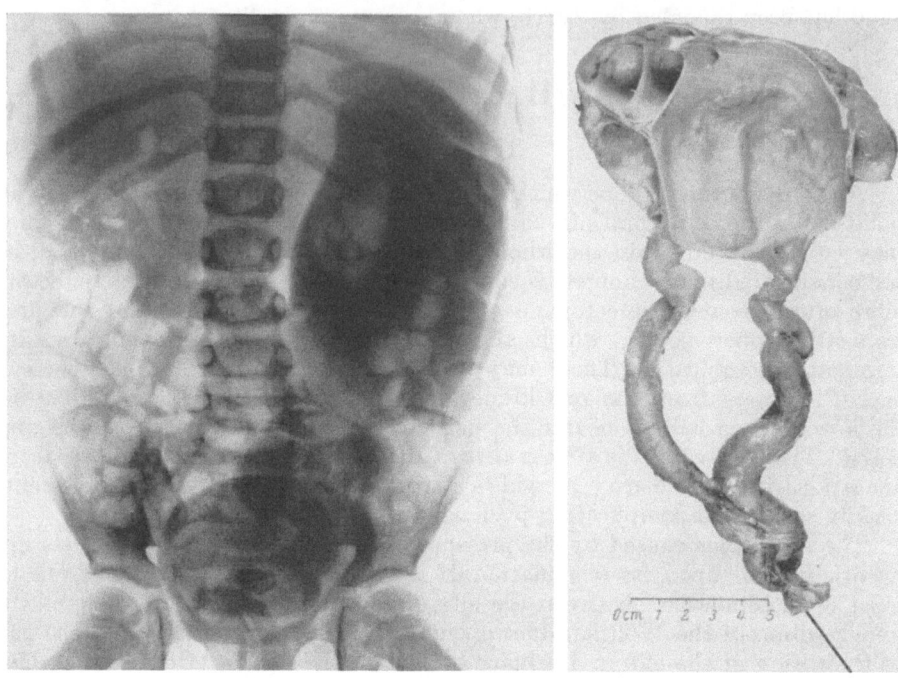

A   B

Fig. 32 A and B. Urethral ectopic ureter with hydronephrosis of the lower pelvis of the same kidney. A Cystogram after micturition in a boy aged 3 years complaining of difficult micturition, and found to have a large residual urine. I.V.P. demonstrated normal right kidney and no function on the left side. Endoscopy showed a wide left ureteric orifice in the normal situation, and a second left orifice in the posterior urethra. Reflux took place only into the lower pelvis (normally placed orifice). B Nephro-ureterectomy specimen. After operation normal micturition without residuum was immediately restored

required, will almost always consist of nephrectomy or heminephrectomy, since conservation of the renal element by re-implantation of the ureter is unlikely to succeed.

3. Urethral and genital tract ectopia in the male

In urethral ectopia the orifice lies at or above the level of the verumontanum, and the clinical features will be similar to those described for the female. When the ureter enters the seminal vesicle or the vas, the symptoms may be due to the development of an inflammatory mass behind the prostatic urethra, or to epididymitis. An additional complication which has been observed is the development of bladder neck obstruction, causing dilatation of the contralateral ureter (cf. SMITH).

In three of my cases pathological complications were not confined to the ectopic ureter; the ureter from the lower pelvis of the same kidney, although opening normally on the trigone, was grossly dilated and allowed free reflux (see Fig. 32). These boys were all brought to hospital with the diagnosis of chronic retention of urine, but it was found that the apparently large residual urine was simply the result of the large volume which entered the ureter at each act of micturition, and which flowed back afterwards. Normal bladder function was in all cases restored by complete nephro-ureterectomy.

4. Ectopic ureterocele

This important lesion has received tardy recognition from urologists and appears in the literature under a wide variety of names; cases have been reported as cysts of the trigone and as double bladders, while MERTZ et al. refer to blind uretero-vesical protrusions which appear to conform to the pattern to be described as ectopic ureterocele. ERICSON has given a full description of the condition, however, and reference should made to his work for a review of the literature.

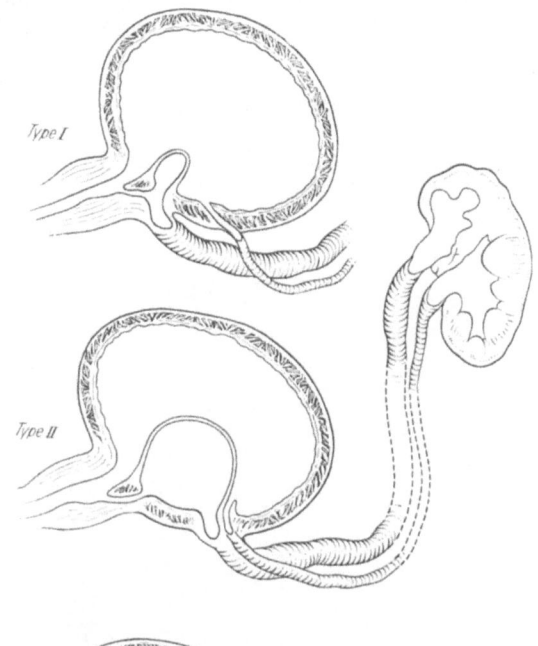

a) Anatomy

The ectopic ureterocele differs in many respects from the simple ureterocele, and in my experience has been the commoner lesion in childhood: sixteen cases have been operated upon in a five year period. The actual ureteric orifice lies within the urethra while the ureterocele is a localized bulge of dilated ureter lying inside the muscular wall of the bladder, but deep to the bladder mucosa (Fig. 33). The ureter, which carries its own muscular

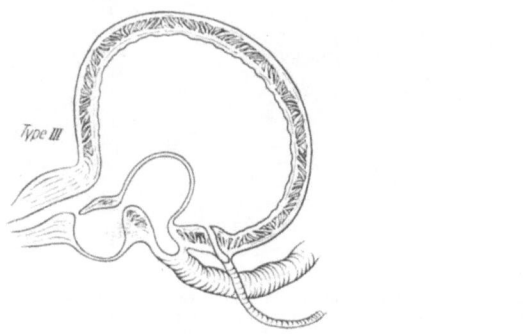

Fig. 33. Diagrams to show the anatomical arrangement in the ectopic ureterocele (see text)

coat, is a little constricted where it passes through the detrusor and again where it passes down through muscle of the internal sphincter to reach the posterior urethra. The findings have varied somewhat and have been classified in three types.

In type I, a small cystic protrusion with a comparatively narrow base is present at the bladder neck, showing on the cystogram as a semi-circular filling defect. At simple cystoscopy with the right angle instrument this may easily be overlooked unless the outline of the bladder neck is carefully followed; the trigone itself and the upper ureteric orifices appear normal. On urethroscopy the swelling is easily visualized and seems to be prolonged down the urethra. This type of ureterocele can prolapse through the female urethra and can cause mild bladder neck obstruction, but does not directly obstruct the other ureters.

In type II there is a broad based cystic protrusion occupying a large portion of the trigone and prolonged down as a ridge in the mid-line of the posterior urethra where the ureter opens through a comparatively wide orifice. The lower pelvis ureter from the ipsilateral kidney is drawn up on the slopes of the ureterocele and the contralateral ureter may be similarly affected. This type of ureterocele may therefore obstruct the lower ends of the other ureters as well as the bladder neck. When bilateral the two ureteroceles may fuse together into a single swelling, but a partition between them persists. At cystoscopy the greater part of the bladder is obscured by the bulging ureterocele, and endoscopic diagnosis is difficult. On the cystogram a large filling defect (Fig. 34) shows well above the bladder neck and to one side of the mid-line, its outline is almost a complete circle.

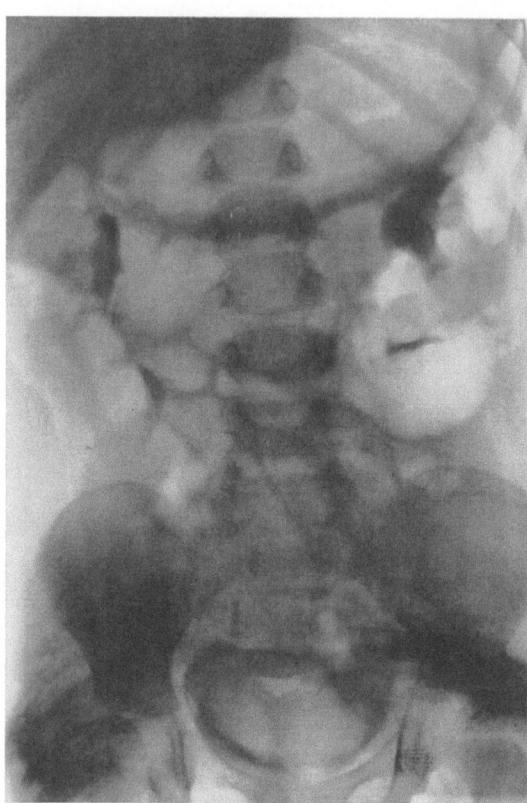

Fig. 34. Bilateral ectopic ureterocele. Intramuscular pyelogram in a girl aged 2 years with pyuria. Only the lower pelves of the double kidneys are outlined, they are displaced laterally by the dilated ureters from the upper pelves. The bladder shadow shows filling defects corresponding to the ureteroceles

Type III is a development of type II in which the ureter as it leaves the ureterocele runs outside the internal sphincter of the bladder and forms a dilated sac behind the posterior urethra. Reflux may occur into the dilated ureter after micturition.

b) Symptoms

In general symptoms are due to the large reservoir of infected urine in the dilated ureter causing recurrent or persistent pyuria (Fig. 35). Difficult micturition due to bladder neck obstruction and prolapse of the ureterocele may also occur, while in type 3 there may be incontinence due to interference with the sphincters. In the case illustrated in Fig. 36, the ectopic ureter, although uninfected became extremely dilated and acutely kinked, causing colicky abdominal pain and a tumour simulating an intussusception.

c) Diagnosis

The condition is usually diagnosed with ease from the intravenous pyelograms: there is the characteristic filling defect in the bladder shadow associated with absent function in the upper element of a double kidney. The bulge in the bladder makes the cystoscopic appearance confusing, but the ectopic orifice can be seen on urethroscopy.

d) Treatment

In most cases the essential measure of treatment is the removal of the dilated ureter and this may be achieved by heminephrectomy and complete ureterectomy. At the same time the ureterocele should be "uncapped" through the open bladder.

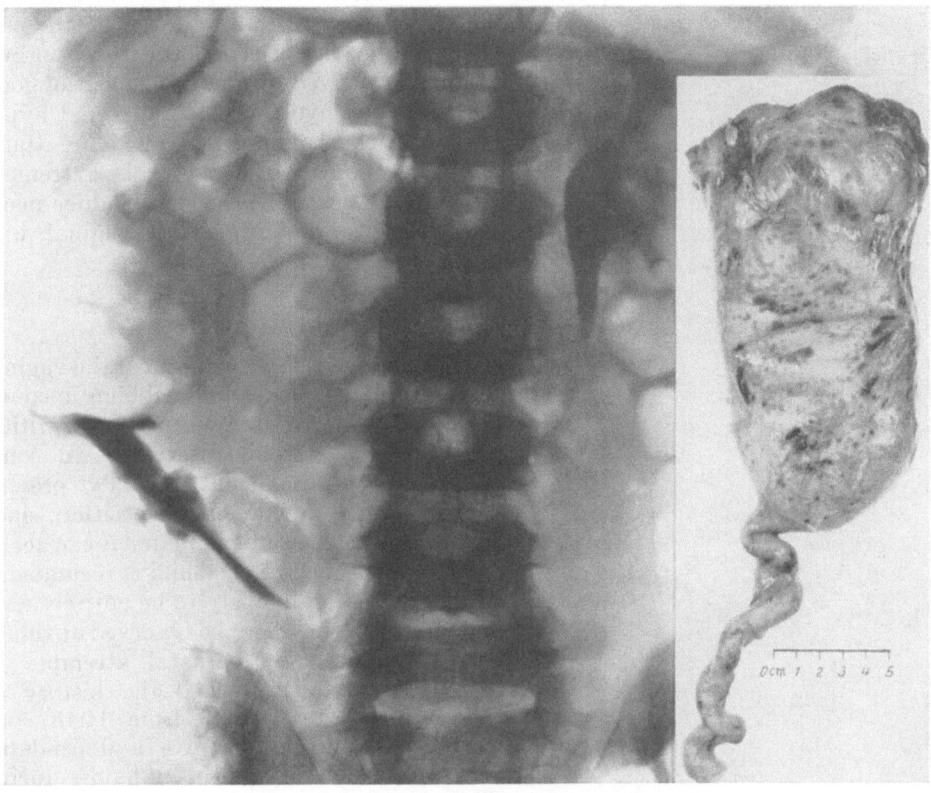

A   B

Fig. 35 A and B. Ectopic ureterocele causing gross dilatation of the upper renal pelvis of the right kidney. A intravenous pyelogram; B heminephrectomy specimen. Girl aged 3 years with persistent pyuria and palpable enlargement of the right kidney. Cystoscopy showed a typical Type I ectopic ureterocele. The lower renal pelvis of the right kidney is displaced but not dilated

Simple opening of the ureterocele cavity by endoscopic diathermy is not satisfactory, as the dilated ureter remains as a reservoir of infection and the renal element associated with the ectopic ureter is so small that it is not worth preserving.

Difficulties arise when the presence of the ureterocele has led to the dilatation of the ureter from the lower pelvis of the ipsilateral kidney: where this dilatation is advanced and the malformation is unilateral, total nephro-ureterectomy has seemed the best solution. In bilateral cases heminephrectomy and excision of the ureterocele has led to the improvement in the function of the lower element but some dilatation persists.

5. Vaginal and vestibular ectopia

In contrast to the other forms of ectopic ureter, vaginal ectopia has received full attention in the literature, and single case reports are very numerous. Apart from the general reviews already mentioned, the papers by ALLDRED and HIGGINS, LANGLEY, SANDMANN, and WILLIAMS may be consulted.

a) Anatomy

The ureteric opening may be found in the vestibule a short distance behind and lateral to the external urinary meatus; more often it is placed higher up the lateral vaginal wall, or even on the cervix uteri. The ureter is occasionally of normal calibre, and served by a renal element of good function, but hydro-ureter and renal hypoplasia are the common findings. At times the lower end of the ureter is extremely dilated, and may displace the bladder neck, or open into a cyst in the vaginal wall (TROLLE, MEADE).

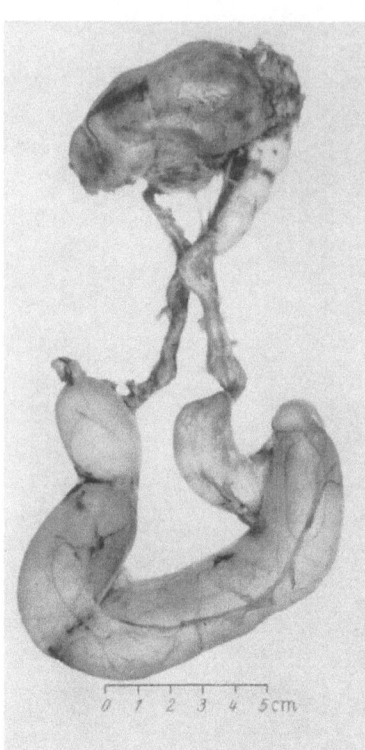

Fig. 36. Right nephro-ureterectomy specimen showing enormous dilatation of the upper pelvis ureter in a case of ectopic ureterocele. The child, a girl aged 3 months suffered severe spasmodic attacks of abdominal pain. The right kidney was palpable and the ureter was felt as a tense, mobile mass in the left iliac fossa. The urine was sterile: cystoscopy showed a typical right ectopic ureterocele, and on intravenous pyelograms the lower renal element only was outlined on the right side, and this was severely hydronephrotic

b) Symptoms

The characteristic symptom of the vaginal ectopic ureter is continual dribbling incontinence of urine despite normal micturition performed at normal intervals. In some children, the incontinence is only present when they are in the vertical position, since when the ectopic ureter is dilated it can act as a reservoir as long as the child is recumbent. Bladder function is likely to be entirely normal, but frequency may be observed at times, perhaps induced by parental attempts to minimize the incontinence; the history of the disorder should date from birth, but mothers do not always give a dependable account of their child's urinary habits during the first two years of life, and a few children undoubtedly have a late onset of incontinence. Where the opening is vestibular the ectopic ureter may be controlled to some extent by the urethral musculature, so that incontinence is not a feature, and intermittent pyuria is the presenting complaint. In the vaginal ureter too, severe infection will modify the symptoms: purulent vaginal discharge in an infant should suggest the presence of an ectopic ureter, while acute obstruction and pyo-ureter may lead to a return to normal control.

c) Diagnosis

On rare occasions the diagnosis may be established by direct observation of the ectopic orifice: the ureter can then be catheterized and outlined by retrograde ureterography. The vagina, however, is a difficult field in which to search for a small orifice, and since the function of the corresponding renal element is poor, little help can be obtained by the intravenous injection of dye. One dye test can be of value in excluding a simple urethral incontinence: the child is catheterized and the bladder filled with a fluid containing indigo-carmine, the catheter is then withdrawn and the vulva carefully cleansed. A white pad is then applied and the child is allowed to run about: if the pad becomes damp with clear urine, a vaginal ureter is certainly present.

Despite the difficulties of direct observation, the presence of an ectopic ureter may be surmised from the ordinary findings of pyelography and endoscopy, and

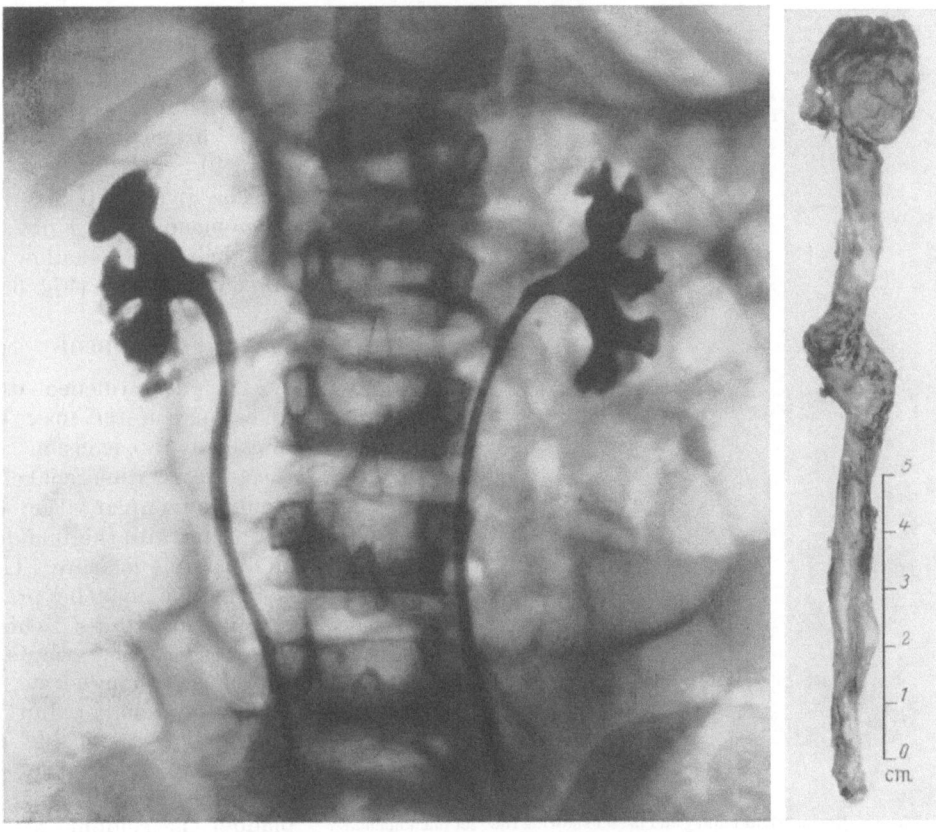

A   B

Fig. 37 A and B. Right double kidney with ectopic ureter. A Retrograde pyelograms in a girl aged 3 years suffering from dribbling incontinence of urine. Two normal ureteric orifices were present in the bladder: on the right side the upper calyx is displaced laterally and contrasts with the opposite kidney. Exploration confirmed the presence of a double kidney, and heminephrectomy was performed. B Operative specimen. Incontinence was completely relieved

it is quite safe to proceed to treatment without having actually catheterized the ureter in question. With the double kidney the presence of a duplication will be recognized from the intravenous pyelogram even if the upper element fails to concentrate the dye (Fig. 37 also see p. 36). Endoscopy then shows only one orifice in the bladder on the side of the duplication, and a retrograde uretero-gram performed with the eye of the catheter just inside that orifice will exclude the possibility of a bifid ureter. It will then be clear that the ureter draining the upper pelvis must end ectopically. It should be remembered, however, that the ectopic ureter like other forms of duplication may be bilateral, and that on rare occasions the ectopic ureter drains a supernumerary kidney.

In ectopic ureter without duplication, absence of one ureteric orifice and asymmetry of the trigone will be noted on cystoscopy, and if the intravenous pyelogram shows a functioning kidney on that side, the ureter must clearly be ectopic. Where no concentration of dye can be seen, the differentiation from renal agenesis presents some difficulty. In these circumstances aortography may be employed to show up the kidney, but where the symptoms leave little doubt as to the presence of an ectopic ureter it may be as well to proceed directly to exploration. The possibility of vaginal incontinence with caudal bifurcation of a single ureter is discussed on p. 40.

The pyelographic "jet phenomenon" must not be mistaken for the shadow of an ectopic ureter (Fig. 38).

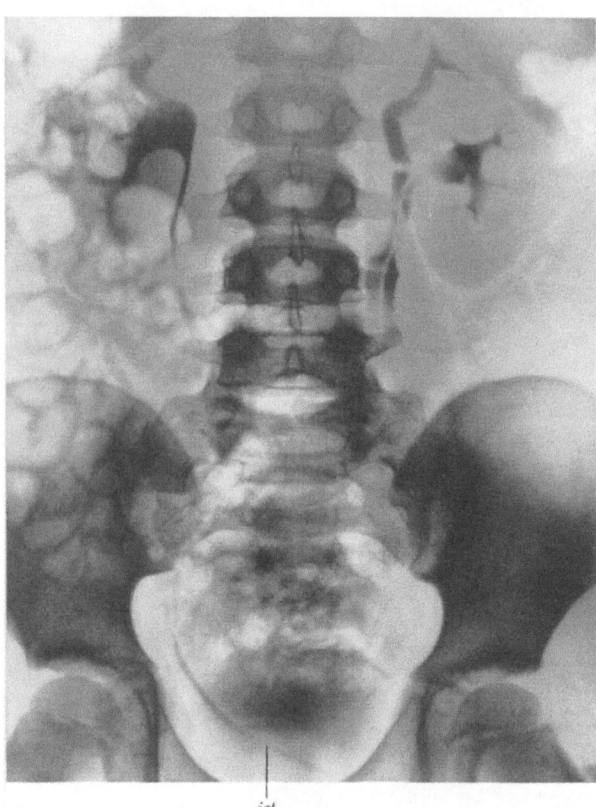

jet

Fig. 38. Normal right kidney and ureter showing the "jet phenomenon". Incomplete ureteric duplication on the left side. Intravenous pyelogram in a boy aged 6 years. The right ureter appears to be unnaturally prolonged, but is entirely normal, and the appearance is due to a jet of radio-opaque urine being propelled into the bladder which contains clear urine

d) Treatment

The incontinence due to ectopic ureter may be remedied by excision of the corresponding renal element, by implantation of the ureter into the bladder or by simple ligature. The last method may be practicable in adults where there is an easy vaginal approach, though it is perhaps unreliable, but it is usually inapplicable to children. Implantation of a dilated ureter into the bladder is seldom satisfactory because of reflux and the liability to infection, but this method may be employed if the total renal function is poor. In almost all cases nephrectomy or heminephrectomy is the treatment of choice, and if the ureter is at all dilated its whole length should be removed. In some instances the presence of the dilated stump in the vicinity of the bladder neck has led to persistence of the incontinence, and in one of the author's cases there was an associated weakness of the urethral musculature, so that control was finally achieved only by the use of the Millin sling procedure (cf. WESSON).

IX. Ureterocele and ureteric prolapse

The ectopic ureterocele, the characteristic form presenting in childhood, has been discussed in a previous section (p. 43); the simple form on a normally

placed ureter need only be described briefly. Full reviews have been given by
BOISSONNAT and by GROSS and CLATWORTHY.

A ureterocele is a cystic dilatation of the intravesical ureter, distending the
short segment lying under the bladder mucosa. In mild cases the cyst fills and
empties with the phases of ureteric activity, and the efflux can be observed cystoscopically as the cyst deflates. The ureteric orifice may be stenosed, but often
appears normal as long as the ureterocele is collapsed. When there is no stenosis,
the development of a ureterocele cannot
be satisfactorily explained, though it
appears to affect a ureter with a long
submucous course, and when, as often, a
double ureter is present, the ureterocele
is almost always formed on the ureter
from the upper pelvis, which opens near-
est the bladder neck. The wall of the
cyst includes vesical and ureteric mucosa
separated by a thin layer of ureteric
muscle.

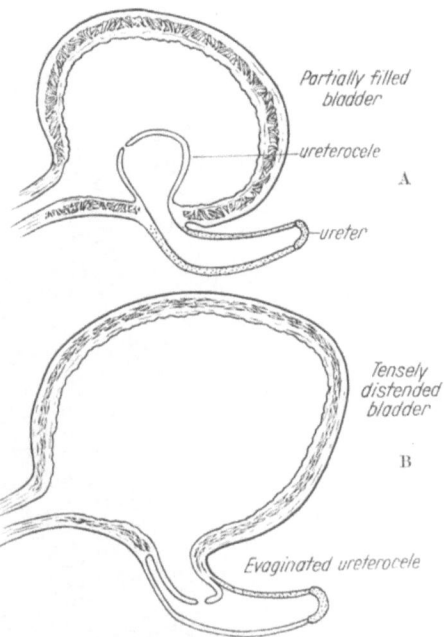

The ureter above the bladder is often
dilated, particularly in its lower third.
The intra-mural ureter, where it traverses
the muscle coat of the bladder, resists
dilatation in mild cases, but ultimately
opens up and allows the cyst to be evagi-
nated when the pressure within the bladder is high. This feature appears to be
characteristics of ureterocele in childhood (CAMPBELL), and findings in one of
my cases are sketched in Fig. 39. When
the bladder is partly filled, and the intravesical pressure is low, the ureterocele
protrudes into the bladder like a balloon;
when the bladder is tightly distended with
fluid, evagination occurs, and the cystoscopic appearance is exactly similar to
that of a vesical diverticulum.

Fig. 39. Evaginating ureterocele. Diagrammatic
para-sagittal sections through the bladder. —
A when partially filled. B when tense. Because
of the wide dilatation of the intra-mural ureter,
the wall of the ureterocele can be blown back into
the ureter, giving on cystoscopy the appearance
of a diverticulum

In mild cases a ureterocele is symptomless: it may, however, produce pain
with the distribution of ureteric colic. The secondary hydro-ureter may predispose
to urinary infection or stone formation, and many cases present with the symptoms
of these disorders. A few are found during the investigation of enuresis, but their
relationship to that symptom is often questionable. A large ureterocele may
obstruct the outflow from the bladder, causing difficult micturition and even
retention. In the female, the ureterocele may prolapse per urethram and present
as a vulval swelling, which is pedicled and can be reduced under anaesthesia.

The diagnosis may be reached cystoscopically or radiologically: the appearance
through the cystoscope is unmistakable to the trained urologist and will only
cause difficulty if the ureterocele is so large that it fills the bladder and obscures
normal landmarks, or if it evaginates. The pyelographic appearance depends
upon the function of the corresponding renal element: when the kidney concen-
trates the dye normally, the ureterocele casts a dense rounded shadow surrounded
by a translucent halo within the bladder area (Fig. 40). When function is poor,
it will show as a circular filling defect.

Endoscopic diathermy incision of the ureterocele wall is a suitable form of treatment when ureteric dilatation is absent or slight. Where there is a complicating hydro-ureter however, simple incision whether endoscopic or performed through the open bladder will leave a gaping orifice which allows easy reflux, and renal pain or infection may be as severe after the operation as before. Prevention of this reflux may be achieved by reconstruction of a sub-mucosal channel of normal calibre; by burying the lowest 2—3 cm. of ureter within the detrusor muscle

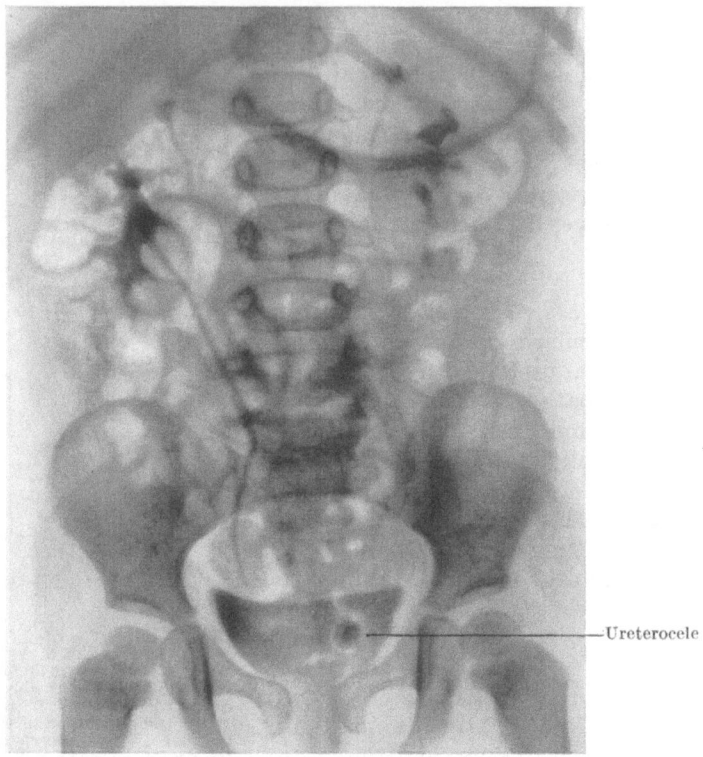

Fig. 40. Bilateral complete duplication of the ureters with ureterocele on the ureter from the upper pelvis on the left side. Intravenous pyelogram in a child aged 2 years with recurrent urinary infection. Within the bladder shadow, the ureterocele is shown by the area of increased density surrounded by a translucent halo

to make a long "intra-mural" course; or by a "nipple reimplant" as described on p. 54. With very advanced dilatation, however, none of these methods is likely to be entirely successful and then a nephro-ureterectomy may be the best treatment for the unilateral case. In double ureters, hemi-nephrectomy is often valuable.

In ureteric prolapse there is no dilatation of the segment protruding into the bladder: it resembles a flaccid and elongated nipple, contrasting with the balloon like appearance of a ureterocele. In three of my cases this type of prolapse has been associated with bilateral mega-ureter without bladder dysfunction, and in none was there any true stenosis of the ureteric orifice. The prolapse could be reduced by traction on the mobilized pelvic ureter, and in one case reduction was maintained by fixation of the ureter within a detrusor tunnel, but no great improvement followed this procedure. GREENFIELD has recorded a very large prolapse in a young boy, who was also suffering from bladder obstruction: the prolapsed portion was excised.

X. Retrocaval ureter

In this rare anomaly, which results from an abnormal formation of the inferior vena cava, the right ureter passes medially behind the cava, and then spirals forwards to resume its usual course. In consequence of the pressure from the vein, the upper ureter and renal pelvis become dilated, but symptoms are seldom noticeable until adult life. Cases presenting in children have, however, been reported by MARCEL, PARKS and CHASE, and CAMPOS; the condition must therefore be borne in mind in cases of right sided hydronephrosis. The diagnosis can be established by retrograde pyelograms, which demonstrate the ureter running towards the midline before turning downwards; if lateral views are obtained the spiralling can also be appreciated. When the kidney is well preserved, a conservative operation is worth while; the dilated renal pelvis should be cut across, the ureter dissected free, drawn through into its normal position and the continuity re-established.

C. Hydro-ureter and mega-ureter

The chronically dilated ureter constitutes one of the commonest and most intractable problems of children's urology. During recent years important new information upon the subject has become available, yet our knowledge of the normal and abnormal physiology of the ureters remains limited, and many forms of pathological dilatation are still unexplained. The term hydro-ureter will be used in this chapter for all forms of chronic dilatation, including those for which a urethral obstruction is clearly responsible, while "mega-ureter" is reserved for the clinical group in which no organic obstruction can be found, and in which ureteric activity appears to follow a characteristic pattern. Secondary hydro-ureter is described in many sections of this volume and will therefore only be discussed in general terms; mega-ureter occurs in two well defined forms, the simple mega-ureter and the mega-ureter-megacystis syndrome, but although typical cases present no difficulty in diagnosis, others are not so easily classified and it may be hard to distinguish the mild dilatation which accompanies infection from the more permanent disorder of function.

1. Normal ureteric function

The physiology of the ureter is discussed in detail in Volume II of this series, but certain specific features are relevant to the problem of the hydro-ureter.

The ureter is a muscular tube whose function is largely independent of the nervous system. The frequency and amplitude of propulsive contractions vary with the rate of urine flow, the pH of the urine, the pressure within the ureteric lumen and other factors, but are little influenced by the sympathetic nervous system (WHARTON) or by drugs acting upon the ganglia or neuro-muscular junctions (LAPIDES). Contractions are apparently initiated by a simple stretch reflex, and though the renal pelvis usually acts as a pace maker, any part of the ureter may respond to stretching by contraction. In transverse sections, the muscle layers appear to be internal longitudinal, circular and external longitudinal, but in fact the fibres are spiral (SCHNEIDER), and where the spiralling is tight the muscle appears circular, where loose longitudinal. There are no intermuscular planes containing ganglia as in the gut, in fact ganglion cells are very scanty, occurring chiefly in the adventitia at the lower end.

4*

The proportions of circular and longitudinal elements vary in the different regions of the ureter, and it is possible to define upper, middle and lower spindles which differ not only in their anatomical make-up but also in their physiological reactions. In the upper spindle, particularly at the pelvi-ureteric junction all layers tend to fuse and the spirals are interlaced: this spindle follows the activity of the renal pelvis and conducts contraction waves downwards, it seldom initiates a contraction. The middle spindle shows a dominance of tightly wound spirals, almost circular, and is more readily distensible. In the foetus and new born child it often appears sufficiently wide to suggest a pathological dilatation (Fig. 1). When subjected to low pressures it will show a conducted contraction akin to peristalsis, whereas with higher pressures it will fill and empty as a single chamber (MURNAGHAN, BEGG). The lower spindle is composed largely of longitudinal elements, and a contraction will tend to shorten it as well as narrow its calibre. Faced with a high intravesical pressure or obstruction at the uretero-vesical junction it will continue to exhibit active contraction for a longer period than the other segments, but as it becomes dilated contractions will no longer obliterate the lumen and urine will pass back through the contraction ring to fill the middle spindle.

II. Radiography and other investigations

In the initial diagnosis and in judging the progress of a case of chronic ureteric dilatation some standard method of investigation is required, for the calibre and activity of the ureter vary greatly with the circumstances. The intravenous pyelogram provides the most satisfactory method provided renal function remains adequate, which is exceptional in the severe mega-ureter. The conditions with regard to fluid intake must be reasonably standardized, however, and since the injection of the contrast medium itself causes an osmotic diuresis and an increased urine flow during the period of the investigation, films are only comparable when exposed at the same interval after injection. (Fig. 139 demonstrates in an extreme case the difference in ureteric calibre consequent upon altering urine flow.) Cine films taken during intravenous pyelography provide the most valuable evidence of function as well as form under physiological conditions, but even with the image intensifier very good renal function is required to give adequate contrast.

In retrograde pyelography the presence of the catheter and the sudden injection of fluid stimulate ureteric contraction, so that in most cases of mega-ureter, the retrograde pyelograms will show a narrower ureter than the intravenous series.

Cystograms frequently outline the ureters by vesico-ureteral reflux, and the force of the reflux during micturition may produce an enormous distension of the ureter, which appears grossly dilated even though the intravenous pyelograms show it to be of normal calibre (Figs. 46 and 47). To obtain a true picture therefore of the progress of ureteric disease, it is vital to avoid comparison of cystograms with intravenous pyelograms; moreover individual cystograms cannot be compared with one another since the degree of dilatation depends upon the volume of the distending fluid and the force of bladder contraction. Cine reflux ureterograms when obtainable give a good contrast and are valuable for ascertaining the functional activity of the ureter (EDWARDS).

Pressure recordings taken through a ureteric catheter were extensively employed by TRATTNER and by JONA in studying the normal ureteric physiology and have been used by Swenson in the diagnosis of mega-ureter. In the dilated ureter, however, they give a very incomplete picture of the functional state.

Electro-ureterography (Hanley) records differences in electrical potential resulting from ureteric activity, but as ordinarily employed, using electrodes on a ureteric catheter, the record is one of movement of the ureter over the electrode, rather than of true electro-myographic changes.

Ureteric activity may be observed by the surgeon during operation, and, when the ureteric orifices gapes widely, by endoscopy, the urethroscope being introduced into the ureteric lumen. Such unstandardized and unrecordable observations make unsatisfactory scientific evidence, but are apt to impress the practising urologist more than graphs and pressure records.

III. Vesico-ureteric reflux

The normal ureter is protected against the full force of bladder contraction by the valvular mechanism of the uretero-vesical junction. No sphincteric muscle has been found to guard this junction, and the intramural ureter is surrounded only by longitudinal muscle fibres, lying chiefly upon the posterior and lateral aspect. It is the obliquity with which the ureter passes through the vesical musculature that is responsible for the valvular action, and the greater the distension of the bladder the more firmly is the valve closed. The valve is least effective towards the end of active contraction of the bladder, and it is at this time that reflux is most likely to occur. The intramural ureter is straightened out by the contraction of the surrounding longitudinal muscle during the ureteric efflux, and if this occurs during micturition reflux is inevitable.

Reflux is more easily obtainable in the experimental animal than in man, owing perhaps to the unusual length of the human intramural ureter (Prather). Graves and Davidoff have given a full description of the phenomenon in the rabbit, in which it can usually be produced by simple bladder distension: they emphasize that the regurgitation occurred as the ureteric orifice opened with the ureteric peristaltic wave, that fresh waves might push back the regurgitated fluid, and that anti-peristalsis played no part in the process. To obtain reflux regularly in dogs, it is necessary to perform a very extensive meatotomy, opening up the whole length of the intra-mural ureter; local denervation of the ureter is without effect (Barksdale and Baker) though of course the neurogenic bladder is very liable to reflux. Auer and Seager demonstrated that rendering the tissues around the ureteric orifice oedematous and rigid by the injection of magnesium sulphate greatly facilitated the production of reflux, and doubtless the same effect is operative in inflammatory lesions.

Reflux is found in a great many conditions in childhood and a general assessment of its significance is hard to give. If micturating cystograms are performed in a large number of cases of enuresis or recurrent urinary infection without pyelographic signs of abnormality, reflux will be found in a small proportion, though it is hard to be sure whether it has any pathological significance. If the film is taken at the height of bladder contraction the ureter will certainly appear dilated, but without cine radiology it cannot be said whether this dilatation is momentary or lasting. It is conceivable that reflux is responsible for rendering the urinary tract liable to recurrent infection, but unless the ureter is large enough to produce a false residual urine it seems unlikely to be responsible for enuresis; it appears therefore that a small reflux may occur in the normal child.

Urinary infection and cystitis undoubtedly predispose to reflux, partly because of the frequency and force of bladder contractions and partly because of the rigidity of the ureteric orifice. The contracted tuberculous bladder provides an extreme example of this type, when reflux may involve the non-tuberculous ureter. Reflux is common in the neurogenic bladder, particularly in the hypertrophied type with urinary infection. Long standing urethral obstructions also exhibit reflux in many cases, particularly when the first investigation is done immediately after decompression of the bladder. A ureter opening into a vesical diverticulum usually allows reflux, which may occur at the time when the urine is returning from the diverticulum to the bladder. Urethral ectopic ureters may fill on micturition, and if a ureterocele has been excised gross reflux is almost invariable. As described later in this section, free reflux is characteristic of the mega-ureter-megacystis syndrome, and may be demonstrated occasionally in the simple mega-ureter, especially if late films are taken (Fig. 132).

Attention has been focussed in recent years upon operations which prevent reflux, and much ingenuity has been displayed in the invention of new techniques. It must first be enquired, however, whether reflux itself is dangerous. VERMOOTEN and NEUSWANGER, working on experimental reflux in dogs, found that ureteric dilatation resulted only when the urine was infected. A slight regurgitation found in the occasional enuretic appears to do very little harm, and some of my cases of mega-ureter-megacystis, in which there is free reflux from a large capacity bladder, have been observed for eight years without evident deterioration of renal function or increase of ureteric dilatation. On the other hand, the simple mega-ureter reimplanted into the bladder in such a way as to allow reflux often deteriorates rapidly if there is a urinary infection. Reflux in the urethral obstructions and neurogenic bladders is usually associated with advanced renal damage. It appears therefore that the dangers of reflux are associated with complicating infection and abnormal bladder function, but since these two factors cannot always be avoided, reflux should be prevented if possible.

Operations designed to prevent reflux may leave the ureter intact, but aim at prolonging its intramural portion by bringing it within the detrusor layer (HUTCH). There is some danger in these that the addition of an obstructive factor will be at least as damaging to the kidney as the persistence of reflux. Other procedures are appropriate for the re-implanted ureter, the most successful being the nipple or cuff type of operation, in which the lower extremity of the ureter is turned back upon itself and sutured to the bladder wall so as to maintain the projecting nipple (see GREY et al.). This type of operation is undoubtedly successful in preventing reflux in the early post-operative stage, and should be employed whenever it is necessary to reimplant a dilated ureter. Follow-up investigations performed a year post-operatively sometimes show that the nipple has disappeared, however, and that the reflux is present as in Fig. 47, and it does not seem that any permanent solution to this problem has yet been achieved.

IV. Hydro-ureter in bladder disorders

In a series of 2,924 post-mortems on children, some type of ureteric dilatation was found in 103, and of these 42 were due to urethral obstructions, usually valves (WILLIAMS). Neurogenic bladder due to spinal cord anomalies, obstructive tumours, and inflammatory lesions accounted for a high proportion and only 10 cases could be placed in the mega-ureter group. In a clinical series the mega-ureters would be much more common, but these post-mortem statistics emphasize the importance of lower urinary obstruction as a cause of ureteric dilatation, and certain general observations as to the type of dilatation are relevant.

Whereas in the adult obstructions hydronephrosis may be more noticeable than hydro-ureter, in the infant the situation is reversed: any obstruction having its origin in foetal life causes a gross dilatation of the ureter, leaving the renal pelvis comparatively small, and at this stage the volume of the distended ureter is often greater than the volume of the bladder. Obstructions commencing in childhood produce an appearance intermediate between the infantile and adult pattern. In the mild cases it is possible to demonstrate that the lower end of the ureter becomes dilated first, and it cannot be claimed that hydro-ureter without hydronephrosis necessarily indicates an intrinsic disease. A ureter which is dilated must also be elongated, and since the two extremities are fixed, elongation involves kinking. In severe cases the kinking is extreme and dense adventitia surrounds the ureter perpetuating the kinks, which in a few cases may lead to secondary obstruction. Cine radiology demonstrates, however, the remarkable ease with which urine negotiates these tortuous channels, and the plastic operations which have been advocated for them (e. g. HINMAN) should be reserved for the exceptional case. More serious is the obstruction which takes place in the lower end of the ureter which always narrows down to a normal calibre as it passes through the hypertrophied vesical musculature;

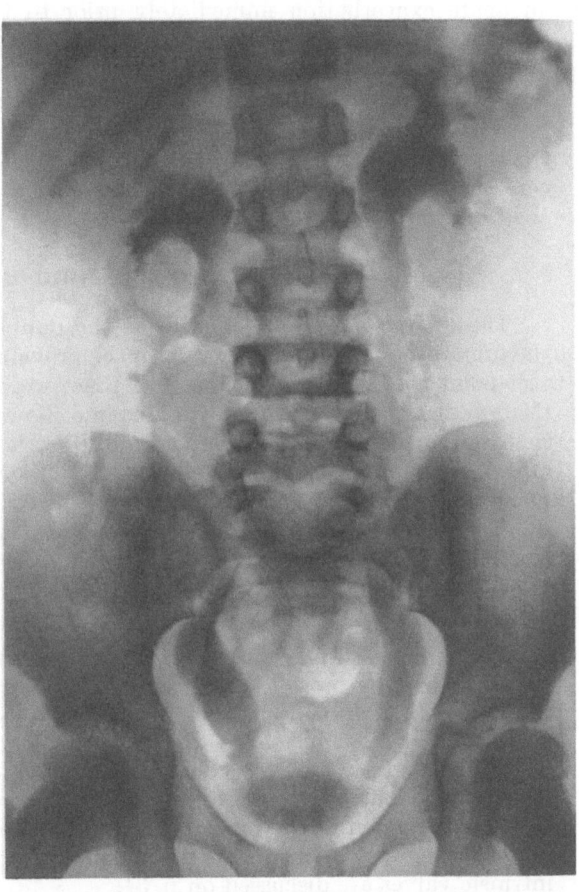

Fig. 41. Hydro-ureter due to "bladder neck obstruction." Intravenous pyelogram in a boy aged 9 years investigated for abdominal pain. Micturition appeared normal, and there was no significant residual urine, but the bladder was heavily trabeculated. The bladder neck musculature was hypertrophied. Trans-urethral resection performed. Slight improvement in ureteric dilatation followed

once the bladder has been allowed to collapse around an indwelling catheter, the dilated ureter may become acutely obstructed and form a palpable abdominal swelling.

The obstructed ureter is hypertrophied and actively contractile in the early stages; gradually it fails, however, becoming incapable of propulsive contractions and possessing only slight elasticity: the hypertrophied muscle is partly replaced by fibrous tissue. Unless there is some additional abnormality, such as a diverticulum, reflux seldom takes place in the early stage but it is characteristic of the advanced case in which cine radiology reveals an almost or completely immobile ureter. Reflux is often unilateral, and the affected kidney is then much more seriously damaged than its fellow; such asymmetrical hydro-ureter is a common finding in congenital urethral obstructions and neurogenic bladders.

A ureter which has become grossly hypertrophied can never return to an entirely normal calibre, and one which has reached the stage of immobility cannot recover at all. Considerable improvement in ureteric dilatation in cases of lower urinary obstruction can only be anticipated therefore when there has been an acute exacerbation immediately prior to the first investigation, and there should be great reluctance to make a double diagnosis of bladder neck obstruction and mega-ureter (BOPPE and MARCEL). We have found no evidence to suggest that a lesion comparable to urethral fibro-elastosis, the pathological basis of the so-called bladder neck obstruction, can affect the lower end of the ureter. From the diagnostic angle it must be noted that bladder neck obstruction occasionally causes hydro-ureter without bladder distension (Fig. 41).

V. Hydro-ureter in other reno-ureteral abnormalities

The dilatation which complicates the double ureter, the ectopic ureter, and the ureterocele, has been discussed in the previous section. From the physiological viewpoint these ureters behave as if there were an obstruction at the lower end (MURNAGHAN), they are hypertrophied and show normal propulsive contractions at first, but later inflammatory lesions and fibrosis occur and they become immobile. Often the termination of such a ureter is stenosed, but some are wide and it must be assumed that their abnormal position leads to inefficient emptying. In some duplications with dilatation it is found that the contralateral single ureter is also dilated, and in these an inflammatory cause is often suspected. Occasionally there is a saccular dilatation of the ureter (WITHYCOMBE) for which a local congenital defect of the ureter wall must be suspected.

A dysplastic kidney, usually infected, is often drained by a slightly dilated ureter displaying more severe kinking than would be expected from the degree of dilatation. Fibrous replacement of the ureteric muscle is evident, and it may be that a developmental disorder is responsible for both renal and ureteric abnormalities. Extremely tortuous ureters, in which the normal spiral arrangement of muscle and blood vessels is unusually evident, are sometimes described under the term "torsion of the ureter" (BERRY) though no explanation is given of the manner in which such an anomaly could arise. Hypoplasia of the ureter and intrinsic valves are discussed on p. 34.

Uretero-vesical stricture is thought by some to be very common (e.g. CAMPBELL) by others to be very rare (e.g. POOLE-WILSON), the criteria for diagnosis being hard to define. All dilated ureters narrow down in the intramural segment and it is difficult to be sure whether the narrowing is sufficient to constitute a stricture. CAMPBELL states that a stricture may be diagnosed when the ureteric orifice cannot be catheterized or when it grips a 3F catheter in the new born, a 4F at four years, or a 5F at eight years. In my experience, however, a ureter which shows no sign of dilatation will sometimes grip such a catheter, while in almost all mega-ureters the ureteric orifice can be passed, although the catheter sometimes kinks and is held up above this point. In the exceptional case, the ureter cannot be catheterized cystoscopically or at operation, and examination of the resected specimen shows that the lumen will admit only a fine bristle, yet the dilated ureter in such cases resembles in every other way the simple mega-ureter of severe degree. CAMPBELL had advocated intermittent cystoscopic ureteric dilatation for cases of stricture and illustrates improvements in the pyelograms following this procedure, but warns of the great danger of introducing infection in such a case.

The ureter from a solitary kidney frequently exhibits a chronic dilatation and is liable to recurrent infection. The pathology of these cases is obscure and treatment must follow the line suggested for mega-ureter.

Congenital extrinsic obstructions due to blood vessels running from the internal iliac artery to the bladder have been described chiefly in adults (GREENE), but I have encountered one undoubted case in a child. The difficulty here is to distinguish, at an operation which inevitably demands some dissection, the extrinsic obstructions from cases in which the ureter has an unexplained supravesical narrow segment, and which seem to fall into the category of simple mega-ureter. PRATHER has suggested that an ectopic testis may obstruct the ureter but there has been little confirmation of this view.

VI. Infections

It is generally conceded that urinary infection and ureteric inflammation may cause a slight ureteric dilatation, akin perhaps to the ileus seen in acute peritonitis. Slight dilatation affecting predominantly the lumbar spindle is quite commonly observed in pyelograms performed during an acute urinary infection; it is not a complete paralysis, for in retrograde pyelograms the stimulation of the injection results in a normal contraction wave. Dilatation of the lumbar ureter is commonly seen below an infected staghorn calculus (Fig. 106).

It has already been noted that urinary infection predisposes to ureteric reflux, and whether infection alone can be responsible for the transient dilatation of the whole length of the ureter sometimes observed in girls is an unsolved problem. I have described (WILLIAMS) five cases in which a mild cystitis, without any bladder contraction, was accompanied by moderate hydro-ureter and reflux in the early stages: chemotherapy alone lead to recovery and later investigation showed normal ureters and no reflux. HEYMAN and MARTIN have illustrated an even more remarkable case of the same type, in which the initial dilatation could be described as gross. MARCEL describes similar cases but emphasizes the large capacity of the bladder, and it may be that this observation indicates that they should be included as mild examples of the mega-ureter-megacystis syndrome.

Whether infection alone can ever be responsible for serious ureteric dilatation or not, it is always a factor which must be borne in mind: it is the complicating pyelonephritis rather than the back pressure effect which is responsible for the deterioration of renal function in serious cases of mega-ureter.

VII. The mega-ureter-megacystis syndrome

It has long been recognized that in some bilateral mega-ureter cases, the ureteric orifices gape widely and the bladder is of large capacity (SARGENT, GREVILLIUS, GROGLER, SCHMUTTE, EISENSTAEDT, LEPOUTRE) but in recent years it has been possible to follow out the natural history of such cases and to define a syndrome to which a purely descriptive title, the mega-ureter-megacystis syndrome, may be applied (WILLIAMS). It is equally common in boys and girls, though it is more difficult to distinguish from bladder neck obstruction in boys.

1. Pathology

Both ureters are grossly dilated with hypertrophied muscle. They are kinked, and narrow at the lower end where they pass through the detrusor although the ureteric orifice appears wide endoscopically. The bladder is large and its wall slightly thickened. No satisfactory explanation of the aetiology of this condition has yet appeared. It has naturally been suggested that an obstruction at the bladder neck or a neurological lesion might be responsible, but a study of the natural history at once demonstrates that these cases do not behave like the lower urinary obstructions or like the neurogenic bladders due to congenital spinal cord lesions. The hypothesis that an overgrowth or gigantism (Exzeß-bildung) might be responsible has received some support (e.g. GROGLER, IRVIN and KRAUS) but it is difficult to reconcile with the failure of function which occurs in some. SWENSON et al. have claimed that the condition is due to a diminution of the number of ganglion cells in the bladder and that it is analogous to Hirschsprung's disease. WYLLIE, reporting 152 cases of the bowel disorder operated upon at the Hospital for Sick Children found no case of significant ureteric dilatation, while in two classical instances of the mega-ureter-megacystis syndrome which I had personally investigated, and which later came to post-mortem, LEIBOVITZ undertook an accurate ganglion count and found no diminution whatever. Any satisfactory hypothesis put forward to explain this condition must take account both of the bladder and ureter abnormalities, for simple reflux can scarcely account for the unusual type of ureteric activity observed on cine radiology.

2. Clinical, radiological and endoscopic findings

The disorder most frequently presents itself as a cause of chronic or recurrent urinary infection, and may appear at any stage of childhood. A few neonatal cases (Fig. 42) are discovered because of palpable distension of the bladder, but usually recover normal micturition, and the element of retention does not appear again until later childhood. Transient acute retention, particularly in the male, during infection or following instrumentation is characteristic, but except in these circumstances difficult micturition and incontinence are uncommon even when enormous bladder distension is palpable. Signs of renal failure appear after some years, perhaps in adolescence or early adult life, in those whose infection cannot be brought under control. Sterile cases may persist unchanged for very many years, and some are only discovered in adult life. Deterioration is sometimes due to chronic pyelonephritis without increase in ureteric dilatation, but in others there is a slow progression towards a retention phase.

Ureteric dilatation is a constant finding and normally involves the whole length of the ureter, often with the renal pelvis. Reflux is almost invariably present on micturition, and usually occurs freely on simple filling of the bladder (Fig. 43), though it may be unilateral. Characteristically the ureteric orifices gape widely, presenting a black hole on ordinary cystoscopy, though distinguished from the openings of diverticula by their obliquity. (Béance congenitale, MARION). The orifices may appear normal in mild cases, though when a catheter is passed through them they are evidently flabby and relaxed. A urethroscope can usually be introduced into the ureter and its activity observed; cine radiology showing the ureter by reflux also demonstrates the motility. In contrast with the late hydro-ureter seen in lower urinary obstruction, active and powerful contractions are seen in the mega-ureter despite its enormous dilatation. These contractions do not always obliterate the lumen, and are not therefore very useful: at times retrograde peristalsis is seen to assist the process of reflux, so that fluid is actively propelled up from the bladder to the kidneys (EDWARDS) in a manner not observed in other conditions.

The bladder is of large capacity quite apart from the fact that a proportion of the fluid injected flows up the ureter. In a child of 6—8 years of age a capacity of 600—1000 ml as measured on cystometry is not uncommon. In children under 3 years accurate assessment is difficult but the increased capacity is evident on cystoscopy to any experienced observer. SWENSON and his co-workers have contributed a number of papers on this subject and fully emphasize the value of cystometry, but do not make any clear distinction between the megacystis and the distended bladder of urethral fibro-elastosis and other lower urinary obstructions. LEIBOVITZ and O'DONNELL discuss this aspect, and demonstrate that the obstructed bladder has a capacity intermediate between the normal and the megacystis. In the megacystis case, the pressure in the bladder in the upper part of the volume range is considerably above normal, a feature which SWENSON suggests must be responsible for back pressure damage. There is often a history that these children hold their urine for very long periods, perhaps all day, and then pass large quantities. Afterwards a second or even a third micturition will still produce a considerable volume of urine. By cine radiology it can be demonstrated that despite their size, these bladders are capable of a powerful contraction which completely obliterates the lumen, and this ability is only lost in advanced cases and during transient acute retention. The contraction is not effective in emptying the urinary tract, however, because a high proportion of the urine flows back and distends the ureter, from which it will return as the bladder relaxes. A second, third or fourth micturition may be necessary to complete elimination of the contrast medium.

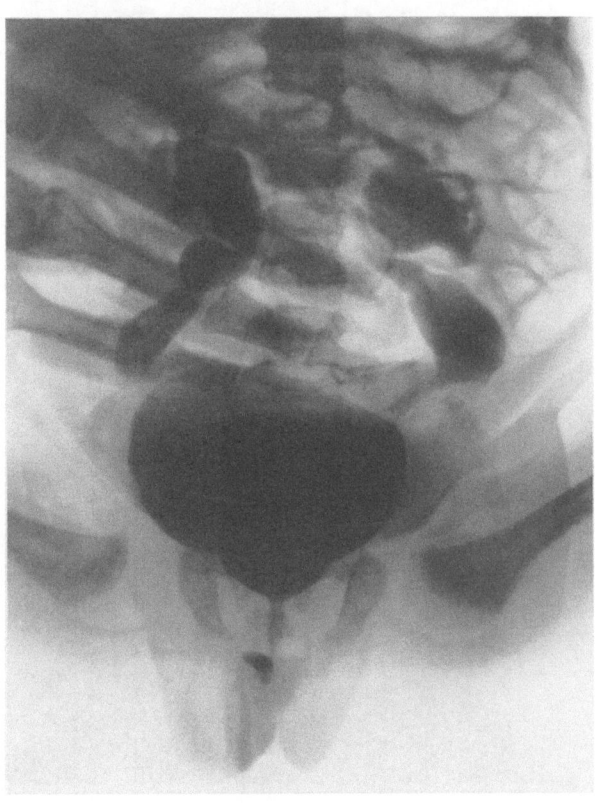

Fig. 42. Megaureter-megacystis syndrome. Expression cystogram in a boy aged 4 months. Shortly after birth, bladder distension had been noticed: thereafter there were no abnormal signs or symptoms. The bladder was of large capacity but normal on cystoscopy. Two years later, the ureteric orifices had become widely dilated

Cystoscopically the bladder, apart from the ureteric orifices, appears normal, and the bladder neck shows no prominence. In advanced cases, especially in boys, mild trabeculation may appear, having usually the form of a few strong bands widely spread out, and sacculation does not occur. The urethra is normal.

3. Diagnosis

The presence of bilateral ureteric dilatation is easily established. The distinction from simple mega-ureter is made from the free reflux on cystography, from the gaping character of the ureteric orifices, and from the increased capacity of the bladder as revealed by cystometry.

In cases which have entered the retention phase, the distinction from bladder neck obstruction is made from the gaping ureteric orifices, and from the observation of the characteristic slow but powerful ureteric contractions, from the absence or mildness of trabeculation, from the high capacity of the bladder revealed from cystometry, and from the absence of fibro-elastosis in biopsy of the anterior urethral wall (p. 74).

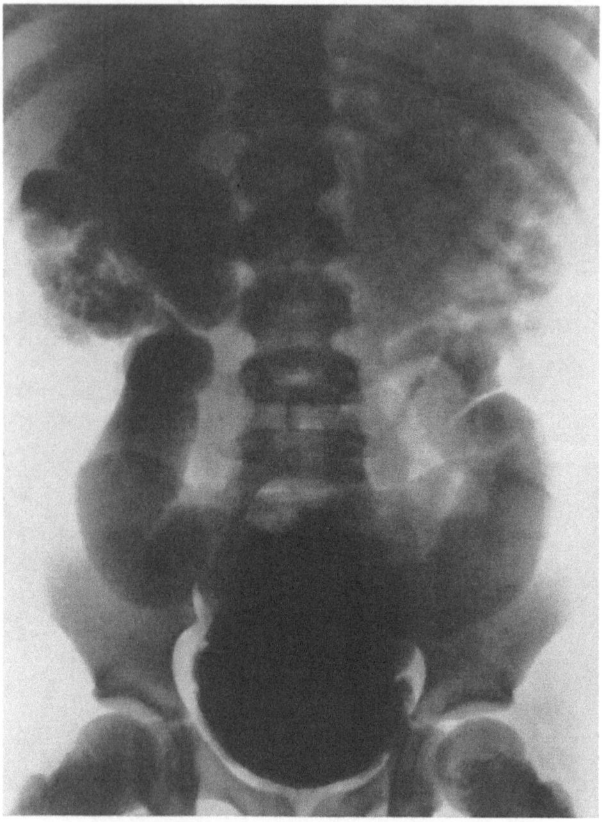

Fig. 43. Megaureter-megacystis syndrome in retention phase. Cystogram in a boy aged 6 years, who was found to have a distended bladder on routine examination. No difficulty in micturition and no incontinence. Cystometry showed a bladder of very large capacity: on cystoscopy the bladder was trabeculated. At operation the bladder neck felt tight: an anterior Y-V plasty was performed. Biopsy showed no evidence of urethral fibroelastosis. After operation he emptied his bladder completely by double micturition

4. Management

Most examples of the mega-ureter-megacystis syndrome are adequately controlled by conservative treatment. The urine must be sterilized by drugs, and if recurrent infection occurs, continuous chemotherapy may be required. The urinary tract must be efficiently emptied so that the intravesical pressure is never high: a regime of double or triple micturition, the second and third acts being performed 5—10 minutes after the first is usually effective, and urine should never be held more than 3 hours by day. Most children will co-operate with this regime if it is sympathetically explained to them, though the younger ones will naturally need many reminders. In ordinary circumstances the ureteric dilatation will not increase during treatment and no operation designed to prevent reflux is desirable.

Attacks of acute retention will subside spontaneously after a period of bladder drainage, but when a residual urine remains, despite double micturition, some attempt should be made to facilitate bladder emptying. SWENSON at first advocated a supra-pubic cystostomy, and though this does ensure effective drainage, it also maintains a chronic infection and is disagreeable to the child. He later employed bladder neck resection, but my own preference is for an anterior Y—V plasty on the bladder neck, and this followed by a double micturition regime has been effective in several cases.

Operations designed to reduce the calibre of the ureter by resection of long strips, combined with a procedure to prevent reflux have been advocated by BISCHOFF, and probably have a place when the actual size of the ureter is preventing sterilization of the urine. Sympathectomy has been performed in a case of this type by GREVILLIUS, with doubtful justification.

VIII. Simple mega-ureter

In this condition ureteric dilatation may be unilateral or bilateral, and the bladder is normal in capacity and function. It occurs in both sexes but commonly presents later in life than the mega-ureter-megacystis syndrome.

1. Pathology

The dilated ureter possesses hypertrophied muscle, with fibrous tissue replacement and sub-mucosal thickening when chronic infection has been present. Elongation and kinking is usual, and the lower end forms a bulb-like dilatation pushed down a little below the level of the intramural ureter, which is of normal calibre. This final kink often produces a valve-like effect which arrests bougies pushed down from above (EVERIDGE) though it is doubtful whether it is responsible for the obstruction to urine flow. In certain cases the narrowing occurs a short distance above the bladder, producing a supravesical segment of normal calibre for which no extrinsic cause can be found. In three of my cases with bilateral simple mega-ureter, such a supravesical narrow segment was present on one side but not on the other, and it therefore appears likely that the same pathology will be found for both forms.

MURNAGHAN has shown in some of my cases that the circular element in the musculature extends abnormally far down into the intramural portion. He has also been able to demonstrate in the excised and isolated organ that contractions are initiated in this lower segment instead of from above. He believes that this abnormal muscular pattern and consequent functional derangement must be responsible for the dilatation.

Many other hypotheses have been put forward to explain the dilatation in the simple mega-ureter. Achalasia (HEPLER) is hardly an explanation but postulates an unknown neuromuscular disorder at the lower extremity of the ureter. Persistence of foetal dilatation seems unlikely, and the foetal ureter shows characteristically greater distensibility in the lumbar region, which does not accord with the bulb-like dilatation of the lower third usual in simple mega-ureter. Dilatation due to the persistence beyond its normal period of Chwalle's membrane (VERMOOTEN) can scarcely be proved or disproved. In general the simple mega-ureter behaves as though it were mildly obstructed, and the cases of definite uretero-vesical stricture are similar, but MURNAGHAN's work as well as SWENSON's (see below) suggests that abnormality of function is the basis.

2. Clinical, radiological and endoscopic features

Once again, a recurrent urinary infection is the most common mode of presentation, but abdominal pain, haematuria, and rarely renal swelling may bring the child to hospital. Pain is seldom as severe as in hydronephrosis due to pelvi-

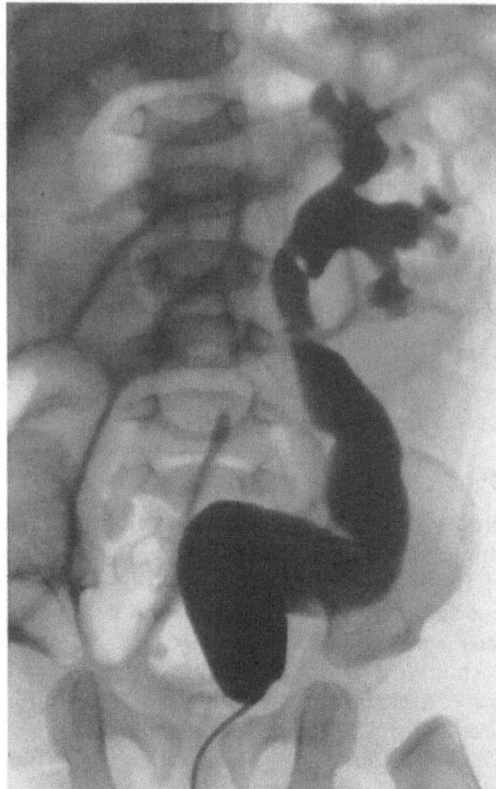

ureteric obstruction, and it is less well localized. Haematuria may be due to complicating stones, which are relatively common, or to infection, but is sometimes unexplained. A few examples are discovered by the routine investigation of enuresis, though unless the urine is infected the megaureter does not appear to have any bearing on that symptom.

Pyelograms show dilatation of the whole length of the ureter (Figs. 44 and 46), often more marked in and sometimes confined to the lower third (Fig. 45). The intramural ureter is always of normal calibre and occasionally a supravesical narrow segment can be defined (Fig. 48). Cine pyelography in most cases shows an

Fig. 44. Unilateral simple megaureter. Retrograde pyelogram in a boy aged 3 months with persistent pyuria and left sided abdominal swelling. I.V.P. showed a normal right kidney, but no secretion on the left side. Bladder normal. Nephro-ureterectomy performed

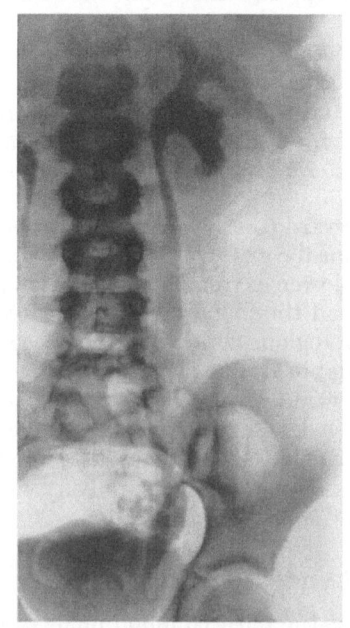

A

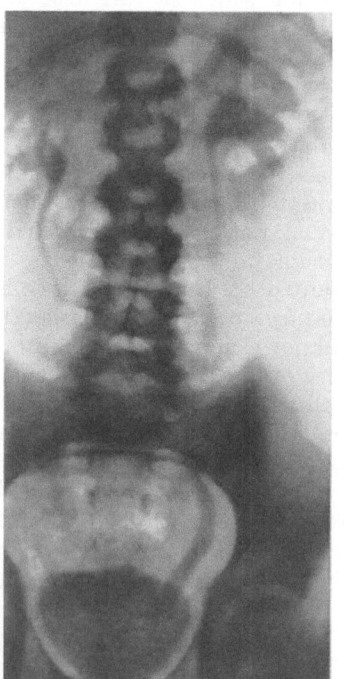

B

Fig. 45 A and B. Simple megaureter. Intravenous pyelograms (20 minute films). A at age of 6 years, investigated after a brief attack of haematuria, no stone found, and no other symptoms. B at age 11 years. No treatment had been given and the boy had had no symptoms. Dilatation unchanged

actively contractile ureter which forces urine down into the dilated segment, but the contraction waves do not completely obliterate the lumen, and the urine

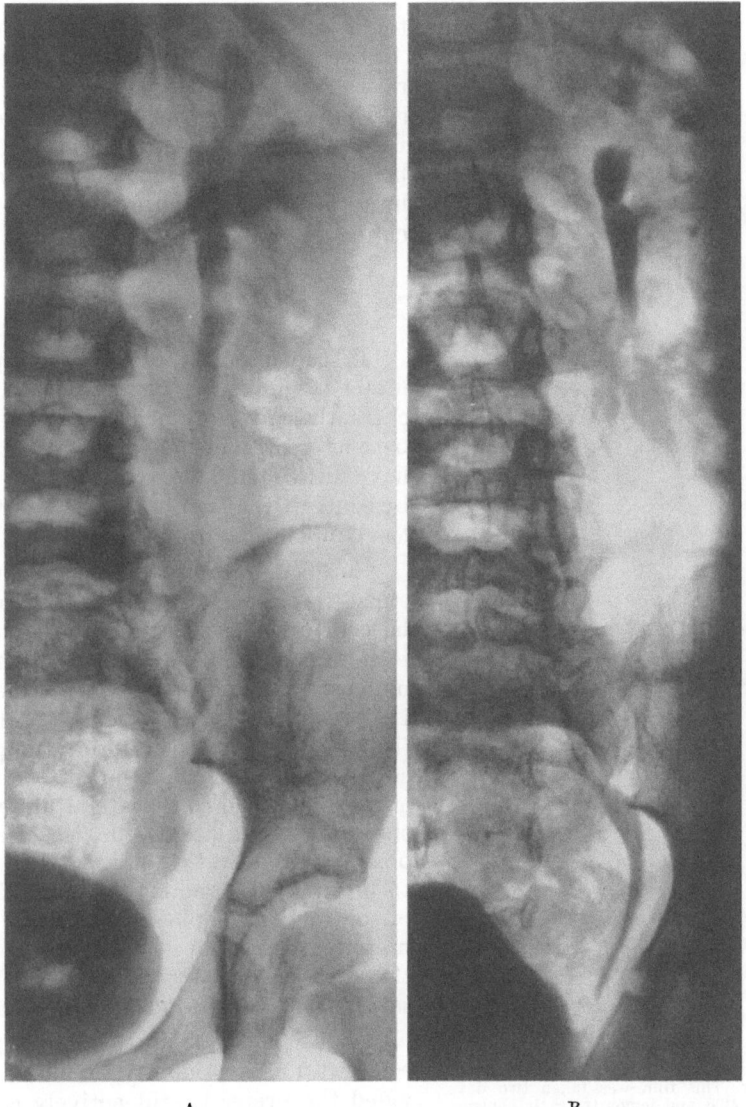

A   B

Fig. 46 A and B. Simple megaureter. Intravenous pyelograms (30 minute films) in a girl aged 7 years investigated for abdominal pain and frequency. A Pre-operative, showing well marked dilatation of the whole length of the left ureter. B Post-operative, eighteen months after "nipple" re-implantation. In the early post-operative period, the nipple prevented reflux and these films suggest that a useful improvement has been effected, but a further cystogram (Fig. 47) shows free reflux into a distended ureter

floods back through the ring into the lumbar ureter. Working with pressure tracings SWENSON has suggested that these ureters are aperistaltic or show abnormal contractions; from cine radiology we find that only very advanced cases lack mobility.

Complicating calculi are rounded, often multiple and freely mobile.

Reflux is unusual but may occur on micturition, when a small amount of bladder urine escapes back into the reservoir of urine in the dilated ureter, quite a different phenomenon from the free ebb and flow of the mega-ureter-megacystis syndrome.

Cystoscopy, cystography and cystometry show a normal bladder unless there is an acute infection. The ureteric orifice is entirely normal, or appears to be raised on a slight pyramidal elevation, suggesting a prolapse rather than a ureterocele. Ureteric catheters pass with ease as a rule, but the differential diagnosis from congenital uretero-vesical stricture presents some difficulties (p. 56).

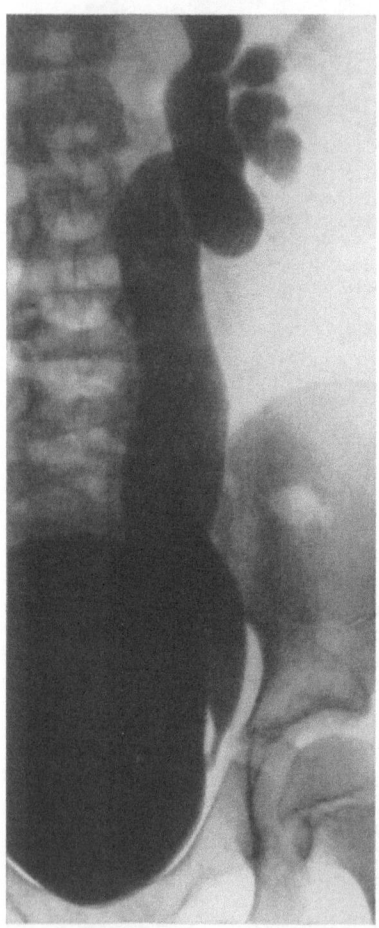

Fig. 47. Simple megaureter (same as Fig. 46). Cystogram showing reflux into the re-implanted ureter. This film was taken two days before Fig. 46 B, and demonstrates the contrast between a ureter under conditions of active reflux from a contracting bladder and the same organ between acts of micturition

3. Management

In the majority of cases, simple mega-ureter requires no treatment other than chemotherapy for urinary infection, they become symptom-free after sterilization and have little tendency to progress (Fig. 45): by contrast the results of operative treatment leave much to be desired.

Surgical interference is indicated when stones are present, when infection cannot be controlled by chemotherapy, and when the dilatation is increasing. When strictly unilateral, the severely infected mega-ureter is best treated by nephro-ureterectomy (leaving as short a ureteric stump as possible), for although it cannot be stated categorially that the contralateral ureter will not show dilatation later in life, this has not been observed. Theoretically it might be desirable to preserve all functioning renal tissue, but in contrast to the plastic operations for pelvi-ureteric obstruction, conservative surgery in the mega-ureter does not give consistently satisfactory results and infection may persist.

In the bilateral cases demanding surgery conservation is evidently essential, and provided the ureter is still actively contractile, excision of the uretero-vesical junction and re-implantation using the nipple technique seems the best procedure. If necessary the calibre of the ureter can be reduced by resection at the same time. Simple end-to-side re-implants have often been followed by free reflux, infection and rapid deterioration of the kidney, and though the nipple may not last it does appear to prevent early deterioration. Extended ureteric meatotomy and side to side anastomosis have seldom proved satisfactory.

When calculi are present in the simple mega-ureter, ureterolithotomy alone is inadequate and a re-implant is usually desirable.

Sympathectomy has little place in treatment, and operations designed to support the ureter by burying it in the psoas muscle (CARLSON) seem doomed to failure.

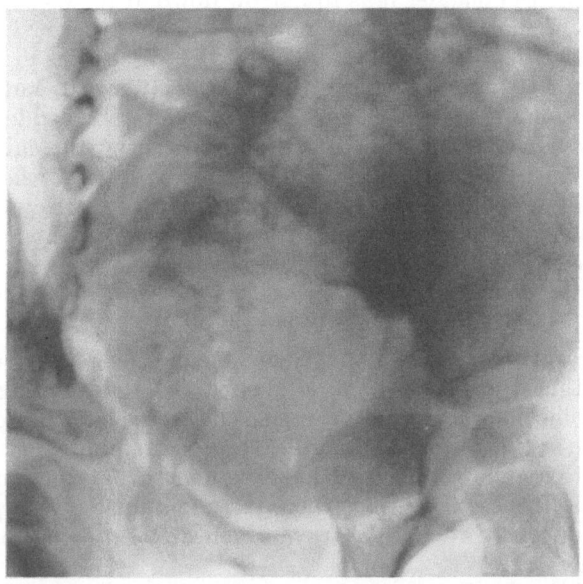

Fig. 48. Simple megaureter with supra-vesical narrow segment. Intravenous pyelogram in a boy aged 1 year, suffering from abdominal pain. The film is taken obliquely to show the abrupt narrowing of the left ureter; the right ureter was grossly dilated and the right kidney did not concentrate the dye. At operation no extrinsic cause of left ureteric obstruction was found, and the right ureter was dilated down to the bladder wall

For the aperistaltic ureter SWENSON has advocated replacement by an ileal loop. His technique includes a preliminary isolation and narrowing of the loop, which is only substituted for the ureter at a second stage. He reports satisfactory results from this method, though in my experience absence of peristalsis in the simple mega-ureter is rare, and the chief cause of renal failure is a chronic pyelo-nephritic process not necessarily influenced by ureteric replacement.

D. Congenital abnormalities of the lower urinary tract

I. Urachal anomalies

During early foetal life the bladder cavity extends up as far as the umbilical stalk, later its apex narrows down to form the urachal canal, which at birth is still connected with the umbilicus. Subsequently the bladder descends into the pelvis, and the urachus which is not more than 5 cm in length (BEGG) is pulled away from its attachment to the umbilicus leaving only the fibrous remnants of the umbilical arteries to connect the bladder to the umbilical region. In consequence of these anatomical facts, the urachus must be severed in order to mobilize the bladder when performing pelvic operations on the new born infant, but not in the older children. Several forms of urachal anomaly may present in childhood.

1. Urinary fistula at the umbilicus

a) Pathology

In some cases the bladder fails to narrow down at its apex, and maintains its attachment to its umbilicus, so that no true urachus is formed. There may thus be a direct vesical fistula at the umbilicus which discharges urine from the time of birth. In other examples, the urachal canal is formed, but remains patent, constituting a small fistulous connection between the bladder and umbilicus. This may be evident at birth, or may open up during the subsequent months, particularly if an obstruction is present. BEGG questioned whether this type of fistula was truly urachal, believing that it arose from a pericystitis and tracking of infection along the plane of least resistance, but in many reported cases, an epithelialized canal has been present.

b) Clinical picture

The umbilical urinary fistula may be wide, and flat on the surface, or it may be hidden within the depth of an inflamed and granulating umbilicus. An associated umbilical hernia is not infrequent. There is little difficulty in diagnosis if the discharge of urine is copious, but less severe examples must be distinguished from persistent vitelline duct, from blind external urachal sinus and from umbilical granuloma. In all these conditions there may be a little discharge of mucus, but the introduction of a probe, or X-rays taken after injection of lipiodol should settle the diagnosis.

Some small fistulae have a tendency to spontaneous closure, but the majority persist until the surgical treatment is undertaken: in uncomplicated cases the wetting may be only slight and many have been reported in which treatment was not sought until childhood was past. In some there is, however, a congenital lower urinary tract obstruction, and although the fistula constitutes some sort of safety valve, it is likely that renal damage is already advanced at the time of birth.

c) Treatment

The state of the urethra and bladder neck must first be determined by radiology or endoscopy: if no abnormality is found, the fistulous track should be excised, and the apex of the bladder closed. Uncomplicated cases have an excellent prognosis. A few examples have responded to simple cauterization (see reviews by DUCLOUX and BLONDIN, HERBST) but the surgical procedure seems more reliable.

2. Urachal cysts

The urachal canal is obliterated at both ends, but remains patent in the middle and accumulates fluid. The cysts may reach a considerable size, and the swelling alone will then attract attention: abdominal pain is also a feature, and infection is extremely likely to occur. Diagnosis may present some difficulty, though the consequent deformity of the apex of the bladder as seen in a lateral cystogram should give a clue. Complete excision by an extraperitoneal approach is the best form of treatment.

3. Urachal diverticulum

An enlargement of the urachus which remains patent at the lower end leads to the formation of urachal diverticulum. This may be an incidental finding at cystoscopy, but several cases have been reported in childhood (CAMPBELL, LADD and GROSS) in which a calculus has formed in this cavity, associated with pain and urgent micturition.

4. Blind external fistula

A small sinus at the umbilicus may lead into a urachal canal which is closed off from the bladder. Infection is likely, and the sinus should be excised or destroyed by cautery.

II. Rare vesical malformations

1. Agenesis of the bladder

Complete absence of the bladder is very rare in the surviving child, and in most reported cases it seems likely that a minute reservoir was present. In the female cases which have been described, the ureters opened directly into the vagina (MILLER) or into the uterus (IGNATESCU et al.); there was naturally dribbling incontinence of urine, and rectal abnormalities were also common. Cutaneous ureterostomy has been advocated as the only satisfactory treatment, though doubtless an ileal loop would now be interposed. LEPOUTRE has reported an example in the male: a boy of 4 months whose ureters opened into the rectum.

2. Duplications of the bladder

True double bladder is most uncommon, although there are a number of malformations which, on superficial examination, suggest a duplication, particularly when an ectopic ureter or ectopic ureterocele forms a very dilated cavity.

The classification of the anomalies proposed by BURNS et al. is generally accepted, and reference may be made to this work for a review of the literature.

a) Complete reduplication

Two separate organs are present, each fed by a ureter and drained by a separate urethra: the penis may or may not be double. Function may be good (NESBIT and BROMME) and no treatment is then required, but in the case of RAVITCH and SCOTT one urethra was abnormal and required excision after anastomosis of the bladders.

b) Incomplete reduplication

The bladder is bilobed, but the bladder neck and urethra single. Infective complications are likely to be responsible for symptoms as in the case of BOISSONNAT, a boy of 4 years with epididymitis.

c) Sagittal septum

The bladder is outwardly single but divided within. In the case of KOHLER multiple septa were present, and rendered function impossible.

d) Frontal septum

A good description of this type is given by MEYER. LAUGHLIN et al. describe a boy of 7 years presenting with incontinence and pyuria in whom a septum was responsible for retention in one half of the bladder. Removal of the septum is clearly required.

3. Hour-glass bladder

The bladder is partially divided by a ring-like constriction into upper and lower compartments, but contracting bladder muscle is present in both, and the condition must be distinguished from the bladder with a large apical diverticulum,

5*

or with very great dilatation of the posterior urethra. ZELLERMAYER and CARLSON have reviewed the reported cases, and although the condition is regarded as congenital it has not been recorded in the young child. Nevertheless two personal cases have been observed which appear to fall into this group. Both had unexplained residual urine, and a well marked waist-line in the bladder: neither was satisfactorily relieved by bladder neck resection, and excision of the upper compartment in one led to a very persistent suprapubic fistula. The nature of this disorder and its treatment are still uncertain.

4. Cysts of the trigone

Cysts arising beneath the trigonal mucosa and causing obstruction to the outflow from the bladder have been described by MICHON et al., and by BOISSONNAT and BOUTEAU, as well as a number of earlier writers. In some cases it

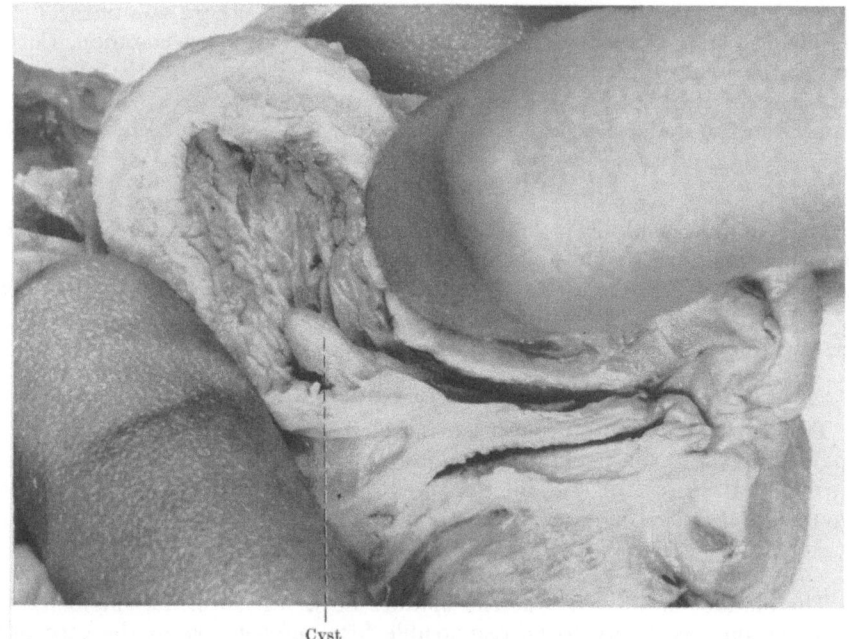

Cyst

Fig. 49. Cyst of trigone. Post-mortem specimen from a girl dying at the age of 5 weeks with urinary obstruction and infection. The child's general condition never permitted a full investigation of her urinary tract, and her only treatment consisted of bladder drainage, and opening of a left peri-nephric abscess. Specimen shows a hypertrophied bladder, and the only obstruction found was a serous cyst projecting up from the trigone

would appear that the cyst has been an ectopic ureterocele, but in others no explanation of its origin can be given. The specimen illustrated in Fig. 49 is from a female child dying as a result of urinary obstruction and infection; the cyst was lined by simple flattened epithelium, and was filled with clear fluid.

In this case, the child's general condition never allowed treatment of the lesion, but clearly suprapubic excision or endoscopic destruction would have been possible in more favourable circumstances.

5. Trigonal curtains

There are a number of cases on record in which a fold of mucous membrane, projecting forward from the trigone, has formed a flap valve partially occluding the outlet of the bladder (CAMPBELL, KOOK et al., LEARMONTH and WATKINS). Both males and females have been affected and the lesion has caused a severe degree of urinary obstruction. Usually the diagnosis was only made during exploratory operation, for the cystoscopic appearance is extremely confusing: excision of the curtain leads to partial or complete relief. POOLE-WILSON has recorded a case in which two valvular folds were attached anteriorly above the bladder neck.

6. Congenital vesico-vaginal fistulae

Fistulae, other than those at the umbilicus, are extremely rare, but SWINNEY has recorded a case of dribbling incontinence in a girl due to a pinhole vesico-vaginal fistula, unaccompanied by any other abnormality. WEBER and SCHOLTZ observed a new-born infant with a similar fistula leading to urinary distension of the uterus and vagina behind an imperforate hymen. KESSELBERG, and ROLLER report utero-vesical fistulae.

III. Vesical diverticula

1. Pathology

It is now usually assumed that vesical diverticula, with the exception of the urachal remnants, are formed only where there is a urinary obstruction, and that if no abnormality is found in the urethra, then a bladder neck obstruction must be present. Thus diverticula would always be regarded as acquired abnormalities. BADENOCH stresses this point, and cites cases in which excision of the diverticulum without bladder neck resection was followed by the development of ureteric dilatation, indicating the persistence of an obstructive factor. It is true that many diverticula are found in hypertrophied, trabeculated bladders with urethral valves or obvious hypertrophy of the bladder neck: they are often found in the male in whom obstruction is relatively common, and only rarely in the female. However, in children, diverticula are also encountered in bladders which exhibit no evidence of obstruction, and HYMAN was able to present cases in which simple excision of the sac, without bladder neck resection, was curative. As a consequence other explanations of the pathogenesis have been sought, and the diverticula are stated to be congenital. The term "congenital" is not accurately defined, however, and may simply imply that the anomaly is present at birth, although the urinary tract presents many examples of acquired lesions which have occurred before birth (see p. 111). There appears to be little anatomical support for the idea that diverticula are congenital deformities in the sense of being active outgrowths of the bladder, for although most are covered with a thin layer of muscle they open through a definite hiatus in the normal detrusor coat.

One of the earliest theories was that of ENGLISCH who believed that there might have been a temporary obstruction to the urethra during foetal life, though this theory would not explain the presence of a diverticulum without generalized trabeculation. CAULK suggested that a blind supernumerary ureter might become dilated and form a vesical diverticulum, an explanation which seemed to fit one of my cases in which a narrow elongated sac, opening immediately behind the ureteric orifice, ran upwards in a common adventitial sheath with the ureter, but this is not the usual picture and the explanation can hardly cover the majority of cases. CHWALLE made a distinction between cases in which the ureter opened into the diverticulum, and others, regarding the former as congenital and the latter as acquired. He suggested that the congenital variety might arise as a result of dilatation behind the occlusive membrane, which as he observed, closes the uretero-vesical junction in early embryonic life (from the 14 mm to the 35 mm stage). However, as will be seen later any diverticulum placed near the ureteric orifice, will draw in that orifice as it enlarges, and the distinction made by CHWALLE does not appear to be justifiable.

A diverticulum consists essentially of a herniation of bladder mucosa, covered only by a thin muscular layer, through a defect in the thickened detrusor coat, and whether a urinary obstruction is present or not, some local weakness in this coat must be presumed responsible for the herniation. It is because the detrusor consists of interlacing bundles of muscle rather than of a continuous sheet that these unsupported areas occur, and although herniation will usually take place only under the circumstances of obstruction and detrusor hypertrophy, if a gross defect of muscle is present, the normal force of bladder contraction will be sufficient to push out a diverticulum. Once a diverticulum is formed bladder contraction will distend it with urine at each attempted micturition, and lead to progressive enlargement. Cine cystography shows that in such a case the bladder is capable of contraction which obliterates its lumen, yet since the urine is driven out into the diverticulum and returns from it with relaxation, a "false" residual urine remains. In these circumstances detrusor hypertrophy may follow and with it the prominence of the bladder neck.

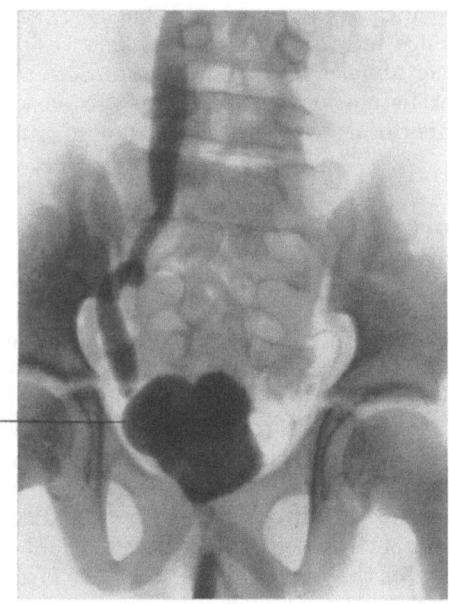

Diver-
ticulum

Fig. 50. Vesical diverticulum with vesico-urethral reflux. Micturating cystogram in a boy aged 8 years with enuresis. There was a defect in the muscular coat of the bladder behind the right ureteric orifice, but mucous membrane only protruded through the defect to form a diverticulum during micturition (see text)

The case illustrated in Fig. 50 was investigated at an early stage of this process on account of persistent nocturnal enuresis. It was demonstrated that when the bladder was relaxed and partly filled, the only abnormality was a slight redundancy of the mucosa behind the right ureteric orifice: with bladder contractions, a diverticulum formed at this point, and drew the right ureteric orifice into the sac. At operation, a localized muscular defect was demonstrated, through which the mucosa could be everted. There was no evidence of urinary obstruction at the time, nor when he was re-investigated four years later. There seems no reason to doubt that in this case, the muscular defect was the primary abnormality. The cystogram of this boy also shows the reflux which occurs into a ureter which is involved in a diverticulum; this reflux is a common though not a constant finding, and it is likely to be one of the factors responsible for ureteric dilatation. Fig 51 illustrates a case of severe unilateral hydro-ureter complicating a diverticulum of the bladder into which the ureter opened, reflux was demonstrated in this case only during the phase of bladder relaxation after micturition. The local anatomy is shown in the inset diagram: this is the usual arrangement in childhood whether a urinary obstruction is present or not, for it appears that the ureteric orifice is less fixed in its position than in adults, and is more easily drawn into the sac. While the most likely site of a muscular weakness is immediately behind and lateral to the ureteric orifice, diverticula also occur at a higher level on the lateral wall of the bladder, and on the posterior wall near the apex.

2. Clinical and radiological features

There is no sign or symptom pathognomonic of vesical diverticulum, for even the classical miction-en-deux-temps may be due to dilated ureters with

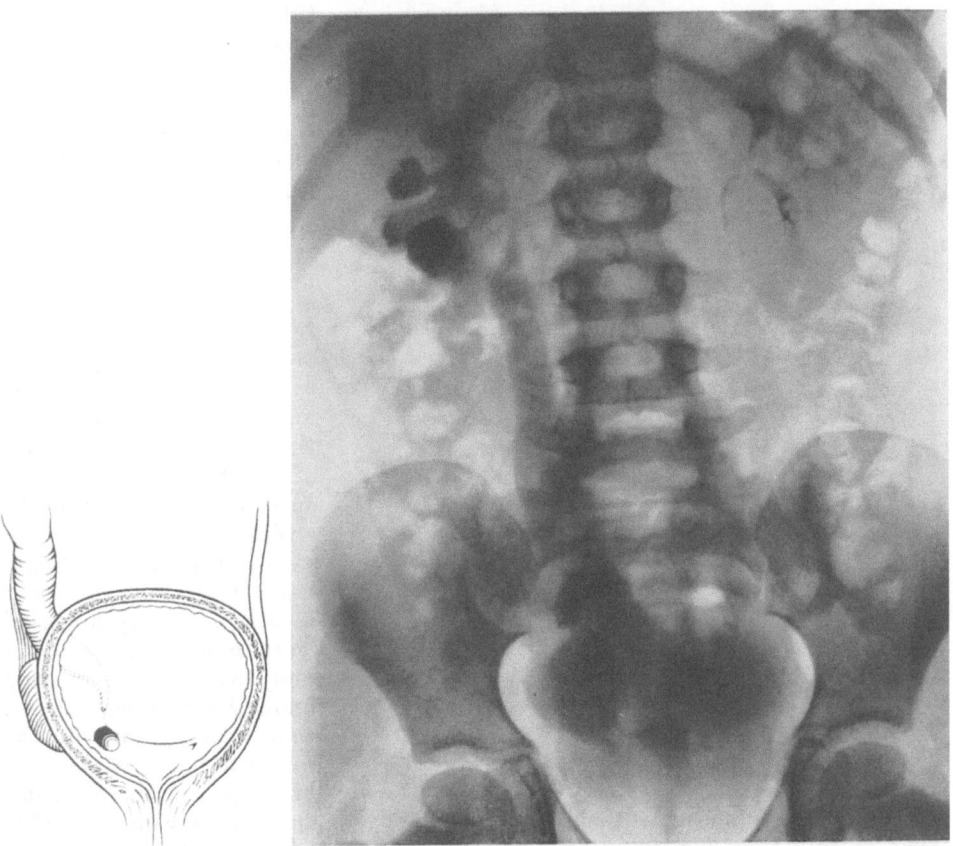

Fig. 51. Vesical diverticulum. Intravenous pyelogram in a boy aged 5 years suffering from recurrent haematuria. Considerable dilatation of the right ureter, which opens into a vesical diverticulum. Normal left kidney and ureter. No trabeculation and no cystoscopic evidence of bladder neck obstruction

reflux. In many cases all the clinical features are those of the congenital lower urinary obstruction, and the diverticulum is a complication found only on investigation. Acute retention with painful bladder distension is, however, more common in cases with this complication.

Recurrent urinary infection is a common mode of presentation in those cases without obvious obstruction: they are symptom-free between attacks.

A diverticulum is occasionally palpable in the abdomen as a swelling distinct from the distended bladder, and it may also be felt on rectal examination. The cystoscopic appearance of the diverticular orifice is well known but may be mimicked by a widely gaping ureteric orifice such as may be seen in the mega-ureter-megacystis syndrome. Such a ureter often shows spontaneous contractions, however, whereas the patency of the diverticulum varies only with the state of the bladder distension and contraction; moreover a urethroscope can be passed into the opening and in a diverticulum the true ureteric orifice can be found on the medial wall.

Cystography is valuable in identifying the presence of diverticula, but special positioning is required. Perhaps the best view is that used in pelvimetry (the "squat-shot") in which the child sits on the plate, leaning forward, and the tube points downwards behind his back. The size of a diverticulum can only be judged during micturition (Fig. 52), since passive bladder distension will not fill the sac to its maximum.

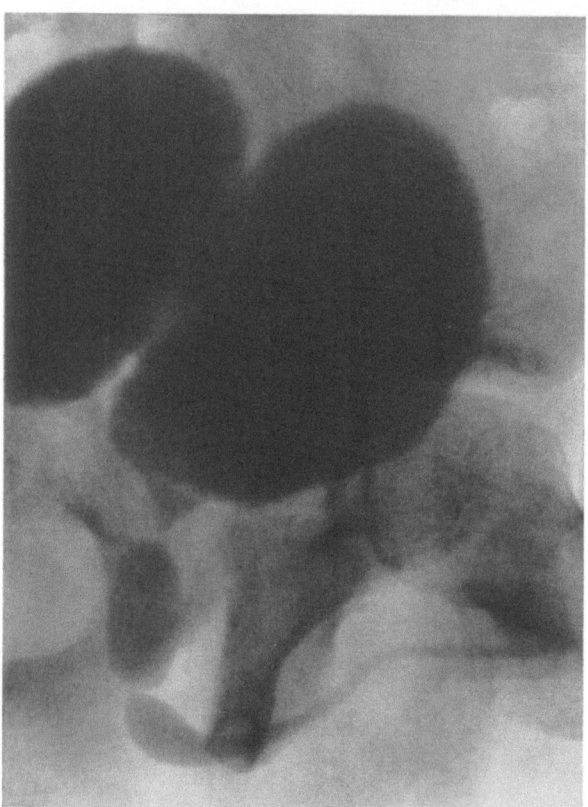

Fig. 52. Vesical diverticulum. Micturating cystogram in a boy aged 8 years with haematuria. There was a valvular obstruction in the urethra

3. Treatment

Small diverticula in which the floor is visible on simple cystoscopy with a right angle instrument, and which occur as part of the generalized sacculation of the bladder require no special treatment: the obstructive lesion must be removed. Large diverticula must always be excised, and recurrent urinary infection is an indication for removing even moderate sized ones. Extravesical dissection with ligature of the mucosal neck of the sac, and repair of the muscular defect is the most suitable type of operation, for the region of the ureteric orifice is easily mobilized in the child. When the ureter opens into the diverticulum, it is sometimes possible to leave it in continuity, excising the redundant portion of the sac and closing the muscle layer, but more often a deliberate reimplantation of the ureter must be undertaken. In the case of a dilated ureter, the implantation must be done in such a manner as to prevent reflux (see p. 54).

IV. Bladder neck obstruction and urethral fibro-elastosis

1. Definition

The diagnosis of congenital bladder neck obstruction has a varying significance in different urological centres, and a failure to appreciate these variations has led to considerable confusion in the assessment of treatment and results. The importance of the "maladie du col" in childhood was first emphasized by MARION, so that the term "Marion's Disease" is now often employed: he regarded the disease as a cause of severe urinary obstruction, mimicking prostatic hypertrophy, in which the bladder neck formed a prominent rim and the urethra below appeared normal. Many surgeons (e.g. BOPPE and MARCEL) have continued to limit the diagnosis to those cases with undoubted evidence of urinary retention; they then find males affected more often than females, and a high proportion of their cases are infants with advanced renal damage. Others have enlarged the diagnostic category to include children complaining of enuresis, or urinary infection, in whom the bladder neck appears hypertrophied, but the signs of obstruction are questionable. Their cases are as often girls as boys, and predominantly in the later age groups, often including a high proportion of adolescents. The advent of endoscopic resection has been chiefly responsible for this development, for while those accustomed to perform open operations for bladder neck obstruction confine that diagnosis to a few seriously affected children, the resectionists find a great many cases on which to exercise their skill. The criteria of diagnosis are seldom clearly defined by the latter group: in EMMETT and SIMON's series it appears that trabeculation was present in only half the total number, that residual urine was minimal in a high proportion, and that no less than one quarter complained only of enuresis, but the bladder neck "looked obstructive" in almost all. Similarly MILLER finds bladder neck obstruction a common cause of simple enuresis in both boys and girls, and makes his diagnosis by rectal palpation against the cystoscope when he can feel the thickened muscle. THOMPSON suggests that bladder neck obstruction is a common cause of recurrent infection, but believes that it often responds to simple dilatation, he appears to regard the obstruction as sometimes due to a mucosal or submucosal change, rather than to a muscular disorder. It is clear that these authors treat many children with enuresis or recurrent urinary infection by resection where others, including the present writer, would employ medical regimes, and the description of bladder neck obstruction as given in this section would not fit the majority of their cases. It is of course, argued that these enuretic children with prominent bladder necks have the same disease as those with chronic retention though in a milder form: the discrepancy in the sex incidence noted above makes this unlikely, however, and it is admitted by all that advanced changes are uncommon in girls or young adult women.

A further confusion has arisen from the inclination of many authors to include examples of neurogenic bladder due to myelodysplasia in the same group as congenital bladder neck obstruction. It is true that in a few cases difficulty arises in differential diagnosis, but my own experience suggests that there is a fundamental difference between the two disorders, and a corresponding difference in what can be accomplished by treatment. The neurogenic bladder is almost always accompanied by other neurological signs, and by a bony deformity of the vertebrae (see p. 128) but the observation of an uncomplicated spina bifida, revealed only by X-rays, is irrelevant and does not assist diagnosis. Furthermore the great majority of congenital neurogenic bladders are expressible, whereas the mechanically obstructed bladder, except in the uraemic infant, can only be expressed under anaesthesia.

The basic difficulty of definition has arisen from the fact that the clinical and, until recently, the pathological diagnosis has been made by a process of exclusion, rather than on any positive finding. The presence of bladder neck hypertrophy associated with signs of urinary obstruction is no certain indication, for it will be equally evident in most distal urethral obstructions, due to valves, diverticula etc.: the bladder neck musculature then hypertrophies together with the detrusor, as a reaction to obstruction, not as its cause. It is only when the urethra itself is apparently normal that the bladder neck hypertrophy is regarded as the primary abnormality, but a diagnosis based on this negative finding is apt to be unreliable, since cases of retention due to mega-ureter-megacystis syndrome (p. 57) and those with large congenital vesical diverticula are apt to be included. A recent advance, described below, in the understanding of the pathology may ultimately clarify this situation.

2. Pathology

MARION stressed the simple muscular hypertrophy found in the region of the internal sphincter, and subsequently many authors have compared the disease to infantile pyloric stenosis, cardiospasm and other sphincter disorders for which the evasive term neuro-muscular inco-ordination has often been accepted as an explanation. Other observers have emphasized the factor of sclerosis: thus CAMPBELL refers to the condition as sub-mucous fibrosis, and although it is admitted that large instruments can always be introduced, the term bladder neck stenosis is sometimes employed. Recently, however, BODIAN has demonstrated a clear cut pathological change described as fibro-elastosis affecting the whole posterior urethra in these children. Working on post-mortem material at the Hospital for Sick Children, and on biopsies of my cases, he finds that the developing prostatic tissue is abnormal in structure and distribution. The normal prostate in an infant consists of simple glandular structures intermingled with plentiful smooth muscle fibres; in the abnormal, glands are rare, while fibrous and elastic tissue predominate; moreover instead of being concentrated in a comparatively short segment of the posterior urethra, this prostatic tissue extends from the bladder neck above to the corpora cavernosa below. The verumontanum is affected by the change, and is often somewhat enlarged. It is postulated that this fibro-elastosis leads to an increased resistance to normal distension, and so to an obstruction to urine flow: detrusor hypertrophy, and with it hypertrophy of the bladder neck musculature, then follows. It must be emphasized that this change has only been demonstrated in the severe obstruction of young males, and it cannot yet be affirmed that it is the invariable pathology of so-called bladder neck obstruction. It is very doubtful whether any such lesion would be found in the numerous cases in both sexes with slight bladder neck hypertrophy described by EMMETT and SIMON. Furthermore, as will be emphasized later, the retention phase of the mega-ureter-megacystis syndrome is responsible for apparent severe bladder neck obstruction in many older children, particularly in girls, and in them no urethral fibro-elastosis is found.

3. Symptomatology

Severe cases presenting in infancy are clinically indistinguishable from urethral valves and other congenital urethral obstructions: they present with a distended bladder, overflow incontinence, and usually signs of renal failure. In later childhood, incontinence, by day as well as by night, a poor stream, recurrent urinary infection, haematuria and abdominal pain may draw attention to the condition. There is no characteristic symptom, and the diagnosis can only be made as a result of urological investigation, carried out in cases of retention along the lines suggested in Section E.

4. Diagnosis

The presence of residual urine, trabeculation of the bladder, and ureteric dilatation usually leaves little doubt as to the presence of an obstruction, and clinical examination should exclude any neurological cause or a mass in the pelvis pressing on the urethra. Vesical diverticula are often associated with urethral fibro-elastosis, but their presence is not a necessary indication of obstruction, for the primary abnormality may be a defect in the detrusor coat, and the diverticulum itself can be responsible for "false" residual urine due to distension during bladder contractions (p. 70).

The bladder neck is seen with a right angled cystoscope as a raised rim posteriorly, and with the urethroscope as a shelf projecting forwards above the verumontanum. The urethra is not dilated, although it may appear wider than normal immediately below the bladder neck.

The urethrograms may be entirely normal (Fig. 53), or the bladder neck hypertrophy may produce an unusual indentation in the urethral outline (Fig. 54). At times the posterior urethra cannot be distended at all, either by micturition or by expression under anaesthetic, and only a thin trickle of dye is seen. Rarely the upper urethra, below the prominent bladder neck is dilated, but tapers down to a point below the verumontanum, an outline

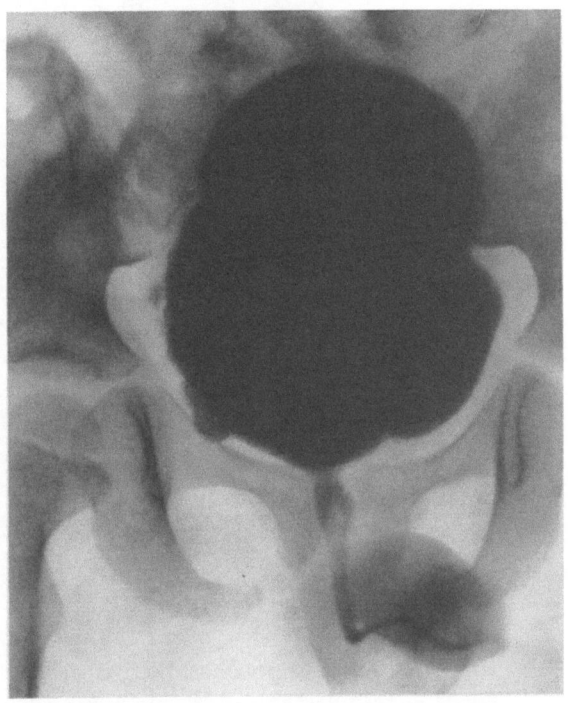

Fig. 53. "Bladder neck obstruction". Expression cystogram in a boy aged 5 years suffering from chronic retention of urine with overflow incontinence. The urethrographic outline is normal. Two vesical diverticula are present. An extensive bladder neck resection was carried out, but there was a long delay in re-establishing micturition

which contrasts with the bulging dilatation due to valvular obstruction. A case of this type, illustrated in Fig. 55, was proved at post-mortem to have the typical lesion of urethral fibro-elastosis, and doubtless a concentration of abnormal tissue in the lower part of the posterior urethra was responsible for the slight dilatation in the upper part.

Some examples of the mega-ureter-megacystis syndrome in the retention phase may closely mimic the fibro-elastosis cases, but differentiation may be made from the following points. The bladder capacity in megacystis is large, usually 800—1,000 ml in children of 8 to 10 years, measured under conditions of cystometry. Trabeculation is absent or slight, represented often by a few strong bands. The ureteric orifices gape, and are usually wide enough to allow the introduction of the urethroscope with which slow rhythmic ureteric contractions may be observed. By contrast in the fibro-elastosis group the bladder capacity is seldom more than 500—600 ml, and heavy trabeculation is the rule, sacculi and diverticula are common: the ureteric orifices are normal unless placed within a diverticulum, and reflux only occurs late, when ureteric contractions have almost failed. A poor stream and incontinence are usual in the fibro-elastosis children, whereas in the megacystis cases it is quite often stated that micturition is normal even when an enormous vesical residuum is present. At operation, the

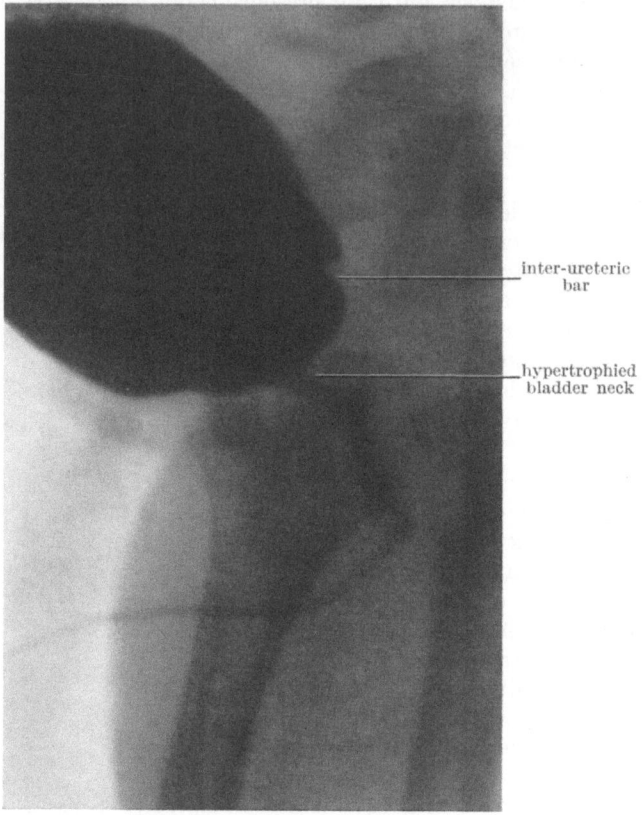

Fig. 54. "Bladder neck obstruction." Micturating cystogram in a boy aged 1 year with chronic retention of urine. The posterior lip of the bladder neck is prominent but the urethra is not dilated. The notch in the posterior profile of the bladder represents the hypertrophied inter-ureteric bar

bladder neck may resist digital dilatation in either group, but it is sometimes surprisingly lax. Biopsy of a long strip of the anterior wall may confirm the diagnosis of fibro-elastosis.

5. Treatment

The management of retention in general is discussed in Section E, the obstructing lesion itself may be dealt with by endoscopic resection or by open operation. None of the methods at present in use is ideally adapted to the lesion, a fibro-elastosis affecting the whole length of the posterior urethra, particularly in the posterior wall. If an open "wedge" resection is performed, a large amount of tissue should be removed, in fact MARION advocated removal of the entire circumference of the bladder neck. In girls there is a definite risk that wide resection, or subsequent attempts to control haemorrhage will result in the formation of a vesico-vaginal fistula, and in them if not in all cases an anterior plastic operation is perferable. I am accustomed to perform a Y—V plasty, centred at the bladder neck, and bringing the V shaped wedge of anterior bladder wall down to widen the urethra. Trans-urethral resection is adequate for many cases, though in chronic retention it is necessary to remove rather more tissue than first inspection might suggest.

In young children and infants with retention, any of these operations may be followed by a period in which micturition is difficult to re-establish since only a part of the fibro-elastosis tissue has been removed: prolonged catheter drainage

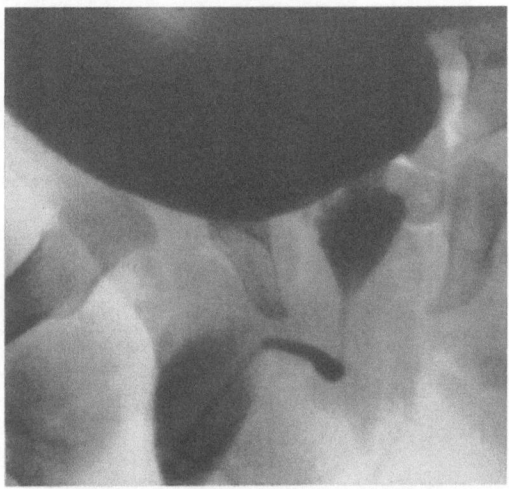

Fig. 55. Urethral fibro-elastosis. Expression cysto-urethrogram in a boy aged 4 months with chronic retention. Films show bladder neck hypertrophy with tapering dilatation of posterior urethra. After death from uraemia, post-mortem specimen showed typical fibro-elastosis

and repeated dilatation may be necessary. Ultimately micturition without residuum is recovered, but then it is often found that some stress incontinence is present: the fibro-elastosis involves a change in the urethral wall which not only presents resistance to normal distension, but when this resistance has been finally lowered sufficiently to allow emptying of the bladder, it damps down the normal elastic recoil. It therefore interferes with the mechanism which maintains continence following closure of the external sphincter in cases where the internal sphincter has been destroyed. This stress incontinence has a tendency to spontaneous improvement in the co-operative child, but where it is very persistent, a plication operation on the urethral bulb may be justifiable.

Diverticula require operative excision, and some of the best results as judged by intravenous pyelograms (Fig. 56) are seen in those cases where diverticula have been removed. The dilated ureters will recover only when the obstruction is treated in its early stages, and often irreversible changes have occurred when the child is first seen. Occasionally operation is required to straighten kinked ureters or to remove an advanced hydronephrosis, for the effect on the upper urinary tract is often asymmetrical.

Recovery of renal function is often better than the improvement in the ureters, but the child will remain liable to urinary infection and therefore to pyelonephritic destruction of the kidneys.

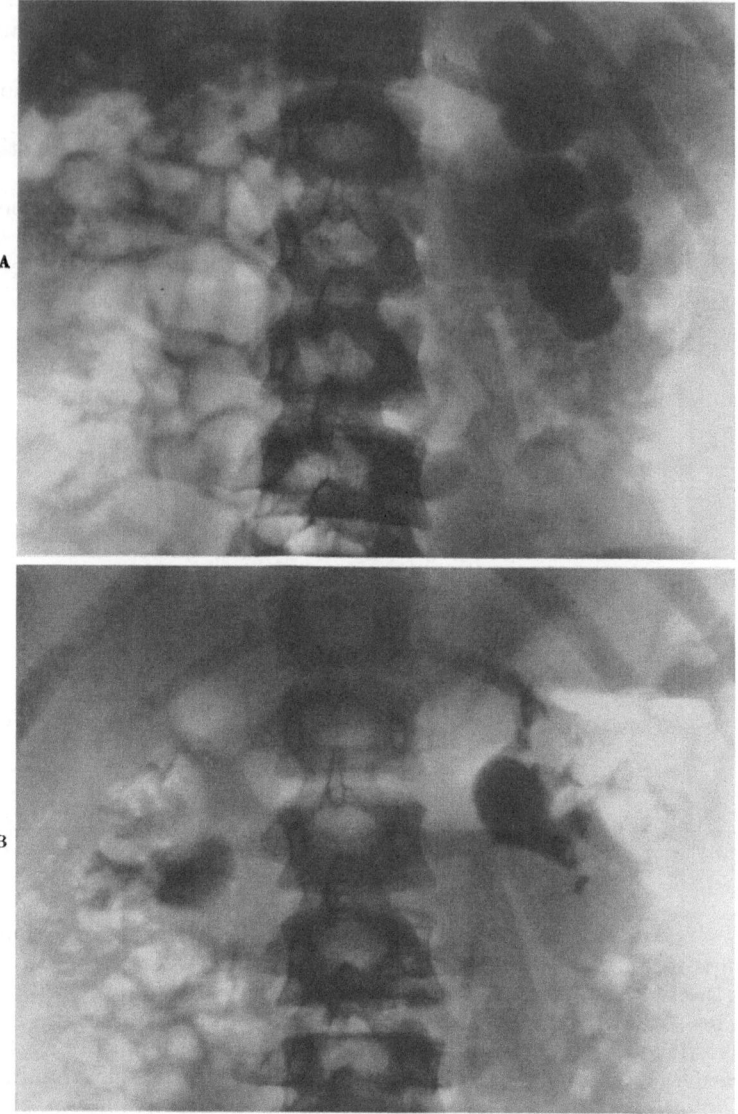

Fig. 56 A and B. "Bladder neck obstruction" with vesical diverticula in a boy aged 10 years. Intravenous
pyelograms A before; B after diverticulectomy and resection of bladder neck

V. Urethral obstructions

1. Congenital obliterations of the urethra

Complete obliteration of the urethral lumen is an important cause of failure
to pass urine after birth: lesser obstructions usually allow an overflow. Obliterations of the posterior urethra are almost uniformly fatal, but if the penile
urethra is affected the prognosis is quite good.

a) Obliterations at the level of the bladder neck

This type is commonly associated with very great dilatation of the bladder,
sometimes causing dystocia, and advanced changes in the upper urinary tract

with either hydronephrosis or renal hypoplasia. The urethra below may or may not be patent, but often gross anomalies of the external genitalia are present. In male cases the rectum often ends blindly in the posterior bladder wall. This type of bladder disorder has been fully discussed by KRUGER: almost all cases have ended fatally, though one observed by the author lived for several days. Treatment is better with-held.

b) Obliteration of the membranous urethra

If no fistulous tract is formed, this type of obliteration is likely to be as destructive of the kidneys as the last mentioned, but an opening may be found at the urachus, into the rectum in the male (MAY), or into the vagina in the female. The obliteration appears to be a localized atresia, and affects all layers of the urethral wall. The anterior urethra is usually patent and instrumentation will indicate the site of the obstruction. It is not possible to lay down any standard line of treatment, which must clearly vary with the precise circumstances.

c) Obliterations of the penile urethra

A large number of cases have been reported (summarized by MENEGAUX and BOIDOT, and DOURMASHKIN) of occlusion of the terminal urethra. Failure to pass urine at birth, with distension of the bladder, has drawn attention to the disorder, but the general condition of the infants has been good. Often no urethral meatus could be seen, yet a process of probing, sometimes prolonged and forceful, has eventually established a channel through to the proximal urethra. In spite of this traumatic instrumentation, these infants appear to have commenced normal micturition soon afterwards, and the upper urinary tract has shown little evidence of dilatation. It seems likely therefore that the urethra was not absent in these cases as some authors suggested, but was temporarily obliterated by epithelial debris. Occlusion of a short segment is commonly observed in cases of coronal hypospadias, but can quickly be remedied by gentle probing, and it may be that in some of the reported cases of absence of the terminal urethra, this type of hypospadiac meatus was overlooked.

2. Urethral diaphragms and strictures

Meatal stenosis is not considered in this section (see p. 244), and apart from that group, congenital strictures are almost exclusively found in the male. In clinical practice it is difficult to make any distinction between a short stricture and a diaphragmatic obstruction, so that these two anomalies are conveniently discussed together. Either may be responsible for a high grade urinary obstruction, presenting at birth or during early childhood, but both are rare, being encountered much less often than urethral valves and in contrast to the valves they constitute an obstruction to instrumentation, as well as to micturition.

Most of the severe forms of stenosis have affected the prostatic urethra, and have often been responsible for death during the first weeks (EHRLICH, CHADWICK and MEADOWS, CROWELL and ANDERSON). A diaphragm with a central perforation (iris diaphragm, YOUNG and McKAY) may be present above or below the verumontanum, and will produce all the secondary obstructive changes commonly seen in association with urethral valves: proximal dilatation of the urethra, detrusor hypertrophy with prominence of the bladder neck, vesical diverticula, hydro-ureter, hydronephrosis, or renal hypoplasia. These cases present with overflow incontinence and uraemia, and will be brought to light by the routine investigation described on p. 114. The urethrogram will demonstrate the level of the obstruction (Fig. 57) and on urethroscopy, the concentric stenosing ring will be found above the external sphincter. A diaphragm is easily destroyed by endoscopic diathermy, but a stricture may require dilatation. Since renal

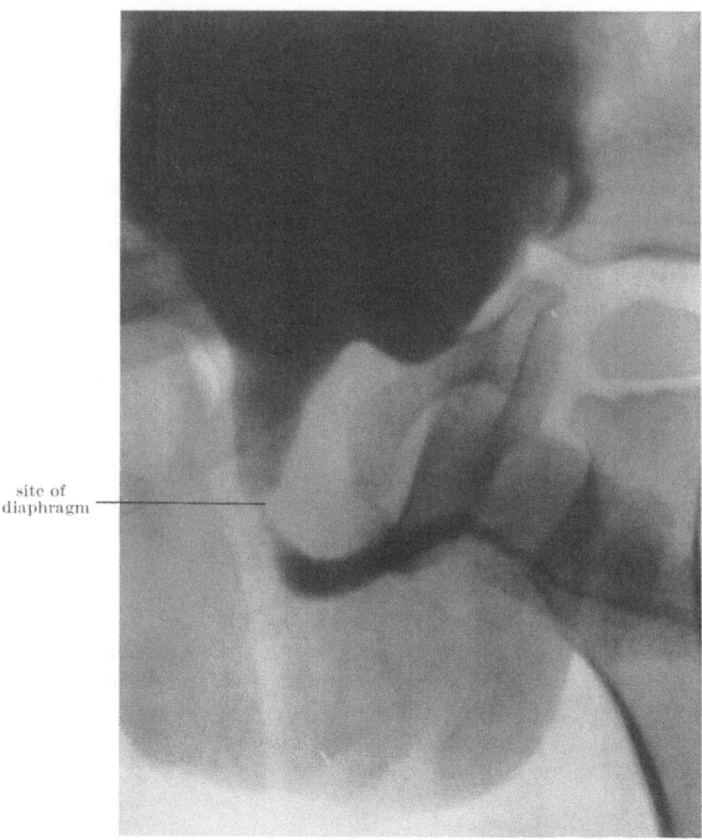

site of
diaphragm

Fig. 57. Diaphragmatic obstruction of the posterior urethra. Expression cysto-urethrogram in a boy aged 3 years with chronic retention of urine. There is annular constriction of the posterior urethra immediately below the verumontanum

damage is usually advanced when the infant is seen, the prognosis is apt to be poor.

A few strictures present in later childhood or in adolescence, but at this age it is often difficult to exclude an acquired lesion. FAGERSTROM, and BUSCH describe posterior urethral obstruction of this type, causing difficult micturition. In their cases dilatation was an adequate treatment. BROWN mentions an anterior urethral stricture in a boy of 10 as a cause of enuresis, and I have encountered a similar case; the diagnosis should be made with caution and the normal narrowing at the peno-scrotal junction must be recognized. Difficulty in instrumentation does not necessarily imply a stricture. Treatment may follow the line suggested for acquired strictures (p. 248).

TSENG reports an interesting case of a diaphragm in the penile urethra, with a fistula immediately distal to it.

3. Posterior urethral valves

a) Pathology

Valvular folds of mucosa are the commonest cause of serious congenital urethral obstruction in the male: in the female their presence is rare and questionable. Although recognized by earlier authors, H. H. YOUNG and his co-workers gave the classical description of the malformation, which has been little improved upon by later observers. He described three main types, illustrated by a familiar diagram given in Fig. 58: in Type I, two folds are raised on the posterior urethral wall, and run downwards and laterally from the verumontanum; in Type II multiple folds run upwards from the verumontanum to the bladder neck; Type III is an iris diaphragm as described in the previous section. Valvular folds may be unilateral, and they may sometimes gain an attachment anteriorly (NESBIT and RAPER). The ridges described as Type II valves may be seen together with Type I, and it may therefore be suspected that the former are secondary formations consequent upon the obstruction, and not a primary cause.

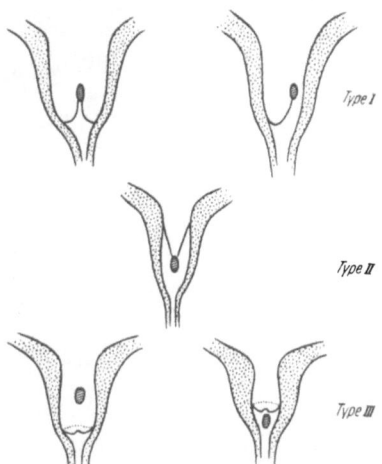

Fig. 58. Congenital valves in the posterior urethra. Diagrams to show the three types originally described by Young

Type I valves are the common findings with which we are here concerned: it will be seen that their situation is the same as the normal low ridges (submontanal folds) which can be seen in the male urethra, and in my opinion they are simply exaggerations of these normal structures. Examination of the urethra in embryos of the 50—100 mm stage shows that during this period very prominent ridges are normal, and a failure of the usual process of regression is presumably responsible for their persistence as an obstructive factor. Valve formation is thus a comparatively minor departure from normal development, and associated malformations, as opposed to consequent lesions, of the urinary tract are uncommon. The similarity of the "valve" to the normal submontanal fold is so close that the obstructive nature of the valve has sometimes been called in question, some observers asserting that bladder neck obstruction is the usual cause of retention but a urethral dilatation ceasing abruptly at the level of the valve is usual, and destruction of the cusps can lead to restoration of normal micturition.

The typical post-mortem appearances are illustrated in (Fig. 59). In order to demonstrate these valves it is essential to remove the entire urethra, and to distend it before fixation. The verumontanum is usually enlarged, and the folds spring from its lower pole, curving downwards and laterally to fuse with the urethral wall at or immediately above the level of the perineal membrane. The posterior urethra is grossly dilated, its wall thickened and muscular. The bladder neck is hypertrophied and stands out as a prominent ridge separating the smooth urethral cavity from the trabeculated bladder. Detrusor hypertrophy is extreme, and may prevent complete bladder contraction; sacculation is usual and diverticula may occur. The ureters are grossly dilated and tortuous, the kidneys hydronephrotic or hypoplastic (p. 111).

b) Clinical features

Many cases of urethral valves present during earliest infancy with vomiting and failure to thrive owing to uraemia. Most of these have distended bladders and overflow incontinence, and clinically it is impossible to distinguish them from many other forms of congenital bladder neck and urethral obstruction. The mani-

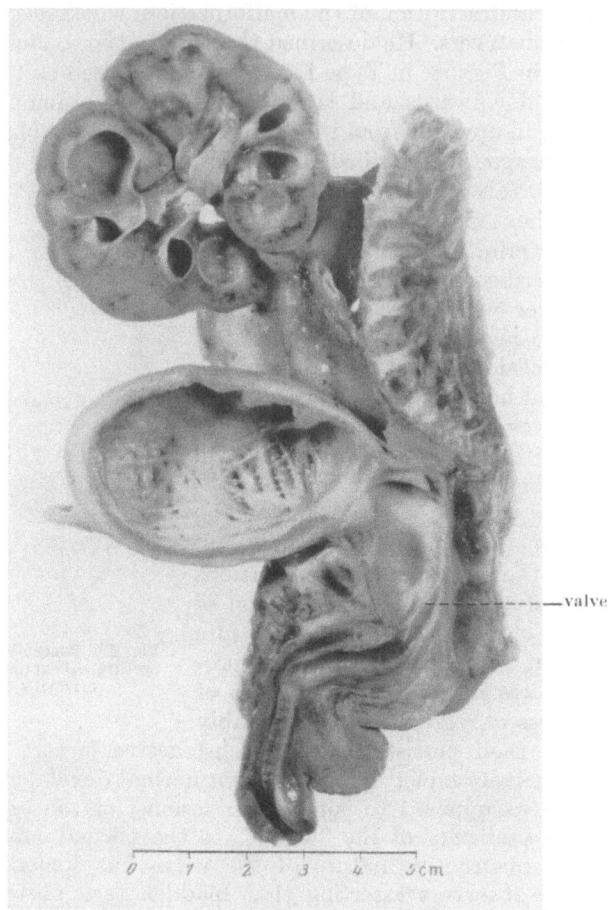

Fig. 59. Congenital valves in the posterior urethra. Post-mortem specimen from a boy dying at 3 days. The posterior urethra is enormously dilated down to the level of the valvular fold

festations of chronic retention are discussed at length in Section E, and only a few special points revelant to urethral valves need be mentioned here. They are present from early foetal life, and symptoms therefore often appear soon after birth, but it is unusual for valves to cause complete retention: overflow is almost always possible.

The bladder is seldom distended above the umbilicus, to which it may be attached, and the renal swellings are often a more prominent feature. With a finger in the rectum, it is sometimes possible to palpate the dilated urethra as distinct from the distended bladder. Rare complications are umbilical urinary fistula, and ascites due to perforation of the bladder.

A valve case diagnosed in early infancy has almost always irreversible changes in the upper urinary tract and a severe degree of renal damage, which may have been incurred before birth: the prognosis is correspondingly poor. In later age groups, difficult micturition and incontinence due to overflow, recurrent urinary infection and haematuria are more common modes of presentation, and the renal damage in these is less advanced. Nevertheless it is uncommon to find true urethral valves without well marked back pressure effects, indeed the mucosal fold can scarcely be said to be valvular unless it causes an obstruction, and in my view valves are a very unusual cause of simple enuresis. CAMPBELL also emphasizes the severity of the obstruction commonly associated with urethral valves.

c) Diagnosis

The diagnosis of chronic retention is made on clinical grounds, the diagnosis of the cause is made by radiology and endoscopy. The radiological methods are discussed and well illustrated by JORUP and KJELLBERG. In infants the expression urethrogram will show a dilatation of the whole posterior urethra, with a narrowed bulb (Fig. 60) and the dilated portion appears in the lateral view to bulge over the distal segment. The bladder neck hypertrophy produces a distinct shelf, and unless the urine is actually being passed or expressed, the urethra may not be filled. In older

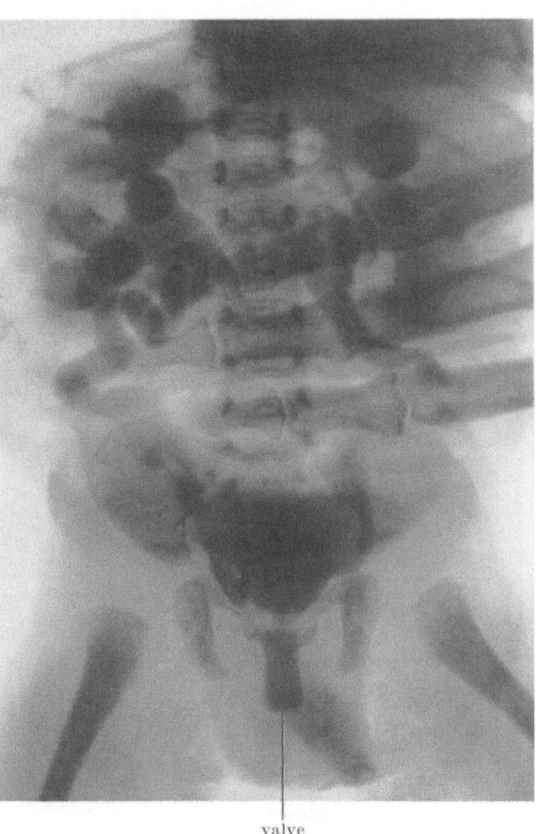

valve

Fig. 60. Congenital valves in the posterior urethra. Expression cysto-urethrogram in a boy aged 3 weeks with chronic retention. The posterior urethra is greatly dilated, with a "bulging" lower end. There is some reflux into the seminal vesicles and free reflux into dilated and extremely tortuous ureters

children, in whom micturating urethrograms are possible the contrast between the dilated and the narrow segment may not be so extreme, but it is always present. The dilated urethra bulges on either side and never tapers towards the obstruction. The actual outline of the valves may be discernible in the antero-posterior view (Fig. 61), but transverse linear filling defects should not be diagnosed as valves unless proximal dilatation indicates their obstructive nature: using viscous contrast media almost horizontal mucosal folds, sometimes multiple, may be outlined in the normal urethra.

On urethroscopy, the valves are best visualized by a direct viewing telescope, they form crescentic folds running downwards from the verumontanum. It is sometimes difficult by inspection of the fold alone to say whether it is valvular, but the condition of the proximal urethra normally gives a clear indication:

it is a widely dilated cavity below a hypertrophied bladder neck. The same fact can often be appreciated with a metal catheter, which although it is not held up by the valves may be difficult to introduce into the bladder because the bladder neck is a comparatively small opening at the top of a wide cavity.

It is preferable to make the diagnosis from the combined evidence of radiology and endoscopy.

d) Treatment

The treatment of urethral valves cannot be separated from the management of chronic retention in general, and biochemical correction and relief of obstruction may take precedence over all other measures (see p. 115).

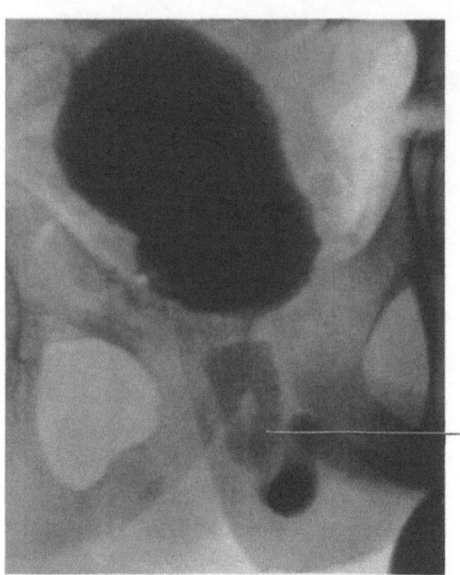

Destruction of the valvular fold may be achieved endoscopically or at open operation. The "blind" rupture of valves by passing a steel bougie downwards from the bladder is in my experience difficult and unsatisfactory: the bougie may not engage the fold or once engaged may cause more damage to the urethral wall than to the valve. Exposure is possible by the retropubic approach, making a longitudinal incision in the posterior urethra, and a good view of the valves may be obtained in this way, but in young infants this approach is difficult and bloody. As will be seen in Fig. 59 the valves are very deeply placed, and remote from the abdominal incision. Endoscopic diathermy is the most satisfactory method to employ: in the small infant a simple pointed diathermy electrode passed through a urethroscope may be sufficient while in larger children a diathermy loop on a miniature resectoscope is preferable. Whenever the anterior urethra does not readily admit the instrument, a perineal urethrostomy should be made, and this opening is conveniently used for an indwelling catheter post-operatively.

Fig. 61. Congenital valves in the posterior urethra. Micturating cysto-urethrogram in a boy aged 8 years, with overflow incontinence. The posterior urethra is dilated, and the filling defect of the verumontanum, with two folds running downwards from it, can be made out

The secondary changes in the bladder and urethra are such that a complete restoration of normal anatomy cannot be expected: Fig. 62 shows the degree of improvement in the dilatation of the posterior urethra. Since in infants the valves are well down in the membranous urethra, their removal may leave an inadequate external sphincter, and as the internal sphincter may have been rendered incompetent by proximal dilatation, a post-operative stress incontinence is not unlikely. This disability is easily overlooked in infancy, but may be troublesome later on, though there is a tendency to spontaneous improvement with the passage of years.

Diverticula of the bladder may require excision, and at times the acutely kinked ureters become secondarily obstructed and require drainage or even nephrectomy. There is always a liability to infection in the damaged urinary tract, and a year of continuous chemotherapy after operation is advisable.

The prognosis depends upon the state of the kidneys: in some there is inadequate renal tissue, and although micturition is restored, a slowly progressive renal failure may be fatal many years later (p. 221).

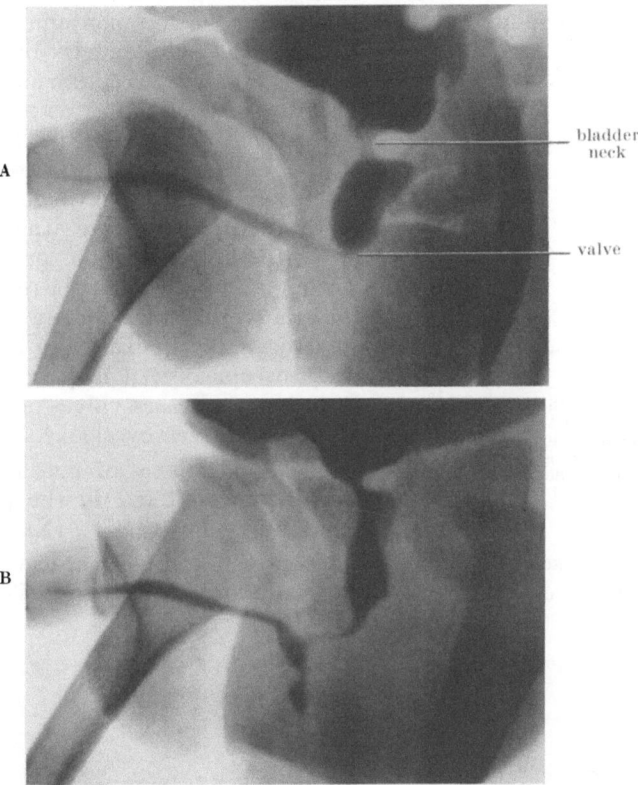

Fig. 62 A and B. Congenital valves in the posterior urethra. Expression cysto-urethrograms (under anaesthesia) in a boy aged 9 months suffering from chronic retention of urine. A Pre-operative. The hypertrophied bladder neck creates a shelf separating the dilated urethra from the bladder; the posterior urethra bulges over the narrow bulbar region. B Post-operative. The posterior urethra has narrowed down and now has a tapered lower end. The perineal urethrostomy opening is not fully healed

4. Anterior urethral valves

A partial duplication or a diverticulum of the urethra may constitute a valvular obstruction (BOISSONNAT), but on rare occasions a simple mucosal fold is responsible. The fold is crescentic and placed horizontally on the ventral wall of the urethra in the region of the peno-scrotal junction. In three personal cases, aged 3, 4 and 9 years, with this malformation, each child presented with difficult micturition, a distended bladder and hydro-ureters, but there was no obstruction to the passage of instruments. The diagnosis will not be missed if a good expression or micturating urethrogram is obtained (Fig. 63) but it is very easy to overlook the valves on urethroscopy since this part of the urethra is seldom inspected with care.

The valve is easily displayed by urethrotomy, and may be cut away. Since there is some danger of its re-formation, sounds should be passed periodically for some months, or an operation similar to that described for urethral stricture by JOHANSON may be undertaken.

5. Hypertrophy of the verumontanum and other rare obstructions

It has already been noted that in the presence of obstructing posterior urethral valves and in urethral fibro-elastosis the verumontanum is hypertrophied.

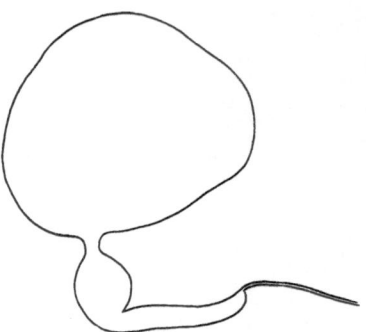

BUGBEE, and subsequently other authors, BALDRIDGE, EMMETT, PILCHER and PRICE, have also described hypertrophy as the primary cause for obstruction in young infants. The aetiology of this enlargement is unknown. In most respects these cases have resembled cases of urethral valves and treatment has consisted in diathermy reduction or resection of the verumontanum. It must be recognised, however, that the verumontanum is a somewhat variable structure, and its exact size is hard to estimate urethroscopically; it may be suspected that in some reported cases valves or other obstructive lesions have been overlooked.

Fig. 63. Anterior urethral valve. Tracing from urethrogram in a boy aged 4 years suffering from difficult micturition and incontinence. Urethroscopy and subsequently urethrotomy demonstrated a crescentic fold at the level of the obstruction

Polypoid masses of muscle tissue are occasionally encountered in the posterior urethra, and may be obstructive (NESBIT and RAPER).

In a few cases with evident back pressure effects on the upper urethra, it must be admitted that no cause of obstruction can be found. The case illustrated

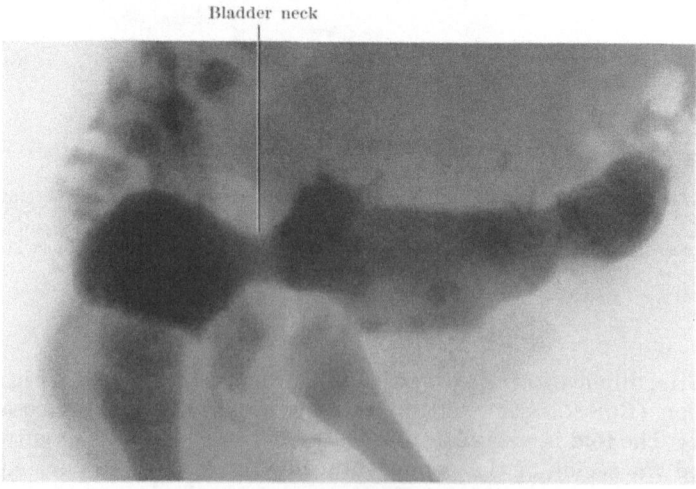

Bladder neck

Fig. 64. Urethral obstruction of unknown origin. Cystogram in a boy aged one week with chronic retention of urine. The bladder is trabeculated and there is an enormous dilatation of the posterior urethra, which fills the entire bony pelvis. No valve or other organic obstruction could be found on urethroscopy or at operation. Died of uraemia aged 6 months

in Fig. 64 showed an enormous dilatation of the prostatic urethra, with hypertrophy of muscle and elastic tissue in its wall, but no cause was discernible at urethroscopy, at open operation, or later at post-mortem dissection.

VI. Urethral diverticula and duplications

1. Congenital urethral diverticula

Congenital diverticula of the anterior urethra are an uncommon but important cause of chronic urinary obstruction in male children, and although they are sometimes associated with severe ante-natal destruction of the kidneys (e.g. TERNOVSKY), many cases are easily and satisfactorily corrected by operation. The diverticula most often occur in the region of the bulb of the urethra; the orifice is comparatively narrow, and the sac is elongated, lying alongside and compressing the normal channel. It often has the appearance of an abortive

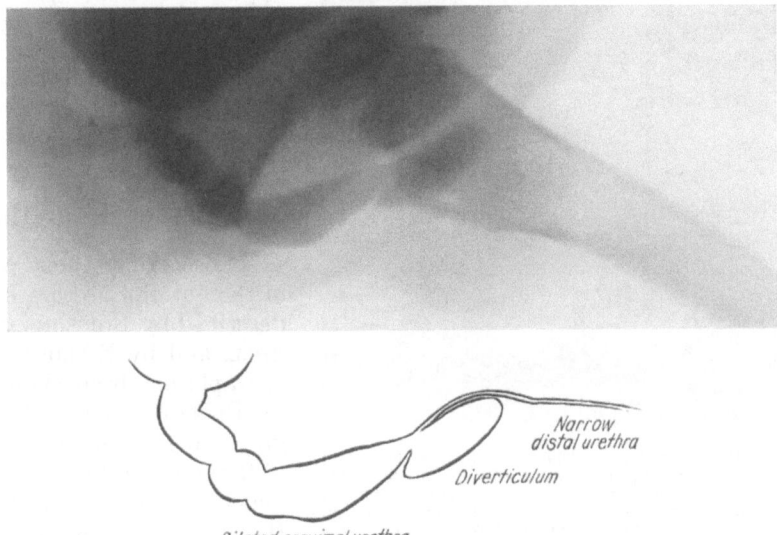

Fig. 65. Urethral diverticulum. Expression urethrogram in a boy aged 2 years with chronic retention of urine. An elongated diverticulum opened from the bulb of the urethra, and compressed the normal channel. Recovery after excision

duplication, and is clearly a congenital malformation rather than a herniation consequent upon a distal urinary obstruction. The sac is distended with each act of micturition, and its enlargement increases the pressure upon the urethra. In the case reported by FORSHALL and RICKHAM the distension was evident clinically, as a swelling in the perineum, but most of the cases of bulbar diverticulum have been discovered only on endoscopy or radiography (Fig. 65) (e.g. GROSS and BILL), a fact which emphasizes the great importance of a complete investigation in cases of chronic retention of urine. The opening may be found only with some difficulty on urethroscopy, but micturating or expression urethrograms will give a clear picture of the condition. Excision of the diverticulum gives excellent results.

A less common form of diverticulum occurs in the penile urethra (Fig. 66), the orifice is so wide that on dissection it is difficult to identify any neck to the sac. This type presents as an obvious enlargement of the penis, and can be outlined by an injection urethrogram. There may be an accompanying meatal stenosis, but it seems likely that the diverticulum is due to incomplete development of the urethral wall rather than to obstruction, and the "megalo-urethra" described below may be simply a severe degree of the same defect.

An enlarged utriculus masculinus might be considered as a urethral diverticulum, and occurs in the intersex group (Section P III). Utricular cysts in the
normal male have been found chiefly in adults (LANDES and RANSOM): MCKENNA
and KIEFER have, however, recorded a case of a boy aged 3 years suffering from
retention of urine and fistulae in the groin as a result of an infected utricular
cyst, while cysts arising in Cowper's glands and causing obstruction have been
described by HOWELL et al. and
by MCKENZIE.

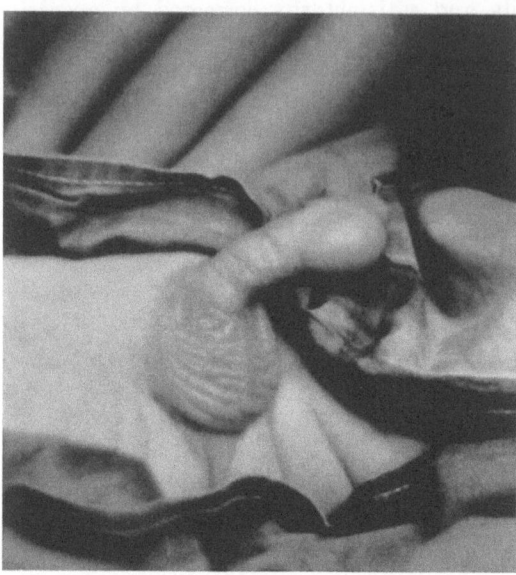

Fig. 66. Urethral diverticulum. The penis during expression of
urine in a boy aged 13 days. The swelling is due to a wide
necked diverticulum of the penile urethra. There was advanced
hydronephrosis, and the blood urea was 110 mgm/100 ml on
admimission: the boy died of uraemia one month after operation

True urethral diverticula in
the female, although sometimes
regarded as congenital, do not
appear to have presented in
childhood. JOHNSON mentions a
cyst in the vagina of a neonate
in discussing urethral diverticula,
but the description of his case
suggests a hydrocolpos.

2. Megalo-urethra

Cases of enormous dilatation
of the anterior urethra have been
described by BOISSONNAT, CAMP-
BELL, and by NESBIT: a further
example has been shown to me
by ELLISON NASH. The penis is
grotesquely enlarged, reaching
well below the knees, it is flabby
and urine can squeezed from it;
the skin is extremely redundant
and the glans entirely hidden. In
NESBIT's case, the corpora cavernosa were present and the deformity seemed
to be an exaggeration of the condition in which a diverticulum is formed
by a defect of the urethral wall (Fig. 66), but in other cases the corpora were
absent, and the penis was simply a bag of urine.

3. Duplications of the urethra

A double urethra is found in complete duplication of the bladder (p. 67)
and in some examples of double penis (p. 239); the malformation may also
occur in less obvious circumstances, and since it may not interfere with normal
function, it is liable to be overlooked. The subject has been ably reviewed by
BOISSONNAT.

The accessory urethra may lie dorsal to the corpora cavernosa, and open on
the dorsum of the penis or on the glans through a broad slit-like orifice somewhat
resembling the meatus in epispadias. If such a urethra is incomplete and uninfected
it will cause no serious symptoms, but where it continues through to the bladder
it may be responsible for dribbling incontinence (GROSS and MOORE). Excision
is a simple matter and curative.

Where the accessory channel is placed between or ventral to the corpora
cavernosa, it may open into the normal urethra either proximally or distally, it
may be blind at one end, or it may terminate on the glans. In hypospadias, an

accessory channel lying dorsal to the normal is comparatively common, but seldom reaches further back than the perineal membrane. Symptoms may be entirely absent, but chronic infection will lead to a peristent discharge, and occasionally there is an obstruction at the junction of the normal and accessory channel, causing chronic retention of urine (HIGGINS, WILLIAMS and NASH). It is often sufficient to lay the two channels open into one another.

Duplication of the membranous urethra alone, causing fatal urinary obstruction has been described by LIBAN. An accessory urethra lying ventral to the normal channel, extending into the perineum and up into the region of seminal vesicles, causing a perineal abscess in a boy of 2 years is reported by RINKER.

Complete double urethra may be a cause of urinary incontinence in the female (MASON-BROWN, DE NICOLA and McCARTNEY), the accessory urethra usually lying behind the normal, and opening on or behind the trigone. Excision of such a urethra is usually required but it may be possible to obliterate it by the injection of sclerosing solutions.

VII. Malformations associated with absent abdominal muscles

1. Definition

There is an interesting and by no means rare syndrome in which congenital absence of the abdominal muscles is associated with malformations of the urinary tract. The disorder affects males almost exclusively: only three females with absent muscles are recorded, and in these the findings were not typical, nor was the urinary tract abnormal (SILVERMAN and HUANG, DE BORD).

The muscular deficiency involves the lower part of the recti, and the lower and medial part of the oblique muscles; sometimes a thin fibrous sheet is found, or even a thin, lax muscular layer, but often there is nothing but fat between the skin and peritoneum. The skin itself is often wrinkled and lies in redundant folds as if it had been stretched, but it seems more closely attached to the fatty layer than in a normal infant (Fig. 67).

In the older, and less severely affected children, this wrinkling is not so marked, but on standing the laxity of the abdominal wall gives them a pot bellied appearance. The umbilicus is often flattened but otherwise normal, and the condition must be distinguished from exomphalos. Bilateral cryptorchidism is a constant finding.

2. Urinary tract pathology

Several surveys of the literature have been published in recent years (MAUER, MEYER, SILVERMAN and HUANG, EAGLE and BARRETT) and reference should be made to these for a full bibliography: it is clear that some malformation of the urinary tract is to be expected in all cases, though its exact nature is inconstant. My own experience of eight cases suggests however, that there is a characteristic disorder of the bladder not found in other conditions. The bladder remains attached at its apex to the umbilicus and may occasionally form a fistula or a diverticulum there; the bladder capacity is usually very large and the detrusor muscle is somewhat thickened, although trabeculation is usually mild or absent. Residual urine is present in some cases, yet in others complete emptying occurs despite the large capacity. The trigone frequently covers a considerable area so that the ureteric orifices appear to be far back on the lateral wall. There is sometimes a tapering dilatation of the posterior urethra as shown in the micturating cystogram (Fig. 68) but no gross abnormality is seen on urethroscopy. The ureters are almost always enormously dilated and tortuous, sometimes but not invariably with vesico-ureteric reflux; one of my cases had normal ureters, however, despite a characteristic bladder disorder. In another there was a ring-like obstruction at the lower end of each ureter as well as the large bladder. Complete obliteration of the urethra with imperforate anus was present in one instance and

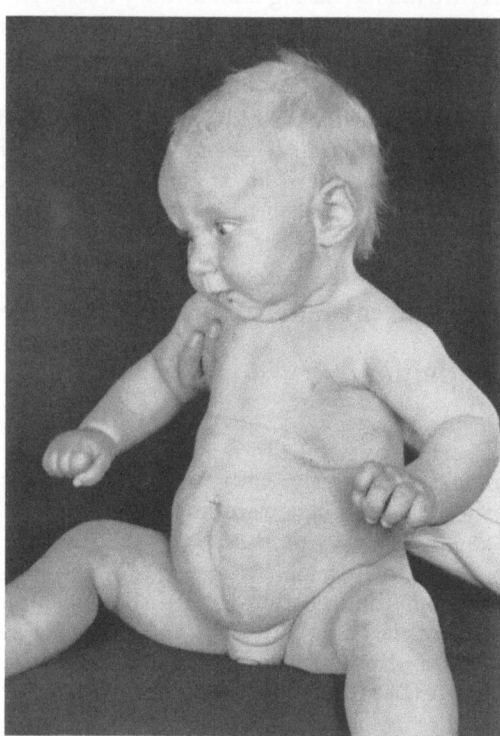

another is recorded in the literature. JAMESON and COOPER have recorded a case in which the ureter from a solitary kidney ended in the seminal vesicle and drained from there into the posterior urethra. It was dilated but there was no evident bladder disorder.

Many hypotheses have been put forward to explain this curious syndrome, though none is satisfactory. Considering the urinary tract alone, the diagnosis of bladder neck obstruction has sometimes been made, while HENLEY and HYMAN, on the basis of microscopy of a few isolated segments, have stated that these bladders are "aganglionic" (see p. 58). In order to connect the absent abdominal muscles with the urinary tract anomalies, it has been suggested that the abdominal muscles atrophy in utero as a result of pressure by the distended bladder. The localisation of the defect appears to support this view but many other children are born with distended bladders, having normal abdominal walls. The converse

Fig. 67. Absent abdominal muscles. Boy aged 6 months. Intravenous pyelograms showed moderate bilateral hydroureter: the bladder was trabeculated but emptied without residuum

hypothesis that a lack of support leads to urinary tract changes seems equally untenable since greater weakness is present in other diseases without any effect on the bladder. My own experience suggests that the typical bladder disorder of this syndrome cannot be interpreted as a simple obstructive phenomenon and that the abnormality of the abdominal muscles is an associated defect of development rather than a cause or consequence.

3. Clinical picture

The appearance and feel of the abdominal wall are unmistakable, and should always indicate the need for urological examination. Some of the children have an imperforate urethra and such advanced renal damage that death during the first days is inevitable; others present with signs of renal failure, or with recurrent urinary infection during infancy. The majority of recorded cases have died from uraemia before reaching adult life, but active treatment of infections is now salvaging a higher proportion. The abdominal laxity itself produces surprisingly little disability and is adequately controlled by a belt.

4. Treatment

The management will depend upon the exact findings of a full urological investigation, and no hard and fast rules can be laid down. In a few cases there

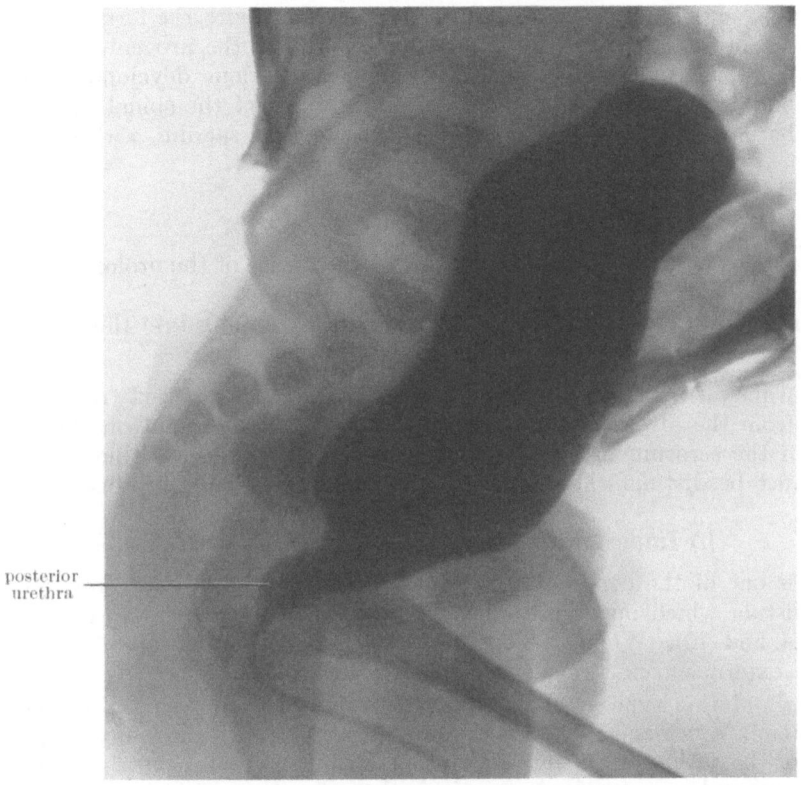

posterior
urethra

Fig. 68. Absent abdominal muscles. Expression cystogram in a boy aged 5 months, with urinary infection and rising blood urea. The bladder was chronically distended, but there was no trabeculation and the posterior urethra shows only a slight tapering dilatation. At the apex of the bladder was attached to the umbilicus. The ureters were also obstructed at their lower ends by diaphragms

may be an indication for operation on obstructed or ectopic ureters, but in the majority treatment must aim at control of infection by chemotherapy and at assisting the emptying of the bladder. DAUT et al. and GREENE et al. have reported considerable improvement following bladder neck resection, though others have not been so fortunate (HENLEY and HYMAN). One of my cases was improved after instrumental dilatation of the posterior urethra, and has remained under control for four years. Orchidopexy may be required.

VIII. Malformations associated with anal atresia: persistent cloaca

The imperforate and ectopic anus is a common problem confronting the paediatric surgeon, and it cannot yet be claimed that the difficulties involved in the restoration of bowel function have been altogether overcome. However, with improvements in technique and the survival of the great majority of these cases, it has become evident that urinary tract abnormalities are frequent and often of importance. This section is only concerned with the urological side of the problem and reference must be made to other works (e.g. LADD and GROSS) for a general discussion.

Anal and rectal atresia result from an early deviation from the normal development, perhaps from an extension of the process of degeneration of the tail gut in the 5—6 mm embryo. This deviation interferes with the formation of the uro-rectal septum, so that a fistulous connection with the urogenital tract is a common complication, and there is apt to be anomalous development of the ureteric buds. Moreover, the atretic process may affect the spinal segments as well as the bowel, resulting in a partial agenesis of the sacrum, with or without neurological disturbance.

1. In the male

Three types of malformation may come to the notice of the urologist.

a) Imperforate anus with a perineal fistula extending into the scrotal or penile raphe

The urinary tract itself is normal, but a narrow epithelialized track extends forward from the atretic lower bowel, and opens at some point on the ventral surface of the scrotum or the penis. Meconium may be seen within this track, which must be distinguished from the rare forms of double urethra.

b) Imperforate anus with recto-urethral fistula

This is one of the commonest types in the male: the bowel terminates in a narrow fistula which opens into the urethra a little below the verumontanum (Fig. 69 A and 70). When the communication is wide, meconium may exude from the external urinary meatus soon after birth.

If cases of this type are treated by a simple incision into the bowel from the perineum, a urinary fistula will result. Urinary continence may be possible because of the action of the internal sphincter, but no rectal control is achieved in this way, and severe colonic inertia is the rule. If a colostomy is performed at birth, and no local operation is undertaken, the recto-urethral communication will remain, and two serious complications are common. There may be a recurrent severe urinary infection usually with chronic pyelonephritis and ultimately renal failure, or a steady leak of urine into the bowel, where urinary salts are laid down in the inspissated masses of faeces, forming "calculi" which may require to be broken up digitally before they can be washed out.

An early separation of the intestinal and urinary tract is therefore desirable, and after abdominal dissection, division of the fistulous tract followed by a "pull-through" of the bowel to form a perineal anus seems the best line of treatment. This operation can be carried out on the first or second day of life, and no colostomy is necessary in such cases. Cases seen later on, perhaps with an established urethro-perineal fistula, may also be treated in the same way by pulling down the mobilized rectum, for any attempt to repair the fistula by local dissection and closure in layers is doomed to failure.

At times, a recto-urethral fistula is associated with hypospadias, so that both bowel and urethra open through a short common channel in the perineum (YOUNG). The same principles of treatment are applicable, and the hypospadias is no more difficult to repair than any other, once the rectum has been brought out through a separate opening.

Children who have had imperforate anus with recto-urethral fistula, and have had a satisfactory restoration of bowel function, may suffer from urinary retention or incontinence. To some of these, the label "bladder neck obstruction" may

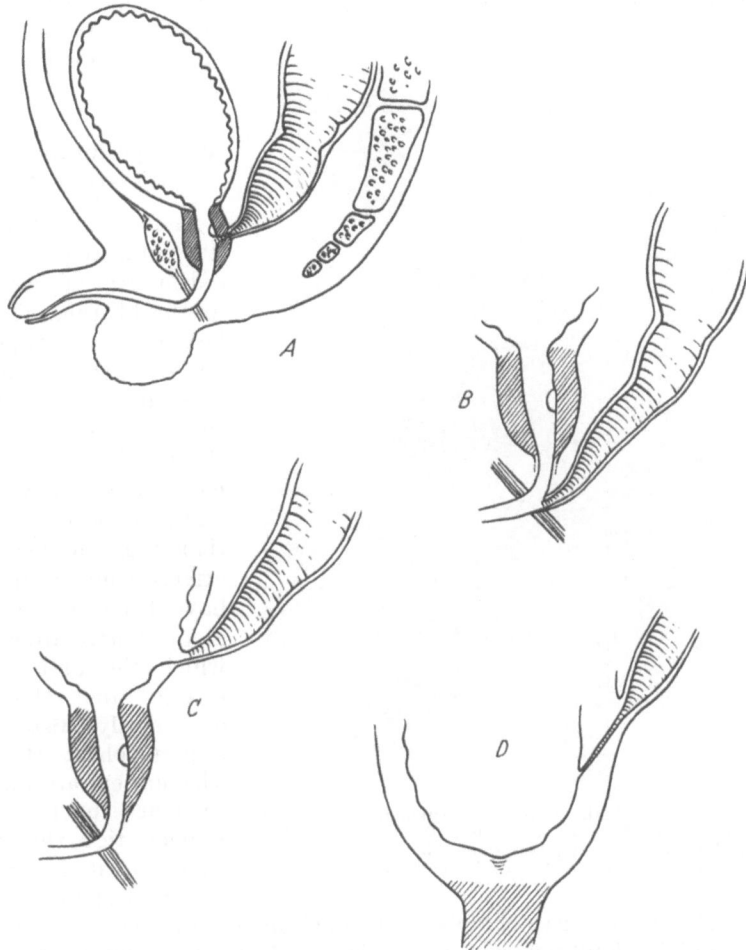

Fig. 69 A—D. Congenital recto-urinary fistulae in the male. Diagrams to show characteristic anatomy: A Common variety with recto-urethral fistula immediately below the verumontanum. B Low fistula, often associated with hypospadias. C Recto-vesical fistula. D Recto-vesical communication in hypertrophied bladder with urethral obliteration

be applied and, though the exact nature of the disorder remains unexplained, some improvement may be obtained by bladder neck resection (SPENCE). In two of my cases, the posterior urethra was unusually long, and the verumontanum was placed at the point where the urethra widened out to form the bladder, having cystoscopically something of the appearance of an enlarged prostatic middle lobe. In such a case, bladder neck resection is impracticable, but an anterior Y-V plasty may be performed and has been of benefit. A neurological lesion may account for some of the cases of incontinence: it may be congenital or acquired. The congenital variety is associated with partial agenesis of the sacrum; WILLIAMS and NIXON have shown that a short sacrum associated with six lumbar vertebrae is comparatively common in cases of imperforate anus, but if three or more pieces of the sacrum are missing altogether, some disorder of bladder function is likely. This type of neurogenic bladder does not differ from that seen with other congenital anomalies of the vertebral column, and is discussed in Section G. Acquired nervous lesions are due to operative trauma to the nervi erigentes: the evolution of the disorder is similar to that found after damage sustained during proctectomy for carcinoma of the rectum (WATSON and WILLIAMS).

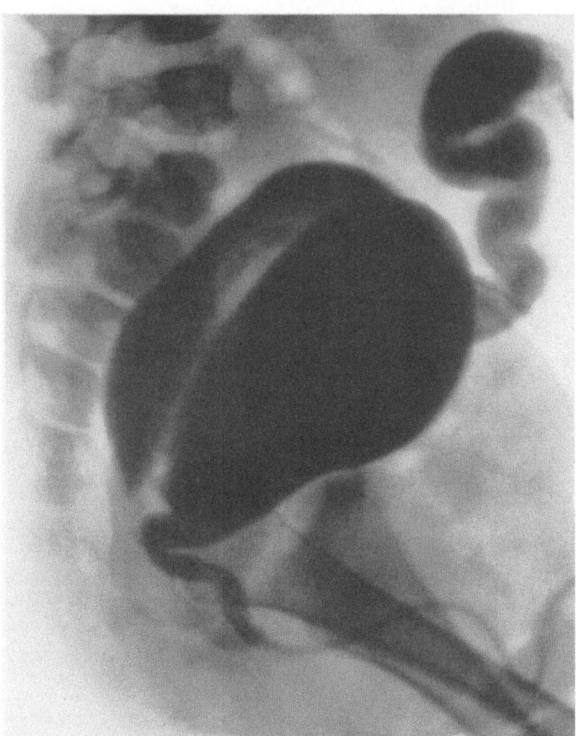

Fig. 70. Atresia ani urethralis. Cysto-urethrogram in a boy aged 2 years with imperforate anus, and a left iliac colostomy. The posterior urethra is drawn sharply backwards at the site of the fistula below the verumontanum, and the dye has entered the rectum

c) Imperforate anus with recto-vesical fistula

This form is rare, though it is not infrequently diagnosed in error in cases of recto-urethral fistula. The opening lies upon the trigone (Fig. 69 C) and the manifestations of an uncomplicated case are similar to those described in the previous section. Treatment may follow the same lines. Associated malformations are, however, comparatively common: many cases have been recorded, dying at or shortly after birth, in which the urethra is also atretic and the bladder enormously distended and hypertrophied (Fig. 69 D). The ureters are dilated and tortuous, the kidneys often hypoplastic: the bowel is narrow at its lower end, and may be lost in the posterior bladder wall. These cases of "giant bladder" have been described in detail by ANDERS, and by KRÜGER, who reach the conclusion that the enormous size of the bladder is due to excessive growth and not to obstruction.

2. In the female

Anal stenosis with a bowel opening in the anterior perineum, or in the vestibule is the commonest deformity. Less often, the rectum opens into the vagina higher up, even in the posterior fornix. Uncomplicated cases of this type do not concern the urologist, but associated malformations may involve the urinary tract. Perhaps the simplest is that described by LOWSLEY, in which an apron of tissue covered over the recto-vaginal and urethral openings, so that a common cloacal cavity was found: the case responded readily to excision of the apron (Fig. 71 A).

A high recto-vaginal fistula may be associated with a large vesico-vaginal fistula, with or without a urethral atresia (Fig. 71 B). Both urine and faeces are thus discharged into the vagina, and severe colonic inertia with "megacolon" is usual. Restoration of bladder function in these is virtually impossible, and a cutaneous ureterostomy or ileo-ureterostomy is advisable.

Several cases are reported in which the urinary, genital, and intestinal tracts empty through a common channel, associated with gross hydrocolpos and hydrometra (Fig. 71 C). The latter presents as a considerable abdominal tumour

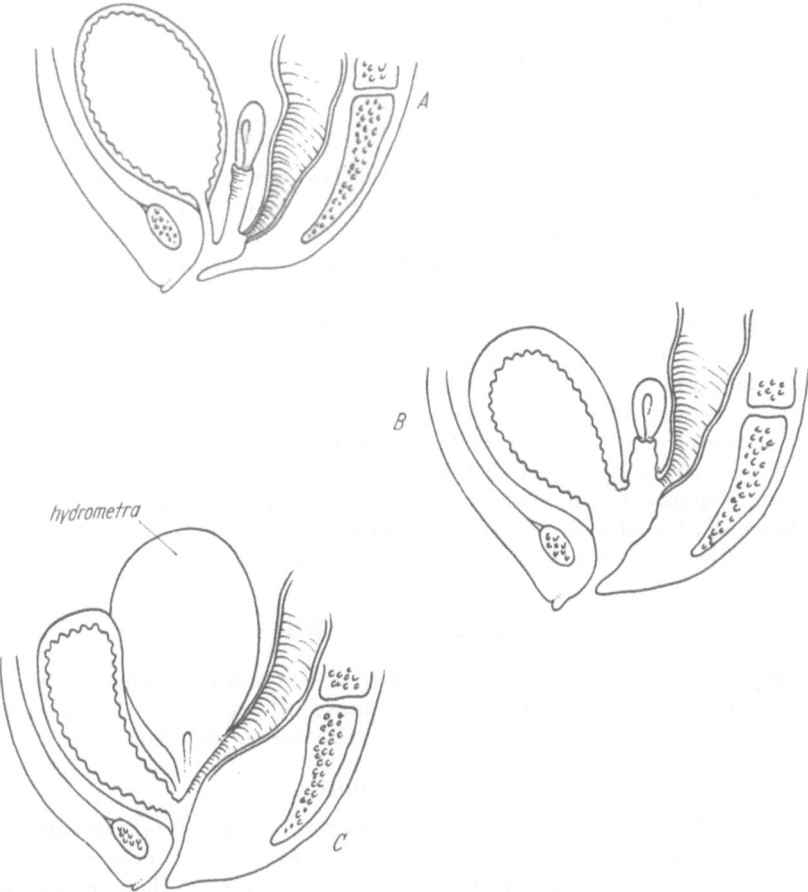

Fig. 71 A—C. Cloacal malformations in the female. Diagrams to show characteristic anatomy. A Covered vagina, with recto-vaginal fistula. B Recto-vaginal with vesico-vaginal fistula. C Cloacal duct with hydrometra

simulating a distended bladder, and in several cases vesical retention has also been present. Associated abnormalities of other organs have proved fatal in most of these cases (MILLER, NORDENFELT).

3. Complex malformations

The term persistent cloaca has been applied to many of the malformations already described, but there are also other unclassifiable cases in which all three tracts, urinary genital, and intestinal end in a common chamber. In these, separation of the pubes and epispadias may also be present or there may be a suggestion of an intersex condition (DE BUYS and CUMMINS, LYNCH and JERVEY). Imperforate anus is also a constant feature of the deformity described on p. 103 as ectopia cloacae.

4. Upper urinary tract anomalies

In all types of imperforate anus, from the simplest to the most complex, upper urinary tract anomalies are common. A high proportion have a solitary kidney (5 out of 15 in SPENCE's series) and a unilateral mega-ureter is a frequent complication. Ectopic, fused and malrotated kidneys may also occur. The relationship of these anomalies to the intestinal malformation is not clear, and they must be treated on their own merits.

IX. Ectopia vesicae and epispadias

Ectopia vesicae and epispadias are the two commonest representatives of a group of disorders characterized by incomplete fusion of the mesodermal elements making up the genital tubercle, anterior bladder wall and infra-umbilical abdominal wall. The embryological mechanisms involved are still not adequately explained: recent discussions of the problem have been published by WYBURN, and by PATTEN and BARRY. The area involved is normally formed at a very early stage by the insinuation of mesoderm from either side into that part of the cloacal membrane which lies adjacent to the umbilical stalk. Failure of this process leads to failure of symphysis of the pubic bones, to failure of complete union of the elements of the genital tubercle, and when the cloacal membrane ruptures, to a midline defect in the ventral wall of the urogenital sinus and its overlying abdominal wall. There is also a shortening of the distance between the umbilicus and the cloacal region: the former is drawn down towards the pelvic region, and the anus is pulled upwards and forwards.

1. Ectopia vesicae

Ectopia vesicae in its classical form is the most frequently encountered malformation. There is a male predominance which is variously as estimated 7 to 1 or 2 to 1, and in my own cases approximates to the latter figure.

a) Anatomy

In the male (Fig. 72) the bladder lies open and everted on the surface of the abdominal wall, and the urethra is represented only by a mucous groove on the dorsal surface of the penis. The bladder itself is smaller than normal and the mucosa, which is continuous round its edges with the skin, often shows squamous metaplasia in its upper part, while the lower part is reddened and polypoid. Irritation of the exposed surface leads to glandular metaplasia and the submucosa becomes considerably thickened so that inversion of the bladder to form a sac may be impossible. The muscular layer is poorly developed and it is continuous laterally with the margin of the rectus sheath. The ureteric orifices are easily identifiable and may be prolapsed. The bladder neck is scarcely recognizable, but the verumontanum is evident in the upper part of the urethral strip. The penis is short and sometimes minute but is comparatively broad: the corpora cavernosa are only loosely attached to one another and the crura are widely separated. The urethral strip is short, cutting the corner between the abdominal wall and the dorsum of the penis, which is therefore upturned. The glans is broad, and grooved dorsally in most cases, sometimes it is divided into two distinct portions. The frenum and penile raphe are normal, and the prepuce is a tuft of redundant skin on the ventral surface. The scrotum is flattened and imperfectly developed: failure of testicular descent is common. The anus lies closely behind the scrotum in the anterior perineum, so that it often faces forwards rather than backwards.

The pelvic ring is incomplete anteriorly and the pubic bones, although fairly well formed, are rotated outwards. The stability of the ring is maintained by a bar of fibro-muscular tissue which is incorporated in the base of the extroverted bladder. This bar doubtless incorporates the homologue of the external sphincter as well as the pubo-vesical ligaments, but its "skeletal" function prevents full muscular development. The rectus muscles are attached to the pubic tubercles and are therefore widely separated at their lower extremities: they are otherwise normal. The umbilical scar, which is low in the abdomen, is closely associated with the apex of the bladder in the majority of cases and a hernia is usually present. This hernia, however, protrudes through a defect in the linea alba, which is distinct from and a short distance above the bladder area. Inguinal herniae are common.

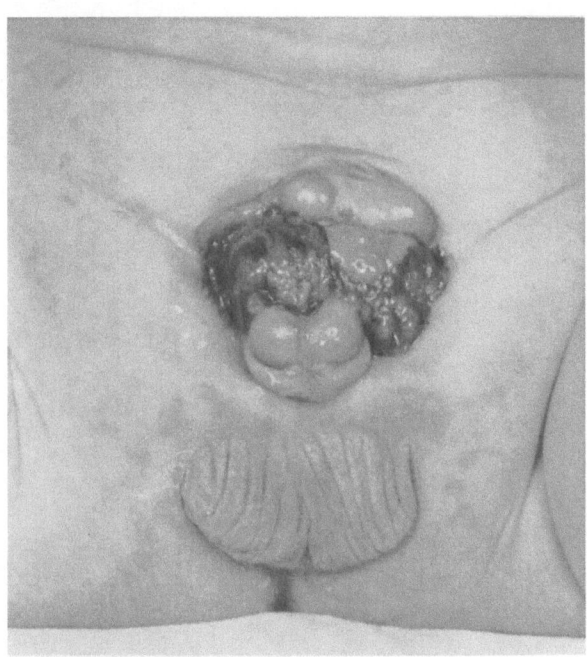

Fig. 72. Ectopia vesicae in the male. Boy aged 17 months

In the female (Fig. 73) the bladder is formed as in the male, but the urethral strip is extremely short. The vagina, uterus and Fallopian tubes are normal, but the vaginal orifice is narrow and lies immediately below the bladder, facing forwards. The clitoris is divided into two entirely separate bodies placed on either side of, and a little posterior to, the vaginal orifice. The anus is drawn forwards in the perineum.

In some rare variants a bridge of tissue may be found across the region of the bladder neck, beneath which a minute channel connects the extroverted bladder above to the urethral groove below. Such a cases was reported by THOMPSON, and I have observed a similar condition in one of DENIS BROWNE'S cases.

A bladder which is complete and continent, but lies immediately beneath the skin of the abdominal wall, pushing forward between separated pubic bones has also been described as a variant of the ectopic bladder by HEJTMANCIK et al., and by GRUBER. A "pubic" umbilicus with an incomplete pelvis but a normal bladder is another occasional finding. GAUDIN and CABOT described a pouting mass of transitional epithelium on the lower abdomen in a boy with a normal urinary tract: they believed that this represented a partial extrophy.

b) Clinical features

The continual discharge of urine on to the surface renders the life of the child with ectopia vesicae a burden to himself and to his parents. The condition is intolerable to most members of civilized communities and treatment is therefore demanded at an early age; as a consequence, opportunities for observing the progress uninfluenced by surgery are limited. MAYO stated that statistics showed that 50% of affected children died before their tenth year, and 66.67% before their twentieth: he gives no information of the source of these statistics, yet this estimate has been repeatedly quoted and regarded as the standard by which the efficacy of treatment should be judged. Observation of untreated children in their early years under modern conditions does not, however, suggest that the

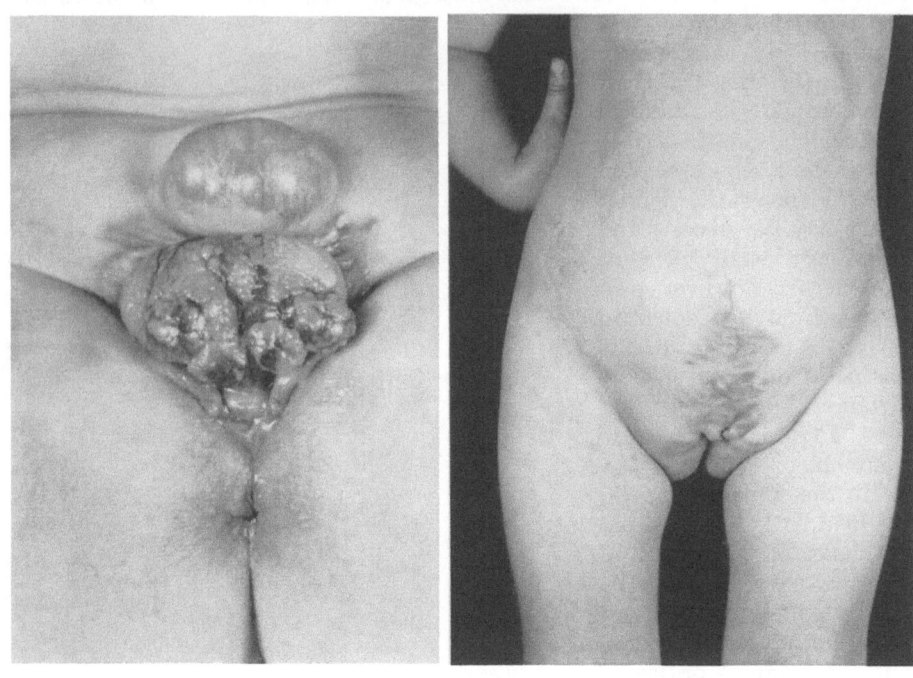

A   B

Fig. 73 A and B. Ectopia vesicae in the female. A at 8 months. B after reconstruction at 2½ years: child passing urine every hour but continent by day

mortality is anything like so high: although there is probably a greater liability to pyelonephritis, and the excoriated and septic condition of the genital area may lower the resistance to other infections, yet these children are far more likely to die of surgery than of any other cause. However, the improvement in the conditions of life rather than the prolongation of existence is the standard by which treatment should be judged.

The typical case of ectopic bladder is an irritable infant who resents interference with the bladder area, for the skin around is sodden and may even be ulcerated. The soreness is increased once the child has started to walk, which he does with a waddling broad-based gait, due in part to the external rotation of the acetubula and in part to an effort to minimize the rubbing of clothes upon the bladder. In later life, the lack of a pubic symphysis is curiously little handicap, and apart from some education in walking, no orthopaedic treatment is required.

Exposure produces in the bladder mucosa a glandular metaplasia, and in time there is a danger of malignant degeneration. McINTOSH and WORLEY find that the average age of onset of carcinoma is 44, the youngest recorded case being 21 years of age. The tumour is an adenocarcinoma with an extremely low rate of metastasis, so that death is almost always due to renal failure rather than to secondaries. There is no evidence to suggest that the reconstructed ectopic bladder is liable to this form of disease.

Ureteric dilatation is a later complication of most untreated cases, probably arising from infection and oedema of the ureteric orifice. It is unusual to see any severe degree during childhood, but on rare occasions an infant is born with a gross hydro-ureter for which a different etiology must be suspected.

Umbilical and inguinal herniae are common and may be troublesome, but rectal prolapse is often a more serious handicap. In some degree it affects most babies with ectopia vesicae, though many recover without assistance. In a few, however, the prolapse appears with the least effort, and although reducible, will recur immediately after reduction. Prolapse is often associated with an incomplete sphincteric control of the anus, doubtless a reflection of the general instability of the pelvic floor, and the widely separated anterior attachments of the levator ani. This weakness has serious consequences if uretero-sigmoidostomy has been performed. On rare occasions, the occurrence of a vaginal anus, or a stenosed perineal anus raises even greater difficulties.

c) Management

The immediate management of a child born with ectopia vesicae is concerned with the protection of the exposed bladder and surrounding skin. It is wise to give the parents a supply of tulle gras, in order to cover the mucosa, and a barrier cream to apply to the surrounding skin. For the first years napkins may be applied in the ordinary way, though plenty of boracic powder is useful for preventing ammonia dermatitis. Rectal prolapse should be reduced as soon as it occurs, and if it is very frequent an encircling subcutaneous catgut suture around the anus is often a help. This will not lead to permanent cure, but may retain the prolapse for long enough to enable the muscles to recover their tone.

With regard to the definitive treatment of ectopia vesicae, there are two basic alternatives, either an attempt must be made to reconstruct a functional bladder, or a cystectomy must be performed with diversion of urine. Reconstructive methods were the first to be given a trial, but fell into disrepute with the apparent success of uretero-sigmoidostomy. The recent recognition of the disadvantages of this operation, however, has led to a revival of interest in reconstruction and a variety of operations have been devised. The review given by Mayo in 1920 shows that almost all the methods now suggested had been tried out in the preceding half century, but it may well be that, as in other branches of surgery, recent advances in technique, in anaesthesia and in control of sepsis will bring to success many of the operations discarded long ago.

α) Reconstructive surgery

These operations are frequently disappointing, but Young, Michon, Sweetser, and Powell have all had successful cases: and in three of mine good but not perfect continence has been achieved. Almost all the successful cases have been girls, for although it might seem that there is very little material with which to form a sphincter, in the female the urethra is not held forward as it is on the penis, and a fuller restoration of normality is attainable. No standard operative technique can yet be recognized, and all surgeons experimenting with this work have made individual variations in each case: for reported details reference should be made to the original articles. My own method is first to isolate the bladder and urethral strip from the surrounding skin, and to mobilize completely the apex of the bladder. Then, keeping close to the bone, the attachments of the

7*

base of the bladder are freed from the pubes, and the tissue so mobilized is brought together in front of the rolled up urethra. The bladder itself is inverted and closed over a Malecot catheter. The transverse bar of rectus sheath and linea alba which lies beneath the umbilical hernia is then mobilized, drawn down and used to join the pubic tubercles. In the male, the urethral strip must be dissected away from the corpora cavernosa and buried between them as in the operation for epispadias. The skin is closed over the bladder by simple apposition or by swinging in flaps.

A saccular bladder is comparatively easy to construct except in those cases in which there is excessive thickening and polyp formation in the vesical mucosa. The difficulty lies in the attainment of continence, and secondary operations to tighten the bladder neck, or to support it by a sling, are often performed. If the bladder is muscular, a moderate degree of stricture may be sufficient substitute for a sphincter, but often the detrusor is poorly formed and contractions weak so that a residual urine is present, and stone formation is a common complication. Vesico-ureteral reflux is also seen in the reconstructed bladder, and where the urethra is narrow may lead to considerable ureteric dilatation. When a saccular bladder has been constructed, but no sphincteric action can be achieved, appliances may be used for the collection of urine in the male, or some form of mechanical device may be used to compress the new urethra, but no satisfactory method has yet been described.

With all its disadvantages and disappointments the reconstructive approach to the ectopic bladder still seems worth pursuing. Even if the urine is ultimately diverted into the bowel, the plastic operations which have reconstructed the abdominal wall will not be wasted. Moreover, these children are for the most part happier without the prolapsing mass of bladder mucosa, and if this is covered in during the first year of life, as is my present practice, urinary diversion may be comfortably postponed until the state of the rectal sphincter is ascertained beyond doubt.

β) Urinary diversion

For many years past, uretero-sigmoidostomy has been the standard method of treatment of ectopia vesicae in Western Europe and America, and it is the only method for which any large series of adequately followed cases is available. In Eastern Europe MAYDL's operation, in which the mobilized and inverted trigone is implanted into the recto-sigmoid has been the more popular, and a recent modification of this has been suggested by GOODWIN and HUDSON which involves splitting the trigone and implanting the ureteric orifices separately into the bowel. The valvular nature of the ureteric orifice is not preserved, however, in most cases, and the MAYDL type of operation has therefore little, if any, advantage over a satisfactorily performed uretero-sigmoidostomy.

The short term results of transplantation are often extremely satisfactory, and the conversion of a wet and miserable child who shuns the company of his contemporaries into a contented one who enters into normal childish activities is a most gratifying experience. The literature is indeed replete with articles recording this satisfactory result, but the few long term studies (e.g. GARRETT and MERTZ, HARVARD and THOMPSON, WILLIAMS and JOLLY, SANDERUD) give a less encouraging view. The biochemical disturbances characteristic of uretero-sigmoidostomy, hyperchloraemic acidosis and hypokaliemia, are well known and need not be described here: theoretically they should be controllable by regular alkali therapy and replacement of potassium. Unfortunately parents are not always willing to undertake a regular attendance at hospital, and in the circumstances of adolescence and starting work, the need for medical supervision is often overlooked and acute biochemical imbalance may occur, or a long-standing mild acidosis lead to bone changes.

The danger of recurring pyelonephritis is always present after uretero-colic anastomosis, and although antibiotics may cut short acute attacks, they have not influenced the development of a chronic pyelonephritic lesion. As a result the renal function of these cases is almost always below normal, and it is ultimately responsible for the death of many. It appears that approximately one third of cases will be dead before they reach adult life, while many of the survivors are undergrown and in poor health. A thirst is always present and may impair the ability to take food.

One further disadvantage of uretero-sigmoidostomy in ectopia vesicae is the weakness of the anal sphincter. A great many of these children do not achieve proper control of the urine in the bowel; they are not continually wet but strains and stresses are apt to produce incontinence, and wetting at night is particularly common. While this wetness is by no means as severe as before operation, yet because the urine is mixed with faeces it is a serious handicap. However, the presence of nocturnal incontinence is often a protection against the development of biochemical upsets.

Thus although uretero-sigmoidostomy always produces an improvement in the child's condition, it is an operation which has many disadvantages, and a search for a better alternative continues. The separation of urinary and faecal streams is undoubtedly some improvement, and a de-functioning colostomy above the uretero-sigmoidostomy has been advocated by some, or the reconstructed bladder may be given an opening into the rectum. The weakness of the anal sphincter is, however, a disadvantage in these cases as in the simple uretero-sigmoidostomy though preservation of renal function is likely to be better. In recent years the cutaneous ileo-ureterostomy has gained some popularity and has been advocated for cases of ectopia vesicae. This operation is undoubtedly followed by good preservation of renal function, and ureteric dilatation which has been present pre-operatively may be reduced. However, it too has its disadvantages: first of all there are sometimes difficulties with the management of the loop itself, and it involves the use of an external appliance which is abhorrent to many parents. It is obviously only suitable for intelligent patients who live in civilised countries where replacement of the bag and its accessories is easy. For the management of ectopia vesicae with incompetence of the rectal sphincter it is probably the best operation yet devised. It should not, however, be performed before the age of 3 or 4 years unless there is a severe degree of ureteric dilatation, because the bag is difficult to manage in toddlers and incontinence in the younger age group is easily managed by napkins.

Simple cutaneous ureterostomy is a much less serious operation than any procedure incorporating an isolated segment of ileum, but it leaves the child with two urinary fistulae, both of which are apt to undergo stenosis. In the infant with serious ureteric dilatation this procedure is valuable and the calibre and tortuosity of the ureters make it easier to perform satisfactorily.

After urinary diversion, a plastic operation is required for the abdominal wall. Where the bladder is small, it may be completely excised, but removal of a large bladder will leave a serious gap in the abdominal wall: it is therefore preferable only to excise the mucosa, and to plicate the muscle layer (HEPBURN). Skin cover should be obtained by rotating inwards broad-based lateral flaps. The urethra should be formed into a tube as in the operation for epispadias, so that there is a channel for semen. The penis although small in children usually develops into a serviceable organ.

2. Epispadias

a) Anatomy

The midline defect is of a lesser degree than in ectopia vesicae, and a saccular bladder is formed beneath an intact abdominal wall. The pubic bones are not united in a symphysis, but a gap of variable extent is bridged by a bar of fibrous tissue lying immediately in front of the bladder neck: in contrast with true ectopia therefore the trigone and posterior urethral wall are not involved in the fibrous "skeletal" structure, and a better development of normal muscular function is permitted. A complete bladder neck is unusual, however, and normal continence is seldom achieved without treatment.

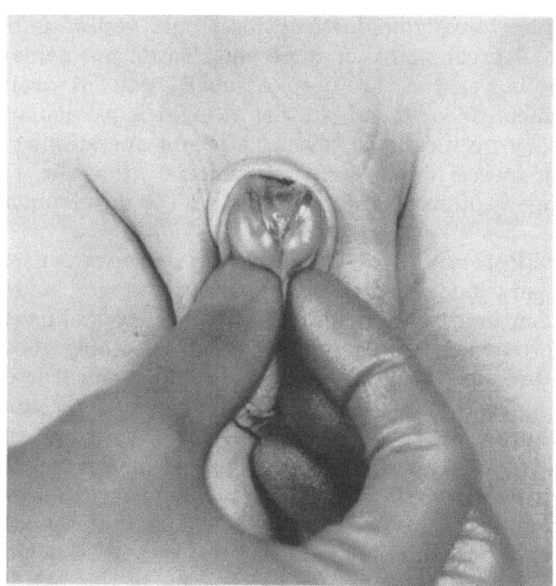

Fig. 74. Epispadias in the male. Boy aged 4 years with complete incontinence

The urethra in the male is a broad but short and straight mucosal strip lying open on the dorsal surface of the corpora cavernosa and disappearing through a broad arch at the base of the penis (Fig. 74). Except in the mildest cases, retraction of this arch brings the verumontanum into view, and beyond this the relaxed bladder neck may be seen. As in ectopia vesicae, the corpora are not attached to one another, and the glans may be bifid. The prepuce is usually represented by a mass of redundant skin on the ventral surface, though in exceptional cases a complete prepuce may be formed.

In the female, the urethra is short and wide: it has characteristically the appearance of a transverse slit, from which a broad strip of mucosa extends forwards to the flattened mons veneris (Fig. 75). The clitoris is divided into two separate bodies lying lateral to and a little behind the urethral opening. The vagina is normal.

b) Clinical features

In mild cases in both sexes, micturition and continence may be normal: the external deformity is then the sole complaint in the male, and in the female the abnormality is likely to pass unnoticed. These cases are exceptional, however, and the great majority have some degree of incontinence, most often a complete lack of control in the standing position although urine may accumulate in the relaxed bladder during recumbency. The severity of the incontinence is not always appreciated by the parents during the first two years of life, and it is wise to be guarded in prognosis. The diagnosis is evident from simple inspection, though it is surprising how frequently the deformity is overlooked in the female.

c) Treatment

Reconstructive surgery, which is of doubtful value in ectopia vesicae, has an encouraging record in epispadias. The repair must aim primarily at the bladder neck, on which continence depends, rather than at the external deformity, and it is important that the first operation, which in the absence of scar tissue has the best chance of success, should be thoroughly and carefully performed. It is wise to postpone this operation until the child is at least three or four years old, when an accurate assessment of the degree of spontaneous control has been made.

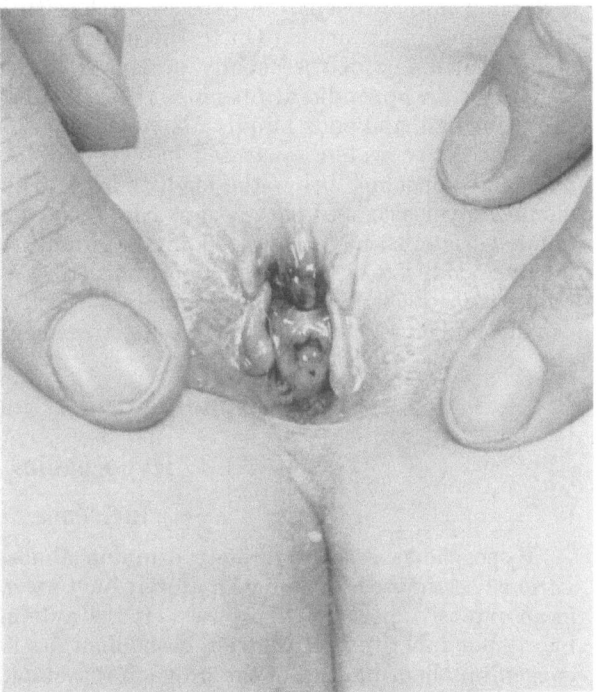

Fig. 75. Epispadias in the female. The external genitalia of a girl aged 4 years with complete incontinence

The essential steps in the operation (see CAMPBELL, DEES) are mobilization of the bladder neck region, which is exposed through a vertical incision severing the fibrous tissue connecting the pubic bones, excision of redundant mucosa at this level, and wrapping round the bladder neck the muscular tissue which lies lateral to it. In the male the urethral strip should be freed from the two corpora cavernosa, and pushed back between them to regain its normal position. In the female (see DAVIS), a similar a operation may be performed, but a sling procedure is often more successful in my experience.

3. Ectopia cloacae

In this rare, but curiously constant, malformation (Fig. 76) the ectopic bladder

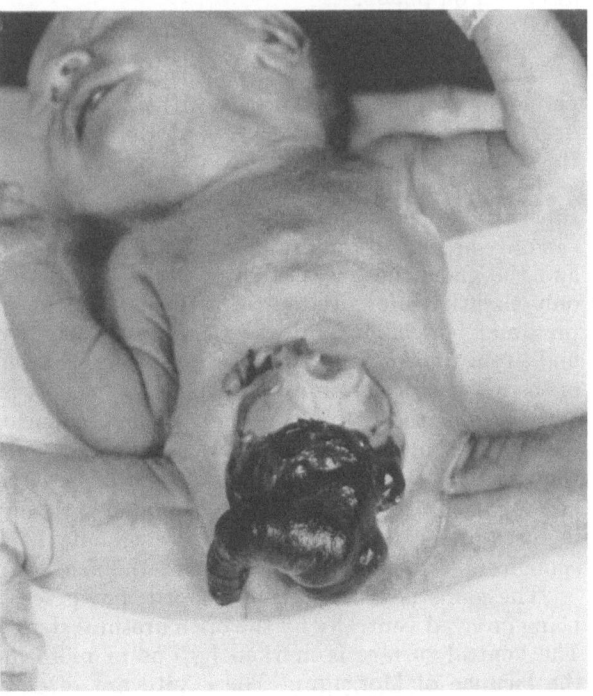

Fig. 76. Ectopia cloacae. Infant aged 1 day. The prolapsing structure is the intussuscepted terminal ileum. An everted bladder area was present on either side of the bowel area. The anus was imperforate

is divided into two separate patches, each with its ureter, between which is an area of intestinal mucosa. On to the upper part of the intestinal area opens the terminal ileum, which is usually prolapsed; on the lower part is a colonic, and sometimes an appendiceal opening, the latter being often double. The colon is short, median, and ends blindly above an imperforate anus. The penis or clitoris consists of two widely separated halves, and the vasa deferentia or Müllerian ducts have openings below the bladder area. There is frequently a concomitant meningomyelocele, and paraplegia. Numerous descriptions of this anomaly, with minor variations, have appeared in the literature, and the works of BRAKELEY, DAVIES, McFARLAND, RUSSELL, HALL et al., may be consulted for a full bibliography. Once seen the anomaly is easily recognized, and although not usually fatal for some days or weeks, treatment is probably better withheld.

X. Hypospadias and allied disorders

1. Hypospadias

a) Incidence

Hypospadias is an extremely common abnormality: its frequency has been variously estimated for clinical material, but CAMPBELL found an incidence of 1:620 in an extensive post-mortem series. It has a definite tendency to run in families, but is not inherited on a strict Mendelian basis. It often accompanies other congenital abnormalities of the urogenital system, and is an integral part of most intersex states, when it represents feminization of the male, or virilization of the female. The so-called female hypospadias is, however, an unrelated condition discussed on p. 268.

b) Anatomy

The basic deformity in hypospadias is the termination of the urethra in the perineum or the ventral surface of the penis at some point proximal to its normal opening. The commonest site is at the coronal sulcus, more severe degrees are the penile, penoscrotal and perineal types.

The meatus itself is often narrow, particularly in coronal hypospadias, though superficial appearances are sometimes deceptive, and the true size of the opening can only be judged by picking up the skin behind it. Between the urethral meatus and the glans there is a strip of mucosa similar to that covering the glans and only slightly differentiated from the skin of the penis, but moist and pink in its proximal portion in perineal cases. Beneath this strip, adherent both to skin and to the underlying corpora cavernosa is a fibrous band, which unites the region of the meatus to the glans, and which being short and inelastic maintains a ventral curvature of the penis (chordee) which becomes very marked on erection. The urethra behind the meatus may be entirely normal, but it is sometimes short so that it is also responsible for chordee: this is particularly the case where chordee accompanies a coronal hypospadias. Some webbing of the skin may also be present in these cases. At times the distal extremity of the urethra is devoid of corpus spongiosum, and lies closely beneath the skin.

The glans penis is well developed, but gives a slightly unrolled appearance, being grooved ventrally by the open urethral strip, and tipped slightly downwards. The ventral surface is marked by one or more blind pits (Fig. 77), representing the lacunae of Morgagni. These pits are often stated to be at the site of the normal external meatus, but this is very rare in my experience, they are commonly proximal to that side, and lead into short ducts lying dorsal to the urethra itself in cases of coronal hypospadias.. Rarely one of these ducts is sufficiently long, reaching well down the penis, to suggest a partial duplication of the urethra.

The prepuce is incomplete in the ventral midline, so that when the preputial adhesions separate and it becomes free of the glans, it retracts to form a "hood" of redundant skin on the dorsum. In a rare variant of coronal hypospadias, the prepuce is complete save for the absence of the frenum, and the urethral meatus has the appearance of a cleft, as if a meatotomy had been performed.

The scrotum is normal in coronal and penile hypospadias, but bifid in the perineal variety (Fig. 78), the two halves being separated by the mucosal strip of urethra. The median raphe extends as far forward as the urethral meatus, though in the coronal and penile types, it is often curiously eccentric.

The more severe degrees of hypospadias border on the condition of male intersexuality, and there is in fact no recognized dividing line between the two. Confusion in diagnosis arises when the penis is very small, when the testicles are undescended and when a vaginal canal is present. HOWARD has pointed out that an enlarged utriculus masculinus, opening on the verumontanum, will be found in many cases of hypospadias; this is of little importance in treatment, but my own experience suggests that a vaginal canal opening into the urethra

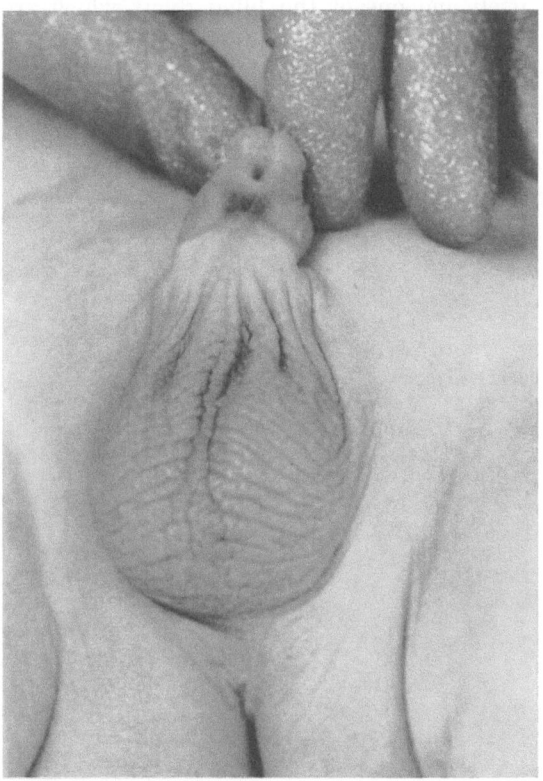

Fig. 77. Hypospadias. The external genitalia of a boy of 2 years, showing a well marked blind pit distal to the urethral meatus

at the level of the perineal membrane is more common and secretions accumulating in it may lead to difficulties in repair.

c) Symptoms

Difficult micturition, a poor stream, and ultimately some incontinence result from meatal stenosis, most marked in coronal hypospadias. Failure to pass urine in the new born due to blockage of such a stenosed opening by epithelial debris is also relatively common.

Difficulty in directing the urinary stream with some tendency to spraying is frequent complaint, it necessitates micturition in the sitting position in perineal hypospadias, though in the coronal variety it is not often a serious disability, nor one which precludes the normal standing position. It leads, however, to a certain amount of embarrassment to small boys.

Difficulty in sexual intercourse will only arise in cases with chordee, and the proximal site of the external meatus is no handicap. In severe cases, difficulties

may arise in the diagnosis of the sex of the infant: this aspect is discussed in
Section P V.

d) Treatment

Meatal stenosis requires a meatotomy, and this operation should be performed
as soon as the condition is recognized. The orifice may often be enlarged without
bringing it to a more proximal position by cutting the septum between the urethra
itself and one of the blind ducts which are so often found lying dorsal to it

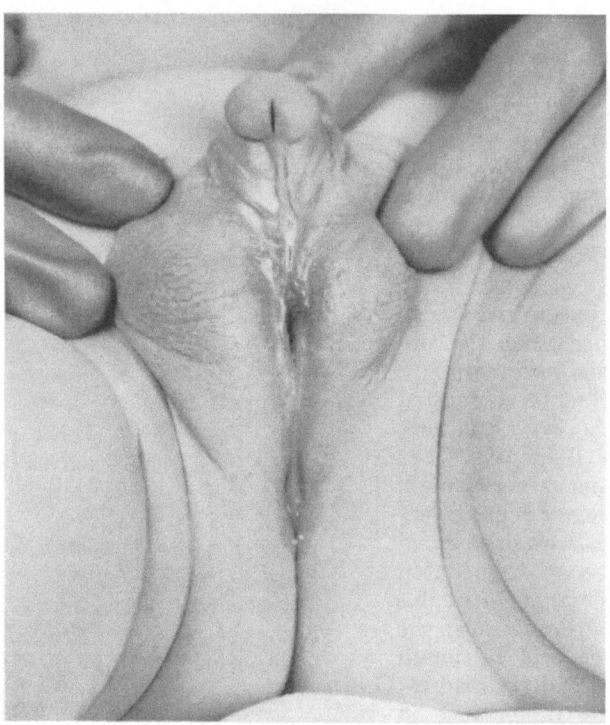

Fig. 78. Perineal hypospadias. The external genitalia in a boy aged 2 years: the penis shows well marked
chordee, and only the right testicle has descended into the scrotum. The opposite testicle was atrophic.
Normal verumontanum seen on urethroscopy

(BROWNE): no stitches are required, but a dilator should be passed for several
days postoperatively. This type of dorsally directed meatotomy often results
in a more easily directed urinary stream.

Coronal hypospadias with an adequate orifice and unaccompanied by chordee
does not require treatment. Operations for such minor degrees of the deformity
are sometimes demanded by parents and advised by paediatricians, largely because
it is believed that it will give rise to a sense of inferiority and to some handicap
in sexual intercourse, but observation of untreated adults lends no support of
those beliefs. Furthermore the results of operation in such cases are often disappointing.

When the urethral orifice is placed further back operation will always be
required in order to produce a manageable urinary stream, and a normal erection.
The two elements in correction must be treated separately, however, since it
is not possible to construct in one operation a straight penis and a full length
urethra. In the first stage, chordee should be corrected: the essential steps being
the excision of the fibrous band uniting the meatus to the glans, and allowing

the meatus to drop back as the penis straightens. The skin correction accompanying this manoeuvre may be accomplished by simple transverse incision behind the glans, which is sewn up longitudinally. The age at which the first operation is performed is not of great importance: it may perhaps allow fuller growth of the penis if it is undertaken early, and any time between second and fourth year seems suitable. It is, however, essential that full correction of chordee is attained before the urethra is reconstructed, and the first stage may require repetition.

Concerning the nature of the second stage of the repair, the completion of the urethral canal up to the tip of the penis, there has been great divergence of opinion, and very many operations have been devised. The details of technique are discussed in another volume of this series, and original descriptions of some of the more popular methods will be found in the works referred to in the bibliography below. It may be emphasized here, however, that it is desirable that the operation should require no further staging; and that it should be completed before the child goes to school (5 years of age in England). Since some co-operation is normally required of a child

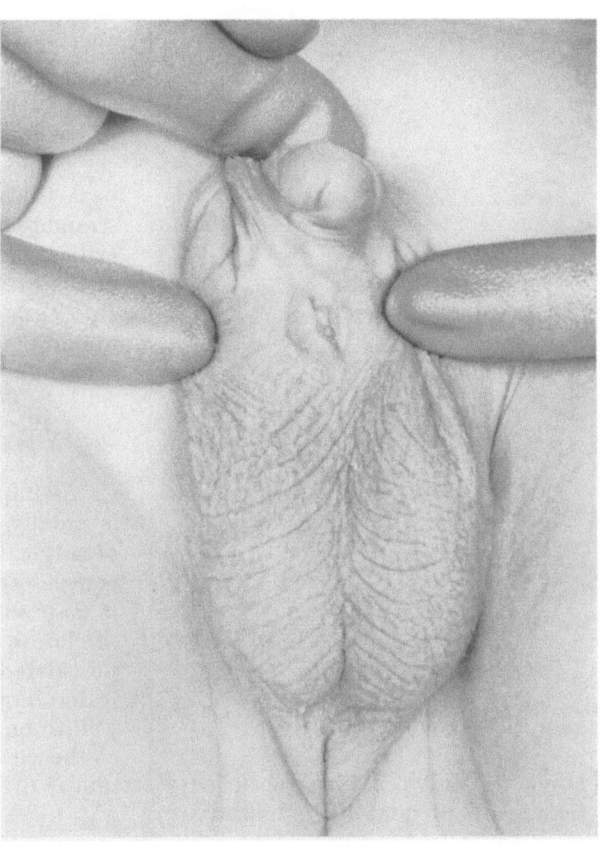

Fig. 79. Short urethra. The genitalia of a boy aged 2¹/₂ years with a severe chordee, but a normal urethral meatus. The urethra lies immediately beneath the skin of the penis, but the sinuses at the peno-scrotal junction do not communicate with it

for this plastic procedure, which necessitates a temporary diversion of urine, it is better to leave it until the child is at least $4^{1}/_{2}$ years old. The operation should not make use of free grafts which tend to form strictures at the site of junction with the original epithelium, and it should not make use of flaps of skin which are later liable to grow hair. The DENIS BROWNE method fulfils all these desiderata, and is suitable for all degrees of hypospadias: it is simple to perform, and has few complications. The OMBRÉDANNE method is simpler still, but applicable only to the minor degrees of the deformity. The CECIL operation is also in common use.

2. Short Urethra

Chordee due to apparent shortening of the urethra, a condition commonly associated with hypospadias, may sometimes be found in cases with a normal external urinary meatus. Often, however, the corpus spongiosum is deficient so that the urethra lies immediately beneath the skin of the penis. In the case illustrated in Fig. 79, there were short sinuses in the skin which did not communicate with the urethra. The diagnosis presents no difficulty, though the distinction must be made from simple webbing of the skin on the ventral surface of the penis.

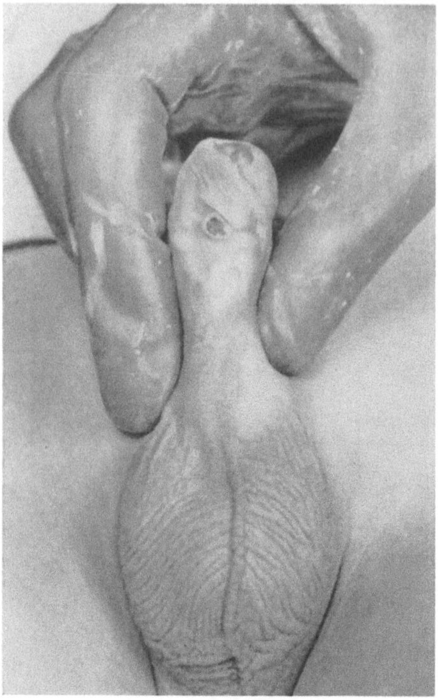

Operative repair should be postponed until later childhood. In the first stage the urethra should be severed in the penis, and the proximal end dissected off the corpora cavernosa, so that it drops back towards the perineum as the penis straightens out. A temporary hypospadiac orifice is established. Reconstruction of the urethra on the lines of the DENIS BROWNE operation for hypospadias is undertaken later when full healing has occurred.

Fig. 80. External urethral fistula (congenital). The penis of a boy aged 7 years

3. External urethral fistula

A simple urethral fistula in the penis is usually an acquired lesion, the result of surgical or accidental trauma. A rare congenital type is illustrated in Fig. 80: it may be noted that although a failure of closure of the urethral folds might be postulated as the cause of such a fistula, it does not lie on the medium raphe, but well to one side. A more common site is at the coronal sulcus. Operative repair is not difficult provided the urinary stream is diverted, and the margins of the fistula are adequately mobilized.

E. Lower urinary tract obstruction

I. Introductory

Whereas in adult urological practice disorders of one organ, the prostate gland, account for a high proportion of all cases with lower urinary obstruction, in children a greater variety of obstructive lesions may be found and in most diagnosis is only possible as a result of special urological investigation. Moreover, while prostatic enlargement may cause both acute and chronic retention, in children these manifestations of obstruction are usually due to different lesions. A complete inability to pass urine associated with a tense and tender bladder swelling is often the result of a minor and easily remediable disorder, such as the impaction of a small stone, or of sulphamerazine crystals, or it may be simply a reflection of severe pain which is experienced or anticipated with micturition. A meatal ulcer is thus a cause of acute retention; the scab formed on the ulcer covers the meatus and urine can only be passed after the stream has torn away this scab. In these circumstances a young child may pass no urine at all while he is awake, and although he is usually very wet shortly after falling asleep, the retention itself causes abdominal pain after a time so that the child is brought up to hospital. Similarly painful micturition resulting from oxaluria and moderate dehydration, occurring perhaps on a hot summer day when the child has eaten a lot of fruit but has drunk little, may go on to acute retention. An accummulation of faeces in the rectum always accentuates this type of retention so that often the administration of an enema will relieve both bladder and bowel. Post-operative retention is seldom a complication of ordinary abdominal operations in children, though acute peritonitis, seen in ruptured appendix, may be responsible (HOFF-MAN): in one of my cases the failure to pass urine was the first localizing sign of appendicitis in a very toxic infant. Severe dysuria amounting to near retention may result also from the instrumental trauma in the male child following cystoscopy.

By contrast with these relatively minor disorders, the causes of chronic retention are commonly of the gravest import: the condition of overflow incontinence associated with a painless distended bladder often indicates serious damage to the renal parenchyma. It is unusual for any long standing cause of mild obstruction to be complicated by an episode of acute retention and, although an exacerbation may be indicated by some pain in the distended bladder, overflow is much more common than a complete cessation of urine flow.

Retention of urine in the new born baby constitutes a special case (which has been well summarized by BOISSONNAT), and at this stage acute retention may well indicate a serious lesion. In the normal infant urine may not be passed for 24—48 hours after birth because of dehydration: this circumstance need not occasion any alarm and can be differentiated from retention by the absence of bladder distension. The commonest cause of true retention at this stage is meatal stenosis with occlusion of the urethral lumen by epithelial debris, in association with coronal hypospadias. The size and position of the meatus render it inconspicious and the infant is often sent to hospital with the diagnosis of absent urethra, yet gentle probing will soon discover the opening and release the urinary stream. This type of occlusion is not associated with renal damage, but true obliterations and other congenital obstructions which cause retention at birth have a very bad prognosis. Cases in which bladder distension has caused dystocia, a rare complication of many forms of obstruction, are always fatal (SAVAGE, GOLDBERGER, EDGECOMBE).

II. Causes of obstruction

1. Intrinsic lesions

A great many malformations of the urethra may be responsible for urinary obstruction and, although these have been described severally in the previous chapter, certain generalizations regarding the type of obstruction are permissible. Posterior urethral lesions cause much more severe back pressure effects than those in the anterior urethra although the actual calibre of the lumen at the site of obstruction is often less in the latter. Thus a meatal stenosis may leave a pin hole orifice from which only a fine jet of urine can be propelled even with straining, but upper urinary tract changes are much less than in the diaphragmatic obstructions of the posterior urethra through which comparatively large bougie can be passed. The earlier the period of foetal life at which the obstruction is formed, the greater will be the disturbance of the upper urinary tract: complete occlusion in the posterior urethra is always an early deviation from normal development, and valve formation must take place quite soon after urine secretion commences: advanced renal changes are therefore the rule with these lesions. Anterior urethral valves must have their origin later in development, and cause a less severe disorder.

Congenital vesical disorders, although not so frequently encountered, may also be obstructive: trigonal cysts and curtains, vesical septa and partial duplications may be mentioned. Ureterocele, particularly of the ectopic variety, produces a mild degree of obstruction to the outflow from the bladder, but often a more severe ureteric obstruction.

Of the acquired disorders, stone (p. 173) is certainly the most important in countries where endemic calculous disease occurs: in these areas impaction of a stone in the urethra is much the most common cause of retention of urine in the male. Impaction may occur in the posterior urethra, or in the penile portion, but seldom in the bulb. Acquired stricture (p. 248) is usually traumatic in orgin and may be responsible for severe hydronephrosis, though the changes will hardly be as advanced as those found in the congenital urethral obstructions.

Neoplastic disease of the bladder (p. 197) and prostate (p. 201) commonly present because of urinary obstruction with overflow incontinence. Prostatic abscess will cause retention.

2. Extrinsic lesions

Any mass in the pelvis will displace the bladder upwards and press upon the urethra. An accummulation of faeces in the rectum is the commonest mass and in the "terminal reservoir" types of idiopathic megacolon (colonic inertia) some urinary obstruction may be present, but is by contrast unusual in Hirschsprung's disease where the colon is loaded but the rectum empty. It is frequently impossible to assess the significance of any intrinsic lesion, such as a doubtful bladder neck hypertrophy, until the rectum has been cleared and kept empty for several days. Mentally deficient children are particularly apt to suffer from severe constipation from an early age and on two occasions cases have been referred to me with a suprapubic cystostomy performed for a retention which could have been relieved by enemata. It should be noted, however, that constipation may be a symptom of chronic renal failure which has resulted from a lower urinary tract obstructions, and that both bowel and bladder dysfunction may result from a central nervous lesion.

Less common and less easily treated pelvic masses may be due to sacrococcygeal tumour (BROWN and BROWN, WOODRUFF and BEGNER), to presacral dermoid, to neuroblastoma and to hydrocolpos: all these may be found in the neonatal period or soon after. At this age I have also encountered urinary obstruction due to haematoma formation and abscess in the tissues behind and lateral to the bladder, perhaps resulting from a descending arteritis of the umbilical artery. Other pelvic masses may be due to duplication of the rectum (LADD and GROSS), hydatid cyst in the recto-vesical pouch (MORRIS), tumours in the female genital tract, or abscesses arising from osteomyelitis of the pelvis or from some visceral infection.

3. Central nervous lesions

The neurogenic bladder constitutes a separate problem from that posed by the mechanical obstruction, and is discussed at length in Section G. It should be remembered, however, that the clinical picture is occasionally confusing and that the pathological sequelae in the upper urinary tract are similar in both disorders. Episodes of acute retention with abdominal pain occur in the neurogenic bladder due to congenital spinal cord lesions and may lead to erroneous diagnosis of mechanical obstruction (p. 130). It is sometimes suggested that a "cord bladder"/may be present without any other signs of nervous disease and CAMP-BELL has described a transient retention in a new born infant as due to cord damage. It is, however, very rare indeed to find a typical expressible bladder without other evidence of neurological disorder.

Poliomyelitis in its early phase is often accompanied by acute retention, indeed this symptom is occasionally the first sign of the disease.

III. Consequences of obstruction

The pathological sequelae of chronic urinary obstruction are well known, and need not be discussed in detail, but certain differences in reaction between the adult and the child may be noted here.

Changes are most marked in the congenital obstructions, and appear to take place with considerable rapidity before birth. The most severe sequelae are seen in infants dying within the first weeks of life. The time of onset of urine secretion in the foetus has not been finally established, probably it occurs between 9 and 10 weeks, and although the elaboration of urine seems to play little part in the regulation of metabolic processes during foetal life, yet obstruction to its outflow will produce results familiar to every urologist. Detrusor hypertrophy is parti-cularly marked, but the bladder is seldom enlarged above the umbilicus, and does not reach the proportions seen in the megaureter-megacystis syndrome (an exception to this occurs with the "giant bladder" associated with rectal and urethral atresia [p. 94]).

The bladder neck musculature participates in the detrusor hypertrophy whenever the obstructive lesion is in the urethra, and the bladder neck therefore forms a shelf which separates the dilated urethra from the bladder cavity: only in the late stages is the bladder neck funnelled. The significance of bladder neck hypertrophy in so-called "bladder neck obstruction" is discussed on p. 74.

Vesical diverticula in the infant usually include the ureteric orifice within the sac: they are first formed at a point of muscular weakness, behind and lateral to the orifice, but draw in the ureter as they enlarge. Good illustrations of this anatomy have been published by HUTCH. A ureter opening into a diverticulum is always dilated, and usually allows reflux.

Ureteric dilatation is much more evident in children (Fig. 81) than in adults, and is extreme in the foetus. The lower end of the ureter is first affected, and the dilatation extends retrogressively. The renal pelvis does not enlarge much more than the upper end of the ureter, but acute kinks are often formed at the pelvi-ureteric junction. Kinking at several points is inseparable from any advanced ureteric dilatation. Ureteric dilatation and hypertrophy is at first associated with active peristaltic activity, but in the later stages when vesico-ureteral reflux occurs, ureteric contractions are absent or sluggish. This state of affairs contrasts with the maintenance of activity despite advanced dilatation in the mega-ureter-megacystis syndrome.

The kidneys are hydronephrotic, but are frequently also dysplastic, and in the new born infant dying of urinary obstruction, the renal mass may be smaller than normal. Scarring with cyst formation (Fig. 82) is common and histological examination of the parenchyma (PUGH) shows persistence of primitive renal elements, as described on p. 13, these changes appear to be secondary to the obstruction suggesting that there is an interference with the maturation of the later generation of the nephrons which normally continue to develop until the time of birth. Hypertensive changes may be found in the renal blood vessels.

Infection is a common complication and leads to an acute suppurative process in the parenchyma or to pyelonephritic scarring. The walls of the ureter and pelvis become thickened and oedematous, and enlarged aortic nodes are common. Venous thrombosis may complicate the picture.

Ascites may be found in neonatal cases (PARROTT, LORD) and appears to be derived from a leak from the bladder, although a gross rupture is not always discernible. The escape

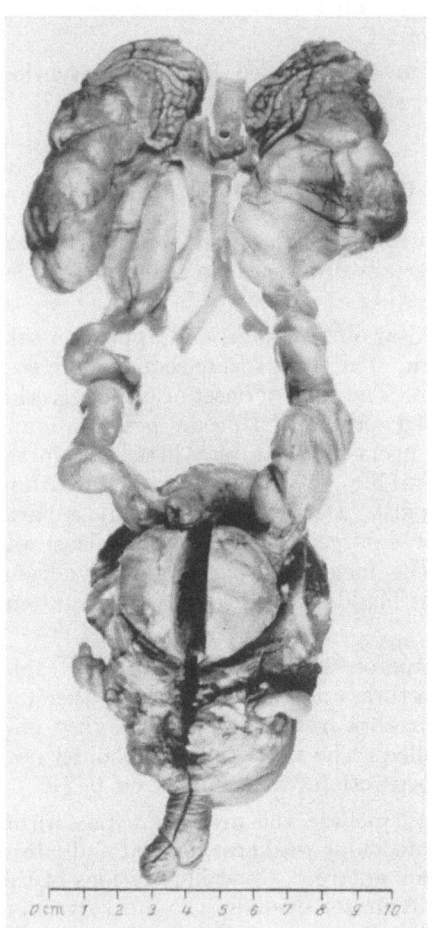

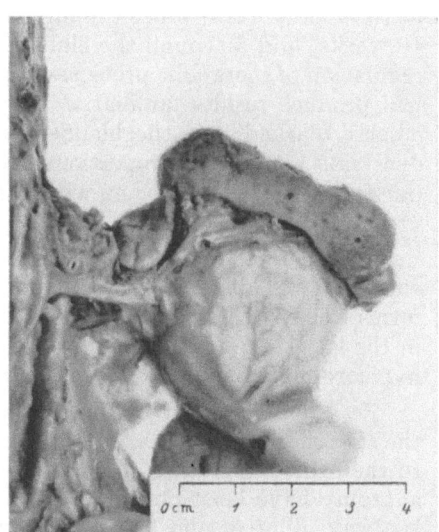

Fig. 81. Upper tract dilatation in urethral obstruction. Post-mortem specimen from a boy dying at 3 years of age with urethral valves, to show dilated and tortuous ureters

Fig. 82. Hypoplastic kidney in urethral obstruction. Post-mortem specimen from a boy dying at 3 weeks with urethral valves. The kidney is small in comparison to the enormous ureter and pelvis, the parenchyma is riddled with small cysts

of urine into the peritoneum, which commences before birth, lowers the tension in the urinary tract and the kidneys may be in better condition in these infants than in other congenital obstructions, although the outlook is very poor unless the condition is promptly recognized. Other fistulae found at the umbilicus or into the rectum may have a similar effect.

In cases dying late in childhood, secondary hyperparathyroidism is usually present, together with renal osteodystrophy, and perhaps deposition of calcium in the soft tissues.

IV. Symptomatology

Acute retention presents an unmistakable clinical picture which can scarcely be overlooked or misdiagnosed, chronic retention on the other hand presents in many forms which do not immediately suggest urinary obstruction. The prominent signs in such cases may be related to bladder function, to complicating urinary infection or to renal failure.

Difficult micturition may be evident on examination but is seldom a specific complaint which is mentioned by the parents. It is most noticeable and most often reported in cases of anterior urethral obstruction due to meatal stenosis, anterior valves or diverticula, but a poor stream is present whenever the obstruction is anywhere proximal to the meatus. A long and redundant prepuce may conceal the forcefulness of the normal stream, but it does not constitute a serious obstruction unless it becomes ballooned at each act of micturition.

Incontinence is much the most common urinary manifestation of obstruction, and although in minor cases this incontinence may mimic a simple "enuresis", the usual type is an overflow. In young infants the use of napkins conceals the normal habit of micturition but in chronic retention the child is always wet and the urine may be seen to be emerging from the penis in a slow drip. In older children with chronic retention, as in the prostatic obstruction of the elderly, nocturnal incontinence associated with day frequency and urgency may be noticed before micturition becomes a continual dribble.

Painful micturition and haematuria are manifestations of complicating urinary infection and seldom occur in the child with sterile urine, but abdominal pain, often severe and colicky, may be due to retention even though overflow continues. Attacks of hypogastric pain associated with the distended bladder are particularly characteristic of cases with vesical diverticula, but pain may also occur in the loin especially when there is reflux into a dilated ureter.

Infection in the obstructed urinary tract produces a severe constitutional disorder and high fever with toxaemia is common: the urine is turbid with pus. In spite of the obstruction antibiotic drugs may well sterilize the urine or at least relieve the acute symptoms for a time; it is therefore of vital importance that the clinical signs of obstruction should be sought at the time of first examination, and full investigation made as soon as the child's condition permits.

Vomiting, with failure to thrive, is the commonest presenting complaint in young infants with congenital lower urinary obstruction and results from renal failure. The vomiting may lead to dehydration, which is accentuated by the obligatory polyuria of the failing kidneys. Acidosis of some degree is usual in the uraemic child, and may be sufficiently severe to cause sighing respiration. The biochemical manifestations of renal failure in obstructions are discussed by ERICSSON et al., and in Section M of this volume.

Constipation is common, and several of my cases were investigated by barium enema, suspected of Hirschsprung's disease, before an estimation of the blood urea indicated the need for urological consultation. Diarrhoea may also occur at times, and gross intestinal distension is a prominent feature of some uraemic infants.

Muscular hypotonia is a symptom in long standing cases, and is probably related to the acquired insensitivity to vitamin D which later manifests itself in renal rickets. Symptoms of hypertension appear in some children.

The children who present with signs of renal failure have usually an overflow incontinence which has been overlooked, but occasionally the micturition appears to be surprisingly normal even though chronic retention has led to advanced hydronephrosis. The prognosis of these infants is naturally very much worse than for the older children whose only complaint is a disturbance of micturition.

Long standing urinary obstruction of a degree insufficient to cause chronic retention does not occasion any characteristic symptoms, for an actual complaint of difficult micturition or a poor stream is uncommon in children. The obstructive element in these cases is only discovered during the routine investigation of children with persistent enuresis, vague abdominal pain, and urinary infection.

V. Diagnosis and management

1. Acute retention

Acute retention presents no difficulty in diagnosis: even in the young infant who cannot indicate the nature of his pain, the dryness of his napkins and the distension of the bladder are unlikely to escape his mother's attention. Sometimes a simple clinical examination will also reveal the cause of the retention, a meatal ulcer perhaps or a stone impacted in the penile urethra, but where no cause is evident, treatment must often precede investigation, so urgent is the need for relief. Since acute retention is often the result of painful micturition, the administration of a sedative and a warm bath may be sufficient to re-establish urine flow, and the cause may be sought later. If the rectum is loaded, an enema will often result in evacuation of both bladder and bowel. When these simple measures are not effective, the urine must be withdrawn by catheterization, but an indwelling catheter should not be required unless difficulty in instrumentation, or subsequent examination reveal the presence of a serious obstructive lesion. The investigation and management in such cases will be the same as for cases of chronic retention.

2. Chronic retention

In this group, chronic obstruction has led to palpable bladder distension and usually to overflow incontinence of urine. In palpating the abdomen of a child it must be remembered that the normal full bladder is an abdominal organ, reaching to the umbilicus or near it, and an adequate opportunity for uninterrupted micturition must be allowed before examination. The presence of a faecal mass in the rectum will render even a partly distended bladder easily palpable. In the infant, who cannot be induced to micturate to order, it is hard to judge whether the distension is due to a residual urine or not, but a fair indication may be gained from the observation of dribbling micturition in the presence of a full bladder. On the other hand, in the infant with congenital obstruction the renal swellings are often considerable, and may divert attention from the comparatively slight bladder distension, so that an upper urinary tract disorder may be suspected even in urethral obstructions.

The palpation of a distended overflowing bladder does not neccessarily indicate an intrinsic urinary tract obstruction and clinical examination can carry the diagnosis a stage further. In the first place, a neurological cause for bladder distension must be sought; usually a meningocele or evident deformity of the sacral vertebrae will betray a spinal cord lesion, but the sensation in the perineum, the tone of the anal sphincter and the tendon reflexes should be tested. The neurogenic bladder is characteristically expressible, whereas the mechanically obstructed bladder can only be expressed under anaesthesia unless the infant is already near coma.

In the older child, an attempt should be made to differentiate between true and false residual urine: the latter term may be used to described bladder distension after micturition which results from the return of urine which has been driven during bladder contraction into distended ureters by reflux. This situation is characteristic of the mega-ureter-megacystis syndrome, and is also seen with large vesical diverticula. The "false" residual urine may be partially or completely expelled by a second or third act of micturition performed ten minutes after the first, and it is seldom associated with overflow incontinence.

Rectal palpation may reveal the presence of an extrinsic obstruction, such as a sacro-coccygeal tumour. In the new born female with retention the vagina must be carefully inspected, for hydrocolpos is a likely cause. Ascites accompanied by anuria in a neonate may be due to urethral obstruction with a leaking bladder.

At the completion of the clinical examination, it will often be possible to say that a state of chronic retention is present, and that it is probably due to an intrinsic obstruction, but it is seldom possible to identify the nature of this obstruction without endoscopic and radiological investigations. However, the infant with chronic retention is in a precarious condition and further diagnostic procedures must be integrated with the urgent problem of treatment. The dangers of infection complicating catheterization, which have been fully recognized for the elderly prostatic, are present in the infant to an equal degree, and the hazards of acute biochemical disturbance are even more perilous. A routine of management is clearly required which yields the maximum diagnostic information with minimum risk, and the routine adopted naturally varies in different urological centres. The general references at the end of this section may be consulted for a full survey, and only my own practice will be described here.

If the urine is overflowing from the distended bladder and the child is not in acute pain, catheterization is not urgently required and certain preliminary investigations are desirable. A clinical estimate should be made of the degree of dehydration from the elasticity of the skin and the state of the fontanelles. An estimation of the blood urea is vital, though the result must be considered in relation to the dehydration, and if possible the serum electrolyte levels should also be investigated. The urine should be examined for pus and organisms.

When the child's general condition is good, the urine sterile and the blood urea only slightly raised (e.g. below 60 mgm/100 ml after correction of dehydration) there is little urgency and a thorough investigation may be undertaken. An intravenous pyelogram should be performed and, if active micturition is possible, a micturating cysto-urethrogram will provide the most valuable data. Endoscopy and operative treatment of the obstructing lesion may then follow.

If the blood urea is raised to 100 mgm/100 ml or over, even though the child's general condition is good, treatment is more urgent. The correction of dehydration and acidosis are often the most immediate requirements, but once these measures are in train, the child should be taken to the theatre and anaesthetized. A metal catheter is then passed, and the bladder emptied. The process of instrumentation itself will give some information, especially in cases of stricture, and once the bladder is empty a tumour in the bladder, prostate or surrounding tissue will be easily palpable. An expression cysto-urethrogram is performed in the manner described on p. 6. The urethrographic appearances in the congenital bladder neck and urethral obstructions have been described in the previous section, and reference should be made to Figs 53 to 65. While the films are being developed the child is placed in the lithotomy position and a cystoscope introduced. In some male infants a perineal urethrostomy will be required for this purpose, but there should be no hesitation in making such an incision. It is important, however, that the anterior urethra as well as the posterior should be carefully inspected endoscopically, for anterior urethral valves and diverticula are causes of

8*

obstruction which are easily overlooked. Once radiological and endoscopic findings are available, it should be possible to reach a diagnosis of the cause of obstruction and a decision as to the mode of treatment. In most cases it is preferable to proceed immediately to removal of the obstruction, and to drain the bladder via the perineal urethrostomy. If a large vesical diverticulum, a bladder tumour, or some other lesion requiring major surgery is found, a catheter may be left in for a day or two while the child is prepared for the operation.

When an infant with chronic retention has a high blood urea, a urinary infection with a persistent pyrexia and is in poor general condition, drainage of the urinary tract, restoration of the biochemical equilibrium and chemotherapy are the urgent requirements, and no attempt should be made to diagnose the exact cause of obstruction. Pyelostomies or nephrostomies are a more effective form of drainage than cystostomy, for the ureters are dilated and tortuous, so they do not always empty satisfactorily once the bladder has contracted around a suprapubic catheter. Bilateral pyelostomy is a simple procedure in infancy, and is tolerated well except in the most advanced uraemia, when a stab cystostomy may be justifiable. An indwelling urethral catheter only provides adequate drainage in girls and in older boys: in male infants the lumen of the catheter must be so small and easily obstructed that it has very little value. Diagnostic investigation and definitive treatment should be undertaken as soon as possible after preliminary drainage, since the use of indwelling tubes of all sorts is ultimately complicated by resistant urinary infection which can only be overcome by restoring normal micturition.

The post-operative management of cases of chronic retention varies considerably in the individual obstructions, but in all the dangers of electrolyte imbalance are great. Estimations of blood urea and serum electrolytes should be made at least on every alternate day during the first week, and appropriate corrective measures should be started without delay. The common disorders are discussed in Section M. Regrettably often, however, in the case of congenital urethral obstruction, the acute disturbances are overcome by careful management, but the blood urea remains high because of irreversible renal damage, and after some months or years the chronic disturbances become evident. Renal osteodystrophy is always a danger in these children, and their vitamin D requirements should receive attention.

The tortuous ureters and hydronephrotic kidneys predispose to later urinary infection, even when the primary obstruction has been overcome. A period of continuous chemotherapy for at least six months after discharge from hospital is desirable and antibiotics should be started immediately pyuria is noticed. Operative measures designed to straighten out the ureteric kinks have been advocated by some authors but have not given satisfactory results in my hands. Similarly operations designed to stop vesico-ureteral reflux are of doubtful value, and when reflux is serious, a regime of double or triple micturition should be instituted as in the mega-ureter-megacystis syndrome.

3. Low grade obstructions

During the investigation of children suffering from incontinence or recurrent urinary infection, but without palpable bladder distension, the possibility of a low grade obstruction in the lower urinary tract must be considered, and it is important to define the criteria on which a diagnosis of obstruction should be based.

The measurement of residual urine has often been regarded as a reliable indication of the degree of obstruction, and has an established place in adult urology. In paediatric work similar measurements are often made without any understanding of their fallibility, and in my opinion far too much importance has been attributed to them. In the very young it is almost impossible to be sure when a complete act of micturition has occurred, and the nervous child who is sent to pass urine while preparations are made for catheterization is often too frightened to make a satisfactory job of it. If residual urine is measured during cystoscopy under anaesthesia, allowance must be made for the period of premedication and cannot be accurate. When reflux is present the residual urine is often simply the volume of the distended ureters and only cine cystography will show whether the bladder was empty at the time of contraction.

YOUNG et al. have introduced a more complicated method of assessing volumes of residuum: they suggest instilling a light solution of radio-opaque oil into the bladder: if X-rays taken 24—48 hours still show oil in the bladder, then no complete contraction can have taken place.

Trabeculation of the bladder when associated with residual urine is good evidence of obstruction, but it must be remembered that any child with severe frequency, even when it is of the enuretic type, will have a slight trabeculation, and this finding alone should not be taken to indicate a hindrance to the outflow of urine.

Diverticulum formation is usually the result of obstruction, but there is good evidence that it is sometimes due to a congenital defect in the detrusor coat (p. 69).

Vesico-ureteral reflux occurs in many conditions, and even in the apparently normal urinary tract. As a solitary finding, it does not indicate obstruction.

Thus although some urologists find minor degrees of urinary obstruction as a common cause of enuresis and recurrent infection, in my opinion such obstructions should only be diagnosed after careful consideration of the evidence and endoscopic resection or intermittent urethral dilatation should be reserved for those with unequivocal signs.

F. Enuresis

I. Normal development

Enuresis, the form of urinary incontinence which is unaccompanied by any major organic lesion, is by far the commonest urological disorder of childhood. The term is difficult to define, since almost all definitions involve acceptance of a particular theory of its causation, but it does not seem useful to follow those writers who include under the heading almost all forms of incontinence, more particularly those which occur at night, for the differential diagnosis of the various forms is of the greatest practical importance. Others define enuresis as a purely functional disorder, but this seems to exclude the possibility that minor organic abnormalities might be present. NASH defines the condition as a persistence or a return to an infantile habit of bladder function, which may result from a variety of causes, and although the implications of this definition are not proven, it does emphasize the clinical importance of analysing the nature and circumstances of the incontinence, the first step in diagnosis.

The normal infant passes urine frequently, and more or less automatically, whenever the bladder is full. Although at this stage conscious control of micturition is lacking, from the physiological viewpoint bladder function is normal, and the term incontinence is not strictly applicable. It is often possible to recognize true incontinence of the dribbling overflow variety from earliest infancy, provided napkins are not allowed to obscure observation. The normal child will pass urine in a good stream and then remain dry for a period, whereas the incontinent one is always wet.

The exact frequency of micturition in infancy varies considerably in different individuals, perhaps from every quarter of an hour to every three hours, and peripheral stimuli may facilitate the reflex action. It thus happens that some mothers succeed in getting their babies to micturate on their pots before and after feeds at a very early age: this is a reflex, however, which will probably break down towards the end of the first year, when the normal conscious control is being acquired. In this later stage, micturition is still frequent and urgent, so that if the pot is immediately available the child will use it, but he is unable to wait after the first desire to micturate until a suitable time. With patient and assiduous training most children acquire diurnal control between 12 and 18 months, though some require up to $2^1/_2$ years. Nocturnal control follows naturally from the diurnal training, and is usually though not invariably acquired later. Training is sometimes temporarily frustrated by the child's natural reluctance to accept the discipline of toilet routine, and a self-willed infant who has been sat on the pot for half an hour without success will often promptly empty his bladder on the carpet: an exasperating circumstance for his mother but of no concern to the urologist.

The infantile bladder habit thus exhibits various stages in its development and enuresis, which is the persistence of that habit, has correspondingly various manifestations, the youngest enuretics having frequency and urgency by day as in early infancy.

The age at which it can fairly be said that the child is an enuretic, rather than a normal late developer is indefinite, and the accepted figures, varying between 3 and 5 years, are dependent upon the practical consideration of when it is useful to start treatment. KLACKENBERG in Sweden found that 87% of children were dry by night at the age of 3 years, and 96% by the age of 6 years. It is, however, never too early to establish beyond doubt that the incontinence is of the enuretic type, nor too soon to advise the mother as to the proper method of training the child, for the treatment of the youngest enuretic is simply a training process.

II. Incidence

Enuresis is well known to be an extremely common complaint, and in the ordinary course of events only a proportion of enuretic children are brought for treatment. The upheaval involved in the evacuation of the great cities of England during the 1939—1945 war revealed the surprisingly high incidence of the disorder. BLOMFIELD and DOUGLAS give figures relating to an unselected group of 5,386 children, whose development is being watched from birth onward. At the age of 6 years 1.8% of boys and 4.1% of girls were wet during the day; this is in keeping with the ordinary clinical observation, the diurnal urge incontinence type of enuresis being particularly common in girls starting school, but the incidence of day wetting falls off very rapidly after this period. At this age (6 years) 11.9% of boys, and 8.4% of girls were wet at night, but 18 months later the incidence had dropped to 8.0% of boys and 6.4% of girls. These figures, which may seem very high, include all cases and only 1.65% of the whole group were wet every night at the age of $7^1/_2$ years. Evidence is not available for a comparable group in later years, but there is no doubt that boys predominate among the older enuretics who have night symptoms only.

The fall in the incidence of enuresis with advancing years seemed very little influenced by treatment in the series of BLOMFIELD and DOUGLAS.

A familial incidence of enuresis is well recognized and FRARY has gone so far as to suggest that it is a condition inherited according to Mendelian laws. At times, however, it seems that a family already innured to the hardships of enuresis does not provide the best training ground for younger children.

Enuresis is more common in institutions caring for large numbers of children than elsewhere. MICHAELS and GOODMAN have discussed its relation to delinquency. It is, however, agreed by most observers that if low grade mental defectives are excluded, there is no direct relationship between enuresis and intelligence.

About 1 in 5 or 6 enuretics have had a period of normal control at the age of 2 or 3 years, but later relapse, often at 4 or 5 years. The late onset cases, however, differ very little from the congenital, and the same aetiological factors apply to both groups.

III. Symptoms and differential diagnosis

In a urological treatise, it is scarcely necessary to emphasize that all incontinence is not enuresis, and that by careful history taking and simple clinical observations it is possible to classify cases under a series of headings which often give a reliable indication of the nature of the basic disorder, and form a starting point for more complex investigations. Such a classification is concerned chiefly with the day symptoms, for it is hard to discover precisely what is happening at night. Moreover, a child who is only wet at night and has no day symptoms at all seldom has any organic abnormality.

In urge incontinence, micturition is frequent, and the desire to void imperative, but no dribbling occurs between the acts. This is the ordinary type of incontinence in the younger enuretics, particularly in girls, though it also occurs in urinary infections, in the neurogenic bladder and in other organic diseases. The simple enuretic form may be distinguished by the sterility of the urine, the absence of other symptoms, and the readiness with which it responds to training: on a regime of regular timed micturition under proper supervision, the enuretic with diurnal urge incontinence will quickly become dry by day.

In dribbling incontinence, the urine flows away continuously, so that the child is wet soon after micturition, if that act is still possible, and a regular timed regime does not make him any drier. Chronic retention with overflow is a common cause of dribbling incontinence which is often present from earliest infancy: when of later onset, the incontinence is often nocturnal at first, as in the elderly prostatic, but diurnal frequency and a poor stream usually suggest the nature of the condition. Dribbling incontinence is also characteristic of the neurogenic bladder due to a low spinal cord lesion; in this, as in overflow, there is an associated failure of normal micturition. By contrast dribbling incontinence due to an ectopic ureter is accompanied by normal micturition. A somewhat similar disturbance has been recorded with double urethra in the female and congenital vesico-vaginal fistula (p. 69).

Sphincter weakness, when the detrusor function is normal, leads to a stress incontinence. In severe disorders such as epispadias all the urine empties from the bladder as soon as the child sits up or stands, though only a little may drain away during the night. Mild stress incontinence with wetting only during active exercise, is occasionally found in girls with no detectable abnormality of the bladder or urethra other than a laxity of the urethral musculature: the symptom often disappears as the child approaches adult life, and its recovery can be hastened by faradic stimulation of the perineal musculature. Some urologists have encountered severe cases of this type in which they believed there was an actual muscular deficiency, and have performed plication or sling operations to support the urethra. A type of stress incontinence may be seen with neurogenic bladder with a low incomplete lesion, and it is common after operations to relieve valvular obstruction of the urethra in infancy.

Giggle incontinence is an affliction of girls of school age, often confused with and occasionally accompanied by stress incontinence. Micturition is normal, and control is only lost when the child dissolves into a fit of the "giggles": a complete bladder evacuation then occurs. No abnormality is found in the urinary tract in these cases, which are often familial. The condition appears to be due to a disorder of the central nervous control, rather than to any peripheral fault, and no effective treatment has been devised. However, the symptom becomes less troublesome as the years go by, and situations no longer seem so humerous as to provoke the uncontrollable giggles.

Enuresis, which is a persistence of, or return to, the infantile habit of bladder function, has several forms; it is never a dribbling incontinence, nor it is precipitated by stress or giggling. It is not associated with a large residual urine, an expressible bladder or a urinary infection.

Four clinical types of enuresis may be recognized:

i) Wetting by day and night, with frequency and urgency of micturition. This form is common in young children, girls more often than boys, and occurs in the congenital as well as the late onset type of enuresis. The frequency is often extreme following the ingestion of fluid, when the child may be passing urine every quarter of an hour, yet the incontinence is always due to urgency rather than dribbling.

ii) Wetting by night only, but some frequency by day. A very high proportion of children with nocturnal enuresis have some frequency, even though they are perfectly controlled by day.

iii) Wetting by night only, with no day symptoms. This type is characteristic of the older child and adolescent, particularly the male, and is often the most difficult to cure.

iv) Wetting by day only, with frequency and urgency. This symptom complex is always suspect, being the least common type of simple enuresis, and mimicked by stress and other types of incontinence due to organic disease.

IV. Aetiological factors

The aetiology of enuresis has been the subject of much research and speculation during the past century, but it cannot be claimed that there is as yet any universally accepted explanation. Almost every observer who has employed some new method of investigation has convinced himself of the cause, which has been demonstrable in a high percentage of his cases; the type of investigation, however, seems to have determined the type of lesion discovered, radiologists find one disorder, endoscopists another, physicians and psychologists others again. All these claims are backed by impressive results obtained by treatment of the lesion described, for it appears that enuresis will always respond to treatment administered with enthusiasm and confidence. The conflicting evidence compels the sceptic to believe that no specific cause can or will be found, but it is perhaps more constructive to suppose that the disordered bladder function may result from a wide variety of factors, which should be sought in each individual case and treated on their own merits. A review of the more widely recognized "causes" must therefore be included here, for although none can have the importance claimed for it by its protagonists, all are likely to be of some significance.

1. Faulty training

Great importance has been attributed to this factor by some authors, though it can scarcely apply to cases in which nocturnal enuresis is the only symptom, for training can directly influence only the diurnal control, and in the ordinary circumstance dry nights will follow. The child with day frequency and urgency can be quickly cured by a strict regime, and it might therefore be said that this disorder is due to a failure of ordinary training, yet in modern circumstances it is often due to a faulty parental attitude rather than to neglect. In BLOM-FIELD and DOUGLAS's series there was a definite social gradient: enuresis was found to be most common amongst the families of manual workers, and least common amongst the professional classes and agricultural workers. Nevertheless, the children of intelligent and well-to-do parents are quite often affected, and if there is a failure of training it is usually due to over-anxiety and to an expectation of perfection at too early an age, coupled naturally with an acute disappointment when the child fails to live up to the high standard set.

2. Psychological disorders

It is a matter of common observation that enuresis is frequent in children with an obvious emotional disturbance. An anxiety state is often present, the child being nervous, worried or frightened, perhaps having just started school and encountered an unsympathetic teacher, perhaps being ill-treated by a step-father. The child who has been sent to an institution, or feels neglected following the birth of a younger brother or sister, the child who has suffered some terrifying physical experience or accident, is frequently brought to hospital for the treatment of enuresis. In a different group are the children with severe behaviour disorders, the truants and delinquents, the psychopathic personalities who are brought up before the courts, and who have often faecal as well as urinary incontinence. In some of these, whose enuresis has been present since birth, it may be argued that the psychological disturbance was consequent upon the bedwetting, and upon the resulting rejection by the parents, but it is equally clear that specialist psychological guidance is necessary once the urologist has assured himself that no organic lesion is present.

These emotional disturbances will be evident to any clinician, but most psychiatrists claim that all enuresis has a psychological basis, and argue that the symptom is only one manifestation, not even a very important manifestation, of a deep-seated disturbance. On this ground they believe that treatment directed to the symptom alone is useless and even harmful (BEVERLY): urological instrumentation or examination of the genitalia will only exacerbate the psychological trauma. This attitude is unlikely to appeal to the urologists, who will naturally draw attention to the many children who have been cured of their emotional disturbances by prolonged psychiatric treatment but still wet the bed. Dreams which include micturition phantasies are held responsible by some, and as might be expected Freudian explanations of enuresis as the equivalent of masturbation or as sexual fears are not lacking (WINNICOT).

A detailed discussion of the psychological theories would clearly be out of place in this volume, but emotional factors can never be ignored in treating enuresis.

All successful methods of treatment include an element of suggestion, a fact which indicates that a psychological adjustment is usually necessary, and the physical methods which are employed should be adapted to the child's emotional status, for instance a system which involves repeated electric shocks whenever the bed is wet is more likely to help a stable adolescent than a nervous five year old.

3. Urinary tract disorders

Urologists have been chiefly responsible for emphasizing the role of minor disorders of the urinary tract in enuresis and the prepuce has inevitably received vigorous attention. WINSBURY-WHITE in a study of 310 cases claimed that 50% of females had vulvitis, and that 70% of males required meatotomy: signs of inflammation at the internal urinary meatus, polyps, granulomata, and mucosal hillocks, were present in 70%, although the urine was sterile in most of these. Other endoscopists of repute have reported similar findings (e. g. CAMPBELL) and claim considerable success as a result of treatment by endoscopic diathermy and dilatation. There is no doubt that children treated in this way remain dry at night as long as they have some dysuria following instrumentation, and since enuresis is ultimately self-limiting in the majority a permanent improvement follows in some.

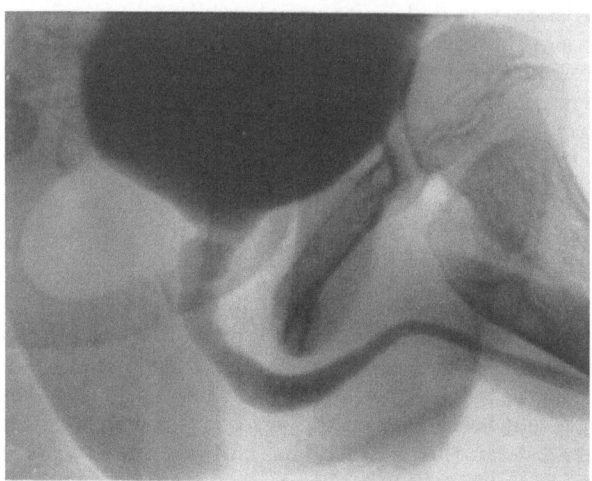

Fig. 83. Enuresis. Micturating cysto-urethrogram in a boy aged 7 years, also suffering from occasional faecal incontinence, and from a definite behaviour disorder. There is well marked transverse line below the verumontanum. He improved on medical treatment

Bladder neck obstruction has been regarded as an important cause of persistent enuresis by MILLER, and many reports of this disease in children include a high proportion of enuretics. It is important, however, to distinguish simple enuresis from overflow incontinence, and in the "bladder neck obstruction" associated with simple enuresis there is usually a prominence of the bladder neck region but only questionable evidence of obstruction (p. 72).

Radiological methods of investigation reveal a different series of abnormalities in the urethra: BRODNY and ROBINS found unexplained stenoses, while FISHER and FORSYTHE demonstrated many cases of urethral valves, though most of these exhibited linear filling defects (Fig. 83) in the urethrogram, but had no proximal dilatation, nor any evidence of obstruction. To the present writer it appears doubtful whether such non-obstructive mucosal folds can be responsible for enuresis, and similar personal cases have recovered without surgical treatment.

Another group to which FISHER and FORSYTHE refer exhibits a dilatation of the upper urethra, with or without a wide bladder neck, so that the urethrogram often simulates that found in the neurogenic bladder (Fig. 84). Similarly it may be demonstrated clinically, particularly in girls, that the urethral musculature is lax, and endoscopically that the bladder neck relaxes when the bladder is full

(SIENKIEWIEZ). Operations to support or plicate the urethra are often advised for this type of case (McFADDEN, GAYET) but have met with variable success. Cine cystography in my cases with an apparently wide urethra has shown normal bladder function, and normal closure of the bladder neck, while a number have improved on conservative treatment. The range of normal urethral distension is considerable, and if the external sphincter is contracted during micturition, the posterior urethra will suddenly balloon out, so that a single film taken at this moment might be supposed to indicate an obstructive lesion. When there is definite laxity of the urethral musculature, it is likely that stress incontinence will be present, as well as urgency.

Abnormalities of bladder function have been extensively studied by cystometry (NASH) and it can be demonstrated that the child with day frequency has a small capacity bladder with many uninhibited contractions. Most of these children will improve with training, and it has been claimed that the gentle distension which accompanies the cystometry will help (STOCKWELL and SMITH), but a few seem to have persistently small bladders, and if they cease to be enuretic they have to micturate once or twice at night.

A thorough investigation of enuretic children

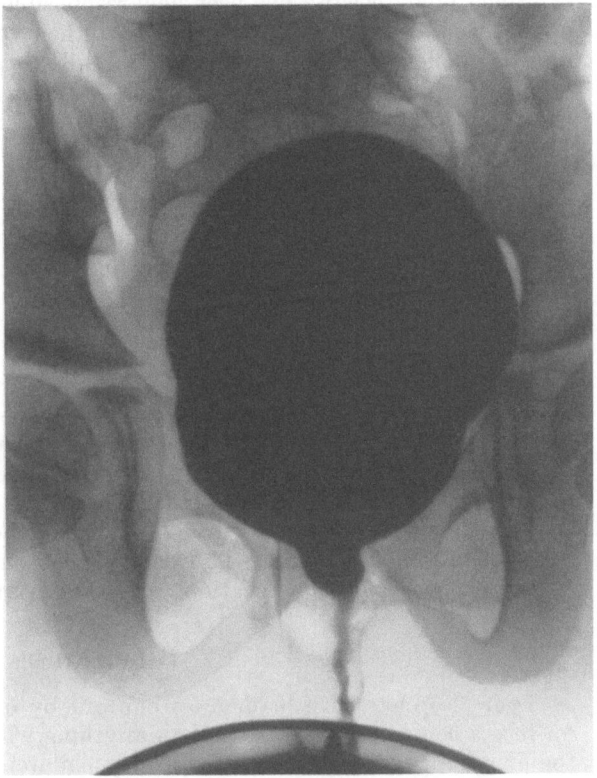

Fig. 84. Enuresis. Micturating cystogram in a girl aged 8 years with persistent enuresis, chiefly nocturnal, sometimes diurnal. The upper urethra is apparently widened, although no abnormality was seen on urethroscopy. Cine cystogram showed a normally functioning bladder, and normal closure of the internal sphincter

will occasionally reveal an unsuspected congenital abnormality such as ureterocele, hydronephrosis, or fused kidney, and in most of these cases it is difficult to establish any relationship between the symptom and the finding. Treatment may be required for these lesions, but is often found to be without effect upon the enuresis.

4. Bowel disorders

Obstinate constipation, and even idiopathic megacolon, is sometimes found in association with enuresis, and emptying the bowel often leads to improvement in urinary control. This type of constipation may occur in emotionally disturbed children, however, and it is not always clear that the bladder disorder is consequent upon the distension of the bowel. In the absence of gross constipation, or of a spinal cord lesion, enuresis accompanied by soiling usually indicates a behaviour disorder requiring psychological attention.

Thread worms may be found in enuretics, and it is reasonable to suppose that the irritation they cause plays a part in the urinary disturbance.

5. Neurological disorders

Spina bifida occulta has been held responsible for enuresis in many cases, and operations to free the nerve roots have had their vogue, as have epidural injections of saline believed to loosen adhesions. While there is no doubt that spina bifida occulta can be associated with myelodysplasia causing a neurogenic bladder (see p. 127) together with other neurological signs, it is very doubtful whether the simple bony lesion has any relation to the usual enuretic type of incontinence. KARLIN has shown that 54% of normal children have a radiologically demonstrable failure of union of the lamina of the fifth lumbar or first sacral vertebra, and that the incidence is no greater in enuretics.

Epilepsy occurs in some enuretics, and an occasional case of diurnal incontinence is due to unrecognized petit mal.

6. Polyuria

A high urinary output renders a child liable to enuresis, and the onset of diabetes insipidus or melitus is sometimes revealed by this symptom. Nevertheless a great many children with polyuria have normal bladder control, often in fact have a bladder of unusually large capacity. It has been claimed (POULTON) that a relative nocturnal polyuria (a failure of the normal diminution of urinary secretion during the night) is responsible for enuresis in a high proportion of cases. The controlled observations of VULLIAMY appear to contradict this view.

7. Other causes

Deep sleep has been blamed for enuresis by many parents and some doctors, for it is a common observation that anything which lightens the sleep alleviates the symptoms. Nevertheless, many dry children sleep very deeply indeed.

Acute infectious diseases sometimes occasion the onset of enuresis after a controlled period, but there does not appear to be a specific factor here.

Allergy has been held responsible by some (POTTER) and among the more fantastic suggested causes are enlarged tonsils and hereditary syphilis.

V. Management

The successful management of enuresis in childhood depends very largely upon the time, care and enthusiasm which can be devoted to each individual case: a brief examination and routine prescription are never sufficient and an initial failure to gain the child's confidence makes subsequent treatment more difficult. The first interview is necessarily prolonged, since it should be concerned with the child's general health, environment and emotional state, it is probably better performed by a general practitioner or paediatrician than by a urologist. It is of course important that cases of overflow incontinence and those with a severe psychological disturbance should be sorted out immediately, but a failure to recognize such cases is usually the result of haste rather than lack of specialist knowledge. A careful history which analyses the nature of the incontinence, followed by a thorough clinical examination and routine urine tests, should eliminate the cases in which the symptoms are due to a gross organic abnormality, and the simple enuretics do not require urological investigation unless they show no improvement on treatment.

Whatever system of treatment is adopted the child must be first of all be assured that no serious disease is present, that there are no terrible consequences to be anticipated and that by his own efforts he can, and will, become perfectly normal. The parents must be instructed to take a reasonable attitude towards the disorder, giving the child every encouragement to improve, yet avoiding dour threats or physical punishments. Any tricks which remind the child of the need for positive effort are valuable, the keeping of calendars and rewards for success for instance; in older children it is reasonable to expect them to help with the washing in case of failure, but they should not be allowed to develop a sense of hopeless inferiority or of rejection by their parents or fellows. The younger child who is feeling neglected by his mother will need extra attention, the older spoilt child needs stimulation in order to become independent, and short stays with relatives or at camp may develop the sense of personal responsiblity.

The sleeping accommodation should be enquired into, and it should be possible for the child to get out to go to the lavatory without fear or difficulty if he should wake in the night. Sharing of beds is sometimes a problem for there is little encouragement to improve if the bedfellow is also enuretic.

Fluid restriction in the evening is almost universally practised in enuresis, and has usually been given an extensive trial before the doctor is consulted. It is difficult to be sure that it is useless.

1. Training and conditioning methods of treatment

The younger enuretic with day frequency and incontinence is most satisfactorily treated by a time training regime (NASH). The child is sent to pass urine at regular intervals by the clock throughout the day: hourly or even half-hourly micturition is necessary at first, but once the routine is established, the interval can be gradually prolonged in successive weeks or months to two or three hours. At this stage the child cannot be relied upon to go to the lavatory without prompting or to get adequate warning of when the bladder is full, it is therefore essential that parent or teacher should insist on a timed interval. Drug therapy may usefully supplement the training but should be regarded only as an auxiliary. On this regime almost all enuretics will become dry by day, and will be able to hold their urine for longer and longer periods: failure to respond is usually due to failure to carry out the instructions. As the bladder capacity enlarges, so dry nights become more likely, but the attainment of nocturnal control often requires much greater perseverance and possibly other methods of treatment. A young child should not be woken more than once or twice at night, for there is a danger that loss of sleep will do more harm than enuresis.

The older child and adolescent with day frequency, but incontinence only at night, may be encouraged to train himself: by voluntary restraint when the urge to micturate is first felt he can increase the effective capacity of the bladder and diminish the frequency. Weekly measurements of the volume held when the bladder is full may stimulate this effort (HIGHAM), and whether because of the physical or psychological effect, dry nights ultimately follow. Once again drug therapy may be employed at the same time.

For the older child who has no day symptoms at all, day training is of little assistance. Regular wakening once or twice at night is sufficient to keep many children dry, and although it does not effect any fundamental cure, it saves a lot of inconvenience and most cases ultimately cure themselves. An alarm clock which forces the child to wake himself is a greater stimulus than a gentle maternal hand, but often the alarm bell wakes everyone in the house except the enuretic himself. In these circumstances a drug which lightens the sleep is advisable.

MOWRER and MOWRER introduced the method of waking the enuretic child by means of an alarm bell which was set off as soon as urine was passed on to a tin foil sheet in the bed; the child must then get out of bed to switch off the alarm and to change the sheets. This system has recently gained popularity and it is satisfactory for the older child without day symptoms who wets the bed only once or twice a night, but wets most nights in the week. After a short time, the child usually wakes before micturition has occurred, but later sleeps through the night without being disturbed. CROSBY modified the method to include an electrode which administered a mild electric shock to the abdominal wall at the same time that the alarm was set off; this apparatus is complicated, and the shock treatment more suitable for adolescents than children.

2. Drug treatment

The most popular drugs used in enuresis are those which lighten the sleep and lessen the frequency of bladder contractions. Belladonna (tincture, minims v each night, gradually increased to the limits of tolerance) is a long established remedy now seldom employed: the atropine in it is believed to act by blocking the post-ganglionic nerve endings in the detrusor, inhibiting excessive tone. Ephedrine is a sympathomimetic drug which has little effect on the detrusor but increases the tone of the internal sphincter: it also has a central stimulant action which prevents deep sleep. Used in the form of Methyl Ephedrine, a dose of $2/_3$—$1^1/_3$ grains three times a day is suitable. Amphetamine has some of the peripheral action of ephedrine, but much more powerful stimulant effect, and very heavy sleepers benefit from its action: 5 to 15 mgm a night may be necessary. Methantheline (Banthine) and Propantheline (Probanthine) are anti-cholinergic drugs which decrease detrusor tone and diminish the frequency of bladder contractions. Probanthine, 15 mgm three times a day, is suitable for a young child with day frequency. All these drugs are best used in combination with the training regime, and two may be used consecutively.

In the nervous frightened child sedation may be more useful than stimulation, and phenobarbitone is valuable as an adjunct to the environmental adjustment which is clearly essential.

Posterior pituitary extract (e.g. "Disipidin" snuff 100 mgm nightly) may be used to reduce the nocturnal flow of urine with effect in some enuretics (MARSON). The effect on renal secretion is comparatively short lived however and doubtless the drug, like other forms of treatment, depends for its success on the element of suggestion.

The spontaneous improvement observed at puberty, possibly associated with the development of the prostate, has suggested the use of hormone therapy to bring about the same effect prematurely. Androgens and pituitary gonadotropins have been employed and success claimed in both boys and girls, but most paediatricians find hormones are no more effective than less dangerous drugs.

3. Surgical treatment

Cases which have resisted training and medical treatment, and which have no obvious psychological complications should be subjected to a complete urological investigation: this may be undertaken earlier in those where abdominal pain, a history of past infection, or dysuria suggest that some organic lesion may be present, and it is better postponed in the case of uncomplicated nocturnal enuresis until other methods have been given an exhaustive trial. The findings of this investigation, together with the bias of the urologist, will naturally determine the treatment given and no universally applicable rules can be formulated. The lesion discovered may have no obvious connection with the enuresis, and must simply be treated on its own merits; meatal stenosis, urethral polyps, and mild degrees of bladder neck obstruction may be treated by dilatation or endoscopic diathermy. Plication operations on the female urethra, or on the bulb in the male should be reserved for older children in whom there is definite evidence of sphincter weakness.

G. The neurogenic bladder

The neurological lesions responsible for disorders of the bladder are as various in childhood as they are in adult life; tumours, traumatic lesions and inflammatory disease all play their part. By far the greatest number of cases, however, are due to congenital spinal cord lesions which are the main topic of this chapter.

I. Congenital spinal cord lesions

The neurogenic bladder is but one aspect of the difficult problem posed by spina bifida in its various forms, and the urologist must of necessity collaborate with those of his colleagues whose interest lies in the treatment of the spinal defect and the limb deformities, while the management of the older children involves a consideration of the forms of schooling best adapted to their capabilities, and of the emotional problems which all too often arise in the severely handicapped. However, the control of incontinence is the most important single factor in fitting these children for a useful existence, and renal failure is the most serious threat to the life of those who have survived the early hazards of meningitis and hydrocephalus.

1. The spinal defect

It is reasonably safe to assume that congenital lesions of the spinal cord likely to cause bladder disturbance are always associated with some malformation of the vertebral column, but the converse is very far from true, and there is very little correlation between the severity of the bony deformity and the nerve lesion. The various manifestations are best grouped according to the clinical and radiological features.

a) Spina bifida cystica

This term may be used to include all those common and obvious defects in the vertebral laminae in which a cystic swelling appears on the surface. In a few cases there may be a simple meningocele involving only the spinal membranes, but these are of little interest to the urologist; the great majority, particularly those in the lumbar and sacral regions are either myelomeningoceles, in which the spinal cord and nerve roots are applied to the walls of the sac, or myeloceles in which the cord is itself exposed and presents an ulcerated surface at birth, though it may later become epithelialized. In all cases the cord is bound down to the level of the defect, and cannot undergo the shortening normally shown in later foetal life. While most cases of spina bifida cystica are diagnosed without difficulty, it must be recalled that in the sacral region myelomeningoceles may be eccentric and deeply placed in the buttock, and on very rare occasions they are anterior and palpable only on pelvic examination.

b) Spina bifida occulta

In these cases there is a failure of fusion of the laminae of the vertebra, but no protrusion of the meninges. The gap in the bone is filled by a fibro-fatty pad and the overlying skin is often thickened, hairy, and naevoid. The cord is bound down to the level of the lesion and commonly exhibits some form of myelo-dysplasia: it may be split into two separate parts (diastematomyelia) or the central canal may be greatly distended (hydromyelia). It must always be emphasized that spina bifida of the lower lumbar and upper sacral vertebrae occurs very commonly without myelodysplasia and KARLIN found this purely radiological evidence of deformity in 54% of normal children who were suffering from no disorder of micturition. Moreover, despite conflicting opinions it seems that this lesion is not a cause of enuresis in cases where there is no other evidence of nerve damage (see p. 124).

c) Other bony deformities

Myelodysplasia may accompany many other types of vertebral malformation in the lumbar and sacral area, and although these cases form a small proportion of the total number of congenital spinal cord lesions they are of considerable importance to the urologist, since the bladder disturbance is commonly their chief manifestation and since there is little external indication of the bony deformity, which is therefore apt to be overlooked.

In sacral agenesis the entire sacrum or its lower elements are absent. Although in severe cases the iliac bones approach one another closely in the posterior midline there is very little orthopaedic disturbance and the deformity may be overlooked unless the sacral area is deliberately palpated (Fig. 85). Some degree of sacral agenesis is common in cases of imperforate anus, and where two or more sacral elements are missing some neurological disturbance of bladder function is to be anticipated, but in cases with the anal deformity a short sacrum often accompanies six lumbar vertebrae, and in that event no interference with the cauda equina will occur (WILLIAMS and NIXON). Partial agenesis may also complicate hemi-vertebrae and complex malformations of the lumbo-sacral junction which defy concise description.

Sacral "scoliosis", in which all the sacral elements are present, but are acutely deflected to one side, is another typical malformation, and one which in my experience has been particularly associated with a late onset of neurological disturbance. In these deformities the conus is not necessarily bound down to the site of the lesion as it is in spina bifida, but fibro-fatty masses of tissue occur in that region and myelodysplasia affects the cord above.

2. Neurological and orthopaedic signs

A considerable, but unknown proportion of cases of spina bifida cystica suffer from a complete flaccid paraplegia: many of these receive no treatment and die within the first weeks or months of life. Often spina bifida accompanies other deformities such as ectopia cloacae which are incompatible with survival. Hydrocephalus, present at birth or developing within the first year is responsible for the death of another considerable group. The cases which present for urological treatment have usually lesser degrees of paralysis though an increasing number of paraplegics are by the use of antibiotics brought through the dangers of infection. In many of the latter group, as CARR has emphasized, the proximal muscles of the lower limbs are sometimes active, and if contractual deformities can be prevented ambulation is possible with the assistance of walking calipers. Talipes

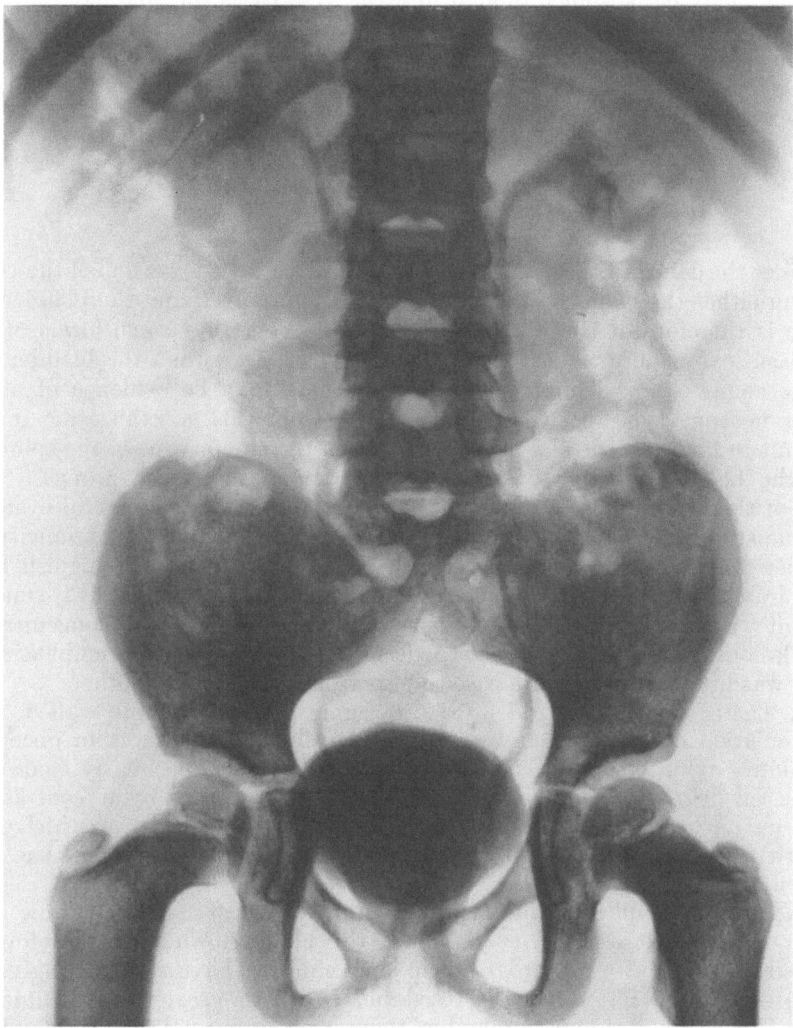

85. Sacral agenesis with neurogenic bladder. Intravenous pyelogram in a girl of 5 years. The sacrum is represented by one small element only

equino-varus and pes cavus are the most common of the minor deformities and provided they are treated early they need not present a serious handicap. Congenital dislocation of the hip is an additional complication in some children. It must be emphasized that many cases with paralytic foot deformities exhibit no disturbance of bladder function.

Anaesthesia of the skin naturally accompanies the motor disorder, and when the foot is involved trophic ulceration is often severe, leading to bone damage. Ulceration of the buttocks and perineum, resulting from pressure and continual wetness are also troublesome. Loss of sensation in the perineum is almost always present in any case in which the bladder is involved, but there are a few of the lower sacral deformities which are exceptions to this rule, and sensation is preserved in the the skin while it is lost in the bladder.

Absence of rectal sensation and paralysis of the anal musculature is usual. The anus may be patulous, though in less severe cases the sphincter is closed at rest but contracts very slowly after dilatation. Faeces accumulate in huge masses in the insensitive bowel causing overflow incontinence. As will be seen later, good management may lead to functional continence, even in the paralysed rectum, and obstinate constipation may be the only sign of the bowel disorder.

3. The bladder dysfunction

a) The natural history

Since the deformity responsible commonly affects the lower end of the vertebral column either the conus or the cauda equina is involved and the bladder disturbance is therefore of the lower motor neurone type, but some forms of myelodysplasia extend upwards from the bony defect, and when the bladder centres in the conus escape complete destruction there may be evidence of an upper motor neurone type of dysfunction. Apart from this generalization it is very difficult to find any correlation at all between the site or type of the spinal lesion and the bladder reaction. Various classifications have been proposed, though none of them is completely satisfactory. McCarrol made a careful cystometrographic study and classified cases according to the spasticity or atonicity of the bladder muscle and sphincter, and in general most authors distinguish between cases in which the obstructive factor is great and those in which it is small. The present writer, reviewing 65 cases of neurogenic bladder due to congenital spinal cord lesions, found it convenient to describe three types, and emphasized that there was little tendency for a case to pass from one type to another.

α) The first type of bladder to be recognized is flaccid, thin walled, without trabeculation and lacking any sensation of fullness. Post-mortem observations on infants dying of other causes show that this type is peculiarly characteristic of the severe myelomeningocele: in the lack of hypertrophy it contrasts with the usual autonomous bladder resulting from traumatic injuries, in which detrusor hypertrophy is often supposed to result from the activity of the intrinsic nervous elements.

In many examples of this type the urethral resistance is very low and the urine dribbles out as soon as it enters the bladder, which is therefore never distended. Still cysto-urethrograms in such children have a surprisingly normal appearance (Fig. 86). When the resistance is a little greater, the bladder has a larger capacity and is expressible, but there is no trabeculation, the bladder neck is flaccid, and the upper urinary tract is normal. There may be a residuum in the bladder after expression which will cause a dribbling incontinence, but a few fortunate children establish a balance between the powers of expression and the urethral resistance so that by periodic emptying of the bladder they can remain dry. This is an accomplishment which requires intelligence and practice, and is seldom achieved until 8 or 9 years of age. The balance will be upset by an attack of cystitis, or by a large accumulation of faeces in the rectum.

Some of the children with this type of bladder suffer attacks of acute retention in which no urine can be passed at all, the bladder becomes tensely distended and causes severe colicky pain. This pain, which is presumably mediated by sympathetic nerve fibres, is not recognized as arising from the bladder, but coincides with hardening of the tumour. Such attacks are precipitated by any type of operation, whether on the spinal cord, the urinary tract or the limbs, but sometimes come on for no apparent reason.

β) Clinically somewhat similar to the first group, but cystoscopically very different are the expressible bladders which show well marked trabeculation, sacculation and a dilated posterior urethra (Fig. 87), often with prominence of

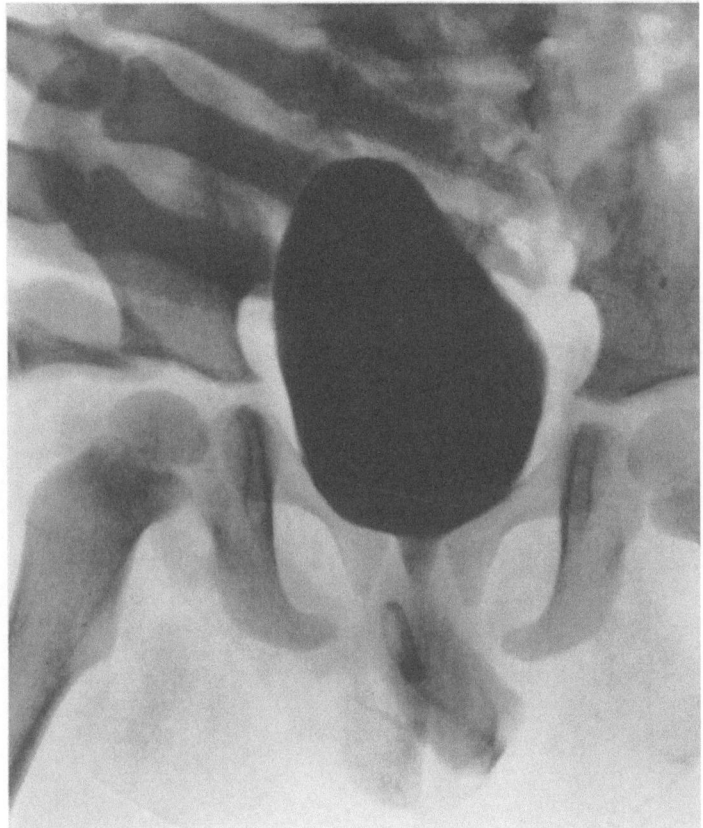

Fig. 86. Neurogenic bladder due to sacral myelomeningocele. Expression cystogram in a boy of 3 years. The bladder has a smooth wall, and the urethrographic outline is not grossly abnormal

the bladder neck as a strong hypertrophied bar. FISTER has reported a case in which the bladder neck became fibrotic and calcified. The sacculations may at times reach the dimensions of diverticula, and be separately palpable, but provided the urine is sterile, complete expression without residual urine is often possible. The upper urinary tract may still be normal or show a slight dilatation. These trabeculated bladders are also subject to attacks of acute retention, and they are a good deal more liable to urinary infection. When infection is present, the urine dribbles continuously, sometimes from a large residuum, sometimes from a small spastic bladder.

At times the trabeculated bladder is associated with severe upper urinary tract dilatation; in cases with gross hydro-ureter, it appears that the dilatation has been present from a very early age and probably develops before birth (Fig. 88). Reflux is common in such cases, but it is unlikely that it is the cause of the dilatation, since unilateral reflux is often seen in the presence of bilateral hydro-ureter (Fig. 89). It can be seen in cine films that these big ureters are unusually rigid and exhibit a striking contrast with the idiopathic megaureters in their lack of movement. Calculus formation is a complication in these cases. With such poor drainage of the upper urinary tract, infection is very liable to occur, and there is a progressive deterioration of renal function. The fact that the

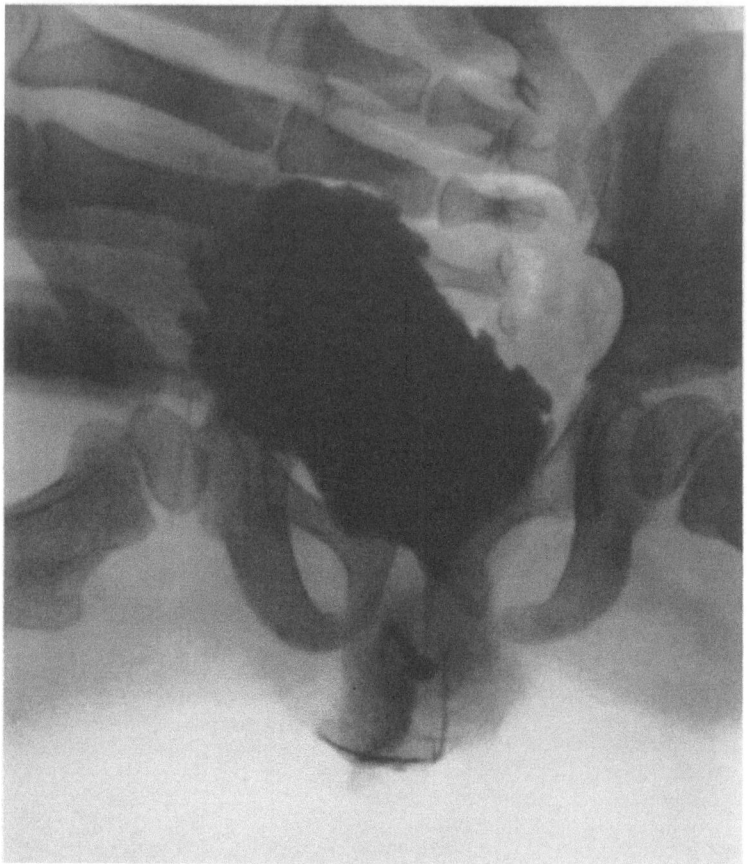

Fig. 87. Neurogenic bladder due to sacral myelo-meningocele. Expression cystogram in a boy aged 3 years. The bladder is severely trabeculated and sacculated, and the upper urethra is dilated. There was little residual urine after expression, and by this means he could be kept dry

kidneys are failing does not, however, affect the degree of continence: all expressible bladders can at times be controlled, and perfect control can be associated with a steadily rising blood urea. It might be supposed that where vesico-ureteric reflux is present, manual expression of the bladder contents would inevitably lead to further ureteric dilatation: fortunately this does not appear to be the case, and this method of management need not be discontinued on these grounds (PRINCE and SCARDINO).

γ) One other form of bladder dysfunction occurs, the type in which some sensation of bladder fullness is present, but as in some cases of disseminated sclerosis, micturition is frequent, urgent and often uncontrollable. Whereas the cases previously discussed may dribble urine in between expressions, these last children will often be incontinent of a large amount of urine at one time, though they never reach the stage of the true automatic bladder. Some residual urine is the rule, the bladder is usually trabeculated and the urethra dilated in the funnel-neck deformity. The upper urinary tract may not be seriously affected. Cystometrograms show a sharply rising curve with desire to void at quite low volumes. Continence may be achieved in these cases by regular timed micturition, so that the urgent desire does not occur.

Two further features of the natural history must be considered: the tendency towards spontaneous improvement, and the occasional deterioration. A number of children will by themselves learn to control their incontinence by frequent micturition as the importance of avoiding the embarrassment of wetness is appreciated, and they will become dry by the age of puberty: this number can be greatly increased by proper instruction, and the improvement is due to good management rather than to any change in the nervous lesion. By contrast an actual worsening of the neurological signs is observed, though much less often, in cases of spina bifida occulta or other bony deformities without meningocele, and may lead to a loss of control in a previously "normal" child; this event may also occur at about the age of puberty, but may be observed many years later. It has been

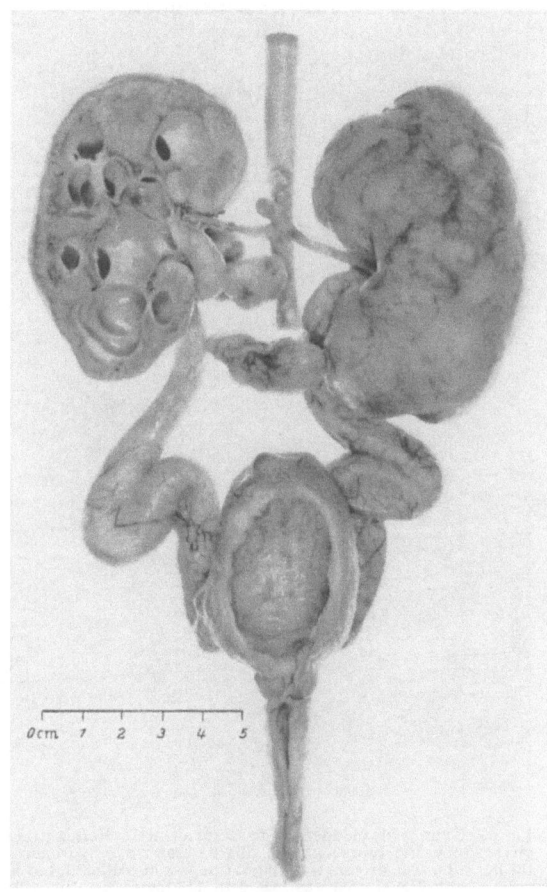

Fig. 88. Neurogenic bladder. Post-mortem specimen of the urinary tract of a boy dying at age of 4 months. There was a sacral meningomyelocele, and a characteristic expressible bladder. Specimen shows the hypertrophy of the detrusor and of bladder neck with bilateral hydronephrosis

attributed to increasing tension on the bands which tether the conus to the site of the vertebral deformity with growth in stature, but in the author's experience has on several occasions occurred after growth has ceased. The onset of a urinary infection is a more frequent cause of loss of urinary control in mildly affected neurogenic bladders, but is not of course associated with a change in the other neurological signs.

b) Diagnosis

In the great majority of cases the combination of urinary incontinence with spina bifida cystica leaves little doubt as to the presence of a neurogenic bladder; some bony deformity is to be expected in every case but difficulty may arise in the lesser lesions and in those who have no other indications of a cord lesion such as a flaccid anal sphincter or perineal anaesthesia. The differentiation from other causes of chronic retention can be made from the ease of expression in the case of the neurogenic bladder: emptying by manual pressure can very seldom be demonstrated in cases of mechanical obstruction except under anaesthesia, whereas the neurogenic bladder is nearly always partly or completely expressible.

Urinary infection, however, or faecal accumulation may temporarily suppress this phenomenon.

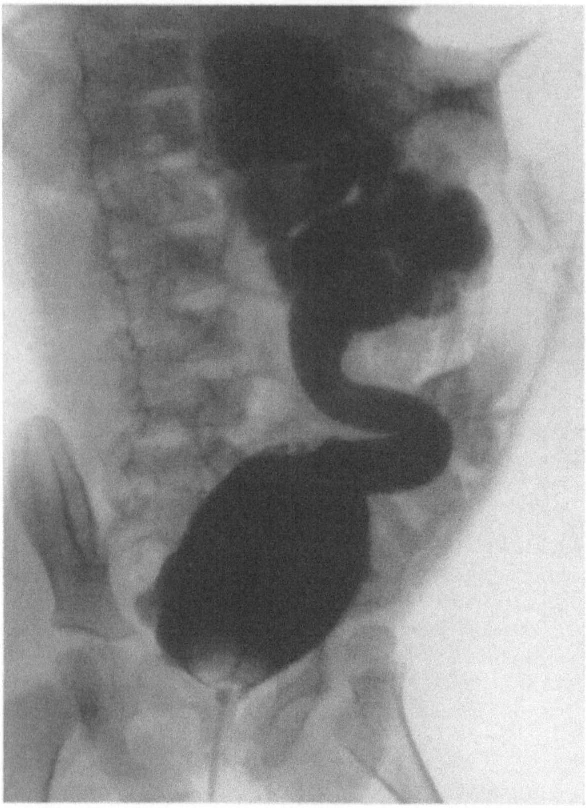

Where there is no retention, the differentiation has usually to be made from the simple "enuretic" type of diurnal incontinence and the failure of the neurogenic case to respond to a course of regular and timed micturition, together with the absence of proper sensation of bladder distension is one of the most reliable indications. These clinical features are of greater importance than the cystoscopic or urethrographic findings, which as already pointed out are very variable. The characteristic type of urethral dilatation is shown in Fig. 87; it will be seen that the narrowing below the dilated segment takes place about the level of the verumontanum, and not as in most cases of urethral valves at the level of the perineal membrane.

Fig. 89. Neurogenic bladder due to sacral agenesis. Reflux pyelogram in girl aged 2 years, shows a grossly dilated ureter and hydronephrosis on the left side. The ureter on the right side was also dilated, but no reflux was present. Blood urea was raised to 115 mgm.-%. Cine films show the ureter to be incapable of contraction

Where the bladder dysfunction suggests a neurological lesion, but the vertebral column is radiologically normal an acquired lesion should be suspected and myelograms will assist in the diagnosis.

c) Treatment
α) Treatment of the spinal cord lesion

This aspect is outside the scope of the present work, but there are certain facts of importance to be noted. The surgical treatment of spina bifida cystica may be desirable for a variety of reasons, but it does not lead to any improvement in the condition of the bladder; it is, in fact, more liable to lead to a deterioration, temporary or permanent, since some nerve tissue in the lining of the sac may be destroyed. There are many tragic cases of children who had normal control until an operation was undertaken for cosmetic improvement of the unsightly swelling on the back, and who were thereafter completely incontinent.

In spina bifida occulta and other bony deformities without meningocele there is a somewhat greater chance of improvement from laminectomy and the freeing of tethering bands, but whereas a number of reports have viewed this proceeding with favour (e.g. MERTZ), in other centres results have been disappointing, and the procedure has been virtually abandoned. Recent deterioration of the bladder condition and of other neurological signs, and particularly the onset of the disorder around puberty, are good indications for neuro-surgical intervention.

β) General management of the bladder disorder

Almost all cases in their early years, and some cases throughout life should be managed conservatively, and a fair proportion of good results may be expected. This aspect has been emphasized by McCARROL, by PRINCE and SCARDINO, and by the present writer, who found that almost one third of his cases were able to achieve sufficient control after the age of 9 years to manage without appliances. The aim is to empty the bladder completely at regular intervals by expression, so that the dribbling incontinence is reduced to a minimum. In the very young this expression must be performed manually by the mother, but soon the child will learn to do it himself, either with his hands or his diaphragm and abdominal muscles.

Regular expression will fail to rectify the incontinence if the urethral resistance is very low, so that the bladder is never distended, or if the resistance is high and a residual remains after the act. The girls with low urethral resistance will almost certainly require surgical interference in the form of a supportive operation or a diversion of urine (see below), the boys may be able to manage with a penile urinal; in neither case is there a danger of hydronephrosis or renal failure. When the urethral resistance is high, it may often be lowered by keeping the rectum empty. The presence of a large accumulation of faeces in the bowel is always a handicap to these children, and must be prevented in order to achieve both rectal and urinary control. Regular bowel actions may sometimes be obtained by the use of aperients, but often enemata are required perhaps as often as twice or three times per week. If the anal sphincter is too flaccid to allow retention of the enema fluid, digital assistance in defaecation may be more effective. Complete expression may also be handicapped by urinary infection and continuous chemotherapy is at times necessary to prevent recurrent attacks.

When after a fair trial of simple measures, there is still a large residuum in the bladder after expression, operations designed to lower the urethral resistance may be undertaken: these are discussed below. Should these procedures fail, a progressive dilatation of the upper urinary tract will often indicate the need for a diversion of the urine from the bladder or from the ureters.

γ) Operations designed to increase the urethral resistance

These procedures have usually been employed in girls, and have on the whole met with very little success. SMITH and ENGEL and later PICKRELL et al. report the use of gracilis transplants, GODARD tried the Goebell-Stoeckell operation which brings down the pyramidalis muscles, EMMETT and HELMHOLZ have plicated the urethra (at the same time resecting the bladder neck). All these operations undertaken in the anaesthetic area are liable to break down, and it is very difficult to adjust the tightness of the urethra to the powers of expression; nevertheless, they have a place in the treatment of children who suffer only a slight degree of incontinence between expressions. SWENSON et al. have recently described an operation for more severe cases of this type, in which the urethra is surrounded by an inflatable rubber cuff, lying in a skin-lined pocket.

δ) Operations designed to lower the urethral resistance

Bladder neck resection, best performed by the transurethral route, has had a considerable vogue in the treatment of the neurogenic bladder, and its use in children has been discussed by EMMETT and HELMHOLZ, and THOMPSON and JACOBSON. In my view it has a limited place in treatment and is indicated chiefly in those boys who have trabeculated bladders with hypertrophied internal sphincters, in whom the bladder cannot be completely emptied by expression. In girls it is unlikely that this measure will assist in the achievement of continence, though it may occasionally be employed in babies where there is a considerable obstructive element. Simple urethral dilatations have been advocated by SMITH and ENGEL, but are now seldom practised.

Presacral neurectomy is said to facilitate the expression of the bladder and successes have been reported from time to time, particularly by CREEVY. Section of the pudendal nerve has been used in traumatic paraplegia, but probably has little place in the congenital cases which are almost always lower motor neurone lesions.

ε) Operations for the diversion of urine

These procedures may be used to secure adequate drainage of a dilated urinary tract, or simply in order to control incontinence by substituting for the urethra a more convenient outlet for urine. In the first case the timing of the operation will depend entirely on the progress of the disease; in the latter, interference should be postponed until it is certain that there is no hope of spontaneous improvement.

The simplest of these methods is suprapubic cystostomy, and where there is a considerable volume of residual urine the immediate results are beneficial, but there are serious disadvantages in the long run. The bladder inevitably becomes infected and contracted around the tube, and despite free drainage from the bladder cavity, progressive ureteric dilatation is often seen; moreover, the fistula is difficult to maintain in a healthy state, and after some years leakage around the tube is likely. When suprapubic cystostomy is used simply for the control of incontinence in girls, it has the additional disadvantage that it is difficult to close off the urethra: simple ligature is never enough and even a carefully performed section with suture of the cut end may break down in the presence of infection.

An indwelling FOLEY catheter in the urethra is a measure which may be mentioned here: it may be a useful temporary expedient, but the likelihood of trophic changes in the urethra is so great that it should not be employed permanently.

Uretero-sigmoidostomy is of little value in the congenital neurogenic bladder, as the anal sphincter is scarcely ever adequate to control the urine, even if faecal continence is good. Cutaneous ureterostomy may be useful, particularly where the ureters are dilated and elongated so that they are easily brought up to the surface; the opening may be made flush with the skin and the urine drained into an ileostomy bag or the ureter may be led up into the skin spout (ureter-penis, THIERMANN). Cutaneous ureterostomy involves less operative risk, but is in every other way inferior to transplantation of the ureters into an isolated ileal loop which drains freely into an ileostomy bag on the abdominal wall. Very satisfactory results may be obtained by this method, as has been reported by JENSEN et al., and NASH. The procedure appears to be equally suitable for the drainage of dilated ureters, or for the simple control of incontinence in girls, though the collecting apparatus is inconvenient in very young children.

ζ) Appliances for the control of urethral incontinence

No satisfactory portable urinal has yet been devised for the female, and where conservative management has failed, diversion to the isolated ileal loop is recommended. In the male, a penile urinal may be fitted as soon as the penis has reached adequate proportions, and where there is no serious degree of urinary obstruction, this method is usually preferred to urinary diversion. A penile clip may be useful in cases where leakage is slight: a special clamp for children has been devised by CAMPBELL, but though a large number of patterns have been tried by the present writer, none has proved ideal. Application of a clip requires a circumcised penis.

II. Poliomyelitis

Poliomyelitis is responsible for acute retention in 10—20% of cases during the first week; in all surviving cases the bladder will recover its function (CLARKE), and disorders of the urinary tract in this disease result chiefly from infection and from recumbency stone formation. It is often necessary to catheterize the child during the period of retention, but this should naturally be avoided if possible. LAWSON and GARVEY have emphasized the value of parasympathomimetic drugs in the treatment of temporary dysfunction.

H. Non-tuberculous urinary infections

I. Incidence

Urinary infections and their consequences constitute a very large proportion of the urological problems of childhood, and although modern drugs have given us an effective weapon against the acute invasions, the slow deterioration of renal function which results from a chronic inflammatory process is still a common cause of death in urinary disease. The urological surgeon is largely pre-occupied with infections complicating congenital anomalies or calculous disease, and the importance of these factors is repeatedly emphasized throughout this volume, yet spontaneous infection of the anatomically normal urinary tract is a common disorder of childhood. Prompt recognition and early medical treatment of such infection will cut short a disease which often leads to renal failure and hypertension in early adult life.

It is impossible to give any estimate of the overall incidence of urinary infections; CAMPBELL reports from New York that they accounted for 0.8% of all children's hospital admissions at his centre, but doubtless statistics would vary considerably from one community to another. Infants in the first year of life are more frequently affected than older children, and at this stage boys are involved almost as often as girls, perhaps even more often in the neonatal period. In later childhood, however, girls are the chief sufferers, and infection in a boy is likely to indicate some more serious disorder of the urinary tract.

A seasonal variation was at one time suspected, the incidence rising with the prevalence of gastro-enteritis, but at present there is little evidence of this in England where epidemic gastro-enteritis is now uncommon. Infections are not passed directly from one child to another, except perhaps in hospital, where ward epidemics commonly affect only those children who have indwelling catheters and drainage tubes.

II. Bacteriology and mode of infection

The organisms most frequently encountered are those included in the group Escherischia coli, named after the German physician whose work first impressed upon the medical world the importance of urinary infections in children. There are, of course, many strains within this group, and in some cases a more precise identification may be required: from the clinical standpoint, it is the sensitivity of the organism to drugs which is of most importance, and this information should be supplied by the laboratory as a routine. Of the other Gram-negative bacilli, Aerobacter aerogenes is a relatively common invader; Proteus vulgaris is particularly frequent in cases of stone formation, but is also regrettably prevalent where an indwelling catheter has been employed. Pseudomonas pyocyanea is another organism more often responsible for secondary than for primary infections. Typhoid, paratyphoid and the dysentery bacilli are occasionally found. Almost all these bacilli are capable, at times, of splitting the urinary urea and producing a strongly alkaline urine which particularly favours the deposition of phosphatic stones. Where the urinary tract is undamaged, however, sterilization of the urine can almost always be achieved with or without the aid of antibiotics: the difficulties in the treatment of Proteus and Pseudomonas infections lie not only in their resistance to drugs but in the abnormalities of the urinary tract with which they are so often associated.

Since E. coli and many of the other infecting organisms are normal inhabitants of the large bowel, it is natural to suppose that the intestinal contents are the source of the urinary infection. Although a direct lymphatic communication between the bowel and the kidney was at one time suggested as the mode of entry, this hypothesis has received little support from anatomical or pathological evidence, and many authors believe that faecal contamination of the external urinary meatus is the most important factor. In infants of the "napkin" age such contamination is easily and frequently observed, particularly in the female, but it remains impossible to prove any causal relationship to urinary infection. A great deal of discussion has centred around the possibility of ascending infection but a full rehearsal of the arguments employed would be out of place in this volume and the works of HELMHOLZ should be consulted. Most urologists are of the opinion that organisms can sometimes ascend from the urethra to the kidney, either via the peri-ureteral lymphatics (WINSBURY-WHITE), or in the urine itself, since inflammation in the bladder may render the uretero-vesical valve incompetent and allow reflux. On the other hand, the fever which sometimes follows instrumentation appears to be due to release of organisms into the blood stream from the traumatized area, and a subsequent pyelonephritis might therefore be due to blood borne infection. At all events, in experimental infections, the effect upon the kidney is practically identical in both ascending and haematogenous infections (KENNEDY) and elucidation of the exact mode of entry of organisms reaching the kidney has little importance to the clinician.

Urinary infections are also due to the Gram-positive cocci: Staphylococcus albus and aureus are both organisms that are pathogenic in the urinary tract, and the latter is particularly likely to be responsible for pyaemic infections of the kidney in cases of osteomyelitis and skin or umbilical sepsis. Both streptococci and staphylococci may be released into the blood stream from infective foci in the throat or sinuses during surgical manipulations and may then initiate a pyelonephritis. DE NAVASQUEZ has argued from experimental evidence in the rabbit that blood borne staphylococcal invasion is often the primary cause of the pyelonephritic lesion and that the damage produced predisposes to the E. coli and other infections more commonly found in clinical practice. Strept. faecalis is quite frequently isolated from infected urine and its mode of entry is doubtless similar to that of the E. coli group.

III. Acute urinary infections

1. Pathology

a) Acute pyelonephritis

A simple urinary infection which responds readily to medical treatment is often described as "pyelitis". It has long been established, however, by the work of CHOWN, HELMHOLZ, and WILSON and SCHLOSS, that an inflammatory process confined to the renal pelvis is exceptionally rare; the lesions almost always involve the renal parenchyma and the term pyelonephritis is to be preferred. Clinically it may even be preferable to speak of pyuria and to avoid any attempt at localization of the infection, but there is no doubt that, although other forms of acute infection may occur, pyelonephritis is much the most common inflammatory lesion of the kidney, either as the only lesion or as a complication of other disorders of the urinary tract such as hydronephrosis or stone.

In acute pyelonephritis the kidney is usually slightly or moderately enlarged.

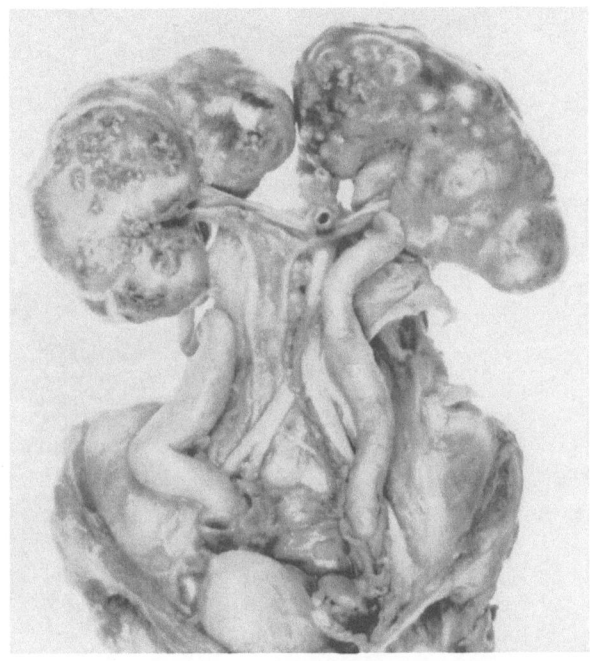

Fig. 90. Acute pyelonephritis complicating a dilated upper urinary tract associated with neurogenic bladder. Post-mortem specimen for a girl aged 2 years

The subcapsular surface is smooth, often congested and may show some yellow abscesses. On the cut surface the pelvic mucosa is seen to be oedematous and reddened and is often covered with an exudate. The parenchyma is swollen and irregularly congested, with radially arranged yellow streaks running from the subcapsular surface to the calyces (Fig. 90). Microscopically, the tubules and interstitial tissues contain pus cells and there are leucocytes in the periglomerular lymphatics, and occasionally in the glomeruli as well. Rarely necrosis of the capillary loops can be seen: the alterative glomerulitis of KIMMELSTIEL and WILSON. All stages of tubular damage are found from cloudy swelling to complete destruction of the epithelium. Not infrequently there is disruption of the affected tubules with the formation of an abscess. Vascular thrombi are frequent.

Pyelonephritis in the new-born infant has been discussed by PORTER and GILES. In their cases, although the typical tubular lesions were present, there were also well marked glomerular changes, with the formation of epithelial crescents. Microdissection studies showed that anomalous nephrons were present, the proximal tubules being short, straight and dilated, and in the opinion of the authors these anomalies predisposed to infection. CLAIREAUX and PEARSON have reported a case of an infant dying at 10 hours, whose kidneys were histologically similar to those described by PORTER and GILES, and were also regarded as pyelonephritic, but as there was no evidence of an ante-natal infection of the foetus, a hypersensitivity reaction was postulated as the cause.

b) Infected hydronephrosis and pyonephrosis

When an acute infection supervenes in a case of congenital lower urinary obstruction in an infant, pyelonephritis may progress to a diffuse suppuration,

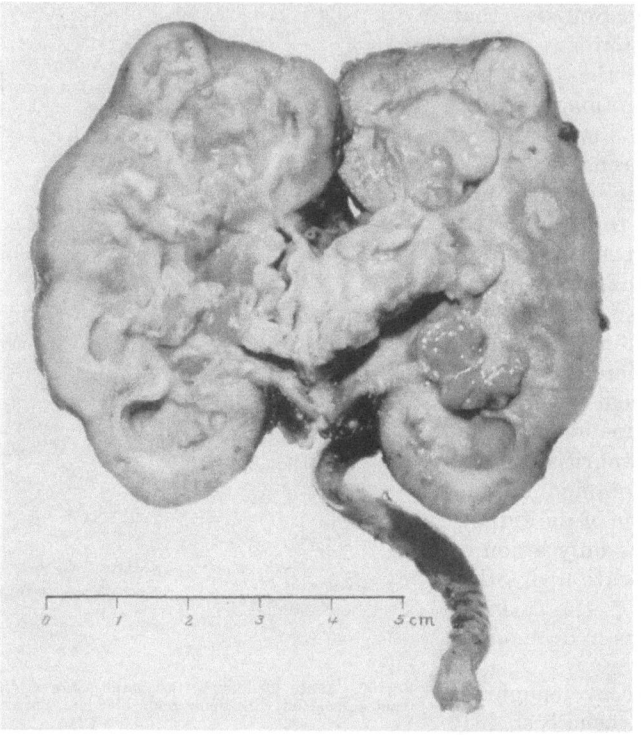

Fig. 91. Pyonephrosis. Operative specimen from a girl aged six months suffering from a persistent E. coli and Proteus urinary infection. Straight X-rays showed a faint opacity in the left renal area, there was no function in in the left kidney on intra-venous pyelograms. The specimen shows an extensive suppurative nephritis with a large clot of congealed pus filling the pelvis. Uninterrupted recovery, following nephrectomy

similar to the "surgical kidney" of the elderly prostatic. There is anuria with rapid destruction of the renal substance. Infection in the dilated urinary passages leads to the formation of large quantities of mucopus and considerable oedema of the ureteric mucosa.

The term pyonephrosis may indicate an advanced suppurative condition resulting from the coalescence of pyaemic abscesses (Fig. 97), but is perhaps better used to describe the condition in which the renal pelvis and calyces become filled with a clot of thick coagulated pus (Fig. 91). This latter phenomenon is not the usual outcome of an infected hydronephrosis, though it may be seen in cases of calculous obstruction of very long standing (Fig. 107). It is a chronic process in the usual unilateral cases, and it seems likely that it occurs when an acute infection is partially checked by chemotherapy. The parenchyma shows advanced pyelonephritic changes, with some perinephric inflammation, and usually with considerable enlargement of the hilar lymph nodes.

2. Clinical features

a) In the neonate

Pyelonephritis is not so common during the first two or three weeks as in later infancy, and as already remarked, may show some unusual features in its pathology. During the first few days of life, normal urine may contain some albumin, red cells and casts, and these should not be regarded as evidence of infection unless accompanied by numerous pus cells. CRAIG found that the onset was often insidious in the neonate: oliguria and anuria occurred with some oedema in severe cases. The temperature is intermittently raised to high levels, but in very sick infants it may be persistently subnormal. Vomiting, diarrhoea, and dehydration are frequent. Jaundice may be the presenting feature in this as in other neonatal infections.

The kidneys may be normally palpable in the newborn and in infection some enlargement and hardening may be discernible. In other respects neonatal infections are similar to those in infants who have passed their first weeks and are discussed in the following section.

b) In the infant

An upper respiratory infection, or an attack of gastro-enteritis may occasionally precede the urinary tract disorder, but usually no such history is obtainable. In some the onset is abrupt with a high swinging temperature, rigors and acute toxaemia; in others it is gradual, the child having been off colour for some time before he is brought to the doctor. Disorders of micturition are seldom prominent and are in any case apt to be concealed by the use of napkins, but the child may cry while passing urine. Vomiting is almost always a feature and intestinal disorders are frequent, constipation being at least as common as diarrhoea. The abdomen is often distended, and at times the infant appears to have some abdominal pain. He is reluctant to take milk or solid food, though he may drink water thirstily. Dehydration is often present and may be severe. In very acute cases there are fits, or perhaps signs of meningeal irritation, though a spinal tap will give clear fluid.

The diagnosis is made on examination of the urine and, in view of the vague nature of the symptoms, it is clear that the urine must be examined as a routine in all infants with pyrexia, or intestinal disorders. A clean specimen is adequate in the case of a boy (p. 3) but a catheter must passed in the girls if an accurate assessment is to be made. The urine shows an excess of pus cells (more than 2 or 3 per high power field) and the cells usually gather in clumps. MASTERS and STANSFIELD have entered a plea for a more accurate estimation of the number of white cells in the urine and advocate the use of a counting chamber as for blood: both authors would regard a count of 50 cells/ml as abnormal and be prepared to make the diagnosis of pyelonephritis on this alone, without bacteriological confirmation. It must be remembered, however, that a febrile and dehydrated infant will always produce a slight excess of pus cells in the urine, and it is wise to allow some elasticity in the criteria of diagnosis: the renal tubular disorders, such as infantile hyperchloraemic acidosis, are usually accompanied by some pyuria, even though there is no evidence of pyelonephritis.

In true urinary infections, the amount of pus may vary considerably from one specimen to another, and during the first two or three days of the pyrexia the urine may contain numerous bacteria but no cells. Urine culture should always be made to confirm the nature of the organism involved. Blood cultures are positive only in very severe cases.

The dehydrated infant with urinary infection will have a somewhat raised blood urea, up to 80 to 100 mgm/100 ml even if no other abnormality is present in the urinary tract. Some degree of acidosis is always likely.

c) In the older child

In the later years of childhood, urinary infections are less severe, and produce symptoms which usually indicate their presence. High temperatures and rigors are common, frequency and urgency of micturition with scalding pain are typical complaints. Sometimes there is considerable renal pain, unilateral or bilateral, or pain may be ill-localized in the abdomen and give rise to the suspicion of appendicitis. Once more the urine will be found to contain pus cells, red cells, albumin and a few casts.

In milder cases, the temperature is little raised, and particularly in girls it may be that a simple cystitis is present without involvement of the upper urinary tract. If in these mild attacks the urine specimen is not obtained immediately, diagnosis may be difficult, for many children have slight dysuria with oliguria during upper respiratory infections, and in girls a simple vulvitis can often lead to pain on micturition, although the urine is normal.

d) Complicated cases

The natural course of an acute urinary infection is towards recovery after one or two weeks, though some symptomless pyuria may persist for much longer, and indicate the onset of a chronic pyelonephritis. In the occasional case, however, there is no immediate response to treatment, and the child's condition deteriorates. This is particularly likely to occur where there is a urinary obstruction, most often in the lower urinary tract; the bladder becomes palpably distended, the kidneys enlarged and tender. Haematuria and the passage of mucopus may be observed, and there is a severe rise of blood urea. With modern antibiotics, even these cases can be temporarily sterilized, but unless free drainage is soon re-established, a fatal oliguria may supervene. Where an upper urinary tract anomaly or a stone is the cause of peristent pyrexia, the unilateral nature of the disorder can usually be appreciated on abdominal palpation and the danger to life is not so great.

3. Management

The treatment of an uncomplicated acute urinary infection consists primarily in appropriate chemotherapy, and in the older child little else is required. In infants correction of dehydration and acidosis may be urgent, and when a complicating urinary obstruction is present, surgical measures may be needed to secure adequate drainage. The great majority of infections acquired outside hospital respond to sulphonamides, and one of these drugs should be started as soon as the diagnosis of pyuria is made from examination of the urine. A wide variety of sulphonamides is available and tablets containing a mixture of drugs have had a certain popularity. In spite of much theoretical argument, there does not appear to be any reliable evidence that a mixture of sulphonamides is superior to a single drug which is readily soluble, and my own preference is to employ Gantrisin (Sulphafurazole 0.2—0.4 gm/Kilo/day, for a small infant, half this dose for larger children, and never more than 8 gm a day). This can be given in tablet form or as a suspension in syrup; it is readily soluble in the urine, no alkalis are required and it has a wide range of action. Sulphacetamide and sulphadimidine are also suitable drugs which can be given in the same dosage. In many cases the urine will clear within two or three days of commencing this treatment, but the full dosage should be maintained for a week, and in infants it is probably wise to continue treatment with half doses for another 3 or 4 weeks to ensure full resolution. The urine should be checked microscopically at the end of the course, and again a month later.

Failure to respond to sulphonamide may be due to the presence of an insensitive organism, or to a complicating abnormality in the urinary tract. The nature of the infection and its susceptibility to antibiotics should be determined by culture and treatment altered accordingly. Penicillin (10,000 units/Kilo/day) is useful only in the coccal infections, which form a minority: when indicated for urinary tract disorders parenteral administration is much preferred to oral treatment. Streptomycin (40 mgm/Kilo/day by intramuscular injection in two doses) is active against many of the Gram-negative bacilli; the course should not be continued for more than three or four days, as resistance to the drug is rapidly acquired and toxic effects may complicate prolonged treatment. Aureomycin, Tetracyclin (10—20 mgm/Kilo/day) and Terramycin (20—40 mgm/Kilo/day) are given orally and are valuable but apt to be complicated by diarrhoea. Chloromycetin (50 mgm/Kilo/day) is put up in a convenient liquid form for children, and provided only short courses are given the danger of aplastic anaemia appears to be remote. Erythromycin (30 mgm/Kilo/day) is probably best held in reserve and used only where no other drugs are likely to be active.

Mandelates have little place in acute infections, though they may be useful in chronic cases with resistant organisms. Mandelamine (MENLEY and JAMES, tabs i—ii t.d.s.) is a convenient compound of mandelic acid and hexamine, and may be administered for long periods without danger of complication.

Nitrofurantin (5 mgm/kilo/day) is sometimes of value where the antibiotics are ineffective.

In many cases antibiotic treatment will sterilize the urine even in the presence of obstruction but continuing pyrexia, or rising blood urea will indicate the urgent need for surgery. In cases of lower urinary obstruction, the bladder will be palpably distended, and micturition reduced to a dribble. No attempt at a full anatomical diagnosis should be made at this stage; the urinary tract should be drained by bilateral pyelostomy in infants, or by suprapubic cystostomy in older children. A simple indwelling urethral catheter is very seldom adequate, and in the very young becomes easily blocked. Once a free flow of urine is obtained, the infection is easily brought under control, and subsequent investigation and treatment should follow the lines suggested in section E.

Upper tract obstructions and calculi are also causes of continued infection, but are usually unilateral and so interfere less with total renal function. Radiological studies are therefore possible in most of these cases, and often nephrectomy or heminephrectomy is the appropriate treatment.

IV. Chronic and recurrent urinary infection

A simple acute urinary infection responds rapidly to treatment, and if pyuria persists or recurs after the acute symptoms have subsided, a full urological investigation should be undertaken as it is likely that some underlying abnormality will be found. In ideal circumstances it might be desirable to have an intravenous pyelogram in all children who had suffered a urinary infection, in order to forestall the possibility of recurrence due to a remediable lesion, but in most hospitals this would involve an impossibly heavy demand upon the X-ray facilities, and the investigation has to be reserved for certain categories. My own practice is to insist on a pyelogram where:

(i) Pyuria persists after adequate chemotherapy.

(ii) The initial infection is very severe, and causes haematuria, enlargement of the kidney, distension of the bladder or a considerable rise of blood urea.

(iii) The infecting organism is Proteus or Pseudomonas.

(iv) Two or more recurrences have been observed in a girl.

(v) Any infection occurs in a boy past the age of 1 year.

Intravenous pyelography is normally the first investigation to be performed, although if the child appears at all ill, a blood urea estimation should precede it as in uraemia the method is unhelpful and not without danger. Cystoscopy, urethroscopy and retrograde pyelograms may be required in some cases.

These investigations may reveal the presence of chronic pyelonephritis without any other abnormality: this disease is discussed in the following section. In many cases a urinary tract disorder will be found, with or without scarring in the kidney itself; the disorder is usually an obstruction or a stone. The various types of ureteric dilatations and duplications are most often recognized because of investigation in cases of recurrent or persistent infection. The pyelograms must always be studied with the possibility of a double ureter in mind, remembering that the corresponding renal element may be functionless, so that the presence of the offending organ has to be surmised from the characteristic deformity of the unaffected pelvis (p. 36). Hydronephrosis, vesical diverticulum or lower urinary obstruction may also be revealed. The management of all these conditions is essentially surgical and is discussed elsewhere in this volume.

While great emphasis must be laid upon the importance of chronic pyelonephritis and urinary tract anomalies, it must be recognized that in girls, particularly during the later years of childhood, it is not uncommon to observe recurrent mild infections in a urinary tract which all investigations indicate to be entirely normal. Some of these episodes may be attacks of simple cystitis, but in others pain and high temperatures indicate renal involvement. Although short-lived and followed by complete recovery, the cumulative effect of a number of these attacks lowers the general health of the child, and interferes seriously with her education. Whether or not treatment is given, attacks tend to cease about the age of puberty, but there is always the fear that the recurrent infections may produce chronic pyelonephritic changes and serious complications in later life. WHARTON et al. analysing the late effects of "acute pyelitis", emphasized the frequency with which such complications were found, but their only serious case was one in which pyelonephritic scarring was clearly present from the time of first investigation, while some of their other "late complications", such as slight dilatation of the lumbar ureter, and slight pyuria could probably be found as often in an unselected group of women. WOODRUFF and EVERETT also found several abnormalities in a group of young women who had had urinary infection in childhood, but many had not previously been investigated and there was no evidence to suggest that these abnormalities could not have been detected at the time of the infection. It is well known that pregnancy is apt to lead to a recurrence of infection in previously damaged kidneys, but HELMHOLZ believes that where the urinary tract is normal, there is little danger to be anticipated. Thus although pyuria may well indicate a serious disorder, a good prognosis can be given for recurrent infections in older girls in whom a searching investigation has revealed no abnormality.

In the management of these cases, every attempt must naturally be made to prevent the recurrences. Attacks are sometimes brought on by exposure to cold, by upper respiratory infection, and by constipation, and where possible these predisposing conditions must be avoided. Tonsillectomy and eradication of other foci of infection is occasionally indicated. Continuous chemotherapy

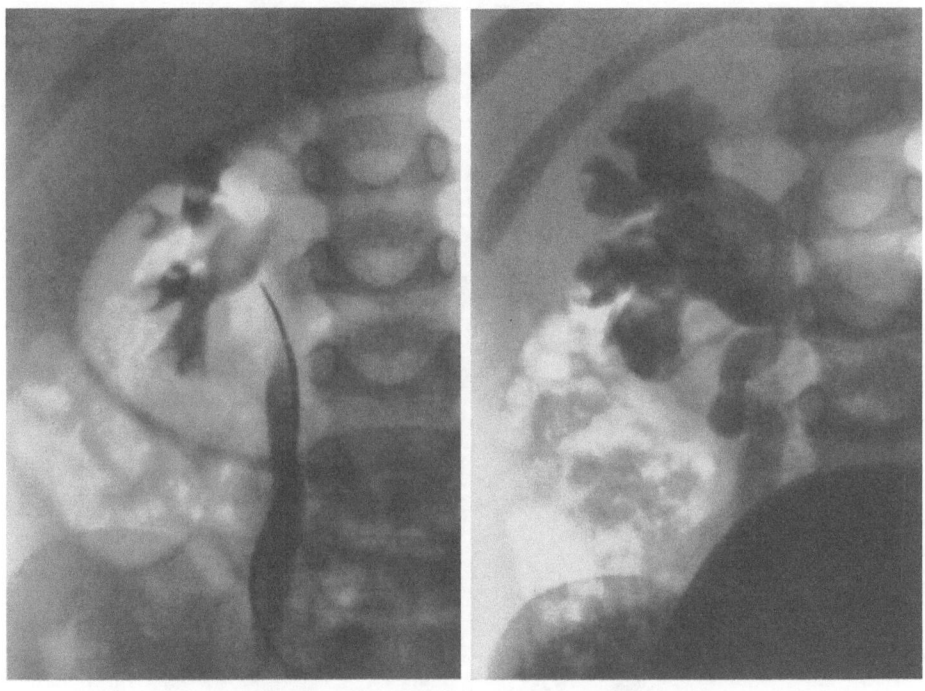

A   B

Fig. 92 A and B. Vesico-ureteral reflux with slight hydro-ureter associated with recurrent urinary infection. A Retrograde pyelogram, B Cystogram. Boy aged 5 years with four attacks of severe E. Coli infection. Cystoscopy and intravenous pyelogram passed as normal. Retrograde pyelogram shows only slight ureteric dilatation, but free reflux is present and causes considerable distension of pelvis and ureter

(p. 149) is the most reliable preventive measure, and may need to be administered for periods varying from six months to two years or more, in fact until the child has grown out of the liability to attacks. When a cystogram shows reflux in an otherwise normal urinary tract, operations to prevent this phenomenon (p. 54) may be undertaken if continuous chemotherapy fails.

V. Chronic pyelonephritis

1. Pathology

Recovery from mild attacks of pyelonephritis may be almost complete though the healing of abscesses will naturally lead to the formation of radial scars, while some tubules may have been altogether destroyed. The changes of chronic pyelonephritis result as often from the scarring left by repeated acute attacks as from a long continued infection, and the chronic disease is an insidious one, the presence of which may be unsuspected clinically until the destruction of the renal parenchyma is far advanced. At autopsy, the kidneys may be so shrunken and scarred that it is difficult to identify the original lesions by naked eye examination, or to distinguish pyelonephritis from congenital hypoplasia.

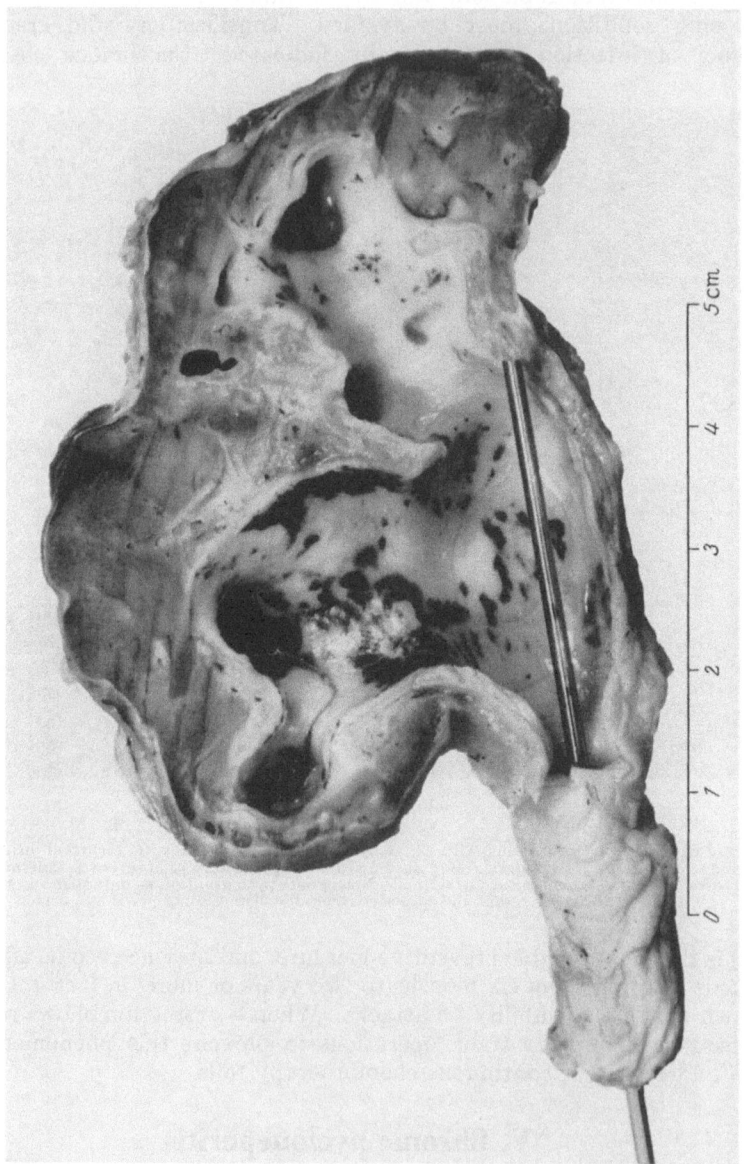

Fig. 93. Chronic pyelonephritis. Nephrectomy specimen from a girl aged 17 years with hypertension. Specimen shows the characteristic scarring of the cortex, and thickened blood vessels

The pathological characteristics of chronic pyelonephritis have been admirably described by WEISS and PARKER. The lesions are irregularly disposed throughout the organ, and almost invariably one kidney is much more severely affected than its fellow. The capsule is thickened and strips only with difficulty, often tearing the underlying cortex. Wedge-shaped scars in the parenchyma pucker the surface and extend in towards the calyces (Fig. 93). The cortex is thinner than normal, and in long standing cases the surviving tissue between the scars hypertrophies and forms raised rounded nodules which grossly distort the kidney pattern: they often undergo fatty change and are then seen as pale nodular zones on the subcapsular surface. Usually the pelvis and ureter are dilated and thick-walled, and in many cases the hilar vessels are more prominent than usual. Microscopy of the scarred areas shows the tubules to be chiefly affected: many are small and atrophic, some dilated with a low epithelial lining. The presence of colloid casts gives these tubules a certain resemblance to the thyroid acini. Often there is a severe lymphocytic infiltration. The glomeruli may appear normal, but there is usually well marked periglomerular fibrosis, and occasionally complete hyalinization. Between the scars the kidney tissue is relatively normal or else shows hypertrophic changes, with dilated tubules and enlarged glomeruli.

In the scarred area vascular changes, consisting of endarteritis of the larger vessels and hyperplasia with hyalinization of the arterioles, are almost invariable and occur as an essential part of the pyelonephritic process. When hypertension supervenes similar vascular lesions affect all parts of the kidney, and perhaps other organs as well; necrotizing changes in the glomerular afferent artery being characteristic.

MARSHALL has drawn attention to the presence of primitive or "dysplastic" elements in pyelonephritic kidneys. Primitive tubules are most easily recognized, not only are they wide, straight and radially disposed, but they also reach the capsule where they curl round to join their glomeruli. In the medulla they have a characteristic collar of fibro-muscular tissue. Proglomeruli, without differentiation of tuft and capsule, and infantile glomeruli, in which the tuft is still compact and invested by a layer of cuboidal cells, are also described. Masses of loose fibrous tissue, hyaline cartilage and angiomatous areas are other "dysplastic" features. It has already been mentioned in another section that these primitive elements are regularly seen in the congenital dysplastic kidney in which secondary pyelonephritic changes are the rule; it has yet to be established, however, that they play any important role in the onset of pyelonephritis in the otherwise normal kidney.

2. Clinical features

Chronic pyelonephritis may follow acute urinary infection, and be itself responsible for recurrent attacks, but in many cases it is an insidious and slowly progressive disease in which no acute episodes can be recognized. Symptoms of a disease which starts in early childhood may not become evident until early adult life, and sometimes an infection which seems to have been eradicated before puberty will recur during pregnancy.

When pyelonephritis occurs as the only lesion, unaccompanied by disorders of the urinary tract, girls are much more frequently affected than boys, and the symptoms are those of recurrent infection, chronic renal failure, or hypertension. In renal failure, growth is retarded and weight lost; the skin is wrinkled and sallow. Thirst and polyuria may be noticed with consequent nocturnal frequency or enuresis. Loss of appetite, nausea and headaches follow. In long standing cases the bone changes of renal rickets appear, and are sometimes the complaint for which the child is brought to hospital. A full discussion of chronic renal failure will be found in Section M, II of this volume: it is an irremediable condition, and treatment can only aim at slowing its progress and relieving the symptoms.

Hypertension (see p. 211) is a complication of some but not all cases of chronic pyelonephritis; no explanation can be given of this selectivity, nor can it be predicted which cases will be affected. The appearance of hypertension greatly hastens the course of the disease, and severe headaches and blurred vision may reduce the child to a pitiable condition.

Although the affected kidney is frequently painful during exacerbations of the infection, there is no clinical sign diagnostic of chronic pyelonephritis, and its recognition has to be made from urine examination, pyelography and history. The urine usually contains a slight excess of pus cells, even between attacks, and a variable quantity of albumin: it is often sterile on culture, for the lesions progress long after the bacterial invasion has been overcome. A few casts may be present. Pyelograms may demonstrate an impairment of function, or an anatomical deformity due to gross renal scarring in advanced disease. Clearly it is difficult by these methods to make a precise diagnosis in early cases, and it is also impossible to distinguish between chronic atrophic pyelonephritis and some forms of congenital hypoplasia.

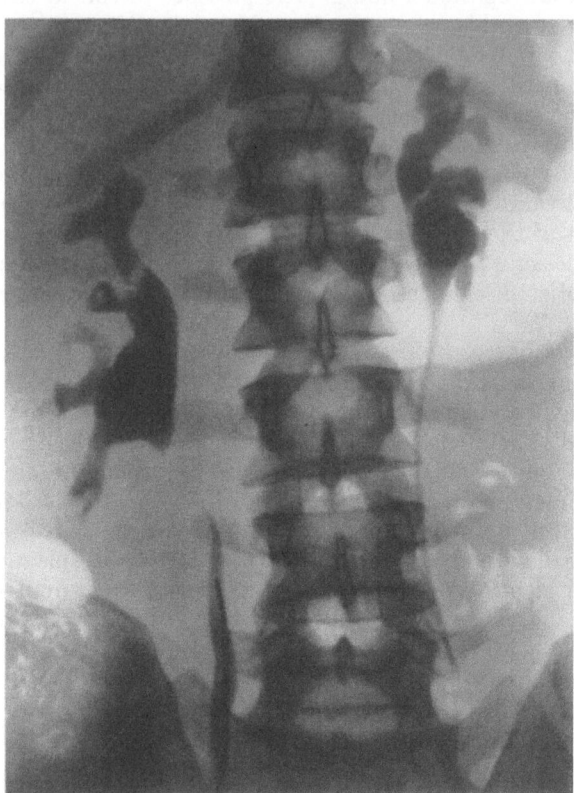

Fig. 94. Unilateral pyelonephritis. Retrograde pyelograms in a girl aged 17 years who had suffered recurrent urinary infections with haematuria since early childhood. Contracted left kidney with marked hypertrophy of the right kidney. Normal blood pressure. Left nephrectomy

3. Radiology

The outline of the kidney should first be studied: the whole kidney is often contracted, and narrowed in the vertical plane (Fig. 94). The surface is rendered irregular by scarring, and is indented in relation to deformed calyces or pyelogenic cysts. This type of indentation must not be confused with the foetal lobulation which is normal up to the end of the first year. When the whole kidney is involved, the pelvis and calyces often appear compressed against the vertebral column (Fig. 95), the pelvis is directed downwards rather than medially and lies in almost the same line as the ureter. Because of the thinning of the parenchyma, the lower-most calyx lies in close proximity and parallel to the ureter. The calyces are irregular, often clubbed (Fig. 96), but sometimes narrow and elongated (Fig. 95, left); the pelvis may appear slightly hydronephrotic, though its enlargement is often apparent rather than real, and is relative to the contraction of the kidney. Hyperplastic areas of the kidney may cause a distortion of the calyces suggesting the presence of cysts.

The function of the pyelonephritic kidney is depressed, but since the lesions are patchy, there may be sufficient number of normal nephrons to concentrate the dye, and therefore to fill the whole pelvis with opaque urine during the intravenous pyelogram. At other times, and especially in extensive bilateral disease, retrograde pyelograms are required. Pyelonephritis is normally a bilateral disease, though one kidney is usually much more scarred than the other. In strictly unilateral disease, the healthy kidney will show a considerable and regular hypertrophy.

ZAPP has claimed that calyco-papillitis with papillary necrosis is a distinctive form of chronic renal infection, common in childhood; he diagnoses it from the

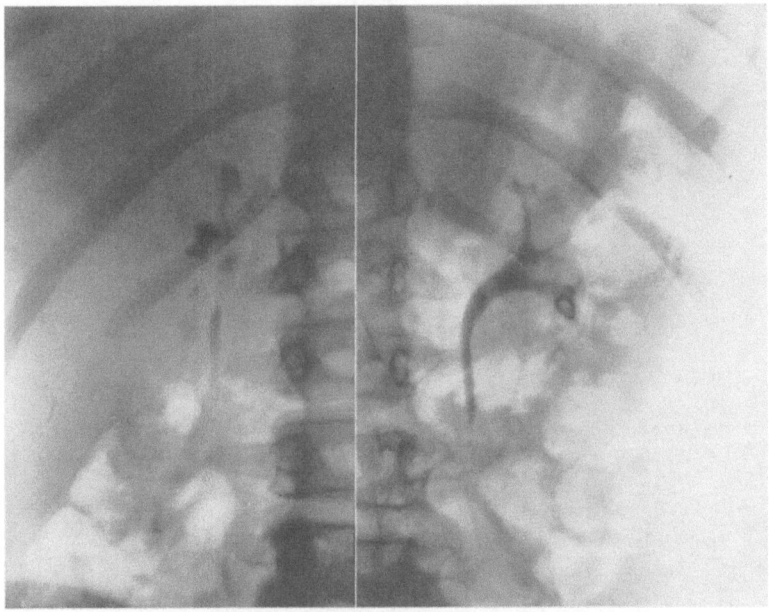

Fig. 95. Bilateral pyelonephritis. Intravenous pyelograms in a girl aged 12 years suffering from recurrent urinary infection and right sided pain. Atrophic pyelonephritic changes in the right kidney; a drawn-out, narrow middle calyx on the left, indicating the presence of scarring this kidney

pyelographic appearance of isolated, blunted and bulbous calyces, but his pyelograms do not show the "ring shadows" seen in the papillary necrosis of diabetic adults, and his view of the pathology does not appear to be supported by anatomical studies.

4. Management

When following an acute urinary infection the changes of chronic pyelonephritis are found in an otherwise normal urinary tract, every attempt must be made to eliminate the infecting organism: an intensive course of antibiotic treatment, followed by continuous chemotherapy should be advised. Small doses of sulphonamide [e.g. Gantrisin (Sulphafurazole) 0.5 gms twice daily] may be required for months, or even years to prevent recurrent infections. Any other foci of infection in the body must be eliminated. In bilateral disease, these measures, together with symptomatic treatment of renal failure (p. 221) and hypertension (p. 215) are all that can be offered: in unilateral disease, which is rare, nephrectomy may be considered. The indications for this operation are hypertension and recurrent acute exacerbations which cannot be controlled by chemotherapy. In hypertension it is vital that the opposite kidney is entirely normal, for if it is at all affected, nephrectomy will reduce the total renal function without curing the disease. In recurrent urinary infection the criteria need not be quite so rigid, and it is sometimes worth removing the worse of two pyelo-nephritic kidneys if complications such as stone or perinephric abscess are present.

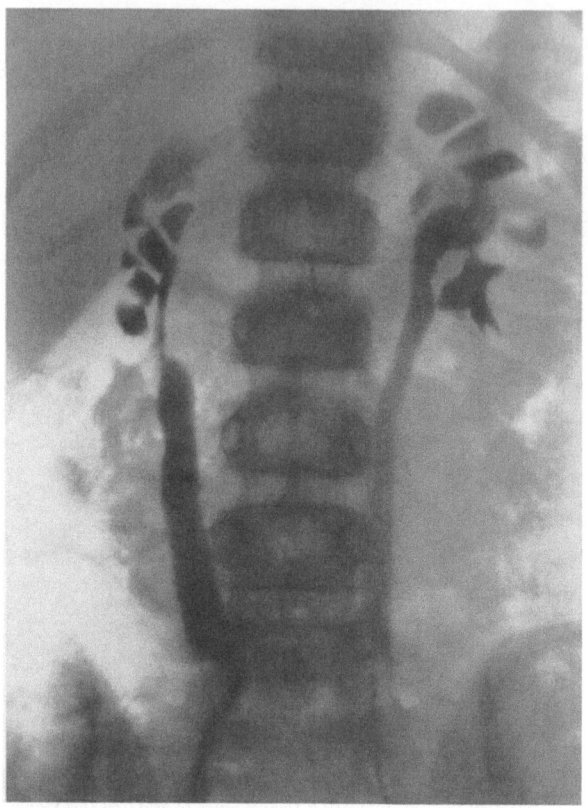

Fig. 96. Chronic bilateral pyelonephritis. Retrograde pyelograms in a girl aged 8 years, who had suffered recurrent urinary infections since the age of 4 years. Steadily rising blood urea but no hypertension. Blunting and distortion of calyces, atrophy of the right kidney far advanced

No advantage will be gained from the removal of a unilateral pyelonephritic kidney if the blood pressure is normal and the infections have been controlled, but heminephrectomy, removing the infected half of a double kidney, is frequently valuable.

VI. Pyaemic kidney; renal carbuncle and perinephric abscess

1. Pathology

The kidney is often involved in generalized blood borne infections, usually due to streptococci or staphylococci. In childhood the primary lesion may be bacterial endocarditis, umbilical sepsis, or osteomyelitis. Abscesses may occur in many organs throughout the body, but not infrequently the kidney is the most severely affected. Being embolic the earliest lesions are seen in the glomeruli or its arterioles, and from a local thrombosis an abscess spreads. Septic infarcts also occur. The kidney is swollen and yellow points of suppuration are seen beneath the capsule. The cut surface exhibits numerous small abscesses (Fig. 97), circular in the cortex, oval and radial in the medulla. The renal pelvis is little affected and it is only late in the disease that pus cells reach the urine.

A renal carbuncle is a localized suppurative process in the cortex, usually staphylococcal, and the result of metastatic infection from superficial sepsis. The affected pole of the kidney is enlarged by the inflammatory infiltration: the centre of the lesion is an abscess which ultimately discharges itself outwards through the capsule into the perinephric space. The pelvis and calyces are seldom involved, though the calyceal anatomy is often distorted.

Occasionally the suppurative process is so extensive that the greater part of both kidneys is involved, resulting in death from toxaemia and anuria (Fig. 98).

Perinephric abscess may arise from rupture of a renal carbuncle, but more commonly, a staphylococcal "metastatic" perinephric abscess is found without evident renal disease: in these it is usually assumed that minute focus in the cortex has ruptured through the capsule, but such a focus is seldom demonstrable. BRUNN and RHODES state

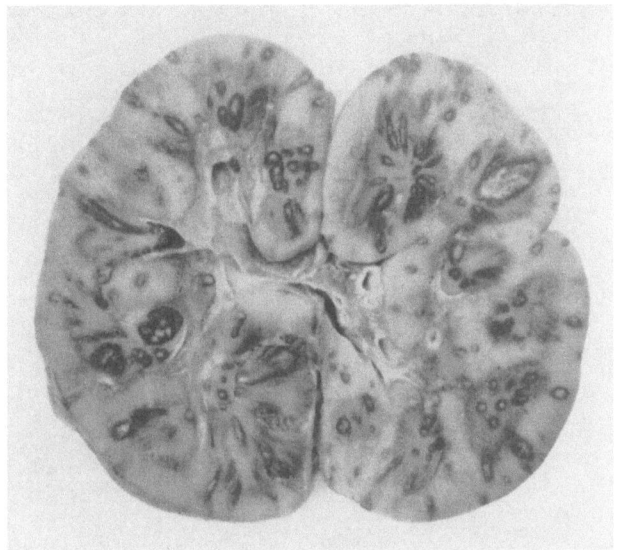

Fig. 97. Pyaemic kidney. Post-mortem from a girl aged 13 months admitted to hospital for investigation of vomiting and low fever. There was a leucocytosis, but urine was normal. Myringotomy was performed for a middle ear infection. The child's general condition deteriorated during the following days, and she died without any signs of a renal disorder

that metastatic perinephric abscess is less common in children than in adults, in contrast to osteomyelitis, another haematogenous staphylococcal infection, and believe that the comparative paucity of the perinephric fat in the young is responsible. SWAN, however, questions this theory and asserts that the incidence of perinephric abscess in children has been underestimated.

Much less commonly perinephric abscess results from the extension of a suppurative pyelonephritic lesion, often associated with stone. An E. coli infection is usually present and the process is a chronic one.

Abscess formation due to penetration of the renal parenchyma by a ureteric catheter has been recorded, but it is an unusual complication of that accident.

Paranephric abscess, a lesion of the space outside Gerota's fascia, is usually a consequence of osteomyelitis of the spine.

2. Clinical features

The multiple pyaemic lesions of bacterial endocarditis produce very few symptoms apart from microscopic haematuria, and are unlikely to come to the attention of the urologist. Carbuncle and perinephric abscess are perhaps less common since the advent of chemotherapy but are still important clinical entities.

The onset of symptoms due to renal carbuncle is slow and insidious: for some weeks the child is off colour, and complains of vague pain in the loin or the abdomen. Loss of weight and pyrexia then become evident, pain is more severe and better localized. Examination at this stage reveals tenderness over one kidney, which may be palpably enlarged but mobile; the urine is normal or contains a few pus cells: the blood count shows a considerable polymorph leucocytosis. On intravenous pyelography there is evidence of a space occupying lesion, usually near one pole, which enlarges and distorts the upper or lower calyx. In the untreated case the suppurative focus will discharge itself through the renal capsule, producing a sub-acute perinephric abscess, with the symptoms outlined below.

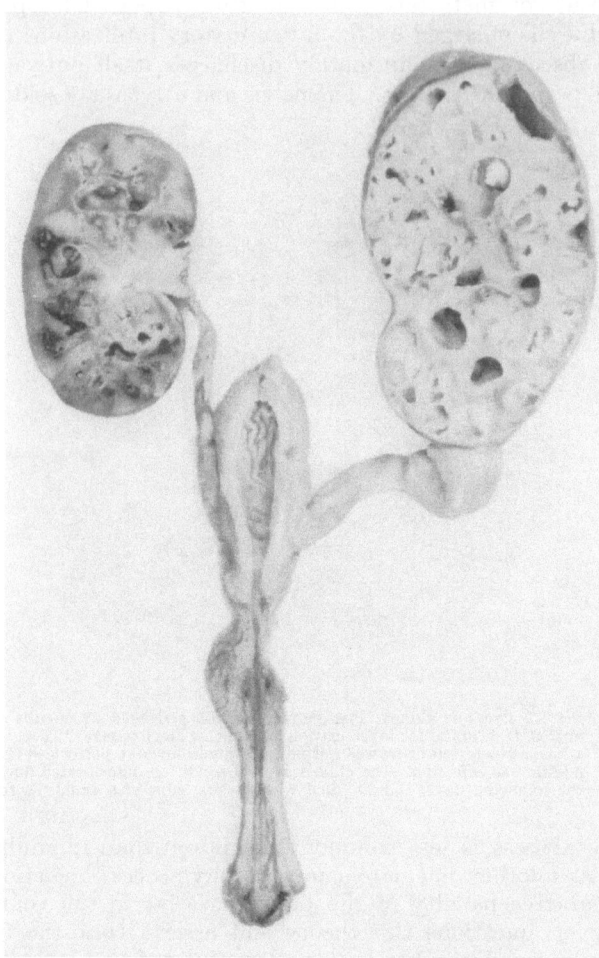

Fig. 98. Acute suppurative nephritis. Post-mortem specimens from a boy aged 3 weeks, admitted to hospital with acute toxaemia and abdominal swellings. Both kidneys were enlarged and hard: they were thought to be polycystic. The boy died shortly after admission. The renal parenchyma is almost entirely destroyed on the left side, and replaced by an enormous staphylococcal abscess

In very acute infantile cases, one or both kidneys may be considerably enlarged and oliguria may be present.

In perinephric abscess the characteristic history is a gradual onset of pain in the loin and limp; the limp is due to psoas spasm, demonstrable clinically by the persistent flexion of the hip without limitation of other movements. The pain is often poorly localized, and on the right side may mimic appendicitis. When first seen, the only physical sign may be tenderness in the flank, later a mass becomes palpable, and finally an oedematous swelling can be observed in the loin. At first there is little pyrexia but when the abscess begins to point, the temperature is high and swinging. Normal urine, and leucocytosis are the rule. X-rays of the abdomen show loss of the psoas shadow and displacement of the kidney (Fig. 99). Cases in which the perinephric abscess complicates a pyelonephritic process are easily distinguished by their association with frequency, pyuria and often an E. coli infection, together with pyelographic evidence of renal disease.

3. Management

In renal carbuncle and metastatic perinephric abscess, it may be assumed that a staphylococcus is responsible and penicillin should be administered in large doses. Drug treatment alone may suffice when the lesion is confined to the kidney, but when a perinephric abscess has formed, drainage through the loin is usually required. Occasionally it has been necessary to open into the kidney to drain the carbuncle, or even to perform a nephrectomy. In most cases the prognosis is excellent, and restoration of a normal pyelogram shows how completely a carbuncle can resolve (HUTCHISON and DAVIES), but in infants the infection may be overwhelming.

The complicated perinephric abscess with chronic pyelonephritis or stone presents a more difficult problem, and treatment must be adjusted to the overall state of the urinary tract. In some cases a nephrectomy is best performed at the same time as the abscess is opened.

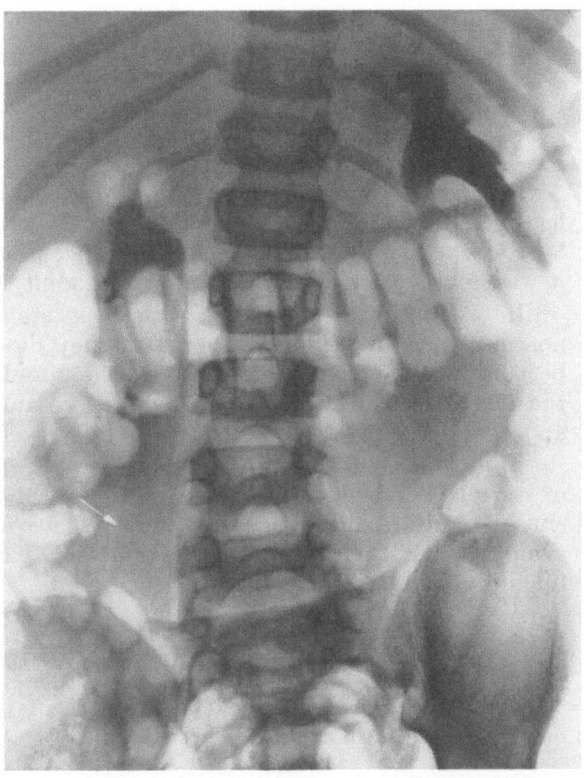

Fig. 99. Perinephric abscess. Intravenous pyelogram in a girl aged 7 years with three weeks history of left loin pain and limp. The left renal pelvis is displaced upwards and outwards and the outline of the psoas shadow (marked by an arrow on the right) is obliterated on the left. Shortly after these films were taken a swelling appeared in the left loin

VII. Cystitis

Acute cystitis is usually one manifestation of a generalized urinary infection, and as such requires no special comment. On rare occasions infection may start in the bladder wall or penetrate it from outside. CAMPBELL has recorded acute lesions due to intramural abscess, to haemorrhagic infarction, and to suppurative thrombo-phlebitis of the bladder wall. Pelvic abscess due to appendicitis or pneumococcal peritonitis may rupture into the bladder, and abscesses arising from osteomyelitis of the pelvis may do the same. The pus is discharged through a comparatively small opening but is very thick, often having the consistency of tooth paste, and may cause retention of urine. The diagnosis is easily established cystoscopically once the bladder has been washed out and treatment should be directed to the primary lesion: the bladder heals surprisingly easily.

Chronic cystitis of particular severity is seen in the sacculated bladder associated with lower urinary tract obstruction or neurological disorder, and in these circumstances it may prove impossible to rid the urine of pus cells. The bladder wall becomes thick and fibrotic and its condition is uninfluenced by removal of the obstruction; the ureteric orifices are gaping and rigid so that they allow free reflux.

Milder chronic infections of the upper urinary tract may be accompanied by the changes of cystitis cystica and cystitis glandularis as in adults. This cystoscopic appearance is particularly common in infected mega-ureters. Malakoplakia is a chronic form of cystitis in which raised yellow plaques are found beneath the mucosa: they are composed of large cells containing "Michaelis-Guttman" inclusion bodies. MORRISON has described a typical example in a six year old girl dying of chronic infection with dilated ureters. Leukoplakia has been observed by CAMPBELL.

Cystitis emphysematosa, in which gas bubbles form beneath the mucosa, has been described in an infant dying of a very acute urinary tract infection by SANES and DOROSHOW. The significance of gas formation was not clear, but it was not associated with diabetes as in adult cases.

Interstitial cystitis (Hunner's ulcer) is stated by McDONALD et al. to be not infrequent in children: the cases they describe, however, appear to have been typical enuretics with day frequency and urgency, and suffered none of the intense bladder pain characteristic of Hunner's ulcer. No other writers appear to have observed the condition in the very young.

Urethro-trigonitis, small granular masses, polyps and bullae on the base of the bladder and urethra, may be observed in children with frequency and enuresis but sterile urine. They may also be found in a few children without symptoms and their significance is doubtful. Treatment when required is light fulguration and urethral dilatation.

VIII. Parasitic and fungal infections

These infections are discussed at length in Volume IX, 2, of this series, and only brief notes are appended here.

1. Schistosomiasis (Bilharziasis)

The schistosomidae are trematode worms which are parasitic in man and pass through their intermediate stages in molluscs or fish. S. haematobium infection is common in children in tropical Africa, Egypt, Arabia and Iraq; the adult worms inhabit the veins of the bladder, prostate and uterus, and ova pass out in the urine. If the ova reach water a free swimming form, the miracidium, then develops which can penetrate the integument of a species of snail (Bulinus) and undergoes further evolution within the viscera of that mollusc. In the next stage a cercaria is formed and leaves the snail, it swims independently in the water, and can enter the unbroken skin of any available human. During the process of penetration the tail is lost and the head enters the blood stream; reaching the liver, the organism attaches itself to the vessel wall and develops into an adult schistosoma. Mating takes place here, the minute female worm being enveloped within the body of the male and thus united they leave in pairs for the bladder where the remainder of their life is spent.

Children bathing or washing in fresh water inhabited by the snail Bulinus are likely to become infected: some irritation of the skin occurs when the cercariae penetrate it, and then there is an allergic phase, during which the child suffers pyrexia, headaches, urticarial rashs and colic. When the fully developed worms have reached the bladder urinary symptoms appear, the most characteristic being terminal haematuria with some frequency and pain on micturition. With severe infestation there will be complaints of suprapubic pain, and perhaps evidence of secondary infection. Spontaneous remission of symptoms is ultimately likely, but may be followed by fresh attacks. The sequelae of schistosomiasis, ureteric stricture, bladder contracture and carcinoma are formidable, but are seen chiefly in adult life.

The diagnosis of schistosomiasis is made by identification of ova in the urine. Several specimens may need to be examined, and the last drops of urine which are passed are most likely to contain the ova. Leucocytosis and eosinophilia are present and a complement fixation test is available. In areas where the disease is endemic it is much the most common cause of haematuria and all children with that complaint should be examined with this in mind; other urological investigations will only be required if schistosomiasis has been excluded. Cystoscopy is therefore not required, but if it is performed it will reveal a number of inflamed areas and small ulcerations. Healing leads to the development of "sandy patches".

The treatment is primarily medical, and surgical measures should not be required during childhood. Antimony tartrate (tartar emetic) is still the most effective drug; it should be administered by daily intravenous injections for 10—15 days. The total dose can be calculated on the basis of 35 mgm/kilo/body weight, and should be divided into daily doses, the first being small and not exceeding 30 mgm. The child should be in bed if possible throughout the course.

Stibophen (Fouadin) can be used intramuscularly in courses of 10 injections administered on alternate days. The total dose for a four year old child should be 15 ml, for an eight year old 25 ml, and for a fourteen year old 40—50 ml, and these doses must be divided appropriately.

Nilodin (Miracil D) is a recently introduced oral preparation given in doses of 20 mgm/kilo/day for 7 to 8 days. Severe side effects are common.

2. Hydatid cyst

The hydatid is the cysticercus stage of the helminth "Taenia echinococcus" a tape worm which spends its adult life in the intestine of the dog. Infection, which is common in certain countries, though not in England or America, often occurs in childhood through the handling of infested dogs, but the cyst may not become evident until adult life. A solitary hydatid may be found in the kidney; it forms a tumour-like swelling, and may destroy the renal parenchyma entirely, or it may rupture into the pelvis, so that daughter-cysts are passed in the urine. The diagnosis may be made as a result of finding these cysts, or calcified ring shadows may be recognized radiologically. The Casoni test is somewhat unreliable. Nephrectomy, provided the opposite kidney is normal, is the only satisfactory treatment.

When daughter-cysts are released into the peritoneum by rupture of a hepatic hydatid, one may settle in the pelvis, and enlarge there, pressing upon the base of the bladder and sometimes causing retention of urine, as in the case recorded by SABADINI.

3. Myiasis

JUNGHANS has recorded the case of a boy of 12 years who excreted in his urine the larvae of Fannia Scalaris, a species of fly. He recovered without treatment.

4. Moniliasis

Moniliasis or "thrush" infection is due to a yeast like organism Candida albicans. It is a relatively common cause of vaginitis in the adult, and may produce a type of napkin rash in infants (p. 243). Generalized thrush infections in which the urinary tract may be involved have become more frequent in recent years, occurring in infants who have received prolonged antibiotic therapy. GERLOCZY et al. describe a three month old infant in whom the renal pelvis was entirely occupied by a mass of greasy substance composed of myriads of monilia organisms. One case of monilial infection has come under my care, a boy with chronically dilated ureters who had had many courses of antibiotics for bacterial infections; he had filamentous structures in the urine for many months, and having resisted all treatment finally cured himself. No specific measures have yet proved satisfactory, though SAREWITZ record the use of Nystatin in adult monilial urinary infection. Generalized moniliasis may be treated with hydroxystilbamidine (5 mgm/kilo/12 hourly) given in an intravenous drip.

5. Actinomycosis

Actinomycosis infection is rare in children, and very rarely is the kidney involved except in continuity with other abdominal lesions. KRETSCHMER and HIBBS have, however, recorded a case and reviewed the subject in detail. In their child there was a long history of loss of weight and pain in the loin; renal enlargement with a filling defect was seen in the pyelogram and the kidney was removed under the impression that a tumour was present. A post-operative sinus formed which discharged pus containing the typical "sulphur granules" but eventually healed after a long course of potassium iodide. A similar and well illustrated case in a boy of 10 years is reported by WILLE-BAUMKAUFF.

I. Urogenital tuberculosis

1. Incidence

Although generalized tuberculosis is relatively common in the young, destructive disease localized in the kidney is characteristically an affliction of early adult life or adolescence. If therefore childhood is deemed to have ceased at the age of 12 years, surgical renal tuberculosis is rare in children, and it is exceptionally rare in infants. The incidence will naturally vary from one community to another with the varying standards of hygiene and nutrition, and with the general level of resistance to tuberculosis: in the past certain writers have been able to refer to a comparatively large series of affected children (e.g. MATHÉ found that children accounted for 10% of surgical renal tuberculosis cases) but nowadays few are encountered, and no new example has attended the Hospital for Sick Children during the past three years. HAWTHORNE and SIMINOVITCH had 9 cases in 57,000 paediatric admissions (Canada 1949); AUERBACH (USA, 1948) in 90 autopsies on tuberculous children found renal lesions in only three.

Most of the cases now recognized occur in children undergoing treatment in long stay orthopaedic hospitals for bone and joint lesions, and few present for treatment primarily on account of urinary symptoms. Because, therefore, of its rarity, and the close similarity between the manifestations in adults and in children, the following description of renal tuberculosis will be brief and reference should be made to Vol. IX of this series for full discussion.

II. Pathology

The tubercle bacillus is believed to enter the body by the way of the respiratory or alimentary system, and forms there a focus of infection which with the involved local lymph glands is known as the primary complex. During this episode there is some disturbance of general health, though few local symptoms. A temporary bacteriaemia occurs during the development of the primary complex and the organisms may settle down in many organs, including the kidney, though active local destruction is unlikely to become evident until a later stage.

Acute generalized (miliary) tuberculosis may result from a rupture of the caseating lymphatic focus into the blood stream and the bacilli so disseminated produce "tubercles" in every part of the body. Until recently this type of generalized tuberculosis was invariably fatal and the "miliary" lesions of the kidney found at post-mortem accounted for a high proportion of recorded cases of renal tuberculosis in childhood. The kidney exhibits a large number of grey nodules under the capsule, and on the cut surface: they are small tuberculous foci composed chiefly of epithelioid cells, and without evidence of caseation. The pelvis and calyces are unaffected by the disease, and the renal papillae remain intact. Miliary tuberculosis produces no urinary symptoms, and cases are unlikely to come under the care of the urologist. Treatment is exclusively medical, and now that effective chemotherapy is available, it can be demonstrated that the miliary lesions are capable of healing.

Blood stream spread also occurs in a less acute form, and is liable to take place at any time in the course of severe local disease in the lungs, lymph glands or bones. Tubercle bacilli are brought to the kidneys through the circulation and produce multiple bilateral cortical foci. The first accurate description of these lesions was given by MEDLAR. They are small and not perceptible to naked eye examination; histologically they consist of leucocytic collections with mononuclear epithelioid cells and no giant cells are present. It is now established that these are the minimal lesions, and that true tuberculous bacilluria, in the sense of bacilli passing through an intact kidney, does not occur.

Healing of these cortical lesions is possible and usually complete: the "surgical" renal lesion arises by extension down the tubules to the medulla. This secondary lesion is commonly unilateral, it is typically a giant cell focus with caseation and frequently ulcerates the renal papilla, releasing its contents into the pelvis. In this way a cavity is formed which may gradually enlarge and extend outwards into the renal parenchyma; complete healing is no longer possible, though scarring and calcification may occur, or the caseous material may partially solidify in closed cavities to form a putty-like substance.

Several ulcero-cavernous lesions may form simultaneously but once tuberculous pus is released into the pelvis secondary spread may take place across that cavity. The mucosa becomes thickened, inflamed, and studded with tubercles. Obstruction of the pelvi-ureteric junction may lead to hydronephrosis and progressive destruction of the renal substance which converts the whole kidney into a tuberculous pyonephrosis.

The ureter becomes a little dilated in early ulcerative lesions and its wall oedematous. Tubercles are formed under the mucosa, and later progressive fibrosis occurs in the muscular coat, which together with fibro-lipomatous changes in the adventitia convert the ureter into a thick and rigid tube. Stricture is particularly apt to occur in the lower end, and if this occurs early, may lead to considerable dilatation of the proximal ureter.

In the bladder the first change is the appearance of tubercles around the ureteric orifice of the affected side; the inflammatory process spreads, and may produce small ulcerations. The bladder muscle becomes spastic at first, but later infiltration and fibrosis of the wall result in a rigid contracted organ. Fibrosis of the bladder neck causing urinary obstruction is seen occasionally.

Tuberculosis of the male genital tract is uncommon in children, though as in adults, it may accompany severe urinary infection. Whether the organisms usually reach the genital ducts from the urine or from the blood stream is uncertain, though the haematogenous type is undoubtedly possible, and it is equally difficult to say whether the prostate and vesicles are affected before the epididymis. Lesions in both the latter sites are found in most cases, though the caseating abscess formed in the epididymis naturally receives most attention. Healing without sinus formation may occur under the influence of chemotherapy, but permanent occlusion of the epididymal ducts is likely.

III. Clinical features and management

1. Cortical lesions

A high proportion of the children now seen with urinary tuberculosis are those already under treatment for a serious lesion elsewhere, usually pulmonary or osseous, who are found to be excreting tubercle bacilli in the urine, but who have no demonstrable pyelographic abnormality. Thus LATTIMER found 12 out of 22 of his cases to belong to this group, and YATES-BELL also emphasizes the high proportion of symptomless cases. As already indicated, the work of MEDLAR and others has demonstrated that these cases cannot be regarded as simple tuberculous bacilluria, and that multiple minute cortical lesions must in fact be present.

The children in this group have no disturbance of micturition attributable to the tuberculous process, but albuminuria, slight pyuria and occasional haematuria occur. The great majority are diagnosed from routine examination of the urine for tubercle bacilli.

Untreated, excretion of tubercle bacilli may continue over a very long period without evidence of destructive renal disease, even in cases where the extra-renal focus is small and healing. No adequate follow-up of this type of lesion has been reported for children, but COSBIE-ROSS has described the progress in adult cases. A few will naturally go on to ulcerative lesions.

The management of these cases is largely the management of the serious lesion elsewhere. Chemotherapy and sanatorium treatment for at least a year are desirable from the renal angle, and should be advised when bacilluria is the only finding. Most cases become tubercle negative in these circumstances, but a few are obstinately persistent.

Since a high proportion of these children are undergoing immobilization treatment for bone and joint disease, it is not surprising that stones are found in association with tuberculous bacilluria in a fair number of cases; occasionally it is the symptoms due to stone which lead to investigation. The stone should be treated on its own merits, and when the tuberculous foci are entirely cortical no sinus will follow pyelolithotomy (YATES-BELL). Nephrectomy is, of course, inadvisable unless the affected kidney is almost completely destroyed, since the cortical tuberculous process is likely to be bilateral and may progress in the contralateral organ.

2. Early ulcerative lesions of the renal papilla

When a caseous focus has developed, and ruptured into the pelvis, symptoms referable to the urinary tract will be present, although they may be overshadowed by the symptoms of a pulmonary or osseous focus. In only a few children is the renal disease the sole clinically evident tuberculous lesion.

The child complains of frequent and urgent micturition; sleep is disturbed by the urge, or there is an onset of bedwetting. Some dysuria may be evident, and at times there is a sudden brisk haematuria. Aching pain in the loin is a common feature, and occasional cases suffer true colic due to clot or debris. Loss of weight, pallor, and sweats are noticed by the parents, often for some weeks before the child is brought to hospital.

On examination there are few physical signs and the temperature is normal or only slightly raised. The urine is hazy and acid, contains albumin and excess of pus cells, but is sterile on ordinary culture media. It is immediately clear that the child is suffering from a chronic urinary infection, and the problem often lies in the differentiation of simple pyelonephritis from the tuberculous lesions, though in known cases of chest or bone disease there should be little difficulty. The Mantoux test is frequently of value in any country where the majority of children are Mantoux negative, for a positive reaction will greatly increase the chances that the symptoms are due to renal tuberculosis, while a negative will obviate the need for prolonged search for tubercle bacilli in the urine.

Intravenous pyelograms in the early ulcerative cases will show the excavation of the renal papilla; the affected calyx is enlarged and fluffy or communicates with a ragged cavity outside the calyceal system. Some calcification may also be present in the adjacent tissue. The renal pelvis and upper ureter are slightly dilated. These signs are almost diagnostic of tuberculosis, but simple coliform infections associated with hydrocalycosis may mimic the typical picture. Bilateral retrograde pyelograms, and collection of separate specimens of urine should be performed to confirm the nature of the disease, and to establish the state of the contralateral organ.

Cystoscopy, at this stage, reveals cystitis with the inflammatory changes and mucosal tubercles localized chiefly in the neighbourhood of the ureteric orifice of the affected kidney. The orifice itself may be rigid and gaping.

Ultimately the diagnosis depends upon the isolation of the tubercle bacillus, and in all suspicious cases, at least three early morning specimens of urine should be examined by microscopy and culture or guinea-pig inoculation.

The management of the early ulcerative lesion is both medical and surgical, and with the recognition of the value of chemotherapy and the sanatorium regime, nephrectomy is seldom urgent and may be avoided altogether. Most surgeons now advocate 3—6 months medical treatment before contemplating nephrectomy even in the clearly unilateral case. During this time the tubercle bacilli may disappear from the urine and healing of the lesion commence, so that the surgery is never required. It is preferable to await healing of any other tuberculous foci present in the body before deciding upon renal surgery, for later infection of the opposite kidney may entirely alter the prospect.

Nephrectomy is indicated, however, for the strictly unilateral case with ulcero-cavernous lesions which cannot be sterilized medically. Partial nephrectomy is a procedure applicable to a few, though the precise extent of the disease cannot always be estimated from the pyelogram. A further prolonged course of chemotherapy should follow, so that the whole treatment is likely to last at least a year. The cystitis usually settles down rapidly once the tuberculous kidney has been removed, and requires no special attention in the early cases when involvement of the lower urinary tract has never been severe. Thereafter, a careful watch must be kept on the urine to give early warning of a recurrence in the opposite kidney.

In bilateral disease treatment is usually exclusively medical though there is occasionally a place for partial nephrectomy, when a cavernous lesion in one pole is accompanied by cortical lesions in the opposite kidney.

3. Advanced lesions

Advanced tuberculous disease is occasionally confined to one kidney, which is excluded from the rest of the urinary tract by ureteric obstruction and con-

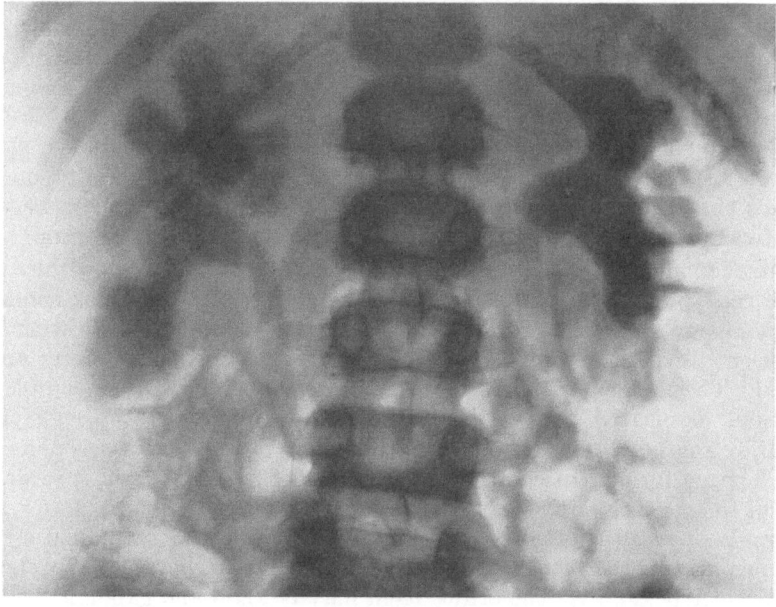

Fig. 100. Right renal tuberculosis. Intravenous pyelogram in a boy aged 14 years with extreme frequency and dysuria. Urine contained large numbers of tubercle bacilli. Bladder spastic and acutely inflammed and catheterization of ureters was not possible. Pyelograms show gross hydronephrosis and cavity formation in the right kidney, mild hydronephrosis on the left. Right nephrectomy performed: frequency much improved and left hydronephrosis returned to normal. Urine rendered tubercle negative

verted into a bag of partially calcified caseous material. Cure is not achieved by this process of exclusion, and such kidneys should be removed.

Much more frequently the advanced lesions involve the lower urinary tract, and often both kidneys. Bladder symptoms are then acute and extremely distressing; ten minute frequency is accompanied by urge incontinence and dysuria. There is an irregular fever, and often considerable loss of weight. Pyelograms show extensive excavation of the renal substance, with ragged cavities and a dilated renal pelvis and ureter; the bladder is small and spastic and there is often dilatation of the opposite ureter in unilateral cases. This dilatation of the uninfected side is at first due to the diminished bladder capacity which results from spasm and oedema and it is therefore recoverable on chemotherapy. Later the bladder becomes thickened and incapable of expansion while the intramural ureter is stenosed, so that the ureteric dilatation can only be relieved by surgical treatment. In the child the ureter becomes dilated much more readily than in the adult, and reversible dilatation is, therefore, much more likely to be seen. It may lead to the erroneous diagnosis of bilateral infection, and the severity of bladder involvement often makes it impossible to pass ureteric catheters to obtain differential specimens. However, the dilated calyces of the healthy kidney are smooth in contrast to the ragged edges of the tuberculous cavities (Fig. 100); in cystograms reflux commonly occurs on the infected, but not on the healthy side, and if the pyelograms are repeated after six weeks on medical treatment, it may be found that the bladder spasm has relaxed, and the healthy ureter has returned to normal calibre. The blood urea is often raised in the acute phase of these unilateral cases, a fact which has been attributed to a tuberculo-toxic nephritis (CAMPBELL), though the pathological evidence for such a lesion is poor. The blood urea, like the dilatation, will return to normal when the disease is controlled by chemotherapy and by excision of the infected kidney and ureter.

As in the early ulcerative lesions, therefore, treatment is both medical and surgical: the greater number of bilateral cases in advanced disease, however will limit the scope of surgery and increase the mortality. Unfortunately even the elimination of the infection by nephrectomy in unilateral cases does not necessarily lead to cure where the bladder involvement has been severe: healing may lead to extreme fibrosis in the detrusor and contraction of the bladder capacity causing progressive hydronephrosis of the remaining kidney. It is rare for this stage to be reached in childhood, but ileo-cystoplasty or diversion of urine will almost certainly be required.

4. Lesions of the male genital tract

Most English and American writers find tuberculous epididymitis very rare in children, and usually accompanied by advanced urinary tract disease and prostatitis, often with multiple cutaneous fistulae.

GARIBALDI and GAMBETTA have emphasized a very different aspect in reporting seven cases of children with hydrocele, which when emptied allowed palpation of a nodular and enlarged epididymis. The fluid withdrawn contained albumin and pus cells, and the Mantoux reaction was positive, but no tubercle bacilli were isolated from the fluid or the urine in the majority. The prognosis was favourable.

IV. Chemotherapy

While the general principles upon which the sanatorium treatment of tuberculosis rests are unlikely to change, new drugs and new combinations of drugs appear with great regularity, so that it is unlikely that any single regime will receive universal approval or even retain its popularity with those who have devised it. Since no large series of affected children is available in any centre, the regime must naturally be based on current practice in adults, modifying only the dosage.

LATTIMER writing in 1955 recommended the following course for cortical lesions:

Streptomycin 20 mgm/kilo/twice weekly in a single injection.

Isoniazid 5 mgm/kilo/day in three doses.

Para-amino-salicylic acid 6—12 mgm/day in 3 doses. The streptomycin should be administered for six months and other drugs for at least a year.

For the ulcerative lesions, the full drug combination should be continued for 12—18 months, and at least 4 months of treatment should precede nephrectomy.

J. Calculous disease

I. Incidence

Vesical calculus was once the most common surgical disorder of childhood, and in some parts of the world it is still a very prevalent complaint, yet in Western Europe and America such calculi are now seldom encountered. This dramatic fall in the incidence of urinary lithiasis has been associated with a change in the nature of the disease so that it becomes possible to distinguish an "endemic" type of calculus from the sporadic form now commonly observed. This distinction must be borne in mind when assessing the statistics relating to stone in children, since any collected series is likely to include a considerable proportion of the endemic cases, and may therefore suggest certain conclusions which are not applicable to the current problem.

Although the relative proportions of the different types may vary, urinary calculi in children do not differ in structure or composition from those found in adults, and for a general discussion reference must be made to Volume X of this work. Children of all ages may be affected, indeed it would seem that some stones must be formed during foetal life: DUGAN reports the passage of urethral stones in infants of 4 days and 8 days of age. In a large collected series WINSBURY-WHITE found the peak incidence to be between the ages of 3 and 10 years, but WINKEL SMITH notes that two thirds of his patients developed their calculi before they were 5 years old, and it is my view that the majority now presenting for treatment begin to form stones during the first two years. BUGBEE and WALLSTEIN comment on the frequency with which stones were found at post-mortem on infants under the age of 12 months, but several of the calculi they describe were very small, and the relation of these minute concretions to calculi causing clinical signs is not established.

Boys are more frequently affected than girls; this predominance is very marked in the case of the vesical and urethral calculi, but is also found in cases of upper urinary tract calculi; thus WINKEL SMITH found the ratio of males to females to be as 3:1.

The symptoms and signs of calculous disease vary with the type of stone as well as with its position in the urinary tract: it will be necessary therefore to consider the problem from both these aspects.

II. Aetiological classification

The precise mechanism of stone formation is scarcely ever clear yet in a number of cases we can identify a predisposing cause. Probably this identification is more often possible in children than in adults: thus MYERS reviewing a series from the Hospital for Sick Children, Great Ormond Street, was able to indicate the predisposing factor in 39 out of 85 cases. Moreover, although no exact pathogenesis emerges, the aetiological groups which can be defined are of considerable importance in treatment and in the prevention of recurrence.

1. Endemic calculi

In any community in which stone is found to be a common disorder of childhood, a characteristic disease pattern appears. The children of the poorest classes of society are chiefly involved, and the male predominance is most marked. The stones are found more often in the bladder and urethra than in the upper urinary tract. The urine is often sterile, and uric acid and urates are the chemical substances forming the greater part of the stones. Modern reports of this type of calculus come from THOMPSON in China, McCARRISON in India, NOBLE, and later PASSMORE in Siam, BRUN in Tunis, BROWN and BROWN in Syria, REYES and FLETCHER in the Phillipines. Thus THOMPSON discusses a series of 3,492 cases of which 25% were under 10 and 45% under 20 years of age; the distribution according to position was as follows: renal, 5 cases; vesical 2,962 cases; urethral 409 cases; preputial 119 cases. Stones were composed of uric acid or urates in 78%. VYAS, however, reports a smaller proportion of urate stones in India. There is no doubt that lack of thorough investigation partly accounts for the comparative scarcity of the upper urinary tract calculi, but this factor cannot be held entirely responsible. LETT has given some interesting figures from the London Hospital which cover the period during which the endemic calculus was becoming uncommon in England; the incidence of stone in the upper tract remained constant, while lower urinary calculi became rare.

Site and sex incidence of urinary calculi in children (LETT)

Year Period	Renal		Ureteric		Vesical		Urethral	
	M	F	M	F	M	F	M	F
1905—09	3	2	3	—	16	1	1	8
1910—14	6	3	10	—	11	5	1	—
1915—19	6	1	1	—	10	1	2	—
1920—24	8	6	1	2	13	—	15	—
1925—29	4	6	1	2	1	—	1	—
1930—35	3	3	2	2	1	—	1	—

In discussions on the aetiology of the endemic calculus many factors have been considered at length in the literature: although this type now occurs for the most part in tropical regions, and dehydration has been suspected as a cause, in times past temperate zones were also affected. The disease has always been rare in Negroes, but otherwise, race does not appear to play an important part, and there can now be little doubt that a dietary defect is the most significant factor. Stone has been common where the diet has been poor and has consisted very largely of cereal foods without the addition of milk or milk products. McCARRISON reviewed in detail the diets in India in regard to the incidence of stone and reached the conclusion that a deficiency of Vitamin A of animal origin was the factor primarily responsible. This author also points out that stone is common where wholemeal bread forms a substantial part of the diet, but is rare where the white loaf has been adopted; he suggests the possibility of a dangerous substance in the former. PASSMORE regards the Vitamin A deficiency theory as untenable in Thailand and again postulates an unknown toxic factor. All authors agree that an enrichment and diversification of the diet will assist in the prevention of stone. There is nothing to suggest that the factor responsible for the formation of endemic calculi is operative in the sporadic cases which are considered in the following sections.

2. Calculi complicating congenital abnormalities of the urinary tract

In the Great Ormond Street series, 25 out of 85 cases fell into this group, and it is clear that congenital abnormalities play a larger part in calculous disease in children than in adults. The stones are composed of calcium phosphate as a rule, though if there is a complicating urinary infection, ammonium magnesium phosphate will also be deposited. Urinary stasis in a dilated passage is presumably

the factor predisposing to stone-formation: the majority of cases are hydronephroses due to congenital pelvi-ureteric obstruction, and mega-ureters without
reflux (Figs. 101 and 102): the stones themselves do not often alter the symptoms
which are due to the primary abnormality, and in treatment the elimination of the
stasis is at least as important as the removal of the stone.

3. Recumbency calculi

Stones may form in the kidney, ureter or bladder as a result of immobilization
and in the past they have been a common complication of osteomyelitis, bone and

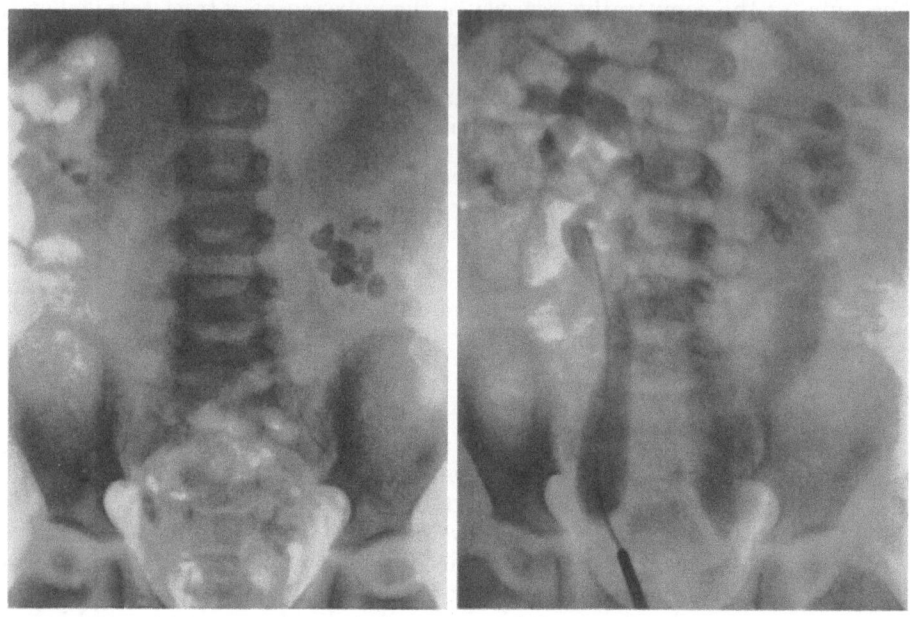

A   B

Fig. 101 A and B. Renal and ureteric calculi with dilated ureters. A Straight X-ray; B Retrograde pyelograms.
Boy aged 3 years suffering from haematuria. Multiple calculi in both kidneys and ureters: the ureteric dilatation
ceased abruptly 1.5 cm above the bladder without evident extrinsic obstruction. Bilateral re-implantation of
ureters into bladder and removal of stones

joint tuberculosis, and poliomyelitis. It is generally believed that stasis of urine
and excessive excretion of calcium consequent upon decalcification of the bones
are the factors responsible, though other mechanisms have been suspected (e.g.
hypervitaminosis D: MAWSON). The concretions usually consist of crystalline
calcium phosphate in the first instance and are formed as a loose "sludge"
in sterile urine, but with the passage of time and the onset of infection, triple
phosphate is added and a true stone is formed. The first evidence of the
disease is often a bout of haematuria following an unusual movement such as
that involved in the change of a plaster cast, or the presence of pyuria may be
noted on routine examination. The sludge may be passed spontaneously with
the resumption of active movements or with diuresis, and with good management
recumbency calculi should not occur. STEVENSON has described the regime of
high fluid intake and the compound pulley suspended beds used in an orthopaedic unit as a prophylaxis, and notes also that the use of aluminium hydroxide
gels has a place in reducing the phosphate output. Once large solid stones are
formed, they must be treated surgically.

4. Foreign body calculi

The natural curiosity of children is apt to lead to the introduction of foreign bodies into one orifice or another, and a wide variety of objects have found their way into the bladder, particularly in the female child. Except in areas where stone is endemic, the presence of a solitary calculus in the bladder should always give rise to the suspicion of a foreign body, but it should be noted that calculi of similar origin can also arise in the upper urinary tract. "Bobby pins" and similar

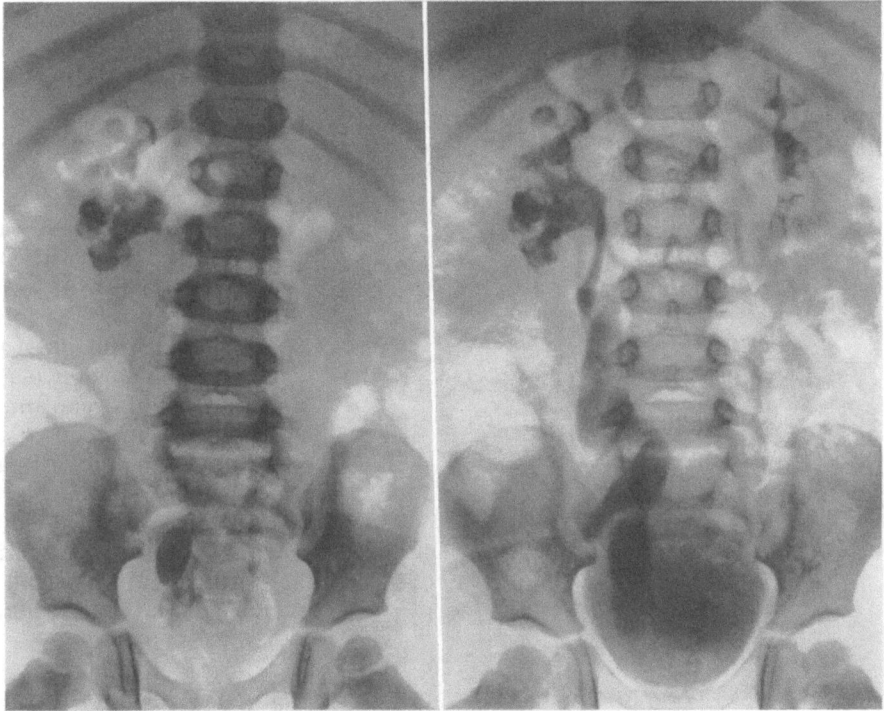

A   B

Fig. 102 A and B. Calculi in kidney and dilated ureter. Plain X-ray and intravenous pyelogram in a boy aged two years with general ill-health, found to have chronic pyuria. Nephro-ureterectomy [performed: stones composed of calcium phosphate

objects when swallowed by small children are apt to penetrate the second or third part of the duodenum, and then come in contact with the renal pelvis or ureter: at this stage they may betray their presence by causing haematuria and a urinary infection, or they may remain symptomless for a long while and be responsible for stone formation and pyonephrosis (BILGER and GREINER). BRATT-STROM has also recorded the ascent of the ureter by grass straws in a 13 year old boy, while penetration from the abdominal wall by needles is also a possibility (BLAINE).

5. Cystine calculi

Although cystine calculi are often regarded as something of a rarity the decrease in the general incidence of stone in children has given them a greater importance, and they may be expected to account for at least 5% of cases in England. They are formed by simple precipitation from urine which contains cystine in high concentration and occur therefore only in subjects with cystinuria.

This is a congenital and often a familial disorder of the renal tubules (entirely distinct from cystinosis, see p. 225) in which there is a failure of reabsorption, and consequently an excessive urinary loss of cystine, lysine and usually arginine. The blood levels of these substances are normal and there does not appear to be any abnormality of cystine metabolism (DENT and ROSE). Some degree of cystinuria may be detected fairly frequently in the general population (1 in 600 normal subjects, LEWIS) but the investigations of HARRIS and WARREN have shown that cases fall into two groups: first those in whom the cystine reaches a high concentration in the urine (500—1,400 mgm/24 hours in adults) and in whom stone formation occurs in about 50% of cases, and second those with lower concentrations in whom stones are rare. The former group were thought to be genetically homozyous for the cystinuria gene and the latter heterozygous; some of the families investigated consisted only of normal subjects and those with high cystine excretion; others showed normal, homozygous, and heterozygous types.

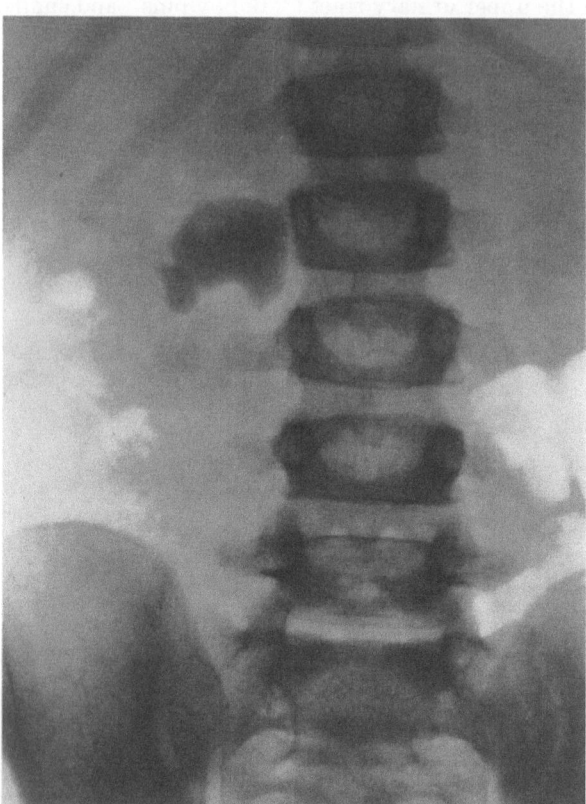

Fig. 103. Cystine calculus. Plain radiograph in a boy aged 7 years investigated for mild abdominal pain. Sterile urine and no history of infection. Pyelolithotomy performed

Cystine stones are first formed in sterile urine, they frequently consist of almost pure cystine, but when secondary infection is present other crystalline or organic material may be added. All are opaque to X-rays and will be evident in any good radiograph, though the shadow is not as dense as that produced by some calcium stones. They may occur at any level in the urinary tract, and small ones are not infrequently passed. When retained in the pelvis, they often assume a dendritic form (Fig. 103). The symptoms of cystine stones do not differ from others similarly placed, but as the urine is often sterile, there is a considerable danger of insidious destruction of the kidney before symptoms appear.

The medical treatment of cystine calculi has been well reviewed by DENT and SENIOR; they have shown that the total daily output of cystine is constant for any individual, but that cystine is soluble in dilute alkaline urine, and that during diuresis existing calculi are reduced in size. Since they find it impossible to keep the urine constantly alkaline they advocate a continuous forced polyuria: so much fluid is taken that nocturnal micturition is the rule, and by drinking during the night the normal nocturnal concentration of urine is avoided. This line of treatment may be the only one required where stones are small and likely to pass spontaneously; it will supplement surgery where the early removal of a vesical calculus or an obstructing renal calculus is required. The arduous routine of diuresis must be continued throughout the life of the patient, since he will always be liable to recurrence if the cystine concentration of the urine is allowed to rise. In some of my cases, children have been kept free from recurrence by continuous alkaline therapy, but regular supervision and frequent X-rays are required.

The relatives, and particularly the sibs, of cystinuric children should be examined, and if their urine contains a high concentration of cystine, even in the absence of stone, a prophylactic polyuria should be advised.

6. Xanthine calculi

Xanthine calculi are exceedingly rare, yet the majority have had their origin in childhood.

They are relatively translucent to X-rays and small ones may not cast a shadow in a plain film of the abdomen. They are associated with an inborn error of purine metabolism resulting in excessive excretion of xanthine (BERMAN, BROWN, DENT and PHILPOT, KRETSCHMER).

7. Calculi associated with nephrocalcinosis

The term nephrocalcinosis describes simply the presence of calcium deposits in the parenchyma of the kidney, and should not be applied to any particular disease process. Microscopic nephrocalcinosis, not demonstrable by clinical radiology, is very common in infants dying of all causes (ANDERSON) and BODIAN has stated that calcium deposits in and around the renal tubules are found in 11% of otherwise normal kidneys in post-mortems on children. Randall's plaques, deposits lying under the epithelium of the calyx, are however less common than in adults. Microscopic nephrocalcinosis of a more severe degree is character-istic of certain pathological states, e.g. Vitamin D intoxication, mercury or sulphonamide tubular necrosis, and idiopathic hypercalcaemia (SCHLESINGER et al.), but in none of these are the deposits sufficient to show up in plain X-rays of the abdomen and in none is nephrolithiasis a likely complication. Radiologically demonstrable nephrocalcinosis is of greater relevance to the present discussion since associated stone may be found; the common causes must therefore be briefly reviewed.

a) Hyperchloraemic acidosis, infantile renal acidosis (LIGHTWOOD et al.)

In this syndrome the infant usually presents with failure to thrive, vomiting, loss of weight, constipation and severe attacks of dehydration. There is a defect of the renal tubular function concerned with the production of an acid urine, and the characteristic findings are polyuria with a persistently alkaline urine despite a low plasma bicarbonate level (less than 18 meq/L after re-hydration). The serum chloride level is raised but the blood urea is only up during attacks of dehydration. LIGHTWOOD et al. found some radiological evidence of calcification in 13 out of 35 cases, but stones in the infantile form, though recorded by ISRAELS et al., are rare and the disease is self limiting provided the child is carried through the biochemical disturbances. There is however, a more severe form of hyperchloraemic acidosis (ALBRIGHT and RIEFENSTEIN) encountered in older children and adults in which the tubular defect appears to be incurable and its effects serious and persistent. Calcium deposits in the parenchyma, chiefly in the pyramids, are clearly seen in X-rays and nephrolithiasis is common. The stones are usually small and pass spontaneously, causing recurrent colic. Most are composed of calcium phosphate, though some urates and oxalates may be found. The urine which usually contains a slight excess of pus cells, is often sterile, but severe pseudomonas pyelonephritis has been described by RUTLEDGE et al.

b) Oxalate nephrocalcinosis

This is a rare but well defined condition (Fig. 104) which has been described by ARCHER et al., DIETRICH, DAVIS et al., MULLOY, NEWNS and BLACK, APONTE and FETTER and NEUSTEIN et al.; it is a familial disorder and ultimately fatal because of renal failure. Affected children have repeatedly passed oxalate stones and post-mortem examination has shown deposition of oxalate crystals in the renal parenchyma. The urinary output of oxalate has been excessive and the blood uric acid has been raised in some cases, even in the absence of renal failure. No effective treatment is known. A familial incidence of oxalate calculi without nephrocalcinosis, and with a comparatively good prognosis has been noted by GRAM and by MYERS.

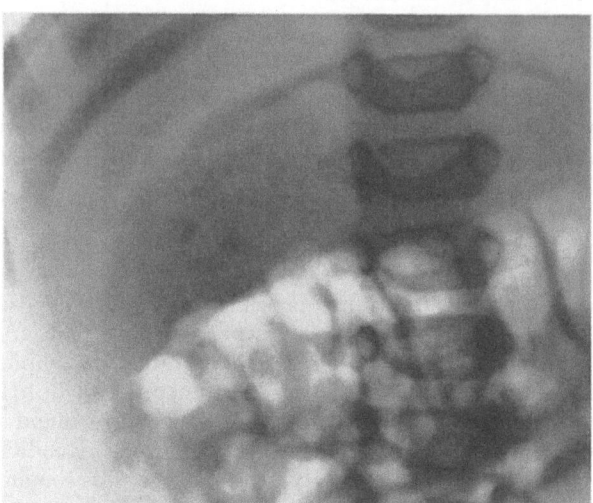

Fig. 104. Nephrocalcinosis. Straight X-ray in a boy aged 6 months. Two months before he had been fully investigated for urinary infection, and no abnormality was then found. Reinvestigation after haematuria showed bilateral nephro-calcinosis with a small stone in the ureter. Urinary output of oxalate found to be enormously increased above average.

c) Hyperparathyroidism

Nephrocalcinosis and nephrolithiasis due to primary hyperparathyroidism are exceptionally rare in children, though a case has been reported in a boy of 13 years by BICKEL. PUGH, and PHILLIPS have recorded younger cases of parathyroid disease without stones.

d) Pyelonephritis, renal hypoplasia and glomerulo-nephritis

Nephrocalcinosis may be found in the chronic forms of these conditions, though it is rarely possible to demonstrate it radiologically.

e) Miscellaneous

PITTS et al. have recorded nephrocalcinosis in a familial form without bio-chemical disturbances; the stones passed were of phosphate composition. NAYLOR has described nephrocalcinosis in hypothyroidism. Some minor degree of nephrocalcinosis is not infequently discovered in children with idiopathic calculi when the kidney, exposed at operation for nephrolithotomy, is X-rayed; the exact significance of this type of calcification cannot be assessed at present.

8. Stones in congenital cystic dilatation of the collecting tubules

DELL'ADAMI and BORELLI have described the formation of stones in a child aged 7 years, with cystic dilatation of the tubules running through the pyramids. The case apparently corresponds with those reported in the French literature as Rein-en-éponge (e.g. LHIZ) and by VERMOOTEN under the term congenital cystic

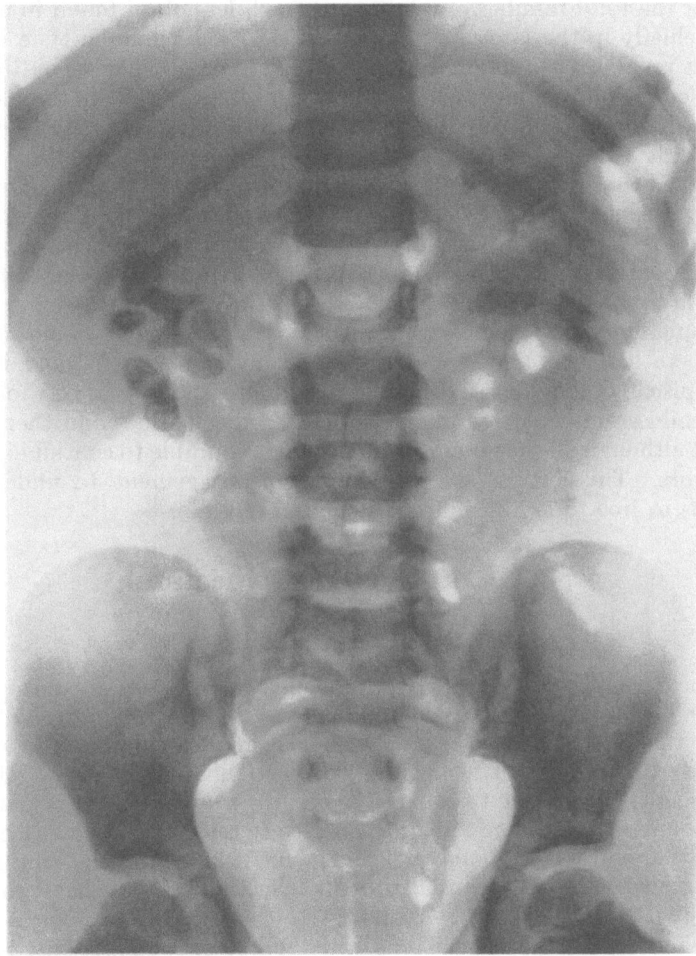

Fig. 105. Multiple phosphatic calculi. Plain X-ray in a boy aged 5 years with pyuria and haematuria. The left ureteric calculus was removed first; at later operations both kidneys were split to remove the calculi from the calyces

dilatation of the collecting tubules. Very little is known about the disease, which has usually presented with haematuria and stone formation in middle life.

9. Idiopathic calculi

When all the known predisposing factors in stone formation have been considered, there remains a large number of cases for which no cause can be found: in the Great Ormond Street series approximately half the total number fell into this group. The stones in these cases were almost always composed of phosphate in various combinations, and oxalate stones were rare; this observation is an inter-esting contrast to that of WINKEL SMITH who reported a comparable series from Denmark, but found that oxalate was the predominant chemical substance in-volved. CAMPBELL, in America, states that in half his cases the stone was composed of phosphate, and in half of urates, so that even in areas where stone is not endemic there appears to be some local variation.

Isolated ureteric calculi, or solitary calyceal calculi, which form a large pro-portion of the total number of adults, are much less often found in children, and are seen chiefly in the later years of childhood. The common type of idiopathic calculus is renal in position, and frequently takes on a dendritic outline. Multiple calculi affecting both kidneys and perhaps the ureters as well are common (Fig.105), and very often appear during the first two years of life. Infection is present in the great majority, Proteus vulgaris being the characteristic organism; occasionally it is observed that a stone develops in a child who has previously suffered a severe pyelonephritis, the first investigations having demonstrated a normal urinary tract. It is reasonable to postulate therefore that pyelonephritis may play some part in the pathogenesis of the stones, perhaps by damaging the epithelial lining of the urinary passages or the lymphatic pathways, perhaps by interfering with tubular function and allowing excessive excretion of calcium. Some of the affected infants have had a previous illness, such as pyloric stenosis, and it is possible that an episode of dehydration may be the starting point of stone formation. At times a child seems to go through a stone forming period, and then pass out of it, so that although all the circumstances seem favourable to continuing deposition, none occurs. This fact is a considerable encouragement to undertake major operations to free the kidneys from stone in early life.

III. Regional classification

1. Renal calculi

All the recognized types of renal calculus may be found during childhood, though the solitary calyceal oxalate stone is rare. In infants the characteristic forms are the dendritic calculus, and multiple small calculi in the renal pelvis and in the calyces, causing little urinary obstruction but associated with a severe pyelonephritis. The symptoms are commonly those of urinary infection with perhaps some pain in the affected loin; cases are often investigated because of the failure of the pyuria to respond to ordinary medical treatment. Surgical removal of this type of calculus is often difficult, the kidney may have to be split to allow extraction, and X-ray pictures of the exposed organ are essential, but conservative surgery is well rewarded and nephrectomy should only be performed where there is advanced destruction of the renal parenchyma in recurrent cases.

Obstructing pelvic calculi cause hydronephrosis or pyonephrosis and are responsible for severe renal pain. A secondary stricture at the pelvi-ureteric junction may result from the presence of such a stone and if uncorrected will cause recurrence. It is quite common to see mild dilatation of the lumbar ureter below such a stone; this dilatation is abolished by stimulation of the exposed ureter and does not indicate any obstruction, it is referred to as lumbar ureterec-tasis (Fig. 106). Occasionally a pyonephrosis develops with the minimum of symptoms and presents as a renal tumour as in the example illustrated in Fig. 107.

Multiple calculi not infrequenly complicate hydronephrosis due to pelvi-ureteric obstruction, either with or without infection. The symptoms are essen-tially those of the obstructed kidney or of the urinary infections. The simple removal of the stone is inadequate, either a plastic operation on the pelvi-ureteric junction or a nephrectomy must be performed, but the presence of stone need not influence the choice of conservative or radical surgery. Stones may also be found in calyceal diverticula and in that situation often require no treatment unless there is a recurrent urinary infection. Anomalous kidneys (malrotated, fused or ectopic) are liable to stone formation even where there is no great dilatation of the pelvis and in unilateral cases nephrectomy is advisable, since recurrence is likely after simple pyelolithotomy.

2. Ureteric calculi

In my experience small calculi in the ureter causing colic are chiefly found in older children; the pain may be characteristic but is often poorly localized, and on the right side may be attributed to appendicitis. CAMPBELL and other American authors, however, indicate that renal colic with the passage of ureteric calculi is not infrequent in infants, and it is interesting to note that in a series from Canada (JACKSON) 9 out of 32 stones were passed spontaneously. Where a stone is held up in the ureter endoscopic instrumentation is not to be advised in children and open operation should be performed.

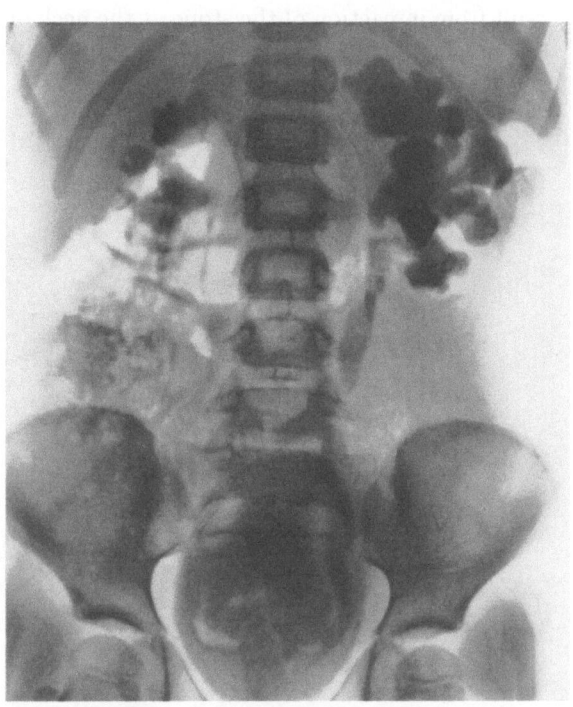

Fig. 106. Bilateral stag-horn calculi with lumbar ureterectasis. Intravenous pyelogram in a boy of 5 years with chronic pyuria and backache. No stone had been passed and there was no evidence of obstruction below the dilated lumbar segment of the ureter. Phosphate calculi treated by pyelolithotomy: later partial nephrectomy for recurrence in lower calyx on the left: plastic operation for acquired stricture of the pelvi-ureteric junction on the right

Large stones forming in otherwise normal ureters may be found in recumbency cases, particularly poliomyelitis (McKAY and BAIRD). Stones complicating mega-ureter are relatively frequent; the mega-ureter is of the type associated with the normal or stenosed uretero-vesical junction, and stone will not form where there is free reflux of the bladder urine. Typical stones are large, rounded and are very freely movable up and down the ureter; they may cause haematuria or a mild pain, but are quite often found during the investigation of pyuria due to the dilated ureter itself. The simple ureterolithotomy is never enough in these cases: the lower end of the ureter must be widened or re-implanted into the bladder, or in strictly unilateral cases nephro-ureterectomy may be the best treatment.

Calculus anuria is a rare but urgent manifestation and has been reported by DEHERRIPON in an infant of three months.

3. Vesical calculi

Stone in the bladder is characteristic of endemic calculous disease, but apart from this is rare and liable to be associated with foreign body or with multiple upper

urinary tract calculi. Symptoms are characteristic: there is a severe pain radiating
into the genitalia with frequency and urgency of micturition. Boys are apt to
grasp the penis to ease the pain, and perhaps to prevent the urge incontinence;
consequent bathing of the hand in urine may lead to ammoniacal dermatitis of
the palm (le signe de la main; BRUN). In a similar way girls often handle the
genitalia and in both sexes masturbation is common. Retention of urine may
result from impaction of the stone at the neck of the bladder, and in small infants,
in whom frequency of micturition is unlikely to be noticed, a distended bladder

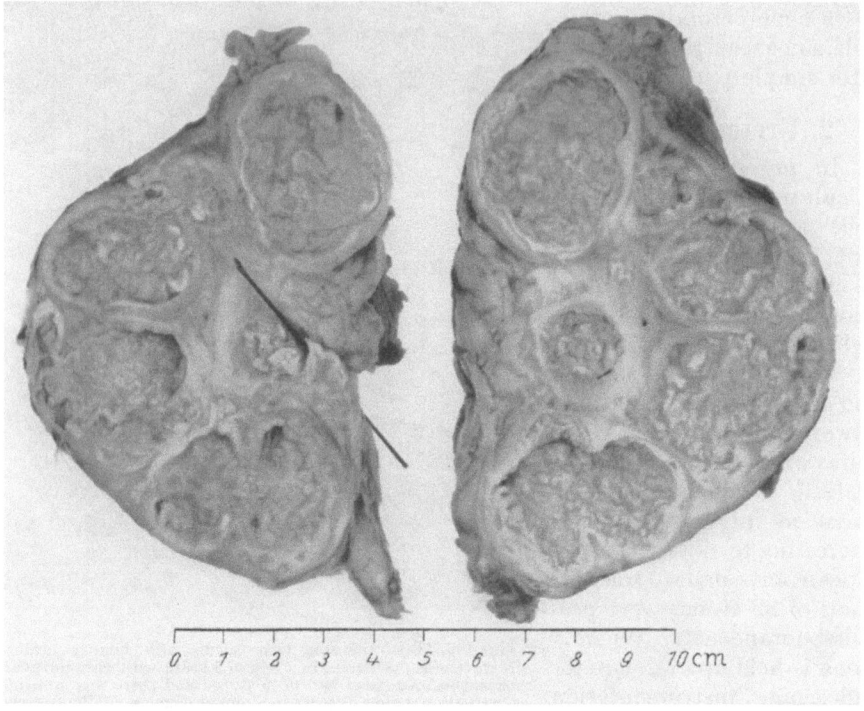

Fig. 107. Calculous pyonephrosis. Operative specimen from a boy aged 4¹/₂ years with a long history of general
ill-health, and a hard renal swelling. X-ray showed several calcifications within the renal area: there was no
function evident in the intravenous pyelogram. Recovery after nephrectomy

is often found. Rectal prolapse associated with strangury is characteristic
(MUKHERJEE) and BRUN describes a case in which the straining produced a
complete uterine prolapse in a girl of three years. When the urine is infected
frequency and urgency become extreme and if the condition is left untreated it
will lead to enormous thickening of the bladder wall, dilatation of the upper
urinary tract, and ultimately to death from renal failure. Stone is an occasional
complication of bladder neck obstruction, in which there will also be hypertrophy
of the bladder (e.g. GOLDBERG) but this manifestation of chronic lower urinary
obstruction has not been common in my practice.

Litholapaxy should only be performed in older children, and only where
there is a small lithotrite available. In general a cystotomy and removal of the
calculus by the suprapubic route is much to be preferred as the possible trauma
to the urethra is thereby avoided. Where the urine is sterile the bladder may be
closed without even an indwelling catheter, provided suturing is accurate.

Stones are particularly liable to form in the reconstructed ectopic bladder; the musculature of such an organ is usually deficient and probably the stasis that results from inadequate contraction predisposes to the stone formation.

4. Urethral calculi

Urethral calculi are common in areas where stone is endemic, but rare elsewhere. Temporary impaction may occur in the posterior urethra, in the bulb or the penile urethra; such impaction causes retention and at times extravasation of the urine as recorded by SUKHAVANAM. Simple manoeuvres usually suffice either to push the stone back into the bladder or to extract it from the penile urethra, but operative removal may be required. In the female urethral impaction is very uncommon, though a case has been recorded by BEGG. Stones in a dilated prostatic utricle have been described in a boy of 3 years by SCHÖNLEBE which radiologically resembled ordinary prostatic calculi.

Diverticula of the anterior urethra may contain a nest of small calculi which are easily palpated from the perineum (BAZLIEL).

5. Preputial calculi

Apart from simple concretions of smegma, preputial calculi may be pure urinary stones which have become imprisoned in the dilated preputial sac behind phimosis, or may consist of a mixture of smegma and urinary salts. WINSBURY-WHITE quotes a case in a child of 2 years, and JOLY has reported a very large calculus in the prepuce of an 8 year old boy.

6. Calculi outside the urinary tract

Stones are occasionally formed in the vagina in cases of urinary incontinence, particularly where there is epispadias in the female and the urine is continually dripping back into the vagina. In atresia ani urethralis where the lower rectum has been defunctioned by colostomy the persistent recto-urethral fistula may allow the urine to trickle back into the rectum, and faecoliths may be infiltrated by urinary salts and simulate true stones.

IV. Management of calculus cases

1. Diagnosis

Except for the actual passage of the stone there is no symptom which is pathognomic of urinary lithiasis, and outside the endemic areas the great majority of cases present with symptoms which might indicate many forms of urinary tract disease. Stones may be palpated in the urethra, in the bladder and sometimes in the lower ureter by rectal examination, and in the same situations they may be visualized at endoscopy. In all other cases reliance must be placed on X-rays, and again with the exception of endemic disease non-opaque calculi are rare. CAMPBELL states that approximately 10% will fail to cast a shadow, but no such stone has been encountered in a series of 85 cases at Great Ormond Street.

Simple diagnosis of stone is never sufficient: every endeavour should be made to identify a predisposing factor and to estimate the secondary effects resulting from the presence of the stone. Intravenous pyelography, bacteriological examination of the urine, estimation of the blood urea and serum electrolytes, and testing the urine for cystine are essential preoperative investigations in every case.

2. Treatment

Active treatment is required in almost all cases, though a few stones will pass without surgical assistance, and even fewer may be safely left in situ. Assessment of the likelihood of spontaneous passage of the stone must depend largely upon the experience of the surgeon and no definite rule can be laid down; much depends upon the shape and situation as well as upon the size of the stone. Where operative intervention is necessary, the operation performed must aim not only at removing the stone but also at eliminating stasis in the urinary tract. Pelvi-ureteric obstruction whether congenital or acquired must be overcome, mega-ureters must be allowed to drain freely into the bladder even at the cost of allowing a reflux. Individual dilated calyces may sometimes require obliteration by partial nephrectomy, diverticula of the bladder or urethra must be excised. Urinary infections frequently require careful treatment, and prolonged chemotherapy.

3. Prevention of recurrence

Where a specific aetiological factor is found corrective measures can often be undertaken with success, as for instance in the control of cystine or recumbency calculi which have already been discussed. In the idiopathic group greater difficulty is encountered: therapeutic diuresis is the only measure which has universal approval now that dietary treatments have largely fallen into disfavour, and in the majority of uncomplicated cases, the recurrence rate at present observed is not so great as to suggest the need for any other prophylactic regime. In the damaged and infected kidneys, however, some precautions are desirable. Acidification of the urine does not entirely prevent the formation of calcium phosphate stones, and in the difficult cases with chronically infected urine, it is very difficult to achieve, because of the activity of urea splitting organisms. SHOER and CARTER were able to show that the administration of aluminium hydroxide gels (Aludrox 20—40 ccs t.d.s.) leads to the retention of phosphate in the bowel, and so lowers the phosphate content of urine. This measure undoubtedly slows the rate of growth of phosphate calculi, and has been of assistance in my cases (ECKSTEIN). Salicylic amide (PRIEN and WALKER) treatment, which aims at chelating the calcium salts in the bowel may also prove useful, but is still under trial. BUTT has advocated the administration of hyalase in order to alter the surface tension of urine, and so to assist the "protective action" of the urinary colloids; in practice, the measure has met with little success, and a daily subcutaneous injection adds considerably to the child's burden.

In children with oxalate calculi, the prohibition of fruits such as strawberries, rhubarb, tomatoes etc., which contain large amounts of these substances may be advisable, and this restriction certainly lowers the level of the urinary oxalates.

K. Neoplastic disease

1. Neoplasms in infancy and childhood

With improvements in nutrition, and with the increasingly effective control of infections, neoplastic disease has now assumed an important place in the list of causes of death during childhood.

Some indication of the prevalence of malignant conditions is given by the following figures taken from the report of BODIAN and WHITE.

Registrar-general's returns of England and Wales 1949

Age Group	Total Number of Deaths Excluding Accidents	Deaths due to Malignant Conditions, including Leukemia	
1—4	3771	343	9.1%
5—9	1411	172	12.2%
10—14	1230	146	11.9%

Tumours treated at the Hospital for Sick Children 1930—1952

Total	390	Ovarian tumours	6
Nephroblastoma	62	Testicular tumours	9
Urogenital sinus tumours	12	Adrenal carcinoma	4

The second table indicates that approximately a quarter of all malignant tumours in childhood come within the province of the genito-urinary surgeon, and the fact that all these are tumours for which surgical treatment is increasingly successful emphasizes the importance of the topics to be discussed in this chapter. In addition, there were 82 cases of neuroblastoma in BODIAN and WHITE's series; the majority of these were sited in the adrenal gland or in the abdominal sympathetic system, and therefore likely to come under the urologist's care. In this group, however, it seems likely that chemotherapy and radiotherapy will ultimately prove more effective than surgery.

Malignant disease in childhood seldom affects the epithelial surfaces, and the long-acting external carcinogenic agents have little influence in initiating neoplastic change. The great majority of the neoplasms are embryonic tumours: they have their origin coincidentally with the development of the normal organs, and frequently exhibit in their histology the various stages of normal differentiation in the tissue from which they arise. Thus in the nephroblastoma, imperfect formation of glomeruli and tubules may be found in the midst of undifferentiated mesenchyme, while in the teratoma, many tissues may appear in varying degrees of maturity. In a sense, therefore, embryonic tumours are congenital malformations as well as neoplasms, but as yet very little is known as to the cause of the departure from the normal line of development. A recent survey by STEWART et al. has demonstrated, however, that malignant disease occurs more frequently in children who were exposed to irradiation in utero during the course of diagnostic radiological procedures such as pelvimetry. It may well be that in the future it will be possible to identify other physical or infective agents capable of producing neoplasia, similar to those already recognized as favouring the development of other congenital abnormalities.

The use of the term "congenital tumours" in relation to the embryonic sarcomata is apt to be misleading, since in the past it has often been applied to tumours which are clinically evident at birth. WELLS has reviewed such cases and finds substantiated examples very rare, although as will be seen, several cases of nephroblastoma causing difficulties in delivery are on record. In relation to the growth of the embryonic tumours, however, the change from intra-uterine to extra-uterine life is not an event of any great importance: the tumours usually remain quiescent until the second or third year.

II. The kidney

1. Nephroblastoma

Nephroblastoma is much the most frequently encountered neoplasm in the genito-urinary system, and has attracted considerable interest from surgeons, pathologists and radiologists: a very large number of papers relating to the topic have been published, and only the more important can be referred to in this article. Although not the first report of the condition, WILMS' description is regarded as classical, and Wilms' tumour has become its common appellation. Recent general reviews will be found in the works of CAMPBELL, GROSS and NEUHAUSER, HARVEY, HUGUENIN and GERARD MARCHANT, SANSONE and ZUNIN, SCOTT (1956) and VUORI.

a) Incidence

Nephroblastoma ranks second only to neuroblastoma as the commonest malignant tumour of childhood, and accounts for approximately 15—20% of deaths from malignant disease during the first four years. It has been recorded at all stages of childhood, and even in adult life, but over 90% of cases present in children under five years of age. It may on occasion be apparent at birth. It shows no predisposition to affect one sex more than the other, and occurs with equal frequency in either kidney: at times it is bilateral as reported by CAMPBELL, BARR and SCHULTE, JOHNSON and MARSHALL, and SCOTT (1955). The last named of these writers has surveyed the literature on bilateral disease and reaches the conclusion that involvement of the opposite kidney is usually secondary and due to blood borne spread from the first, but many cases without distant metastases are on record, and there are even a number of survivors reported (e.g. GROSS and NEUSHAUSER; RICKHAM; PETERSON and JOHNSON). An origin in multiple foci may therefore be suspected, and there is some suggestion of discrete tumours in one kidney at times. A familial incidence is rare, but has been described on several occasions (MASLOW; FITZGERALD and HARDIN), and three or four members of the family may be involved.

There are numerous descriptions of nephroblastoma arising in kidneys exhibiting some congenital malformation: a double kidney, a horse-shoe kidney (e.g. ROSE and WATTENBERG, MCGINN and WICKHAM) or a polycystic kidney (FEENEY et al.). The tumour may be discovered as an incidental finding at operation for the malformation, but more often it is the growth which has been responsible for symptoms. Although the multiplicity of reports might suggest that the anomalous kidney was more liable to neoplasia than the normal, this is by no means established, and in the Great Ormond St. series, congenital abnormalities were not found more often than would be expected in a random sample.

An interesting observation has been made by BJORKLUND, who noted that many cases of nephroblastoma showed hemi-hypertrophy of the whole body, and this phenomenon has been observed in other tumours. The significance of the observation is not clear, but it does suggest that infants with hemi-hypertrophy should be regularly examined during the first years of life.

b) Pathology

A full discussion of the pathology would be out of place in this volume, and it will only be necessary here to describe briefly the features which are of particular interest to the clinician. The tumour, because of the many histological pictures which it may present, has received a multitude of names: adenosarcoma, renal embryoma, embryonal sarcoma, and congenital mixed tumour being the most widely used and the most appropriate; it is generally believed, moreover, that many malignant tumours of the kidney formerly described as sarcomata of a particular tissue, such as myosarcoma or chondrosarcoma, are in fact usually nephroblastomata, and that if sufficient search were made, the characteristic tissues would be found. The following account is based on the review of a series of cases at the Hospital for Sick Children reported by BODIAN and WHITE.

The tumour arises within the substance of the kidney, and after a quiescent phase enlarges rapidly, compressing the surrounding renal parenchyma, and thinning out the overlying tissue. There appears to be a well formed tumour capsule in most cases, and local invasion of surrounding tissues is a rare and late

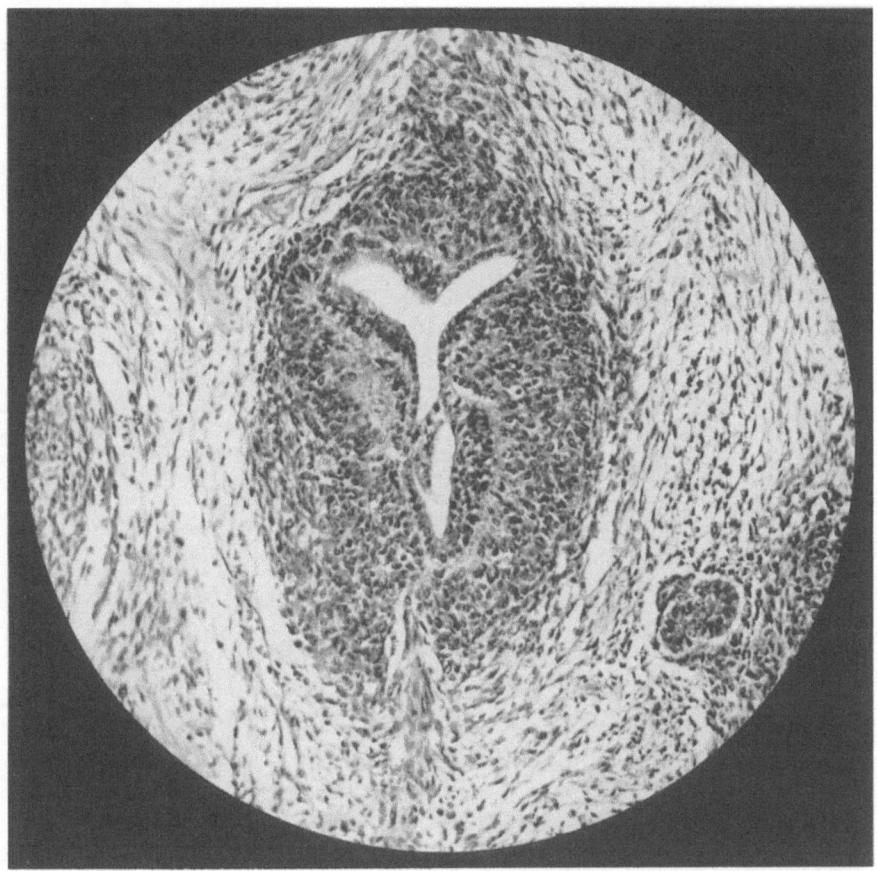

Fig. 108. Histology of nephroblastoma. Section of a nephroblastoma showing an island of epithelial blastema surrounded by young mesenchyme. The morphology of the tubule enclosed in the blastema suggests that it is of collecting type (i.e. a ureteric outgrowth) and hence not derived by differentiation from the blastema (× 140)

development. Occasionally, when the tumour has its origin close to the surface of the kidney, expansion tends to extrude it from the kidney substance and it takes on the appearance of an appendage; this type is sometimes described as an "extra-renal" tumour. The tumour tissue is soft and white, with firmer fibrotic areas; necrosis and haemorrhage are common and may lead to a cystic appearance.

Histologically the bulk of the tumour is composed of undifferentiated embryonic tissue, either embryonic mesenchyme or renal blastema (Fig. 108). The mesenchymal elements may be differentiated in areas to give rise to collagenous connective tissue, to smooth or striated muscle (Fig. 109), to cartilage, or osteoid material. Developing renal tubules are frequently found, and a few tumours consist very largely of such tubular structures (Fig. 110): differentiation of glomeruli occurs but is less commonly seen. Developing tubules may be occasionally of the collecting tubule type and derived from the ureteric bud tissue, not from the metanephros; mitoses are frequently observed in the derivatives of the renal blastema, but not in the mesenchymal elements. Attempts at subdivision of the nephroblastoma cases in histological sub-groups have not been very successful,

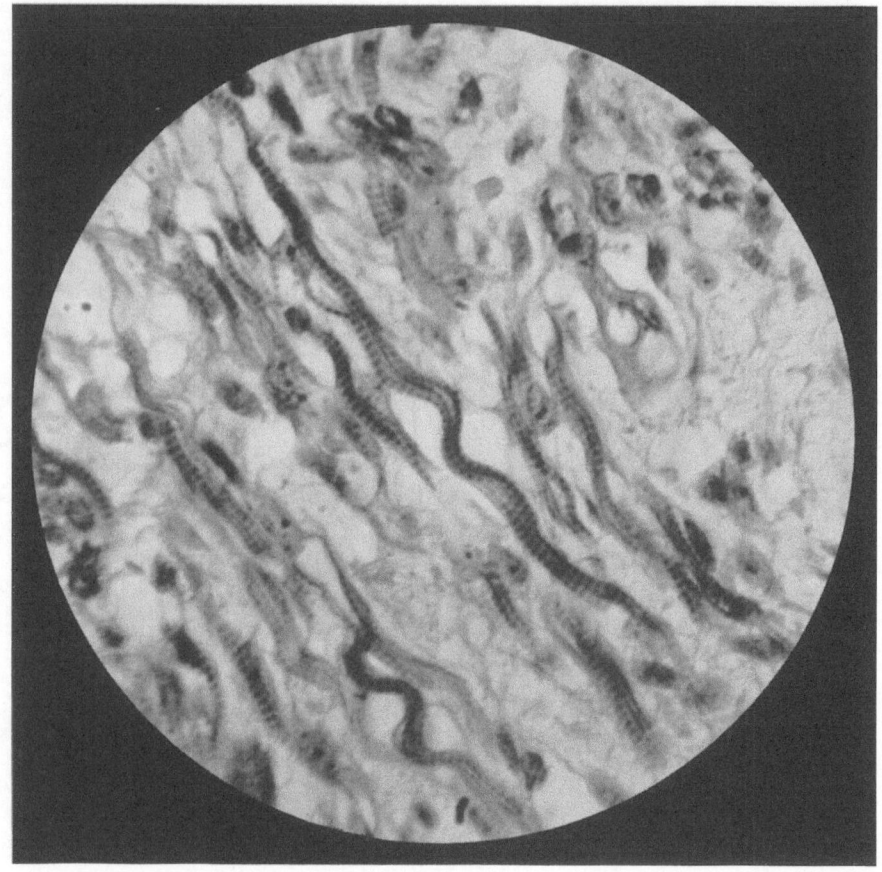

Fig. 109. Histology of nephroblastoma. Well developed rhabdomyoblasts differentiating from mesenchyme, in a nephroblastoma. This form of heteroplasia is not uncommon, in contrast with the occurrence of cartilage

but WHITE has noticed that tumours with a high proportion of differentiated tubules, and those with a papillary appearance and exhibiting an epithelium of the pelvic type with many collecting tubules are more common in the younger infants and appear to carry a better prognosis.

Spread of the tumour is chiefly via the blood stream, and metastases are first found in the lungs and liver. In contrast to the adrenal neuroblastoma, secondaries in bone are very uncommon. There may be direct and continuous invasion of the renal vein, and cases have been seen in which there was a solid column of tissue leading up through the inferior vena cava into the right atrium. The early appearance of a secondary in the epididymis of the left side is occasional evidence of direct venous spread. Lymph gland involvement in this tumour has probably received less attention than it deserves, and if a regular dissection of the hilar and para-aortic glands is made, neoplastic tissues will often be found. Local extension of the tumour into the retroperitoneal tissues, or across the peritoneum is an uncommon and late finding: even less common is spread via the urinary tract, though this has been recorded by FERRIS and BEARE, and by WATKINS.

The histology of the metastases is in general similar to that of the primary, though there may be rather less differentiation.

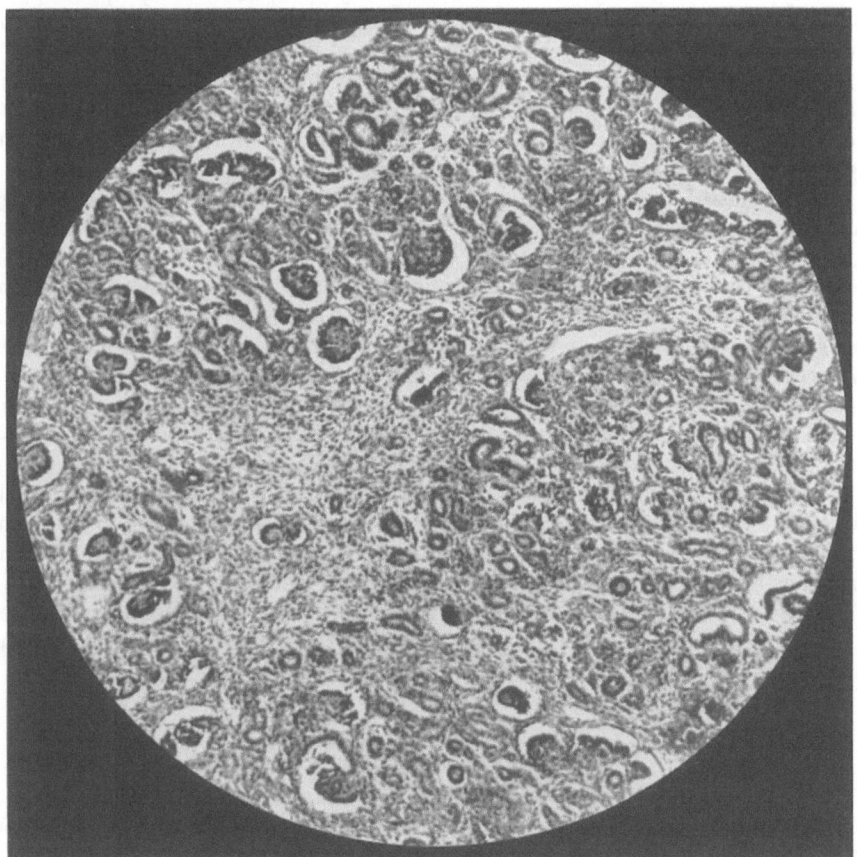

Fig. 110. Histology of nephroblastoma. Section of nephroblastoma found at autopsy in a male infant of two months. There is an advanced degree of differentiation of tubules and glomeruli, which are embedded in immature mesenchyme (× 120)

c) Clinical features

The onset of a tumour in the renal parenchyma is silent, and most nephroblastomata have reached a considerable size before their presence is recognized: the finding of an abdominal mass is in fact much the most frequent mode of presentation, pain and haematuria being later, and less common features. The general condition of the child is often good when medical advice is first sought, despite the large size of the tumour mass, but later loss of weight occurs, due to vomiting and loss of appetite as well as to the growth of the tumour. Anaemia is a common problem in the later stages. In a few, the first symptoms are those of the metastases in the lungs, though this is much less frequent than in the case of the adrenal neuroblastoma. The predominant clinical features may now be considered severally.

α) The abdominal tumour

In more than two thirds of the cases in the Great Ormond Street series, general swelling of the abdomen or localized abdominal mass was the first abnormality noticed, moreover even where other symptoms first drew attention to the disease, a tumour was palpable. Although cases have been recorded (e.g. CAMPBELL) in which the tumour was an incidental finding at operation, it is probably true to say that all those causing any symptoms are palpable provided adequate relaxation is obtained, and this fact emphasizes the very great importance of careful, and gentle, abdominal palpation in infants. The tumour may vary from the size of a golf-ball to a mass which fills the entire abdomen: the majority are more than 12 cm across; it enlarges forward into the abdomen, bulging across the mid-line and up under the costal margin; it extends back into the lumbar region and is palpable bimanually, but is not so liable to form a protruding mass in the loin as the adrenal neuroblastoma. The consistence varies from stony hard to tensely cystic, and the surface is smooth or coarsely lobulated. The smaller tumours exhibit the usual mobility of the normal kidney, the larger ones seem fixed even though infiltration of surrounding tissues is not present. The tumour can usually be distinguished on clinical grounds from splenomegaly, from ovarian and hepatic tumours, from choledochal cysts and from tuberculous peritonitis, but great difficulty may be experienced in differentiating the various causes of renal swelling and pyelography is sometimes required to establish the diagnosis. Hydronephrosis is probably the most common cause of the enlargement of the kidney; when unilateral and tense it will closely simulate neoplasm, though it is apt to vary somewhat in size from day to day, and when very large transillumination may be possible. Pyonephrosis is comparatively rare, but resembles tumour even more closely (see Fig. 107). Polycystic disease is likely to be bilateral, but other forms of cystic disease may mimic nephroblastoma so closely that only examination of the excised specimen will decide the issue. Spontaneous venous thrombosis in the neonate may cause haematuria associated with a palpable enlargement of the kidney, but nephrectomy is required in these cases (see p. 230), and the diagnosis may be decided at operation.

β) Abdominal pain

Pain is seldom severe except when the tumour has ruptured, but a mild complaint may be the symptom which leads to examination of the abdomen. A more continuous aching pain is evidence of local spread. Vomiting may accompany the pain, and result from the disturbance of the digestive tract consequent upon its displacement by the tumour mass.

γ) Haematuria

The incidence of haematuria has varied considerably from one series to another; in the writer's experience it has occurred in approximately one third of the cases. Many authors regard this bleeding as due to rupture of the tumour capsule into the renal pelvis, and therefore believe that the symptom indicates a poor prognosis: however, bleeding can certainly occur from the compressed renal substance adjacent to the tumour, and thus may be of value in drawing attention to an early growth. In the case illustrated in Fig. 113 the haematuria was accompanied by elevation of the blood urea, and by passage of casts, so that it was at first attributed to glomerulo-nephritis; yet on careful palpation the tumour mass could be felt. The loss of blood is seldom great, and cannot be held responsible for the development of anaemia.

δ) Spontaneous rupture

This event has been described by TANNER, and by other authors: it has occurred in the Great Ormond Street series. There is a sudden onset of severe abdominal pain, and in all cases laparotomy has been performed for suspected perforation of an abdominal viscus. The peritoneum is found to contain blood and tumour tissue: the outcome is invariably fatal even if the child survives the immediate dangers, and if nephrectomy is performed. Since however, rupture may occur in benign tumours which cannot be differentiated at the time of operation, treatment should always be undertaken.

ε) Hypertension

In many cases the blood pressure in nephroblastoma is never recorded before operation under sufficiently controlled conditions, but various authors have drawn attention to the occurrence of hypertension in association with this tumour: Silver noted it in 7 out of 8 cases. In most the blood pressure has fallen to normal after removal of the tumour-bearing kidney (e.g. MOONS and RUCH) or after radiotherapy (BRADLEY and DRAKE) and the subsequent appearance of secondaries has not led to any recurrence of the hypertension. This fact suggests that a compression of the kidney tissue is responsible, but BRADLEY and PINCOFFS have reported a case in which the blood pressure did rise again in the presence of metastases. It is possible, however, that in this case the opposite kidney was involved, for no detailed examination was made. In one of the writer's cases reported by COX and SMELLIE, the child was first admitted to hospital for investigation of hypertension, and the tumour was found on routine pyelography.

ζ) Varicocele

Distension of the spermatic veins may be seen as a late complication, but this is not an early sign.

η) Dystocia

When it occurs in the foetus, nephroblastoma may cause difficulty in delivery, and even obstruct labour. Many of the infants affected have succumbed (JOSEPHS) but where an accurate diagnosis is made, and nephrectomy is carried out within the first few days of life, long survival is quite possible (SILVER, BERNHEIM).

θ) Metastases

The symptoms of metastasis are naturally variable: pallor, wasting and dyspnoea are the most common. The liver may be enormously enlarged with secondary deposits; ascites is comparatively rare. Deposits in the lung may cause cough and haemoptysis, and a pleural effusion is often found.

d) Radiological diagnosis

Although the clinical examination is often sufficient to indicate beyond doubt the need for exploration, and if possible nephrectomy, an intravenous pyelogram should always be performed to confirm the diagnosis and to assess the state of the contralateral kidney. A chest X-ray should also be a routine procedure.

The plain films of the abdomen will show an extensive soft tissue shadow, often displacing the intestines to the opposite side. Calcification may be seen within the tumour, though it is not as common in nephroblastoma as in neuroblastoma.

The intravenous pyelogram will usually show some evidence of excretion of dye in the affected kidney: complete absence of function is more characteristic

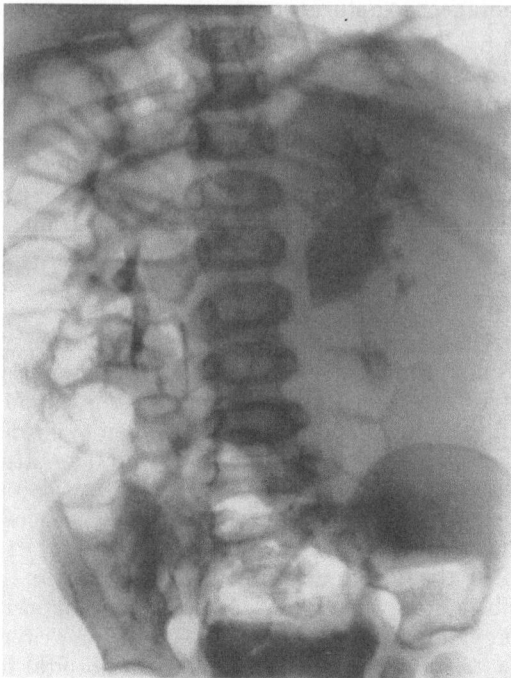

A

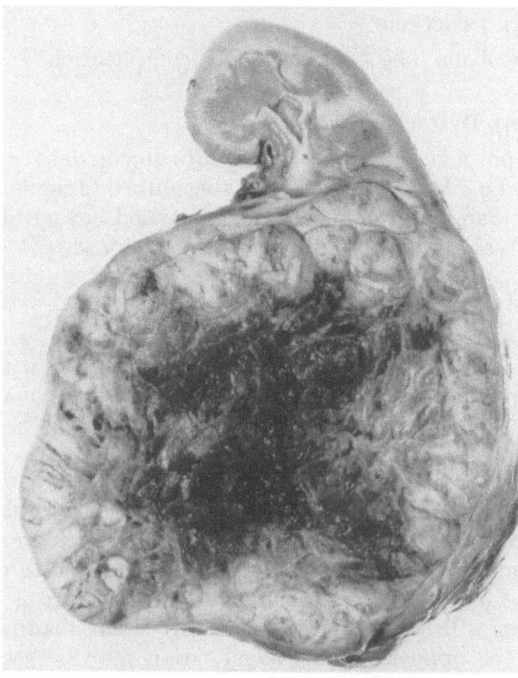

B

Fig. 111 A and B. Nephroblastoma. A Intravenous pyelogram in a boy aged 3 years with abdominal tumour. The pelvis and calyces of the left kidney are splayed out over the surface of a tumour. B Operative specimen

of advanced hydronephrosis or the multicystic kidney. The shadow of the pelvis may, however, be grossly distorted and displaced, so that it is not at first recognized. Lateral views are of assistance. There is no typical pyelographic appearance of tumour, but most cases exhibit one of the forms illustrated:

a) The whole pelvi-calycine system appears enlarged, and is flattened out on the surface of the tumour mass (Fig. 111).

b) There is a localized distortion of one pole of the kidney, with a filling defect in the calyces of that pole (Fig. 112).

c) A filling defect in the renal pelvis, and hydronephrosis of a distorted pelvis (Fig. 113).

d) The pelvis is represented by a bizarre shadow at a point remote from the normal position (Fig. 114).

Retrograde pyelograms are seldom required, since if there is a functioning contralateral kidney, exploration will be necessary in all cases. When the clinical findings suggest the possibility of hydronephrosis, however, and the intravenous series is inconclusive, retrograde pyelography may be helpful, and it will certainly be indicated if there is a suspicion of bilateral disease.

Even after pyelography, differentiation from benign tumours, simple and multi-locular cysts, may be impossible, while adrenal neuroblastoma may still cause confusion. The latter tumour displaces and distorts the upper pole of the kidney, though it is unlikely to obliterate any calyces.

e) Treatment

Until recent years the controversy regarding treatment of nephroblastoma concerned the relative merits of surgery and radiotherapy: all contemporary writers agree, however, that both methods should be employed, and differ only in timing of the procedures. It is true that surgery alone could in the best hands yield encouraging results, and credit must be given to LADD and his fellow workers at the Boston Children's Hospital for showing that the great majority of tumours could be successfuly removed. GROSS and NEUHAUSER summarizing the results of that hospital show that the survival rate was brought up from 14.9% in 1914—1930 period to 32.2% in the 1934—1939 period, by immediate nephrectomy. Improvements in anaesthesia and in methods

Distorted lower calyx

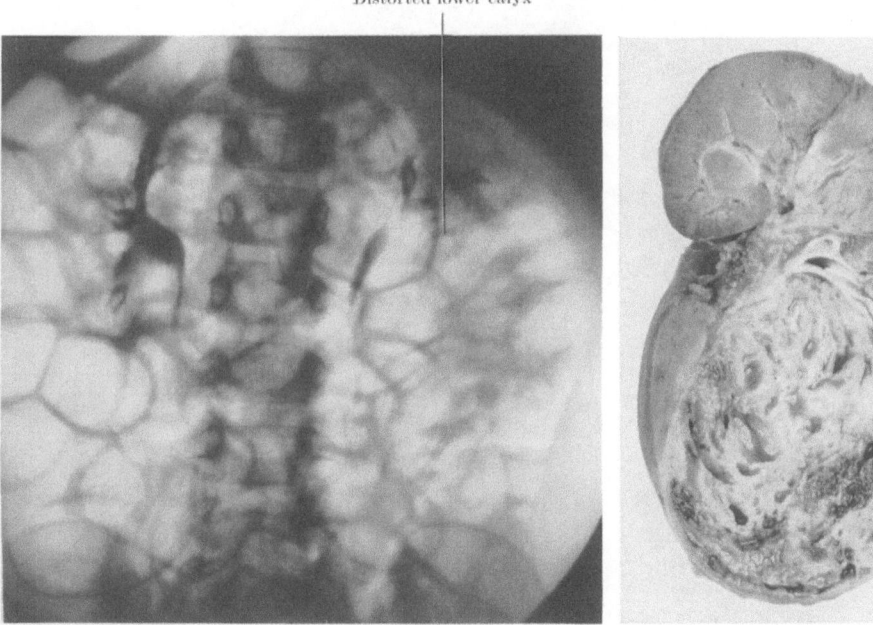

A   B

Fig. 112 A and B. Nephroblastoma. A Intravenous pyelogram from a boy aged 2 years with haematuria, and a palpable left kidney. The lower calyces of the left kidney are displaced by a tumour of the lower pole. B operative specimen

of resuscitation minimized the operative risk, and better exposure through long abdominal incisions improved access and allowed early ligature of the vessels with complete clearance of the regional glands. The same writers report, however, that the survival rate was still further improved to 47.3% in the 1940—1947 period by the addition of post-operative irradiation.

The protagonists of irradiation alone (e.g. DEAN) were never able to produce any considerable series with comparable survival rates, though "cures" have undoubtedly been effected. NESBIT and ADAMS, BIXLER et al., DICKEY and CHANDLER, and SAUER report long term survivals with biopsied tumours: in the case of the last author the growth became extensively calcified and could still be felt 10 years later as a hard mass. ADAMS and HUNT, on the other hand suggest that many of the survivors were in fact suffering from neuroblastoma, which they regard as a more radio-sensitive tumour.

The excellent results reported from Boston have influenced a great many surgeons to favour the programme of immediate nephrectomy followed by early post-operative irradiation. This method is employed by the author, and HIGGINS has reported from the Hospital for Sick Children a 40% $2^{1}/_{2}$ year survival since

that programme has been followed. The child is admitted to hospital as an
emergency, and pre-operation investigations are confined to pyelography, chest

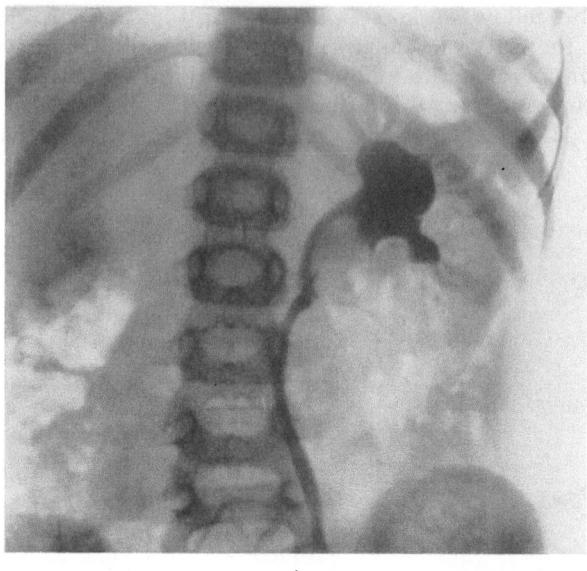

A

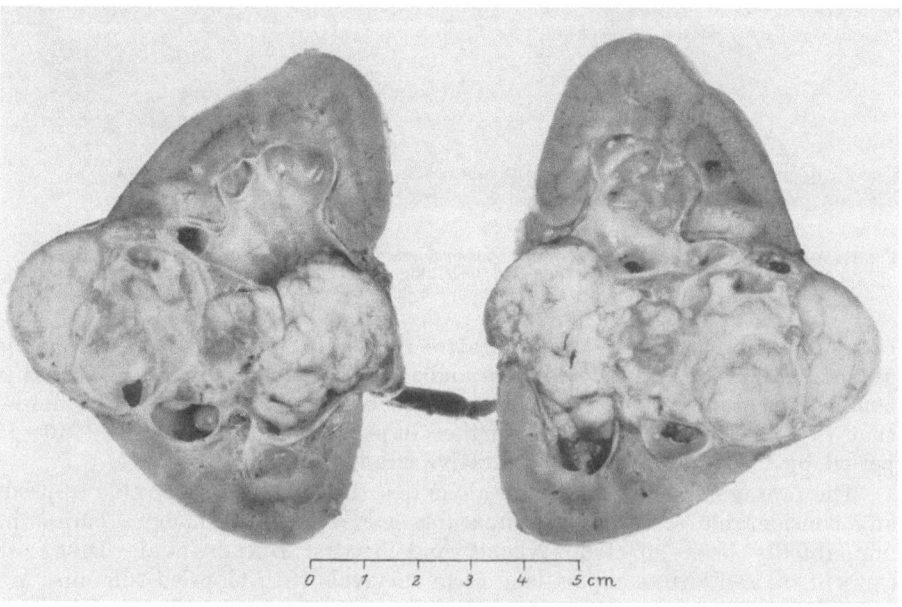

B

Fig. 113 A and B. Nephroblastoma. A Retrograde pyelogram, B Specimen from a boy aged 5 years presenting
with painless haematuria. The mass was only palpable under anaesthesia

X-ray, and blood counts and grouping. Extensive palpation of the tumour is
not allowed, and the child is kept at rest, as it is believed that increasing the
tension within the tumour will facilitate metastasis. Nephrectomy is undertaken
as soon as preparations are complete, and is carried out through a long transverse

incision in the upper abdomen, cutting both recti. The colon is reflected back, and the vessels are ligated before the tumour is mobilized. The para-aortic glands are cleared. Radiotherapy is started as soon as the child can comfortably be moved to the X-ray department, usually within the first week. The tumour bed, and lymphatic glands received 2,000—2,500 R, during the course of 4—6 weeks, (WILLIAMS, HIGGINS and BODIAN) administered through two ports. No disturbance of wound healing has been encountered.

In many clinics, pre-operative radiotherapy is administered as a routine (e.g. KRETSCHMER, RUSCHE, PRIESTLEY and BRODERS), and it is believed that this procedure renders nephrectomy an easier and safer operation. Nephroblastoma is normally very susceptible to irradiation, and rapid shrinkage may occur within two or three weeks of commencing treatment: the tumour continues to shrink for some time after completion of the course, and nephrectomy is therefore usually undertaken after an interval. A further course of radiotherapy can be administered post-operatively. The disadvantages of pre-operative treatment are that metastasis may occur during the course, that the tumour may prove radio-resistant, and that

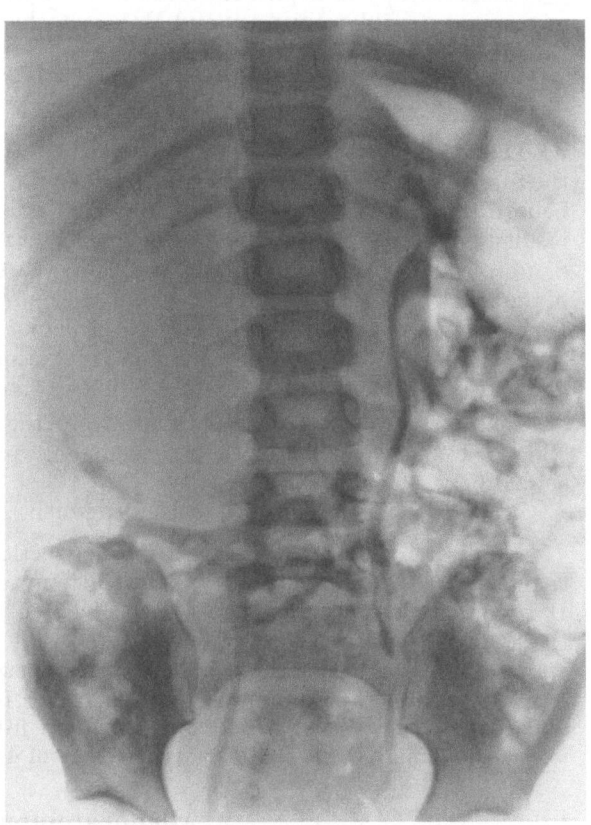

Fig. 114. Nephroblastoma of the right kidney. Intravenous pyelogram in a girl aged 3¹/₂ years with large abdominal mass. The right renal pelvis is displaced downwards and distorted by the tumour. Nephrectomy. Death from metastases within one year

the diagnosis may be incorrect, so that a child with a non-malignant condition is subjected to a heavy dose of irradiation. Moreover with skilful surgery, immediate nephrectomy, though difficult, is possible in almost all cases where metastasis has not occurred, and carries a very low operative mortality. Bilateral cases have been treated by nephrectomy and heminephrectomy combined with radiotherapy (RICKHAM).

While radiotherapy has undoubtedly improved the results of treatment in nephroblastoma, the method itself is not without danger, particularly if high doses are used (GARRETT and MERTZ, GROSS and NEUHAUSER). Irradiation of the tumour or tumour bed is apt to lead to damage to the epiphyseal centres in the iliac crest, and more important, in the vertebral column, where it may result in scoliosis (WHITEHOUSE and LAMPE). Irradiation of a wider area in order to include abdominal lymphatics may lead to irradiation nephritis, and ultimately to death from uraemia (GROSSMAN; SMITH and WILLIAMS). Treatment of the

chest may cause pulmonary fibrosis, and a death from this cause is reported by
KERR and FLYNN, so that prophylactic irradiation of the lungs is not advisable;
nevertheless, the risks may be worth accepting since long term survivals after
partial removal of the abdominal tumour (NESBIT and ADAMS) and after the
appearance of lung secondaries (GARRETT and MERTZ) are on record.

Chemotherapy in nephroblastoma has not yet had sufficient trial to make an
assessment possible: JOHNSON and MARSHALL have had some encouragment from
the use of nitrogen mustards.

f) Recurrence

The majority of fatal cases show evidence of recurrence or metastasis within
the first year of observation, and die within a few months. Most authors therefore
believe that a 2 or $2^1/_2$ year survival period is a fair criterion for assessment of
results, but much later recurrences may occur. FEENEY et al. report re-appearance
of growth at 7 years; FALKINBURG et al. at 8 years (in a case in which involvement
of the renal vein was found in the original specimen) and RITTER and SCOTT at 10
years. Early recurrences are likely to be found in the abdomen, and doubtless
represent tumour tissue left behind at operation in the tumour bed or lymph
glands. Later recurrences often show first in the lungs.

Temporary relief may be obtained from the irradiation of recurrences, but
where these are multiple, such treatment only prolongs the child's suffering and
should be withheld.

g) Prognosis

Almost all the authors quoted in this section have given figures regarding
their survival rates, and HARVEY has attempted a summary of these results.
It is doubtful however, whether such collective surveys give any true picture of
the situation, and it may simply be stated that under the best possible circumstances, with present methods of treatment, between 40 and 50% of cases should
survive 2 years. The prognosis is much better for the younger children (GROSS
and NEUHAUSER report an 80% survival in infants under 12 months), and it
is correspondingly bad for those over the age of 4 years.

2. Adenocarcinoma

In the last century, many of the renal neoplasms of childhood were reported
as hypernephromata, but with the growing realization of the protean nature of
the histology of nephroblastoma, these cases ceased to be recorded, and adenocarcinoma was regarded as a disease of exceptional rarity in childhood. During
recent years, however, several examples of this tumour have been described in
children of all ages: the present writer has operated upon two. CLINTON-THOMAS
and ROBINSON record a child of 10 years with orbital metastases simulating
Hutchison's syndrome, and give several references to earlier papers. BEATTIE;
CURRIE, and JOHNSON and MARSHALL have also discussed cases, all of which
have been fatal. The presenting symptoms are abdominal tumour and haematuria, and the exact nature of the tumour is not likely to be suspected until the
nephrectomy specimen is examined.

3. Papillary tumours of the renal pelvis

Transitional cell neoplasms are exceptionally rare, and it is not unlikely that
some of the recorded cases were papillary forms of nephroblastoma. SCHLAPIK

describes a case in a boy of 13 years: THOMAS in a girl of $3^1/_2$ years, and HIGGINS et al. in a girl of 18 months. All have been malignant tumours.

4. Hamartoma and other benign tumours

A hamartoma is defined as a tumour-like overgrowth of one or more tissue elements normally present at the site: growth of the tumour is co-ordinated with growth of the body as a whole and regression may occur. There is a tendency to include under this designation lesions such as angioma and fibroma formerly described as benign tumours, but in the kidney the most important hamartoma is found in the tuberous sclerosis complex.

Tuberous sclerosis is a congenital disorder of which the cerebral symptoms are the most common manifestation, and which is likely to be fatal in early adult life: there is a nodular gliosis causing epilepsy, mental deficiency and ultimately increased intracranial pressure. The skin of the face exhibits a characteristic rash, adenoma sebaceum, around the nose and cheeks. Tumour-like nodules are found in the heart (congenital "rhabdomyoma"), the lungs and the bones. The renal lesions are multiple and commonly affect both kidneys: nodules containing smooth muscle, fat and blood-vessels are scattered through the cortex, and tend to grow outwards away from the kidney. They may be responsible for haematuria, particularly after trauma, and can cause a deformity of the pyelogram which arouses a suspicion of malignancy: MOOLTEN gives a full description of such a case in a 15 year old girl. LE BRUN et al. comment upon the frequency with which hamartomata cause retro-peritoneal haemorrhage. PRATT-THOMAS describes a case in the new-born. The diagnosis may be suspected from the co-incidence of a renal lesion with adenoma sebaceum or epilepsy and mental deficiency: there is very little likelihood of subsequent malignancy (though it is on record) and the bilateral nature of the condition suggests that treatment should be conservative.

ZANGEMEISTER reports that fibromata, in a microscopic form, are not un-common in the infant's kidney, but they are extremely rare as large tumours. LANGHÖF operated upon a girl of 11 years with a huge abdominal mass which proved to be a fibromatous hamartoma attached to the front of the kidney, while in reviewing the literature on fibroma, KRETSCHMER found two reports of affected children.

Leiomyoma attached to the kidney in a neonate is described by ZUCKERMAN et al. and CONSTANCE has reported a case in which "benign" rhabdomyomata destroyed both kidneys in an infant of one year.

Haemangioma of the kidney, sometimes regarded as an important cause of "essential haematuria", is seldom reported during childhood, although many cases of unexplained bleeding are subjected to exhaustive and repeated investigation. A cavernous haemangioma causing a filling defect in the pyelogram of a girl of 7 years was removed by McLEAN and MATTHEWS, and another in a boy of 14 by SWAN and BALME.

Lymphangioma in the kidney of an infant is discussed by HIGGINS et al. True teratoma is reported by McCURDY.

5. Lymphosarcoma and leukaemia

Both kidneys may be infiltrated by leukaemic or lymphosarcomatous deposits, producing a great increase in size and a characteristic pyelographic appearance closely resembling that seen in adult polycystic disease, though with better preservation of renal function (MILLICHAP).

III. The adrenal gland and retro-peritoneal space

1. Neuroblastoma

The adrenal medulla is developed from cells derived from the neural crest, which also gives origin to the sympathetic ganglion cells. A variety of tumours

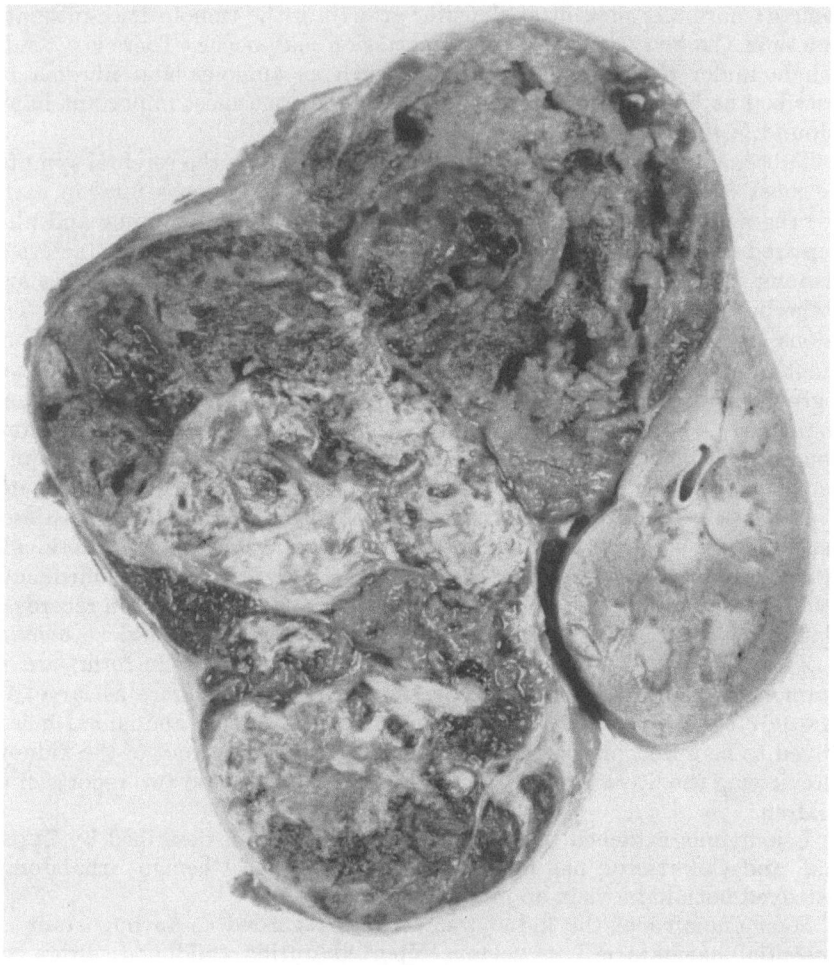

Fig. 115. Adrenal neuroblastoma. Specimen removed at operation from a boy aged 2¹/₂ years who presented with a large abdominal tumour. Intravenous pyelography showed a distorted and displaced left renal pelvis. The specimen demonstrates the typical distortion of the upper pole of the kidney

may be derived from these cells: the malignant neuroblastoma, the benign ganglioneuroma and the adrenaline secreting tumour, the pheochromocytoma. All of these tumours may arise in the adrenal itself, or in the abdominal sympathetic chain, but in the gland the malignant neuroblastoma is the only common type, and is in fact the commonest tumour of childhood. BODIAN and WHITE have reviewed 94 cases of neuroblastoma seen during a 30 year period at the Hospital for Sick Children; they found 41 in the adrenal gland and 24 in the adjacent sympathetic system. Seventy-seven of these cases presented during the first four years of life.

Neuroblastoma (Fig. 115) is a rapidly growing tumour which quickly infiltrates surrounding tissue planes, it becomes fixed to neighbouring organs, and surrounds the great vessels. Blood stream metastasis occurs early to the liver, the lungs and the bones, and is often responsible for the first symptoms. It has been customary, although no longer very useful, to recognize "Pepper's syndrome" in which hepatic secondaries are the predominant feature, resulting sometimes from

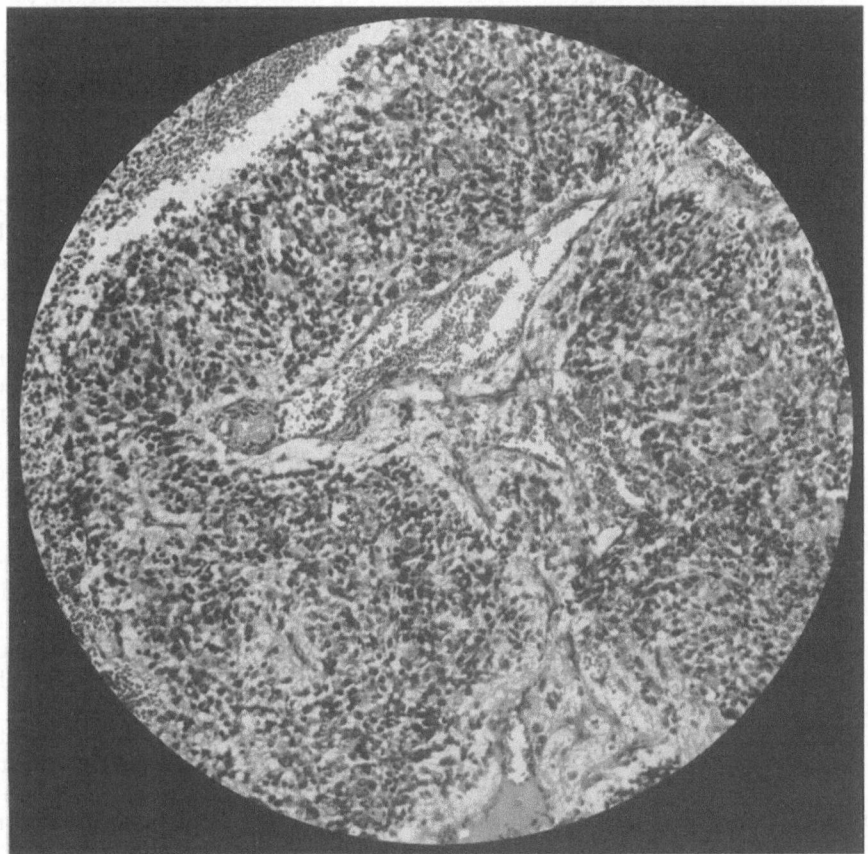

Fig. 116. Histology of neuroblastoma. Section of a neuroblastoma arising in the adrenal. The component neuroblasts are very primitive with deeply staining chromatic nuclei and small cell bodies, but there is some development of delicate axonic processes which in places are aggregated to form areas of delicate fibrillary structure (× 120)

direct invasion by a right sided growth, and characteristic of the young infant, and "Hutchison's syndrome" in which orbital metastases first draw attention to the disease. Solitary secondaries in the long bones are sometimes the first sign, and have often been mistaken for primary bone tumours.

The tumours exhibit in their histological structure the various stages of differentiation seen in the normal development of the sympathetic nervous system. In the most primitive, and the most malignant, there are closely packed small cells with dark-staining nuclei, and only a thin rim of cytoplasm; these tumours exhibit no evident structure, and have often been regarded as retro-peritoneal sarcomata. In tumours with greater differentiation the nuclei are larger and vesicular, the volume of cytoplasm increases, and may form fibrillary material composed of sprouting axons (Fig. 116). Arrangement of the cells to form pseudo-rosettes is common.

The urologist is chiefly concerned with the adrenal neuroblastoma which presents as an abdominal swelling and simulates nephroblastoma. The neuroblastoma has certain clinical characteristics which may make distinction possible, and radiology may give further help, but at times only laparotomy will give the final answer. The adrenal tumour arises high up under the costal margin, tends to cross the midline, and is seldom mobile. It is hard and its surface finely lobulated. The disturbance of general health is more severe than in most renal tumours and the child has often a low fever and anaemia. Clinically or radiologically detectable metastases are present in about two thirds of cases when first admitted to hospital.

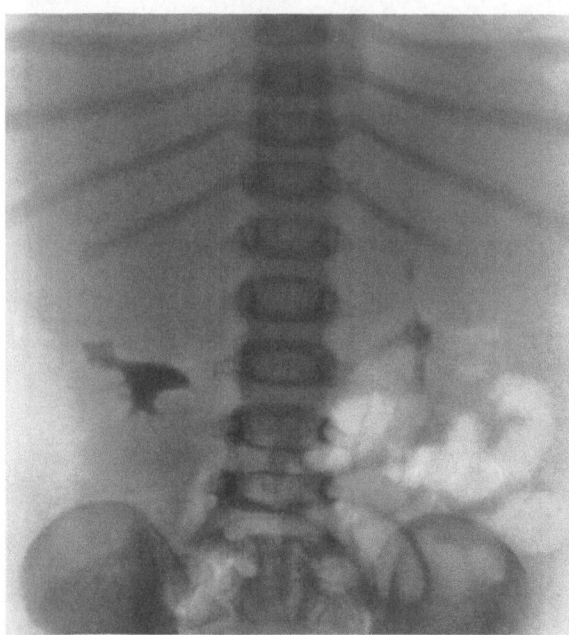

Fig. 117. Neuroblastoma of right adrenal gland. Intravenous pyelogram in a boy aged 1 year with abdominal tumour. The upper calyx of the right kidney shows the characteristic deformity due to adrenal tumor

On X-rays some calcification within the tumour shadow is commonly seen, taking the form of a coarse stippling or flocculent masses, or occasionally of ring shadows. This appearance may, however, be mimicked by calcification in adrenal haematomata (WILLIAMS) and in adrenal cortical tumours. Calcification also occurs in nephroblastoma and pyelograms must be performed to complete the differential diagnosis. In neuroblastoma the renal pelvis is displaced downwards, and slightly distorted; the upper calyx may be elongated as shown in Fig. 117.

The rapid growth and early dissemination of neuroblastoma results in the death of the great majority of affected children within a year of the first appearance of the symptoms. However, in a small minority the growth undergoes spontaneous regression, and the child is restored to health. Sometimes the regression takes the form of a maturation of the tumour cells, so that the growth acquires the characteristics of ganglioneuroma (CUSHING and WOLBACH) and persists indefinitely as a partly calcified mass: in other cases the tumour appears to be completely re-absorbed. Examples of this curious phenomenon have been recorded by WYATT and FARBER, by LADD and GROSS, by BODIAN and WHITE, and several other authors, though no satisfactory explanation has been put forward. The possibility of regression is nevertheless a great encouragement in the management of apparently hopeless cases, and treatment may be surgical, radiological or chemotherapeutic. In the absence of metastasis, it is probably always wise to explore the abdomen in adrenal neuroblastoma, and it is often necessary in order to confirm the diagnosis. Radical excision is sometimes possible, though very much less commonly than in nephroblastoma; a biopsy should be taken in the inoperable cases. The tumour is radiosensitive and radiotherapy should be employed post-operatively: it is also of value in relieving pain where secondaries are already present. The technique of radiotherapy is discussed by WITTENBORG. Small doses, not exceeding 1,000 R are most valuable. Many chemotherapeutic drugs have been employed, particularly the nitrogen mustards, but the most successful, when employed during the first year of life, appears to be Vitamin B_{12} (BODIAN and WHITE), 1—2 mgm should be administered daily for several weeks.

Neuroblastoma arising in the abdominal sympathetic chain is often slightly less malignant than the adrenal tumour, and follows the pattern of the ganglioneuroma described below, save for its more rapid evolution.

2. Ganglioneuroma

This is a slow growing and benign tumour which may by pressure upon surrounding organs cause serious symptoms. It arises from the abdominal sympathetic chain, usually below the kidney, or very rarely from the adrenal gland and spreads into the adjacent tissue planes (GLASSER et al., STOUT). Many cases present with an abdominal tumour fixed to the posterior abdominal wall, displacing the kidney upwards and ureter forwards or outwards. Sympathetic paralysis may be detectable from the warmth of the ipsilateral lower limb. The tumour mass may surround the great vessels, and there may be small but dangerous prolongations through the vertebral foramina into the spinal canal, which produce pressure on the cord and ultimately perhaps paraplegia. Growth in this tumour may be very slow, or may cease altogether, leaving the child with a large palpable mass, but no symptoms. Treatment should consist when possible in surgical excision, and an approach may have to be made by laminectomy, as well as by laparotomy. Involvement of the tissue planes surrounding the great vessels may make complete excision impossible, but in view of the nature of the growth, partial excision may still be of great value.

3. Pheochromocytoma

Pheochromocytoma is a very rare tumour arising from the adrenal medulla or from the sympathetic ganglion cells, and is responsible for a high output of adrenaline and noradrenaline which causes an elevation of the blood pressure.

Although a tumour with frequently fatal consequences, most examples of pheochromocytoma are from the pathological standpoint benign tumours; they are usually small and may, particularly in children, be multiple (CAHILL and ARANOW).

The cells resemble those of the normal adrenal medulla, and exhibit in varying degrees the characteristic chromaffin reaction. The tumours and the formalin fixatives in which they are preserved turn brown from the oxidation of contained adrenaline: a rich brown colour is obtained with potassium bichromate.

In a few cases concomitant evidence of Recklinghausen's disease, particularly the patchy skin pigmentation, is found.

The characteristic clinical history is one of paroxysmal attacks of severe headaches, pallor, palpitation and trembling. During the attacks, the blood pressure is considerably raised, the systolic level perhaps rising above 200 mgm of mercury; at the same time hyperglycaemia is also found in adults but seldom in children. After the attack, collapse and profuse sweating occur, sometimes with polyuria, causing frequency or enuresis. The attacks may at first be infrequent, and between them health may be unaffected, but with time they follow one another more rapidly, and the blood pressure is constantly raised. A sustained hypertension has in fact been more common than paroxysmal attacks in children, and sweating may be the chief complaint.

All cases of hypertension in children should be thoroughly investigated, and if no renal cause is found evidence of the presence of a pheochromocytoma should be sought. The most satisfactory evidence appears to be the excessive urinary output of adrenaline and noradrenaline estimated according to the method described by VON EULER and HELLNER. Other methods of diagnosis have included the precipitation of a hypertensive paroxysm by the intravenous injection of histamine phosphate (ROTH and KVALE), a somewhat risky procedure, and the characteristic reduction of blood pressure which can be obtained by the use of adrenergic blocking agents. GOLDENBERG and ARANOW recommend the use of benzodioxane (0.25 mg/kg body weight) which will terminate a paroxysmal attack, or bring down a persistently raised blood pressure for three to five minutes. Phentolamine (Rogitine) is probably the most reliable drug (HELPS et al.); 2—5 ccs should be injected into a saline intravenous drip.

If these tests suggest the presence of pheochromocytoma, the problem of localization still remains. When situated in the adrenal the tumours are seldom large enough to be palpable (though one such was recorded by SNYDER and VICK); they may be clinically demonstrable in the neck, and straight X-rays may reveal their presence in the chest, but localization of the abdominal tumours is very difficult. SNYDER and RUTLEDGE have demonstrated the value of aortography in this connection, and a number of investigators have employed, with variable success, radiography after peri-renal insufflation of air.

The treatment of pheochromocytoma is clearly excision of the tumour, but this has proved to be a hazardous operation. As soon as the tumour is handled, there is an enormous output of adrenaline and noradrenaline, and a sudden hypertension which may be disastrous; the immediate injection of phentolamine into one intravenous drip should, however, control this effect. Later when the tumour is removed, the blood pressure is apt to fall to a dangerously low level, with results that have often proved fatal. A second, noradrenaline drip should be employed to maintain the pressure at a safe level in the first post-operative hours.

4. Adrenal cortical tumours

Tumours derived from the adrenal cortex may be either benign or malignant, and histologically the distinction is often difficult. In most the tumour cells closely resemble those of the normal adrenal cortex, but in others there is extreme cellular pleomorphism, with numerous mitoses (Fig. 118). The latter phenomena may be observed in well-encapsulated growths, with a low recurrence rate, as well as in the locally infiltrating examples, so that the prognosis is hard to assess from the histological findings. The great majority of such tumours are discovered because of their hormonal effects, but some do not appear to be active in this respect, and present as large abdominal masses simulating adrenal neuroblastoma or even nephroblastoma; they are then likely to be invasive and inoperable, whereas the hormonal tumours are often discovered at an early stage, when still small and easily removed.

The usual form of endocrine disturbance is an androgenic stimulation, causing isosexual precocity in boys and virilism in girls (Fig. 119). The general somatic growth is stimulated, and the child appears much older and tougher than his or her contemporaries; the skin exhibits acne, pubic hair is plentiful, and the penis or clitoris is enlarged. In boys this type of development can be distinguished from true precocious puberty by the absence of spermatogenesis, and the infantile size of the testicles. The 24-hour output of 17-ketosteroids is always raised in both boys and girls, in carcinomata it may reach 150—200 mgm, but much lower figures are found with small adenomata and in a 3 year old girl operated on by

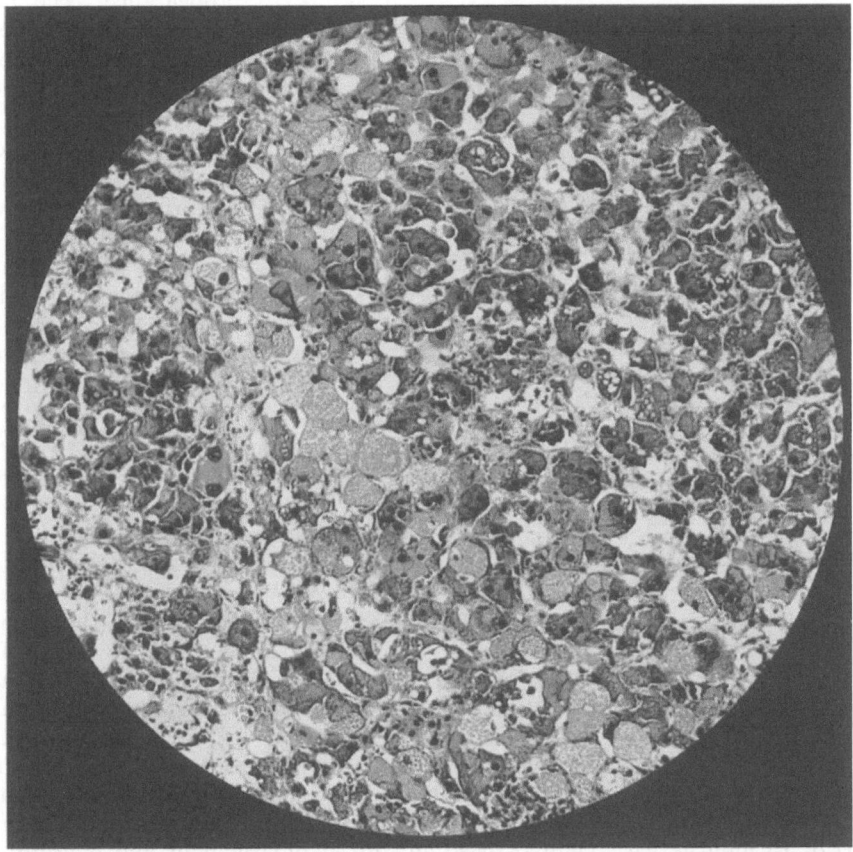

Fig. 118. Histology of adrenal cortical tumour. A section of an adrenal cortical tumour which led to precocious pubertal (feminising) changes in a girl aged 5 years. The cells are large and polymorphic, with abundant, dense or granular cytoplasm, and nuclei which vary considerably in morphology and are sometimes multiple. Despite the bizarre cytology, the tumour was probably benign

the author only 5 mgm were excreted. In both sexes the differential diagnosis between adrenal tumour and hyperplasia has to be made, though the presence of a palpable mass will sometimes render this easy. Hyperplasia always causes signs evident at birth in girls (see female pseudohermaphroditism), but although tumour development is a post-natal phenomenon, signs may appear very early. Hyperplasia is much less common in boys, but its age of onset is more variable and gives no certain lead. The administration of cortisone however, will cause a fall in the 17-ketosteroid output in the hyperplasia cases (see p. 276) but has no consistent action in tumour (WILKINS 1950). PATTERSON believes that a high output of dehydro-iso-androsterone is characteristic of tumour rather than hyperplasia, and describes a test of this substance. His conclusions have not, however, received universal support. Pregnanetriol excretion is raised in hyperplasia but not in tumour.

The second important endocrine phenomenon encountered in adrenal tumour is CUSHING's syndrome, which in childhood is almost always due to an adrenal disease, and most often to a tumour (JOLLY). These children exhibit a striking obesity of the face, trunk and abdomen, but not of the limbs. There is a particularly prominent pad of fat at the back of the neck, giving a "buffalo hump" appearance. The face is plethoric, the skin marked by acne, and the bodily hair plentiful; in the uncomplicated case, however, there is no abnormal growth of the penis or clitoris. Muscular weakness is common, contrasting with the abnormal strength found in the androgenic cases. Hypertension is the rule and may reach very high levels. Classically the 17-keto steroid output is normal, but the 11-17-oxy-corticosteroid excretion is consistently raised.

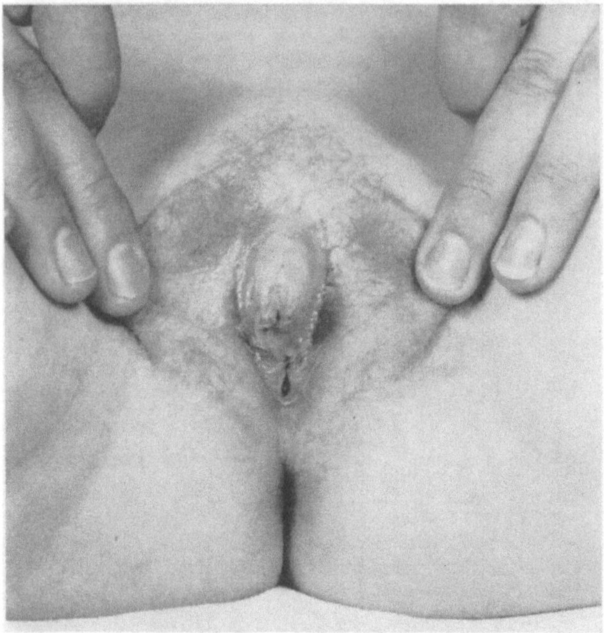

The third, and least common effect is feminization: this has been described in boys (HOLL, WILKINS 1948) causing growth stimulation and gynaecomastia, and girls

Fig. 119. Adrenal cortical adenoma. The external genitalia of a girl aged 5 years. Considerable growth of pubic hair, and enlargement of the clitoris

(Fig. 120) with precocious pubertal changes (KEPLER et al.). In the many girls with this type of response, there have also been signs of CUSHING's syndrome or some androgenic effects as well. Thus, HIGGINS et al. describe a girl of 15 months with vaginal bleeding, breast enlargement and overgrowth of the clitoris. After removal of an adrenal cortical carcinoma the breasts and genitalia returned to normal, and the present state of the child, 10 years later, is satisfactory. GARRETT records cases in which the androgenic and CUSHING's phenomena occurred together, and a similar case has been observed at the Hospital for Sick Children. The mixed endocrine response is at least as common as the simple types described.

No tumour responsible for hyperaldosteronism has yet been recorded in a child, though HOLTEN and PETERSEN report a girl aged 13 with adrenal hyperplasia with increased output of aldosterone causing hypertension and potassium depletion.

Once the presence of an adrenal cortical tumour is suspected, investigations should be aimed at localisation. An intravenous pyelogram is most useful, since it will often show the corresponding kidney to be displaced downwards, and sometimes a calcification in the tumour itself (Fig. 121). Peri-renal insufflation of air or aortography may be of assistance, or palpation at laparotomy may be preferred. The recent interest in adrenal surgery for malignant diseases has drawn attention to the fact that both adrenals can be often adequately exposed through a high oblique abdominal incision (AIRD and HELMAN) and if the operator is using this approach, the question of localization may be decided at operation. In the simple androgenic or feminizing cases excision of the tumour bearing adrenal gland is clearly required, and the post-operative management is usually

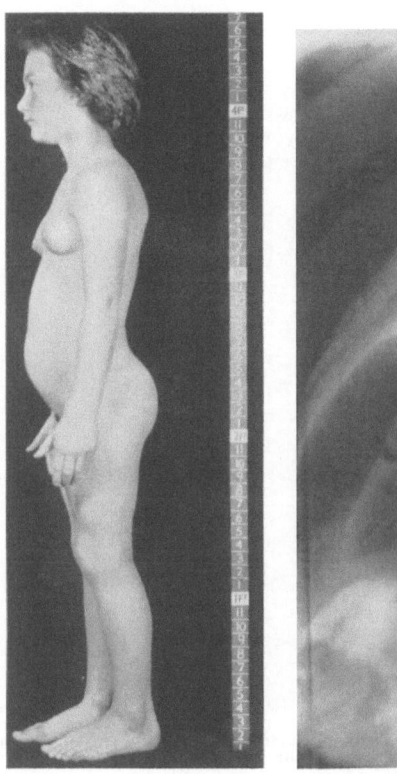 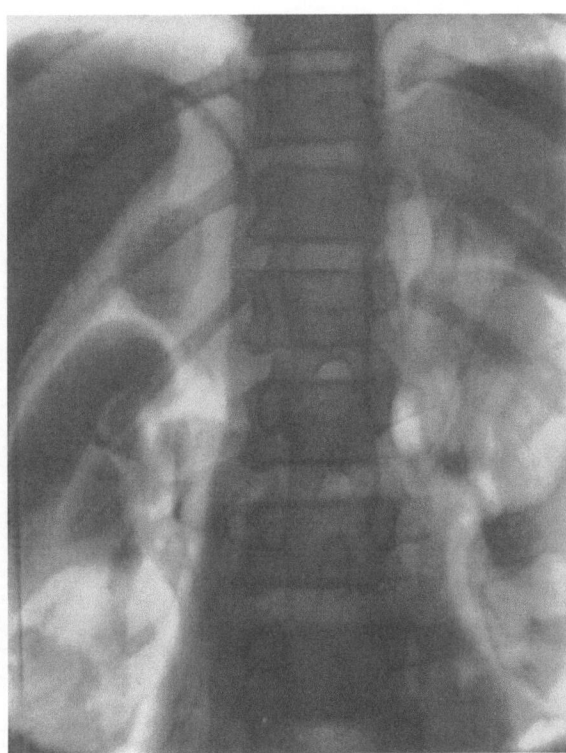

A   B

Fig. 120 A and B. Feminizing adrenal cortical tumour producing precocious puberty in a girl aged 5 years. A Clinical photograph showing breast enlargement. B Retroperitoneal air insufflation X-ray outlining tumour. The bone age was 12 years; excretion of 17 ketosteroids and of oestrogens was raised; menstruation had occurred on three occasions. Adenomatous tumour removed at operation. Hormonal levels returned to normal and menstruation ceased. General clinical improvement and shrinking of breasts followed

straightforward. In the Cushing's cases, however, biochemical disturbances are to be expected after excision of tumour, and have in the past frequently proved fatal, since the contralateral adrenal is atrophic or absent. Cortisone replacement therapy, and careful electrolyte control should enable a greater proportion of these cases to be brought through the hazards of operation in the future. In Cushing's syndrome where bilateral adrenal hyperplasia is found, sub-total adrenalectomy followed by cortisone therapy appears to be the most satisfactory treatment; where the adrenals are normal, pituitary irradiation may be advisable.

5. Adrenal haematoma

A note on adrenal haematomata is conveniently included in this chapter, since on occasion there may be difficulty in distinguishing these lesions from true tumours.

Although the cause is not known, bilateral adrenal haemorrhage of slight degree is not a very uncommon finding in post-mortems performed on neonates, and the lesion may certainly be responsible for adrenal cortical failure. In later childhood, haemorrhage and acute failure may complicate many severe infections, particularly meningococcal septicaemia (WATERHOUSE-FRIDERICHSEN syndrome). The treatment of these conditions is exclusively medical, but on rare occasions in the neonatal period, a unilateral severe haemorrhage occurs in which the danger

Calcified tumour

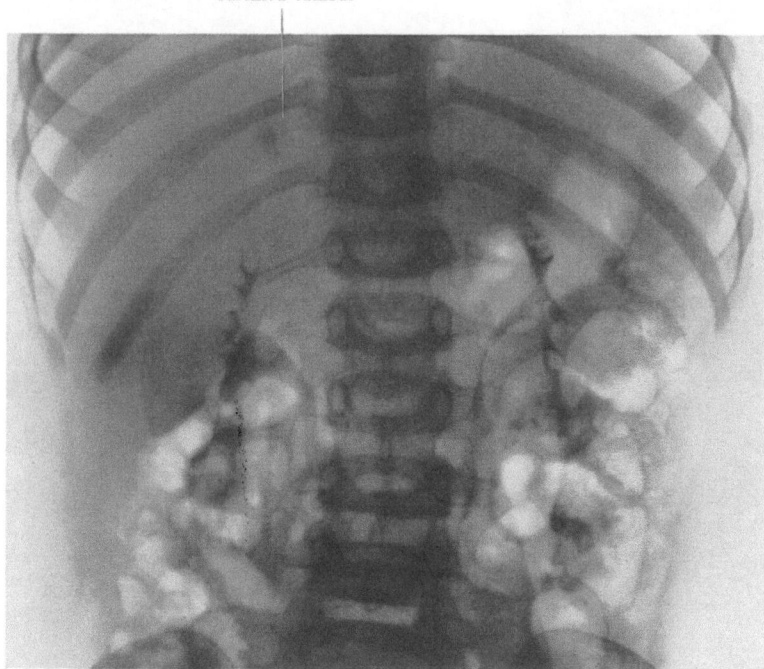

Fig. 121. Adrenal cortical adenoma. Intravenous pyelogram in a girl of 2 years with signs of virilism. There is a calcified area in the right adrenal area

arises not from adrenal cortical failure, but from the loss of blood from the circulation. A number of these cases has been reviewed by EMERY and ZACHARY: an infant during the first week of life is noticed to be pale and irritable, a lump is then felt in an upper quadrant of the abdomen which simulates a renal or adrenal tumour. Often the child dies suddenly before treatment can be given, but on several occasions laparotomy has been performed revealing blood in the peritoneum, and a haematomatous mass which has been excised. Although the clinical diagnosis may be difficult to make, it is important that the disease should be recognized at operation, for clearly only haemostasis is required.

Calcification takes place rapidly in an old haematoma, and probably the majority of opacities seen in the adrenals of children are due to this cause: tuberculosis must be very rare. If the haematoma is large, and displaces the upper pole of the kidney, the differential diagnosis from adrenal tumour may be difficult or impossible, though the history of a severe infection may give a clue. In the case illustrated in Fig. 122 exploration seemed indicated (WILLIAMS). Small cysts which may be found incidentally in the adrenal probably also result from old haemorrhages.

6. Retro-peritoneal teratoma

Although rare the retro-peritoneal teratomata form a distinct group and ARNHEIM was able to collect 44 cases from the literature including 3 of his own.

Over half the cases occurred in infants under one year of age, and although only three exhibited malignant changes 13 had died. The tumours may be attached to the kidney or free, and they are not infrequently bilateral. Most have presented with an abdominal tumour, and displacement of the pyelographic shadow. Calcification and bone formation may occur. Exploration is often essential to establish the diagnosis, and radial excision, although difficult, should always be undertaken. ARNHEIM, whose papers should be consulted for references to earlier literature has also reported a series of "combined pelvic and retro-peritoneal teratomata" in which the mass was palpable both in the abdomen and in the pelvis. KRETSCH-MER discusses retro-peritoneal lipo-fibro-sarcoma.

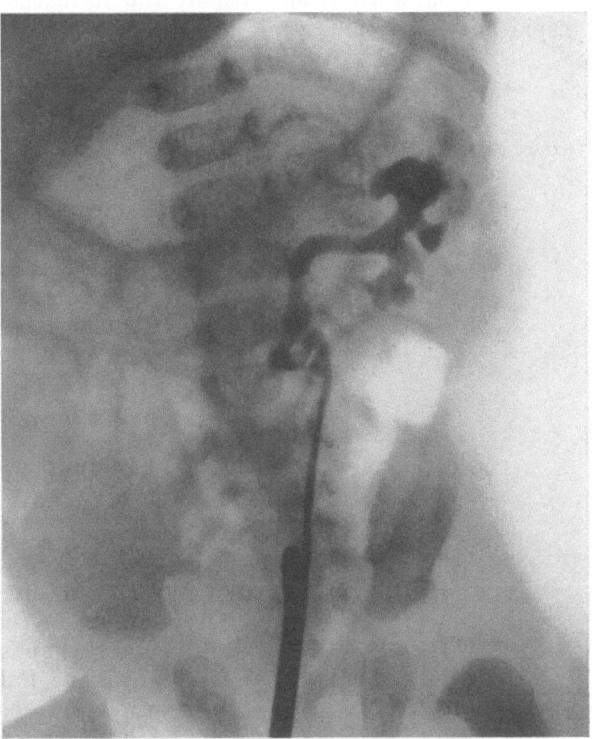

Fig. 122. Calcified left adrenal haematoma. Retrograde pyelogram in a boy aged 3 months, who had had a very severe E. coli urinary infection and meningitis when 3 weeks old. The upper pole of the kidney is displaced outwards by a partially calcified mass (some pyelo-tubular backflow is also shown); exploration undertaken to exclude the possibility of adrenal neuroblastoma revealed an organizing haematoma

IV. The bladder

1. Rhabdomyosarcoma

The most common type of bladder tumour in infancy and childhood is an embryonic growth which exhibits some tendency to differentiate striated muscle cells and is therefore designated a rhabdomyosarcoma. A tumour with a similar histology and behaviour may arise in the prostate or in the vagina, and it is perhaps better to consider the growth as an "embryonic sarcoma of the urogenital sinus" (WHITE). In case reports, which are numerous, these tumours are often described as myxomata, myxosarcomata or fibromyxosarcomata, and in many cases the myxomatous appearance is the most striking feature, the rhabdomyoblasts being poorly differentiated and easily overlooked. Reviews of this topic have been published by CAMPBELL, KRETSCHMER, HENRY, KHOURY and SPEER, MOSTOFI and MORSE, PEZZOLI. Cases have occurred at all stages of childhood, but most commonly in the first 4 years: in a few the tumour was present at birth.

In the bladder, rhabdomyosarcoma takes a polypoid form often described as sarcoma botryoides: pearly grey, fleshy lobules arise from a broad area of the bladder wall, most often from the base but sometimes from several centres, and fill the bladder cavity. (Fig. 123). Ulceration isuncommon but the neoplastic process may extend in the submucosal layer both within the bladder and along the urethra or lower ureters. When the disease has spread from the vulva, there may be a flat infiltration without the formation of the polyps Growth is fairly rapid but is for some time confined within the urinary tract, neither breaking through into the surrounding tissues nor metastasizing: most of the affected children die as a result of urinary obstruction and sepsis without secondary deposits.

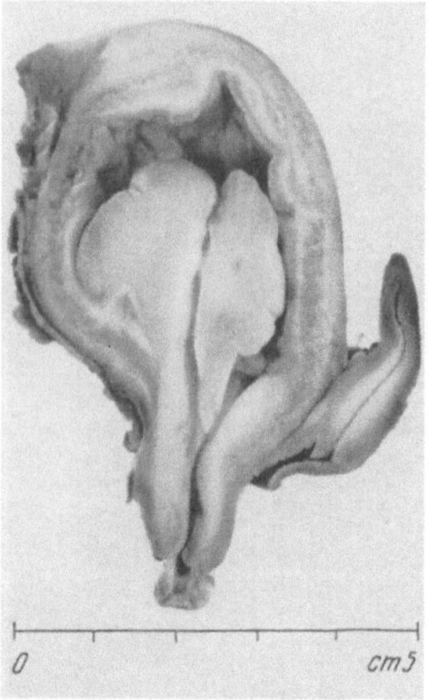

Histologically the tumours exhibit embryonic mesenchyme represented by fusiform or stellate cells embedded in a mucoid ground substance (Fig. 124). Differentiation of these cells towards collagenous connective tissue cells, and towards striated muscle fibres may be seen; all stages of rhabdomyoblast formation occur, from strap-like cells with a single nucleus, to large multinucleate cells with distinct cross striation.

Clinically the symptoms which first draw attention to the condition are frequency, painful and difficult micturition sometimes going on to retention, pyuria and later haematuria. In direct contrast to carcinoma the bleeding in rhabdomyosarcoma is almost always a complication of infection, and is not an early sign. Pain due to the bladder distension may be severe. In the female the polyps may prolapse through the urethra, or break away and pass spontaneously. Where the onset of the disease occurs before or immediately after birth, the obstruction may lead to the formation of umbilical urinary fistula (HUNT, KHOURY and SPEER). On examination a firm mass is found arising from the pelvis, which

Fig. 123. Rhabdomyosarcoma of the bladder. Operation specimen from a girl aged 11 months, who presented with retention of urine. The tumour formed an easily palpable mass, and the diagnosis was confirmed by endoscopic biopsy. Total cystectomy with urethrectomy and hysterectomy. The entire anterior vaginal wall was removed, but a recurrence developed on the posterior wall, and secondary deposits appeared after one year

does not entirely disappear after catheterization. Intravenous pyelograms are likely to show some dilatation of the ureters, and cystograms (Fig. 125) demonstrate the characteristic lobulated filling defect. Cystoscopically, the grape-like appearance of the polyps is unmistakable, though the flat submucosal infiltration may be difficult to recognize.

Although some benign bladder tumours are discussed in the following section, and cure has occasionally followed local removal of a rhabdomyosarcoma (HIGGINS et al.) it is wise to assume that all bladder tumours in infancy are malignant, so that treatment should be urgent and radical. For confirmation of the diagnosis of rhabdomyosarcoma, trans-urethral biopsy with a resectoscope is a simple procedure, or if this instrument is not available, a polyp can be torn off with crocodile forceps. The growth is not sufficiently susceptible to irradiation to make this form of treatment worth while; moreover, since there is often infection and always obstruction, radiotherapy is likely to cause a considerable deterioration in the symptoms and in the general condition of the child. The treatment should consist in immediate total cysto-prostatectomy, with removal of the bulb of the urethra and the lower ends of the ureters in continuity with the bladder, as there may well be an extension along these channels. In the female, the entire urethra should be removed, and in view of the likely multicentric origin of the tumour, total hysterectomy and colpectomy should also be advised. The ureters may be

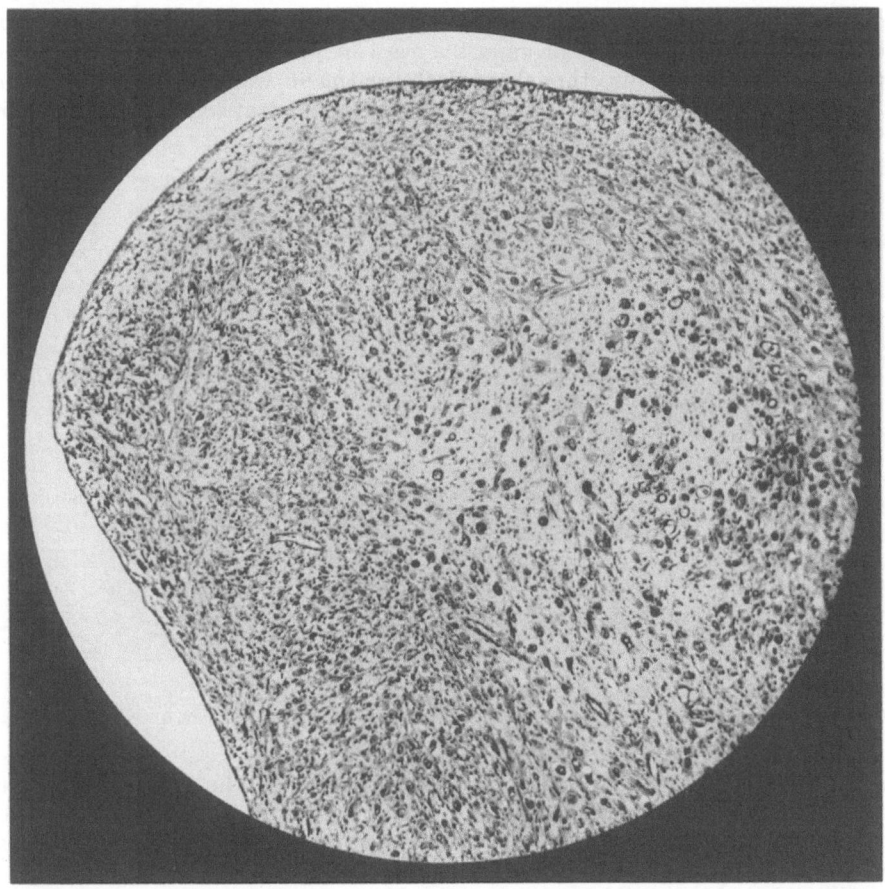

Fig. 124. Histology of rhabdomyosarcoma of the bladder. Section of a polypoid tumour involving bladder and prostate. The field includes a portion of a polyp, showing the submucous situation of the neoplastic tissue. The latter consists of an embryonic mesenchyme in which there is plentiful differentiation of plump and strap-like rhabdomyoblasts. Whilst the term rhabdomyosarcoma is in common use for such a tumour, it is suggested that embryonic sarcoma is a more appropriate designation ($\times$ 55)

implanted into the sigmoid colon at the same operation, or drained on to the skin: small infants stand up well to the one stage procedure.

Most reports give a depressing view of the prognosis in this condition, but HIGGINS, reporting four cases from the Hospital for Sick Children had three survivors, and two of these are still alive seven years after operation. Four further cases have been treated recently. Satisfactory results have also been reported by SLOTKIN and DAVIS.

2. Other bladder tumours

A number of myxomatous or fibromatous tumours have been reported (RIDLON, MEADE, GANEM and AINSWORTH) in which the local removal of the polypoid mass has resulted in a permanent cure, and the exact status of the neoplasms is not always clear. LANGE has described a pedunculated myoma which was responsible for a severe haemorrhage, but which was easily removed. A spindle cell sarcoma was removed by partial cystectomy by FEGETTER from a girl of 10 years, with 12 years survival (HENRY).

Haemangioma of the bladder is rare, and though it more often presents during adult life, it is probably a congenital condition, and may well be encountered in childhood. BALLLENGER et al. report a case in which haematuria commenced at the age of 6 months, though radical treatment was not undertaken until 27 years. RATHBUN, CAMPBELL, and HIGGINS et al. illustrate cases of haemangioma

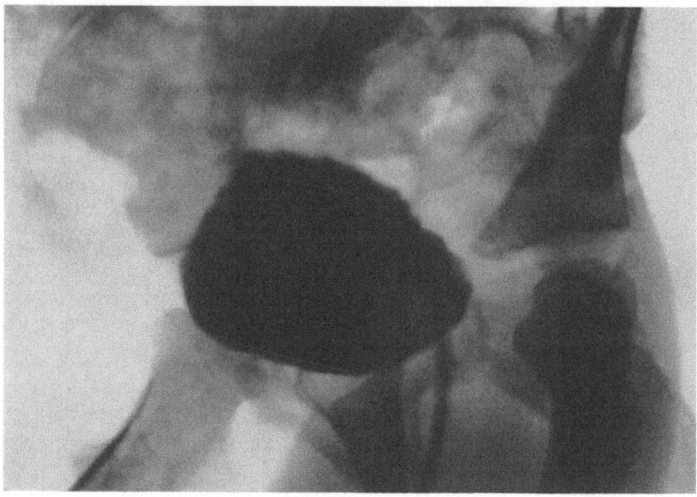

Fig. 125. Rhabdomyosarcoma of the bladder. Cystogram in a boy of 3 years with retention of urine, showing lobulated filling defect at the base of the bladder. Total cystectomy performed; well and free of recurrence 4 years later

in children: painless and profuse haematuria has been the chief feature, while haemangiomata on the skin, or in the rectum have on several occasions led to the correct diagnosis. Cystoscopically the haemangiomatous tissue may be easily recognisable, but the appearance may at times suggest a solid tumour. Removal of the growth by partial cystectomy has been the most satisfactory form of treatment, but when the base of the bladder is involved diathermy coagulation should be tried before resorting to radical surgery.

Neurofibromatosis may on rare occasions affect the bladder; in the 7 year old boy reported by KASS there was a large tumour arising in the perivesical tissue causing ulceration and haematuria. The diagnosis was suspected from cutaneous nodules and pigmentation. The disease is also recorded by CHALKLEY and BRUCE.

Tumours arising at the apex of the bladder may be derived from the urachus: cases of this nature in children have usually been sarcomata. SHAW has reported an interesting example in a boy aged 6 years, who presented with acute abdominal pain and haemoperitoneum: the growth was a spindle cell sarcoma.

Epithelial tumours are exceptionally rare in children and the only adequately described case appears to be that reported by LOWRY et al., a boy of 6 years with painless haematuria who was found to have a pedunculated, low grade transitional cell carcinoma.

V. The prostate and urethra

Tumours arising in the prostate during childhood are almost always embryonic sarcomata and although fibrosarcoma, lymphosarcoma and leiomyosarcoma, are recorded, the common form is the rhabdomyosarcoma of a type similar to that already described for the bladder. LOWSLEY and KIMBALL reviewing the subject found that one third of all cases of sarcoma of the prostate occurred under the age of twenty. Reviews and case reports concerned with children will be found

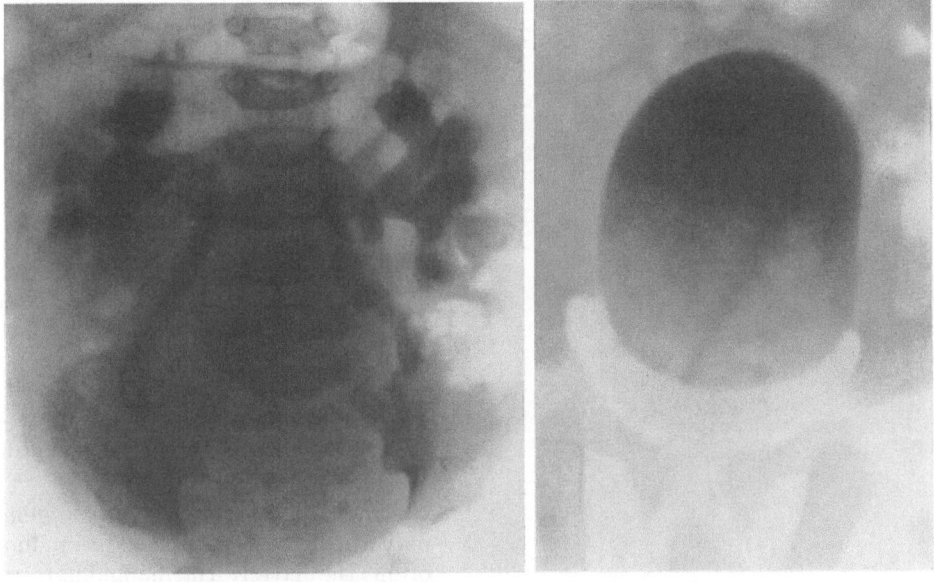

A   B
Fig. 126 A—C. Rhabdomyosarcoma of prostate. A Intravenous pyelogram; B cystogram; C (see overleaf)

in the works of GMELIN, HOLMES and COPLAN, MERTZ et al., WALLGREN, and TZOVARU and VASILESCU.

In the prostate the tumour takes a solid form, but if it escapes into the bladder or the urethra it may become polypoid. Spread may occur in the urethral wall as in the bladder tumours. Growth is rapid and causes urinary obstruction which may be fatal before metastasis has taken place.

Difficult and painful micturition is the common mode of presentation, and the bladder is found to be chronically distended. An enormous enlargement of the prostate is palpable on rectal examination, it is smooth and tense, but feels cystic and is easily mistaken for prostatic abscess. Cystograms show the upward displacement of the bladder, and a dome-like filling defect at the base (Fig. 126); the urethrograms demonstrate a displaced and distorted urethra. The size of the mass renders endoscopy difficult, but if the base of the bladder is infiltrated, the white tumour tissue may be seen beneath the mucosa.

Bladder drainage is often urgently required and after catheterization the diagnosis can usually be made on clinical grounds. The absence of fever, and other signs of infection will suggest tumour rather than abscess, and for confirmation an exploratory needle may be inserted immediately before operation. Treatment should take the form of radical cysto-prostatectomy, as in the bladder tumours, but cure has not yet been achieved in this disease. Some writers have advised radiotherapy, but there has been little evidence of any beneficial effect from this treatment.

A very slow growing tumour, described as a plexiform neurofibrosarcoma has been recorded by HESS; it infiltrated the base of the bladder and perineum, but was known to have been present for seven years at the time of writing.

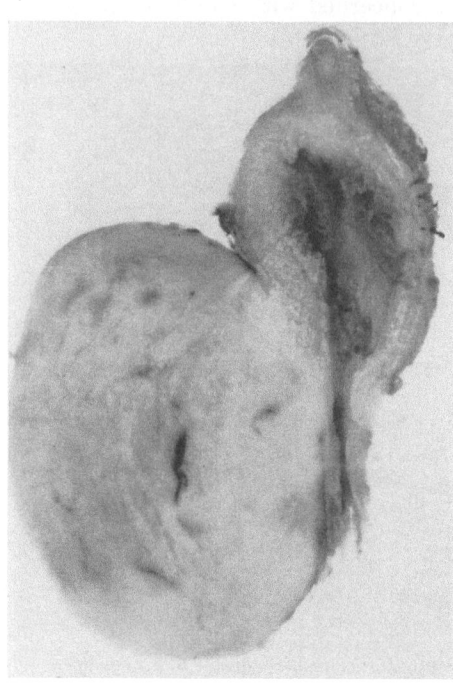

True neoplasms have not been found in the urethra during childhood, though small polyps in the region of the bladder neck and verumontanum are not uncommon both in symptomless and in enuretic children. On rare occasions such polyps may attain sufficient size to cause dysuria.

c

Fig. 126 Cooperation specimen from a boy aged 3 months. The child presented with retention of urine: the enormous prostatic enlargement was palpable per rectum and per abdomen. Total cysto-prostatectomy. Death 8 months later with widespread metastases

VI. The penis and scrotum

A papillary adenocarcinoma of the glans penis in a two year old Indian boy has been described by KINI; the growth developed beneath the foreskin and followed the usual adult pattern. The condition is exceptionally rare in children and appears to be unknown to most Western authors.

Haemangioma and lymphangioma may affect the penis and scrotum, more often the latter. Haemangiomata are often small and unnoticeable at birth, but either spread or fill out during the first few years: in the scrotum they may reach a considerable bulk (Fig. 127) without causing any serious symptoms, and many receive no attention until adult life. Excision of the entire mass is the most satisfactory form of treatment (WINSLOW). Small haemangiomata may be observed on the surface of the glans (Fig. 128), they usually cause no symptoms, and should not be interfered with unless bleeding occurs, when superficial cautery may be applied. An enormous haemangioma involving the whole genital area has been described by MATTHEWS, the penis was enlarged to such an extent that it reached the infant's feet. Treatment of such an extensive lesion is a matter of great difficulty, and in this case a fatal air embolism occurred during attempted excision.

Lymphangioma presents as a soft circumscribed swelling attached to the skin of the scrotum. It is unsightly but causes little inconvenience. The mass may be excised completely with the overlying skin, and does not show any attachments to the testicle: if it is extensive it may have to be dissected away from the skin, though no satisfactory plane of cleavage will be found.

Congenital elephantiasis of the penis and scrotum without lymphangioma is described by ZSCHAU.

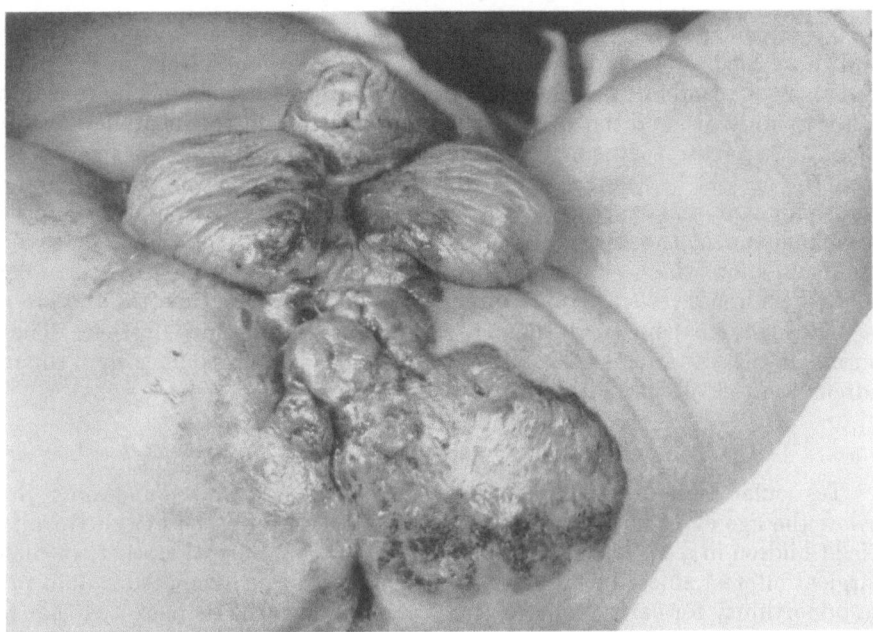

Fig. 127. Haemangioma: the perineum of a new-born infant

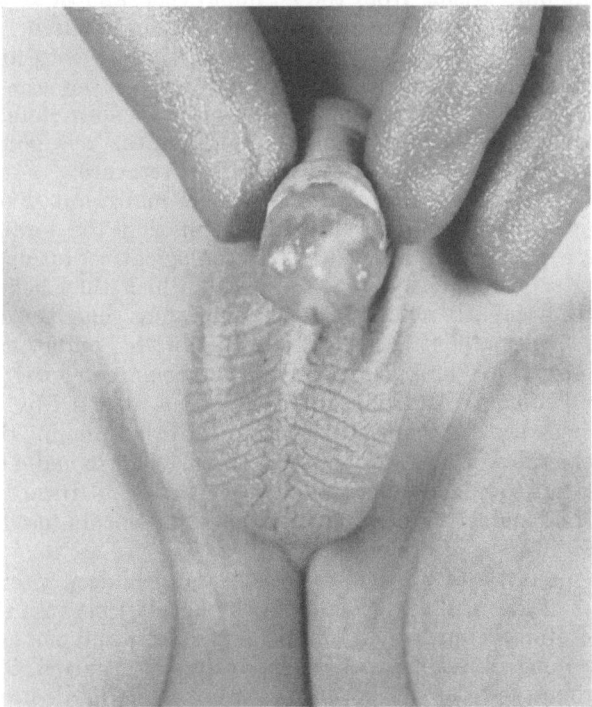

Fig. 128. Haemangioma of the glans penis. Boy aged 4 years, without symptoms

VII. The epididymis and spermatic cord

True neoplasms are very seldom seen in the epididymis or cord during childhood, and those reported have been similar to the growths found in adult life. BURROS and MAYCOCK, and SUNDARASIVARAO have described benign adenomatoid tumours of the epididymis, and the latter has traced their origin to the Müllerian vestiges found at that site. HIRSCH records a rhabdomyosarcoma of the spermatic cord in a 16-year-old boy, and finds references to the same tumour in infants: it was malignant and responsible for metastases. THOMPSON found a symptomless haemangioma in the cord and GUEKDJIAN operated upon a case of cavernous lymphangioma which simulated inguinal hernia.

Some adrenal rests are quite often found in the spermatic cord, and are particularly likely to be seen during operations for undescended testicle. They are normal in this situation (see CULP), but may become enlarged in cases of congenital adrenal cortical hyperplasia.

VIII. The testicle

Testicular tumours are uncommon in children; DEAN found only 8 cases below the age of 14 in a series of 500, and only 10 were seen at the Hospital for Sick Children in a 27-year period. These tumours are nevertheless of considerable surgical interest since the ease with which they may be diagnosed should present an opportunity for early and effective treatment: it is to be regretted that in the past the malignant nature of the lesion has sometimes been recognized only after some delay, or even after attempts to tap a suspected hydrocele.

The pathological classification of testicular tumours is complex and disputed, and a detailed discussion of the problem is outside the scope of this work. Of the common tumours arising from the germinal cells, almost all may be classified as teratomata, since seminoma is exceptionally rare in children. A teratoma may be composed of well differentiated "adult" tissues, often with formation of cysts containing epidermal elements: these are much more often seen in infancy than at any other time, and they are benign tumours. RUSCHE noted 9 cases of this type in a series of 12 testicular tumours, and JULIEN has given an incidence of a little over 25% in cases collected from the literature.

Teratomata composed of immature tissues are malignant (Fig. 129), and may exhibit such overgrowth of one cellular element that the teratomatous nature is difficult to recognize: this has led to terminological confusion. MAGNER et al. describe an "adenocarcinoma with clear cells" which they believe represents a type of growth peculiarly characteristic of infancy, but BODIAN and WHITE believe that these clear cells are typical undifferentiated embryomatous cells, and that the tumours should be included in the teratoma category (Fig. 130).

A Sertoli-cell tumour (Androblastoma) has been reported by CULP et al., and is believed to be a benign neoplasm. Interstitial cell tumours though rare have attracted considerable attention because of their hormonal effects: they are usually benign, but some have been bilateral (REZEK and HARDIN) and in adults late recurrence and metastasis are known. ROSENTHAL encountered a haemangioma of the testis in an infant of 3 months.

The great majority of testicular tumours in children present during the first three years of life, and are brought to the hospital because the parents have discovered a scrotal swelling. The tumour is painless, and the general condition of the infant is good unless secondaries have already occurred. The mass is often three or four times the size of the normal organ, it is hard, heavy and smooth or slightly lobulated. Cystic areas may be palpable, and occasionally there is a little fluid in the tunica vaginalis: the consistency and the failure of transillumination, however, should distinguish tumour from hydrocele. The skin may have a faintly bluish tinge as in torsion; the absence of pain will normally prevent any confusion with that disorder, but occasionally haemorrhage into the neoplasm will produce temporary pain and pyrexia. The epididymis is unaffected and can

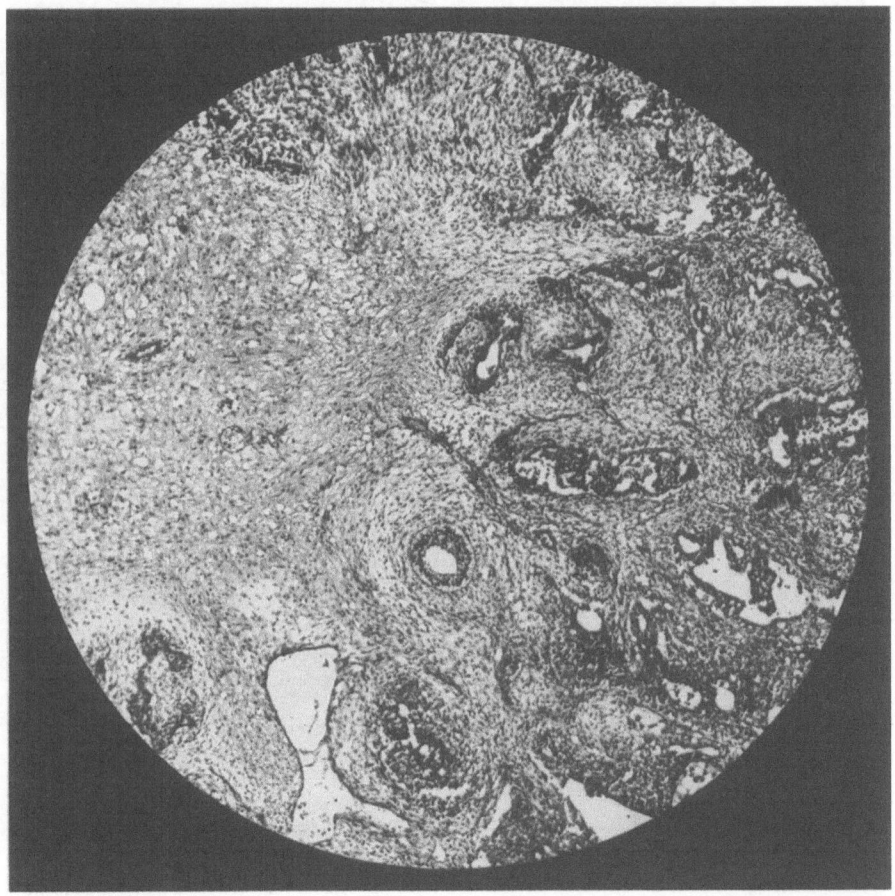

Fig. 129. Histology of teratoma of testis. Section of a malignant teratoma of testes, showing immature mesenchyme (which in other areas contained developing cartilage) and irregular masses of primitive epithelial blastema, one of which has differentiated into a tubular structure. The tumour was removed from a boy of 13 years, 17 months after orchidopexy. He was alive and well 5 years after surgical excision (× 55)

be felt separate from the tumour mass. Involvement of the inguinal glands only occurs when the growth has extended into the scrotum, but nodules may be found within the spermatic cord. Palpable lymphatic secondaries in the para-aortic and epigastric nodes may be the most prominent feature, which has sometimes suggested a diagnosis of nephroblastoma. Malignant glands may also be found in the mediastinum and in the supraclavicular fossa. Blood stream metastasis to the lungs follows lymphatic spread.

Where the tumour involves an undescended testicle (e. g. GORDON-TAYLOR and WYNDHAM) some difficulty may be experienced in the diagnosis of an inguinal or pelvic mass, though the absence of the testicle from the scrotum should give a clue.

Hormonal effects are seen chiefly with interstitial cell tumours though slight gynaecomastia has been observed with adenocarcinoma (MATASSARIN). The interstitial cells are capable of producing large amounts of androgens, and of stimulating precocious sexual and somatic development. POMER et al. have given a recent review of reported cases, and reference should also be made to the works

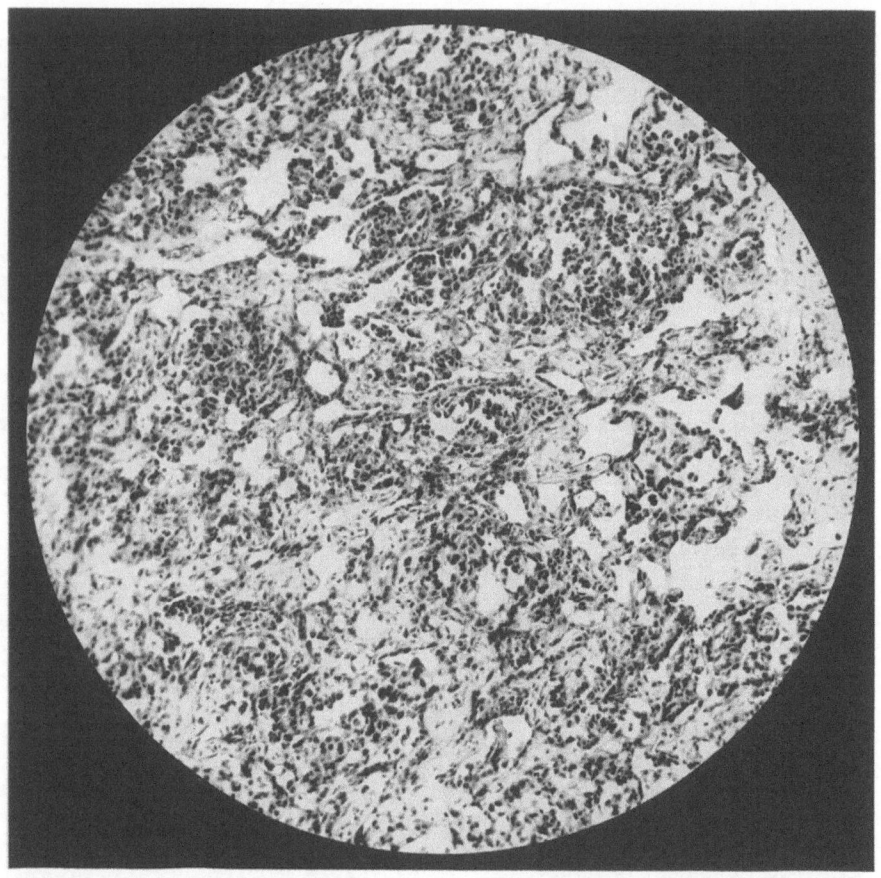

Fig. 130. Histology of teratoma of testes. Section of a testicular tumour removed from a boy of 18 months, who died from pulmonary metastases 13 months later, despite post-operative radiotherapy. Although frequently called embryonal adenocarcinoma, this type of tumour appears to be an extremely primitive form of teratoma; the delicate acino-papillary epithelium is believed to be the primordial tissue of such neoplasms, and may be seen alone or with more differentiated components in this or other sites

of NEWNS, BLUNDEN et al. and THAMDRUP. The growth and muscular development of the child is advanced, pubic hair appears, the skin is marked by acne, and the voice deepens. The penis grows to adult proportions, and erections occur, but the opposite testicle remains small, and there is no spermatogenesis. The tumour is often comparatively small, and is therefore apt to be overlooked (JOLLY); it may even be supposed that the small testicle is the pathological organ, since the size of the tumour bearing one is more in keeping with the size of the penis. The androgen excretion, as measured by the 24 hour output of 17-keto-steroids, is considerably raised. Orchidectomy will lead to a fall in this figure, unless the opposite testicle is also affected (REZEK and HARDIN), but regression of clinical signs of precocity is slow or may not occur at all.

In cases of congenital adrenal cortical hyperplasia, both testicles may be enlarged, and contain cells which resemble those found in the reticular zone of the adrenal. The affected children are suffering from precocious puberty (see p. 293) and the enlargement of the testicles may lead to a misdiagnosis of the true cause.

While the diagnosis of testicular tumour should not present any difficulty to the surgeon, it must be realized that no clinical distinction can be made between the benign and the malignant teratomata. Pre-operative irradiation for all cases is therefore advised by some writers (e.g. DEAN), but this may well involve unnecessary destruction of the opposite testicle. Needle biopsy has been advocated (GUILLEMINET and FOURRIER) but carries a considerable risk of disseminating the growth, and there can be little doubt that immediate orchidectomy should be the treatment for all cases without evidence of metastasis. The spermatic cord should be severed high up in the inguinal canal and if nodules are palpable along the spermatic vessels within the abdomen a more extensive dissection may be justifiable (GROSS). The decision regarding post-operative irradiation follows a study of the histology of the tumour; treatment is not required in cases of adult teratoma or interstitial cell tumour. Because of the comparatively high proportion of benign forms, the overall prognosis of testicular tumours is good, only two out of 12 cases died in RUSCHE's series, and only two out of 9 in the Great Ormond Street series (BODIAN and WHITE). DOYLE's review however, gives a gloomier picture for "embryonal carcinoma".

IX. The ovary

If simple follicular cysts are included in the category, ovarian tumours in childhood are probably not as rare as testicular tumours, and a large proportion are benign. COSTIN and KENNEDY have published a comprehensive review, and collected 200 cases from the literature: approximately one third of reported cases were stated to be simple or multilocular cysts, one third dermoids and the remainder sarcomata and carcinomata. The last group, however, probably includes tumours which would now be classified as dysgerminomata or as granulosa cell tumours.

Ovarian cysts and tumours may present at all ages; a bilateral case has recently been encountered in a neonate at the Hospital for Sick Children, but the average age is considerably higher than in testicular growths. They cause lower abdominal pain, and nausea, or simply present as large abdominal swellings. Torsion, however, is common with all histological types, and has occurred in about a third of the cases reported in childhood: the complication causes acute lower abdominal pain and collapse; a tender swelling is palpable in the pelvis, but diagnosis is usually made only at laparotomy (TAYLOR).

Simple and multilocular cysts require little comment, though it may be mentioned that sexual precocity (see p. 294) has been associated with a simple follicular cyst on one occasion at least (KIMMEL). Cystadenoma appears to occur only after puberty.

Teratomata may sometimes be diagnosed radiologically because of included bone or tooth formation. Malignant changes are rare in this group, but in a few instances there is isosexual precocity.

Dysgerminoma affects chiefly older children, but is much more common than its equivalent seminoma in boys. It is a tumour particularly liable to occur in association with pseudohermaphroditism, and genital hypoplasia. The malignancy of this growth is variable, and irradiation should always be advised even when the excision appears to have been complete.

Granulosa-cell tumour is characteristically associated with isosexual precocity, and a very high excretion of oestrogens. Most cases have presented with early development of the breast tissue and menstruation, though in one reported in a child of 14 weeks, the abdominal masses were the chief feature (ZEMKE and HERRELL). As in the dysgerminoma group, the malignancy of these tumours is variable and cannot be predicted from the histology.

Theca-cell tumour has been reported only once (GORDON and MARVIN), it was responsible for menstrual discharge in a child of one year.

Arrhenoblastoma is a tumour of later life, but has been recorded in a girl of 13 years, causing amenorrhoea, enlargement of the clitoris and deepening of the voice (FLANNERY).

Ovarian tumours which cause symptoms in childhood are almost always large enough to be palpable on careful bimanual pelvic examination, and doubt as to the diagnosis will be settled at laparotomy. In view of the high proportion of benign forms, simple oophorectomy and salpingectomy should be performed unless there is clear evidence of spread of malignant disease; a decision as to radiotherapy should be made after histological examination of the excised tumour.

X. The vagina and uterus

The characteristic vaginal tumour in children is the embryonal rhabdomyo-sarcoma of the type already encountered in other derivatives of the urogenital sinus, the bladder and prostate, but it has long been known from the grape-like appearance of its lobules as a "Sarcoma Botryoides". McFARLAND gives an excellent review of the pathology, while SHACKMAN has recently summarized the clinical findings and lists relevant papers. As with other embryonic tumours it occurs predominantly in the first three years of life, though it is also encountered in older girls.

The tumour arises from the vagina or labia and forms fleshy polypoid masses which protrude through the vulva, though their origin may be as high as the fornices. Ulceration of the exposed lobules may occur, and infection may lead to haemorrhage and purulent vaginal discharge. Pain is not a prominent feature of the early stages. The polyps are easily curetted away from the vaginal wall, but recurrence is rapid and after a time infiltration of neighbouring structures may be found; pressure and involvement of the urethra will be responsible for retention of urine. In the case illustrated in Fig. 131 there was a sub-mucous infiltration by tumour cells of the whole urethra and lower part of the bladder, which was not evident on endoscopy. Dissemination to the local lymph glands may follow, the inguinal glands being involved in vulval growths, the pelvic and aortic in more deeply placed tumours. More distant metastasis only occurs if the local disease has been brought under control, and many cases have died as a result of cachexia and urinary obstruction.

The diagnosis should be made without difficulty since there is no benign lesion which produces multiple polypi arising from the vaginal wall, and biopsy is easily performed. The myxomatous appearance of lobules must not deceive either surgeon or pathologist, the growth is always malignant and must be treated by radical surgery. Radiotherapy has no useful effect. ULFELDER and QUAN were the first to report successful radical excision of uterus and vagina, and later SHACKMAN described a case in which cystectomy had been performed at the same time. The value of the cystectomy lies chiefly in the more radical nature of the operation, removing the entire field of potential tumour growth, but if the urinary diversion employed is a uretero-sigmoidostomy a satisfactory outcome may ultimately be vitiated by the complications of that procedure.

BODIAN and WHITE have described four children, between 8 and 12 months of age, who presented with a blood-stained discharge from the vagina, and in

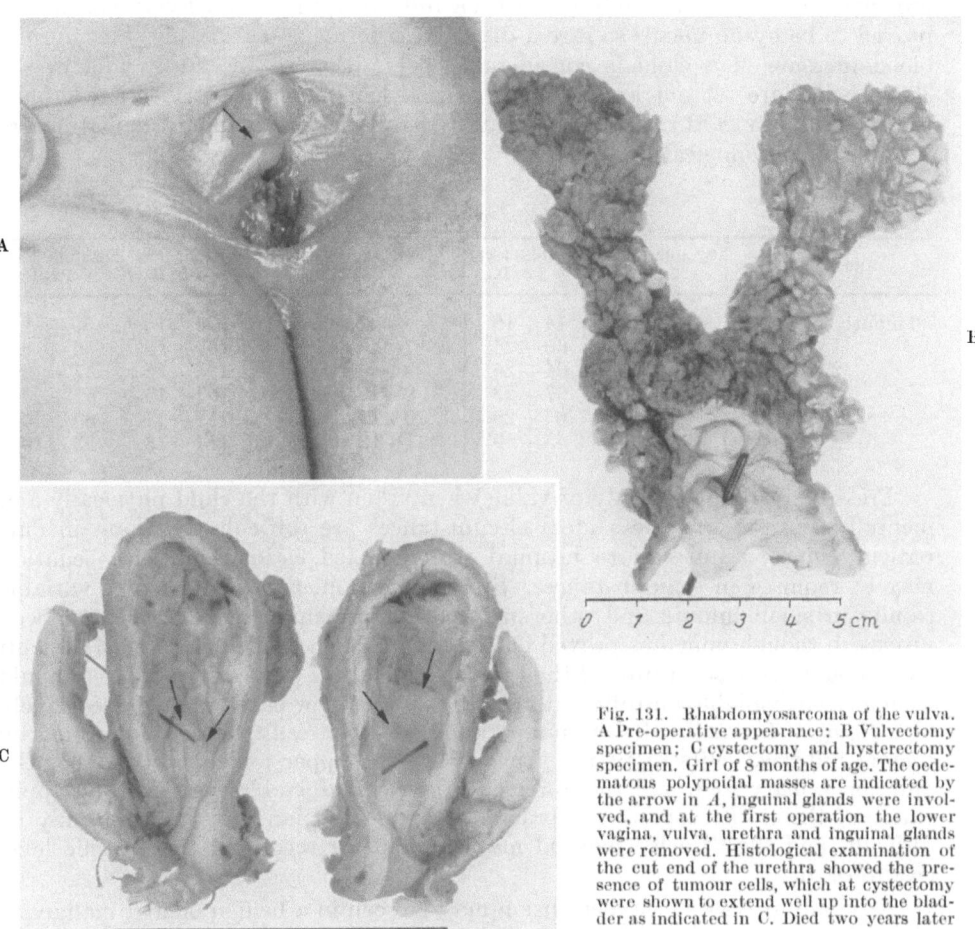

Fig. 131. Rhabdomyosarcoma of the vulva. A Pre-operative appearance; B Vulvectomy specimen; C cystectomy and hysterectomy specimen. Girl of 8 months of age. The oedematous polypoidal masses are indicated by the arrow in *A*, inguinal glands were involved, and at the first operation the lower vagina, vulva, urethra and inguinal glands were removed. Histological examination of the cut end of the urethra showed the presence of tumour cells, which at cystectomy were shown to extend well up into the bladder as indicated in C. Died two years later

whom a carcinoma of the vagina was found. The tumours arose from the vagina or vaginal portion of the cervix, they were composed of cells of epithelial origin with acinar or acino-papillary arrangement. The authors suggest that these tumours may have arisen from Gaertner's duct. Spread occurred to local lymphatic glands, and all cases were fatal within three to nine months of the onset of symptoms.

True carcinoma of the cervix uteri is exceptionally rare in children, but POLLACK and TAYLOR were able to collect from the literature reports of eleven cases under the age of 10 years. A case of adenocarcinoma of the body was recorded in a child of 2 years of age (LOCKHART). Abdominal tumour and vaginal bleeding were the presenting signs.

L. Hypertension

I. General observations

It is only within comparatively recent years that the importance of blood pressure estimations in children has been fully recognized and hypertension has proved to be by no means so rare a disorder as formerly supposed. The normal blood pressure of a child is considerably below that of the adult, and in the Table below are set out approximate normal levels for the various age groups (after HAGGERTY et al.): variations greater than twice the standard deviation are considered pathological.

Normal blood pressure in children

Age group	Systolic level ± 2 S. D.	Diastolic level ± 2 S. D.	Age group	Systolic level ± 2 S. D.	Diastolic level ± 2 S. D.
6 month — 1 year	80 ± 16	44 ± 16	6 — 7 years	100 ± 15	56 ± 9
1 year	89 ± 29	60 ± 25	7 — 8 years	102 ± 15	56 ± 8
2 years	99 ± 25	64 ± 25	8 — 9 years	105 ± 16	57 ± 9
3 years	100 ± 25	67 ± 23	9 —10 years	107 ± 16	57 ± 9
4 years	99 ± 20	65 ± 20	10—11 years	111 ± 17	58 ± 10
5—6 years	94 ± 14	55 ± 9	11—12 years	113 ± 18	59 ± 10

Pressure readings are only of value when taken with the child physically and mentally at rest, and these ideal circumstances are difficult to obtain in out-patient clinics: admission to hospital and repeated estimations with sedation may be required in some instances. Sphygmomanometry is apt to give variable results in small infants and other methods of pressure estimations have been proposed, though none has proved entirely reliable. It is important that the cuff used should cover two thirds of the length of the upper arm, different sizes should therefore be available for different age groups: a narrow cuff will give deceptively high figures. If small cuffs are not at hand, reliable results may be obtained by folding full-sized cuffs to fit the arm so that the upper folded part reaches the anterior axillary fold, and the lower edge gives comfortable space for the application of the stethoscope to the brachial artery. In infants auscultation may be difficult, and the "flush" method may be used for recording the systolic level (REINHOLD).

As in adults, cases of hypertension may be seen in a benign or in a malignant phase, but in the great majority of children the first is short, lasting no more than two or three years, while the second is, if untreated, uniformly fatal within 18 months. In contrast with adult disease, however, a cause can be assigned for the hypertension in almost all cases. It is true that essential hypertension has been discussed by a number of authors, yet with increasing knowledge the number of cases which can be allotted to this category diminishes. The cases described by COURT, by TAUSSIG and REMSEN, and by ZUELZER et al., were examples of essential hypertension in its malignant phase with the secondary pathological changes in the kidney of malignant nephro-sclerosis. Clinically they were indistinguishable from the much more common examples of primary renal disease; they all suffered from haematuria and some from terminal renal failure, but at autopsy only the vascular lesions and their sequelae were found. HAGGERTY et al. have discussed the clinical diagnosis of essential hypertension and describe several cases. SOBEL believed that mild degrees of essential hypertension were quite often encountered and that a very labile blood pressure in the young preceded more serious trouble in later life; supporting evidence for this view has yet to be produced.

Of the known causes of hypertension, renal disease is by far the most common and is the main topic of this section, but in order to clarify the diagnostic problem, the extra-renal causes may be briefly listed.

Hypertension is characteristic of CUSHING's syndrome (p. 194) and is often found in other varieties of adrenal cortical tumour or hyperplasia (p. 276). It is seldom the chief cause of symptoms in these cases and its origin will not be in doubt.

Pheochromocytoma (p. 191) is a tumour manifesting itself almost entirely through its effects upon the blood pressure, it cannot be diagnosed by clinical examination and must be sought by appropriate investigations (p. 192) in all hypertensive children where the kidneys are normal. It should be noted that pheochromocytoma in the young produces the paroxysmal form of hypertension less commonly than the sustained form. Ganglioneuroma has been described as a cause of hypertension by ENGELSON et al.; hyperthyroidism and acrodynia are other rare associations, but are unlikely to cause diagnostic difficulty.

Coarction of the aorta causes a considerable difference between the blood pressure in the upper and lower limbs, and in the former hypertensive levels may be reached. Simple palpation of the femoral pulse will usually indicate the need for investigation of the vascular arrangements.

II. Renal hypertension

Although renal disease is recognized as a potent cause of hypertension, the precise mechanism by which it produces this result is very far from adequately explained. On the basis of Goldblatt experiments it is usually believed that renal ischaemia is in some way responsible, and clinical support can be found for this view. Nevertheless the relationship of the two processes cannot be a simple one, and much of the experimental evidence conflicts with the view that the ischaemic renal tissue produces a hypertensive factor. A discussion of the theoretical aspects of the problem would be out of place in this volume, which is concerned only with the clinical manifestations; a recent brief review of the experimental data is given by FLOYER.

1. Pathology

Hypertension may accompany the following renal lesions:

a) Glomerulo-nephritis

In the early stages of acute glomerulo-nephritis (Ellis Type I) the blood pressure often rises steeply but falls again after a few days with equal rapidity. In the later, chronic stage of this disease hypertension is again a feature: it may be symptomless for some years but then enters a malignant phase and at autopsy the changes of necrotizing arteriolitis are found to be super-imposed upon the nephritic process. A mild degree of hypertension may also accompany the nephrotic form of chronic nephritis (Ellis Type II), if it is entering an azotaemic phase, which is likely to be fatal.

b) Chronic pyelonephritis and renal hypoplasia

This category includes the largest and, from the urological viewpoint, the most important group of hypertensive children. However a large number, probably the majority, of children with chronic pyelonephritis have no disturbance of their blood pressure and the selective factor is unknown. WEISS and PARKER believed that there was a significant relationship between the degree and type of vascular change in the kidney and the onset of hypertension, but other observers find vascular changes in all cases of pyelonephritis, and regard the necrotizing arteriolar lesions characteristic of hypertension as the result rather than the cause of that disorder.

Clinically, hypertension is most often found with the contracted kidney, which may be due to atrophic pyelonephritis or to congenital hypoplasia: a distinction between these two processes is seldom possible, and it is therapeutically unprofitable since the treatment and prognosis is the same in both. It may be debated whether hypertension can be produced by the small but otherwise normal kidney (miniature kidney, p.14); HUTCHISON and MONCRIEFF reported a case with so-called "primary hypertension" in which one kidney was only one third of the size of its fellow but otherwise normal, a finding which might suggest that uncomplicated hypoplasia carries some risk, but at the time of this and other early reports the possibility that minor degrees of renal arterial stenosis could cause hypertension was not appreciated and such a lesion is easily overlooked. That hypertension can occasionally result from pyelonephritis without contraction of the kidney is demonstrated by the case reported by KOBAYASHI and SAKA-GUCHI.

Pyelonephritis is commonly a bilateral disease, producing scattered lesions throughout both kidneys, but it is on occasions confined to one organ, or even to a small segment of kidney tissue. It is clear from the study of these latter cases that the factor producing hypertension bears no direct relation to the secretory capacity of the kidney and it must be recognized that a kidney which is scarred but still capable of concentrating the dye on intravenous pyelography may well be responsible for a rise in pressure. Removal of a unilateral pyelonephritic kidney will in the early stages reverse the tendency to hypertension, but where the blood pressure has been raised for a long period, and secondary arteriolar changes are present in the opposite organ, no improvement will follow nephrectomy.

c) Hydronephrosis

Hypertension is uncommon in the group of diseases resulting in hydronephrosis and usually occurs only when pyelonephritis is present as a complication. Nevertheless sterile hydronephrotic kidneys may be responsible and there is even a suggestion, from the autopsy findings in infants dying within a few days of birth from lower urinary obstruction, that hypertension can occur in utero. Bilateral hydronephrosis is apt to be associated with uraemia, and no treatment is effective in such cases.

d) Vascular lesions

Direct interference with the main renal artery is uncommon but may occur in the case of aneurysm or congenital stenosis. HOCK and JONES, HOWARD et al.; and SNYDER et al., have all recorded cases of aneurysm of the renal artery producing hypertension during childhood, with cure following nephrectomy. When the aneurysm has a partially calcified wall, casting a ring shadow on X-rays, the diagnosis presents little difficulty, but the "berry" aneurysms on one side of the artery in SNYDER's case were only demonstrable by aortography. The secretory activity of the kidney and its ability to concentrate dyes may be little affected by this vascular change.

LEADBETTER and BURKLAND found a curious plug of muscle tissue in the artery leading to a pelvic ectopic kidney in a hypertensive boy: the kidney was otherwise normal but nephrectomy was curative.

POUTASSE et al. have recently described an idiopathic and probably congenital bilateral stenosis of the renal artery. This lesion is only detectable by aortography but these writers have brilliantly demonstrated its causative relation to hypertension in a boy of 15 years: a by-pass of the stenosed segment using a freeze-dried homograft brought the blood pressure down to normal. Since the stenosis is very easily overlooked at nephrectomy it seems likely that this lesion was involved in some of the cures reported to follow removal of a small, or poorly functioning, but histologically normal kidney (e.g. HIGGINS et al., GRIFFITHS).

It must be recognized that in unilateral arterial stenosis, as in the WILSON and BYROM experiments, the affected kidney is protected from the hypertension, and is histologically normal, whereas the contralateral organ shows arteriolar lesions (ISAACSON and WAYBOURNE).

Ligature of aberrant arteries during operation for hydronephrosis must often produce an area of renal ischaemia, yet reports of consequent hypertension are surprisingly rare, and often questionable (e.g. ØSTER). Probably only partial arterial obstruction causes hypertension and ligature produces complete obstruction.

Venous thrombosis is apparently also capable of producing hypertension if recovery of renal function occurs (PERRY and TAYLOR).

e) Injury and perinephric haematoma

MATZNER and SOBEL have both recorded hypertension of rapid onset following rupture of the kidney, cured in both instances by nephrectomy. It is postulated that the perinephric haematoma acts like the cellophane envelope in PAGE's experiments and compresses the kidney. I have seen transient hypertension after heminephrectomy which may have resulted from the same mechanism.

f) Tumour

Nephroblastoma is often associated with hypertension, though this is symptomless and usually unrecorded (see p. 181). In one of my cases, however, it was the observation of hypertension during the investigation of general ill-health which led to pyelography and the discovery of the tumour. The pressure falls after nephrectomy and seldom rises again with the appearance of secondaries, so that hypertension is probably due to the effects of the tumour upon the kidney. BRADLEY and PINCOFFS record an exception: a case in which recurrence of tumour was accompanied by recurrence of hypertension but the possibility of contralateral renal involvement was not excluded in this case.

g) Miscellaneous causes

Polycystic kidneys, renal lithiasis, tuberculosis and amyloidosis are all associated with hypertension on rare occasions.

2. Clinical features

Except where an acute lesion is involved, such as tumour or acute glomerulonephritis, the onset of hypertension is gradual and the resting systolic pressure does not at first exceed 120—140 mm Hg. In this phase the child may be symptom free or there may be some falling off of general health with vomiting and occasional headaches. Clinical examination will reveal nothing other than the rise of pressure, and the eye grounds appear normal. After a variable period the blood pressure tends to rise more steeply, perhaps to a systolic of 200 mm Hg; headaches become severe and disabling, and there may be some blurring of vision. The ophthalmoscope shows retinal haemorrhages and exudates. Later still, in the true malignant phase, haematuria will occur whatever the primary lesion, together with haemorrhage from the nose and bowel. The child becomes almost blind and papilloedema will be observed. Cardiac failure with pulmonary oedema and severe dyspnoea follows and may be fatal, although spontaneous temporary remissions are still possible. Many of the children suffer attacks of hypertensive encephalopathy, with convulsions and coma, and these may be the first evidence of the disease in some. Abdominal pain and intestinal distension are due to the formation of multiple necrotic ulcers in the ileum, which may bleed or perforate. Although there is considerable variation from case to case, the symptoms are in general proportional to the elevation of blood pressure, and the more steeply it rises, the shorter will be the duration of the illness.

3. Investigations

In a disease with such an extremely poor prognosis, it will be clear that the fullest investigations are justifiable, for in the early surgical correction of the causative lesion lies the only hope of cure. Except where the clinical findings suggest an extra-renal cause the first investigations should be examination of the urine and intravenous pyelography. The X-rays will immediately reveal a tumour or hydronephrosis, or may suggest the presence of pyelonephritis. In the latter case the films must be carefully scrutinized in order to decide whether the disease is unilateral or bilateral; examples of the typical deformities of the pelvis and calyces are illustrated in Figs. 93 to 96 and 132; the outline of the kidney substance must also be traced, for scars in the parenchyma may show here and nowhere else. Where renal function is poor, retrograde pyelograms and differential analysis of kidney urine may be helpful. In doubtful cases, and where intravenous pyelography shows no definite abnormality, aortography should be undertaken: this may demonstrate abnormalities of the renal artery, and will also give a clearer outline of the whole renal shadow. Incidentally it may also localize a pheochromo-cytoma (p. 192). In chronic glomerulo-nephritis the function of both kidneys is poor, but there is no significant deformity of the pelvi-calyceal system.

4. Management

The cases presented to the urologist fall into two main groups: first those children with symptoms related to the urinary tract disorder in whom hyper-tension is discovered on routine examination, and second those who have attended the paediatrician because of hypertensive symptoms and who are referred for urological investigation. Those in the first group, with the disease still in its benign phase, have naturally the better prognosis, but the surgical management is similar in both groups: permanent cure can only be achieved by excision of the affected renal element and no fall in blood pressure can be expected as a result of conservative procedures aimed at securing better drainage of the urinary tract, even though these may be indicated for other reasons. Nephrectomy is therefore clearly indicated in unilateral cases of hydronephrosis, stone, tumour, tuberculosis or rupture. The same treatment may be applicable in cases of abnormalities of the main renal artery, although the work of POUTASSE et al. already referred to demonstrates the possibility of correction by arterial grafting.

Unilateral pyelonephritis is a tantalizing problem to the surgeon; since the first report of BUTLER in 1937, there have been many published records of successful nephrectomy (though mostly with inadequate follow-up), yet in the experience of any individual the failures have greatly outnumbered the successes even when all precautions in establishing the normality of the contralateral kidney have been observed. The failures are undoubtedly due to the inadequacy of our methods of detecting pyelonephritic changes unaccompanied by gross scarring, and to the secondary vascular lesions which occur in long standing hypertension. Since the progressive failure of the renal excretory activity is also a danger in pyelonephritics, nephrectomy should be restricted to those with a normal blood urea in which all available tests including renal biopsy indicate the opposite kidney to be free of disease, and those in which the affected organ is so small and functionless as to be of no value to the child. The operation itself is usually simple and free from complications; only where there has been cardiac failure or encephalopathy is pre-operative medical treatment required. In the successful case, the pressure will fall immediately, or at least within 48 hours; in others there is not infrequently a transient fall followed by a slow rise, though it is sometimes months or years before the original level is reached. HILLEBRAND suggests that there is a possi-

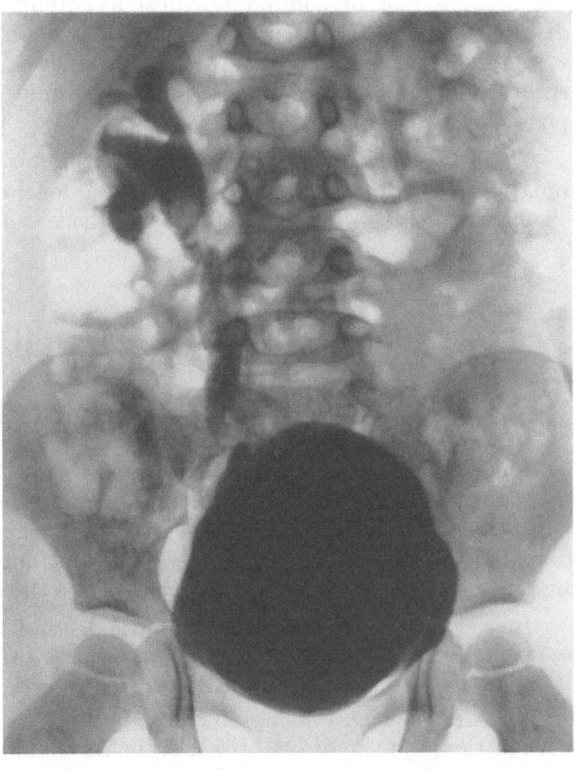

Fig. 132. Simple megaureter with chronic pyelonephritis. Late cystogram taken two hours after filling the bladder. A boy aged 4 years suffering from hypertension and chronic urinary infection. I.V.P. showed no secretion by the right kidney, and the ureteric orifice on this side could not be catheterized. On cystography there was no immediate reflux, but the ureter was filled in the late films. Nephrectomy resulted in a fall of blood pressure to a normal level: it has remained low for one year

bility of late improvement following nephrectomy, though this is not the experience of most observers.

The treatment of bilateral disease and "failed nephrectomy" is largely medical: sympathectomy has little place in the treatment of hypertensive children, and sub-total adrenalectomy is a procedure yet to be fully evaluated, though PICKERING et al. report a partial success in a child. Hypotensive drugs are often of great value; they are capable of reducing the blood pressure in renal disease at least as efficiently as in essential hypertension (WILSON and ABRAHAMS), of alleviating symptoms and prolonging life, but permanent cure cannot be obtained by their use. Any of the drugs used in adult hypertension may be administered to children in appropriately reduced dosage; hexamethonium bromide and

Ansolysen (Pentolinium tartate) are administered by injection, Serpasil (Reserpine) can be given by mouth. The dosage is determined empirically, and the child must be in hospital during the trial period. The first dose should be very small (Hexamethonium bromide 10 mgm, Ansolysen 2 mgm, Serpasil 0.1 mgm) and the effect on the blood pressure must be carefully followed; the final dose employed may be 10 times these figures but increases should be given cautiously and under observation.

A full drop to a normal pressure should not be aimed at for this will involve too great a risk of sudden postural hypotension. Side effects such as bowel disturbances are often tiresome. Because hypotensive treatment is essentially symptomatic treatment, it is probably unwise to employ it in the symptomless case, but if a sudden rise of pressure gives warning of the approach of the malignant phase the drugs should be started.

According to WILSON and ABRAHAMS the duration of life in medically treated renal hypertension is closely related to the level of blood urea: uraemic cases are sometimes made worse by hypotensive drugs and deteriorate rapidly.

M. Renal failure and allied disorders

I. Acute renal failure

Children are, in general, little exposed to those hazards, such as crush injuries and obstetric complications, which are common causes of acute renal failure in adults, but are much more liable to episodes of severe dehydration producing renal damage: the circumstances of the onset of anuria are therefore often different but the general principles of management are the same at all ages.

In the new-born a period of anuria lasting 24—48 hours after birth is not abnormal, and requires no treatment. Cases of bilateral renal agenesis seldom live long enough for the anuria to cause concern.

Birth trauma and neonatal asphyxia may lead to a considerable rise of blood urea in the following days: JONSSON believes that this is due to a type of "lower nephron nephrosis", though urine secretion does not cease in these cases. McCANCE has demonstrated, however, that in the neonate the urea clearance rate is low, and that the ingested protein is largely used in tissue building at this stage: should this process be halted or reversed by a traumatic episode protein catabolism will lead to a sharp rise in blood urea levels even in the presence of normal kidneys. This explanation is probably correct for some cases, but the problem of clinical diagnosis in the uraemic neonate is still confused, and some infants who ultimately recover completely have firm and slightly enlarged kidneys when first seen.

This section is principally concerned with cases of anuria or extreme oliguria due to organic renal or ureteric disease, but it must be emphasized that dehydration and salt depletion, frequently the result of gastro-enteritis, may lead to severe oliguria and to a considerable rise of blood urea. These effects (pre-renal uraemia) are due to circulatory renal failure; they are in the early stages unaccompanied by histological change in the kidney and are easily reversible if the deficiency in water and electrolytes is made good; if allowed to go unchecked, however, the circulatory failure will lead to renal tubular necrosis which is discussed below.

1. Pathology

a) Acute tubular necrosis

This lesion, which has gone under a variety of names such as "lower nephron nephrosis", "crush syndrome" or "haemoglobinuric nephrosis" may result from a variety of insults, and especially in children it is by no means easy to identify the particular cause. The precise local pathology has been clarified by the work of OLIVER et al. and later by DARMADY. Where the disorder is primarily a failure of the circulation, whether local or general, the changes are described as "tubulorrhexis"; degeneration and desquamation is found at various levels of the nephron, often with complete disruption of the basement membrane, and the formation of tubulo-venous anastomoses. The glomeruli remain intact, and there are usually some nephrons which escape damage altogether. Where the primary disorder is one which releases large quantities of pigment into the circulation, as in acute haemolytic anaemia and mismatched blood transfusion, pigment casts are found in the tubules. It seems unlikely that these casts cause serious obstruction, though their presence may perhaps be an additional embarrassment to the kidney. The interstitial tissue is oedematous and may be infiltrated by inflammatory cells.

Where a toxin, such as one of the metallic poisons, is primarily involved, all the nephrons will be affected but the damage may be confined to a specific level of the nephron, often the proximal tubule, and epithelial desquamation may occur without rupture of the basement membrane. However, the general action of the toxin may itself result in circulatory failure, while carbon tetrachloride and other organic poisons are capable of producing a local vascular disorder, so that tubulorrhexis may occur. In sulphonamide poisoning the lesions are the result of hypersensitivity rather than toxicity.

Anuria results partly from the failure of glomerular filtration due to the circulatory disorder, and partly because of complete reabsorption of the filtrate which enters the interstitial tissues from the ruptured tubules. The process of repair begins within a few days, however, and in many cases an adequate functional recovery is possible through epithelial regeneration and through hypertrophy of surviving elements. At first tubular function will be inefficient; urine excreted will be isotonic with a plasma ultrafiltrate and will contain such substances as amino-acids and glucose. With time, however, normal urine will be elaborated though urea clearance levels are likely to remain below normal.

b) Acute glomerulo-nephritis

RUBIN states that anuria or extreme oliguria occurs in about 5% of the cases of acute glomerulo-nephritis in children. The tubules remain intact and fatal cases are very rare.

c) Bilateral renal venous thrombosis

Bilateral venous thrombosis (p. 230) and symmetrical cortical necrosis (p. 229) are relatively common causes of anuria in the neonatal period: their pathology is discussed elsewhere and recovery is unlikely.

d) Suppurative nephritis

The rapid destruction of the parenchyma which occurs in bilateral metastatic suppurative lesions (p. 150) will produce anuria for the short time of survival. Acute pyelonephritis supervening in kidneys already severely damaged by hydronephrosis may have the same result, often the terminal event of congenital lower urinary obstruction.

e) Ureteric obstruction

Calculous obstruction of both ureters, or of a solitary ureter, is rare. Obstruction by sulphonamide crystals has been comparatively common during the past 15 years, but its incidence is decreasing rapidly with the employment of more soluble drugs. Sulphapyridine, sulphaguanidine, and sulphamerazine have been the most serious offenders. This type of anuria may be the result of tubular necrosis as well as of ureteric obstruction and both causes may be operative in the same case. The ureters themselves become oedematous, inflamed, and are friable if handled; the obstructing sludge is composed of epithelial cells and debris as well as sulphonamide crystals. Sulphamerazine sludge may block the urethra rather than the ureters on occasions.

2. Clinical picture

The clinical picture at the onset of acute renal failure is dominated by the disorder which causes it, and anuria itself produces so little disturbance that it is often impossible to find out exactly when the last urine was passed. Thus the child may be severely shocked after operation or injury, or extremely dehydrated as a result of gastro-enteritis. There may have been a blood loss due to injury or haemolytic anaemia, and perhaps the additional complication of a mismatched blood transfusion. A clear history of the ingestion of some poisonous substance may be obtained, often a chemical in ordinary household use which the toddler has tasted out of curiosity or even when such a history is not forthcoming, a toxic origin may be suspected from the coincidence of sudden vomiting, diarrhoea and collapse with the anuria. In the case of sulphonamide renal failure, the dosage has usually been excessive, and the fluid intake has been severely limited by vomiting or lack of nursing. The drug has often been administered for an upper respiratory infection, and in these circumstances it may be subsequently difficult to distinguish between sulphonamide anuria and acute glomerulo-nephritis, though oedema and hypertension will suggest the latter. Haematuria preceding the final cessation of urine flow occurs in both. Acute tubular necrosis is a painless condition, and when there is a complaint of an ache in the loin or of ureteric colic, an obstructive cause should be suspected. Renal venous thrombosis in the neonatal period is accompanied by a sudden enlargement of the kidneys, and often by haematuria; symmetrical cortical necrosis is symptomless and rapidly fatal. Anuria resulting from acute infections in an old case of lower urinary obstruction is easily recognized. Anuria may very rarely follow bilateral retrograde pyelography; the use of sodium iodide is usually blamed, but diodone has been responsible where there was a sensivity to that substance (CAMPBELL).

It must be emphasized that in many cases of anuria in childhood, the cause cannot be precisely identified: urine flow ceases in the course of some respiratory or gastro-intestinal disturbance which has not produced severe collapse. Drugs have been administered in ordinary doses, and hypersensitivity is not established. Full descriptions of such cases are given by PRATT, and CARRÉ and SQUIRE: the pathology is assumed to be acute tubular necrosis, and the illness follows the usual course of that disease. BULL et al. were the first to give a comprehensive description of the various phases of the disease in adults, and to draw attention to the fact that many of the lesions are recoverable if the patients can be kept alive until renal function returned. The onset phase has already been described, it is followed by the anuric phase, the early diuretic and the late diuretic phases.

During the early part of the anuric phase, there may be few clinical findings and the child appears surprisingly well. Nausea and vomiting occur later, often provoked by the unpalatable diet offered. The child usually remains alert and bright despite the rise of blood urea, but if anuria persists, drowsiness, disorientation and convulsions may appear. Oedema, whether pulmonary or subcutaneous, is due to excessive ingestion of fluid and does not occur in properly treated cases. Hypertension of mild degree is found in a few. Normocytic anaemia is a constant feature in cases of acute tubular necrosis, even when the primary disorder does not entail blood loss or destruction, though these factors will accentuate the condition.

On a normal diet, the blood urea will probably rise by 50—100 points each day, its rate of increase can be halved by a high calorie, protein free diet. Acidosis accompanies the uraemia, but the most dangerous biochemical change is the rise in serum potassium, which has caused a fatal termination due to cardiac arrest in several reported cases. Low sodium and chloride figures may accompany the rise in potassium due to a shift of ions between the intra-cellular and extra-cellular compartments. Resumption of urine flow may be noted after three or four days, but recovery may still occur after a much longer duration of anuria or extreme oliguria, periods up to 3 weeks being recorded in adults.

In the early diuretic phase, small quantities of urine are passed containing albumin, glucose, amino-acids, and perhaps casts. During the following three or four days the urinary volume rises rapidly; urine concentration is low, but because of inefficient tubular function its electrolyte content is variable and may be high. The blood urea falls steadily but during the diuretic phase the dangers of acute biochemical disturbance are great. Rapid loss of fluid will cause sudden dehydration with hypotension and collapse. Loss of sodium or chloride potassium may all produce acute disturbances, and in the case of potassium the fall in serum level is due not only to the urinary loss but to a shift back into the intracellular compartment. The total renal function gradually returns to normal or near normal levels, but albumin is found in the urine for many months after the anuric episode. Only in the most severe cases of tubular necrosis is there a permanent impairment of renal function, or any persistent hypertension.

The common causes of death due to acute renal failure are:
a) An irremediable renal lesion.
b) Overhydration during the anuric phase.
c) Hyperkaliaemia during the anuric phase.
d) Dehydration and electrolyte loss in the diuretic phase.
e) Complicating infection of the urinary tract or elsewhere.

3. Management

It is likely that some form of treatment will already be in progress when anuria is first noticed, such as resuscitation for shock, blood transfusion for haemolytic anaemia, stomach washouts and the administration of antidotes for poisoning. The onset of anuria does not lessen the need for these measures, and despite the dangers of overhydration, it is vital that initial dehydration and blood loss should be made good, for in this way the circulation will be most rapidly restored to normal.

Diagnostic measures are largely concerned with the elimination of an obstructive factor: a straight X-ray of the abdomen for calculi should be routine, and if there is any suggestion of renal or ureteric pain, cystoscopy and ureteric catheterization should be carried out. In sulphonamide anuria, such catheterization is probably always wise, although acute tubular necrosis may be present as well as, or instead, of ureteric obstruction. The ureteric orifices in the obstructive cases are reddened and oedematous: a plug of yellow sludge can be seen within the orifice or can be brought down by passing the catheter in and out a few times. Indwelling catheters are seldom useful, and if blockage recurs after the plug has been released pyelostomy is preferable. There is often an element of spasm in the obstruction and when one ureter has been unblocked, both kidneys often start secretion. Other surgical measures aimed at starting the urine flow are seldom of value and have been largely discarded: spinal anaesthesia or novocaine block of the renal pedicle as advocated by BARTHÉLEMEY may occasionally be useful in calculous or sulphonamide obstruction, but not in acute tubular necrosis. Decapsulation of the kidney has failed so often that it should no longer be advised. Similarly medical treatment with diuretics in the presence of severe tubular damage is without theoretical justification or practical advantage.

The fundamental principle in treatment is the maintenance of the biochemical state of the body fluids as near to normality as possible until renal function returns. No more fluid must be administered than leaves the body, and the rate of protein catabolism must be reduced to the minimum. No protein is given in the diet, and a high calorie intake is supplied to spare the breakdown of body tissue.

Thus provided the child is not in a state of dehydration, the fluid during the anuric phase must be restricted to rather less than the amount of insensible loss, as estimated by daily weighing (insensible loss = body weight loss + weight of food and water intake — weight of urine, vomit and faeces). Although standard figures have been given for the insensible loss in basal conditions (1 gr/kilo/hour for infants; 0.8 gr/kilo/hour for bigger children) in the circumstances of anuria, loss will be perhaps twice as great. PRATT for instance found that a 7 kilo baby required 300 ccs per day. Some loss of weight should be allowed, however, since it is impossible to provide a fully adequate calorie intake. Calorie requirements for infants are 100 calories/kilo/day; for older children 75 cals/kilo/day, and should be given in the form of a peanut oil-glucose (1:4) mixture emusified with acacia in the calculated volume of water. This is distinctly unpalatable and is best administered by a continuous intragastric drip, together with vitamin supplements (but not fruit juices containing potassium). Vomit should be collected, strained and returned to the drip. In some cases the consequent gastric disturbance is too great to allow the continuation of this method, and instead a 10 to 20% glucose solution is given via a polythene tube into the superior vena cava. This may be maintained for some days.

These conservative measures should suffice until urine flow recommences and although the blood urea will rise to very high levels other electrolytes may remain within the normal limits. In general, variations of the sodium chloride and bicarbonate figures during anuria may be ignored, but overhydration and hyperkaliaemia may demand active treatment. Methods of artificially relieving these accumulations have included extra-corporeal dialysis (the artificial kidney), peritoneal lavage, and exchange transfusions. The first mentioned requires a highly expert team and can only be employed in a special centre; its use in the child has been reported by MATEER et al. Peritoneal lavage in children has been described in detail by SWAN and GORDON, who believed it to be of great value although hazardous. Exchange transfusion may be more easily applied to small children than in adults, but the complications are many. Serum potassium levels may be reduced by the use of ion exchange resins (e.g. ZEOCARB 555) but their administration presents many difficulties in infants as the material is hard to introduce through a small intragastric tube. MacDONALD and ROBINSON report the successful use of Amberlite XE (20 mgm/day) in older children.

Great precautions against infection must be observed. Indwelling catheters should not be employed, and some routine antibiotic cover may be given. In general a single large dose of antibiotic at the onset will suffice for many days, since in the absence of urine flow little will be lost. Non-toxic antibiotics such as penicillin may be given continuously.

Once the diuresis commences, the output of fluid must be carefully watched, and full replacement ensured: an intravenous drip is almost always required at this time. Serum electrolyte estimation should be carried out daily and any exceptional losses replaced without delay. Extra potassium is often needed, and should be supplied as a routine in the form of fruit juices. This phase is perhaps more dangerous than the preceding one, but reactions are so variable that no hard and fast rules can be laid down.

II. Chronic renal failure

1. Aetiology

A very large variety of renal diseases may at times lead to a gradual deterioration of total renal function, and the clinical or biochemical changes which ensue depend more upon the age of onset and rapidity of progress than upon the nature of the renal lesion.

During the first and second year of life, chronic renal failure is most often due to congenital lower urinary obstruction with consequent hydronephrosis and hydro-ureter, or to congenital renal hypoplasia. These lesions continue to be found throughout childhood and adolescence, but in later years bilateral mega-ureter, chronic pyelonephritis, chronic glomerulo-nephritis, and polycystic disease are important causes, while many other forms of renal disease, such as lithiasis, tuberculosis, amyloidosis, peri-arteritis nodosa are occasionally responsible.

The disorder of renal function is very similar in the advanced stages of all the diseases mentioned and is for the most part irreversible. The number of functioning nephrons is in all cases reduced, with consequent retention of nitrogenous waste, while damage to the survivors may be responsible for unusual losses of electrolyte.

Many authors have commented upon the frequency with which dilated ureters are found in chronic renal failure (e. g. ELLIS and EVANS), and often neither clinical nor post-mortem examination has elucidated the cause of the dilatation. Undoubtedly some of these cases are lower urinary obstructions and others mega-ureters, though often pyelonephritic changes have produced more damage than the urinary stasis. There is often a suspicion, too, that the extreme polyuria may lead to some enlargement of the urinary passages: this can be proved in cases of diabetes insipidus, but is not established in cases of renal disease.

2. Clinical course and biochemical changes

Chronic renal failure is an insidious process which does not proclaim its presence by any urgent sign, and often by the time symptoms have become apparent to the child and his parents, destruction of the renal tissue is far advanced. The mechanism by which the clinical manifestations are produced cannot be fully explained, the simple accumulation of urea in the body fluids is certainly not the important factor, but where possible the signs will be described in relation to the biochemical aberrations.

The growth of the child is retarded, and the milestones of the infant's development are reached after some delay. His gain in weight is slow, he does not lift his head, sit up or walk until many months after the normal child. The limb muscles are often hypotonic, sometimes even to a degree where a myopathy is suspected. When the failure is of late onset, growth retardation may not be so marked, but sexual infantilism is a feature of those who have passed the normal age of puberty.

The bone changes and consequent limb deformities are often the presenting complaint: they are not seen before the end of the first year, and are most marked in those very slowly progressive disorders which are fatal only in early adult life. The complexity of the "renal rickets" problem is such that the topic has been allotted a separate section (p. 224).

The skin is sallow, dry and wrinkled, sometimes it is deeply pigmented. Anaemia is almost always present: it is normochromic and normocytic, and its cause is unknown. Haemorrhages from all mucous surfaces may occur in the terminal states, or when acute infections complicate the picture.

Thirst and polyuria are characteristic symptoms, the urine is extremely dilute and often has a specific gravity as low as 1002 or 1003. In the advanced stages of failure, urine remains isotonic with a plasma ultrafiltrate, the specific gravity is approximately 1010 and cannot be altered by varying the fluid intake. It is, of course, the inability of the kidneys to produce a concentrated urine which causes the high fluid intake, and if infection or gastro-intestinal disturbances interfere with this intake, the loss of body water will lead to dehydration. This in turn results in circulatory renal failure which will, if uncorrected, be rapidly fatal. Plentiful fluids are essential therefore to the well-being of these children, but the polyuria itself may cause frequency and enuresis which are troublesome.

The blood urea in these cases is always raised, and though for long periods it may be very little above the normal limits, it is extremely labile and a minor infection or slight dehydration may send it rocketing up from 50 to 150 or 200 mgm/100 ml in the course of 48 hours. Levels of 70 or 80 are compatible with apparent good health in many children with chronic renal failure: some go much higher without serious symptoms, and terminally levels of 400 are not uncommon. The blood urea is, therefore, only of value in assessing the state of the kidney if a series of estimations is available: not only are temporary variations common, but extra-renal factors, such as sudden acceleration of protein breakdown, may be responsible for a rise.

Vomiting is frequent in renal failure at all ages, the infant is particularly hard to feed, and very reluctant to take solid food. Constipation is a common complaint, and hard dry stools are doubtless often the counterpart of polyuria. Diarrhoea occurs from time to time in seriously ill cases. Intestinal distension is often seen in the infants with lower urinary obstruction.

Headaches are an occasional symptom, though they are seldom severe unless there is an associated hypertension. Severe acidosis is the normal accompaniment of uraemia, causing deep hissing respiration and later coma, while a mild depression of the serum bicarbonate is often found in symptomless cases. The acidosis results from loss of the sodium ion and retention of phosphate and other anions (Fig. 133). Sodium may be lost into the stools in diarrhoea, or temporarily into the intestinal contents in cases of gross intestinal distension, but a tubular failure is chiefly responsible. There is an impairment of the mechanism of excreting hydrogen ion, and of manufacturing ammonia in order to conserve the fixed bases, and sodium is therefore lost in the urine. At times this tubular loss of sodium may be extreme, and dominate the entire clinical picture, leading to collapse and circulatory renal failure as in Addison's disease: this "salt-losing" syndrome was first described by THORN et al., and has usually been reported in adults. Similar specific loss of potassium due to pyelonephritis is rare, and some of the earlier recorded cases are now recognized as examples of primary aldosteronism

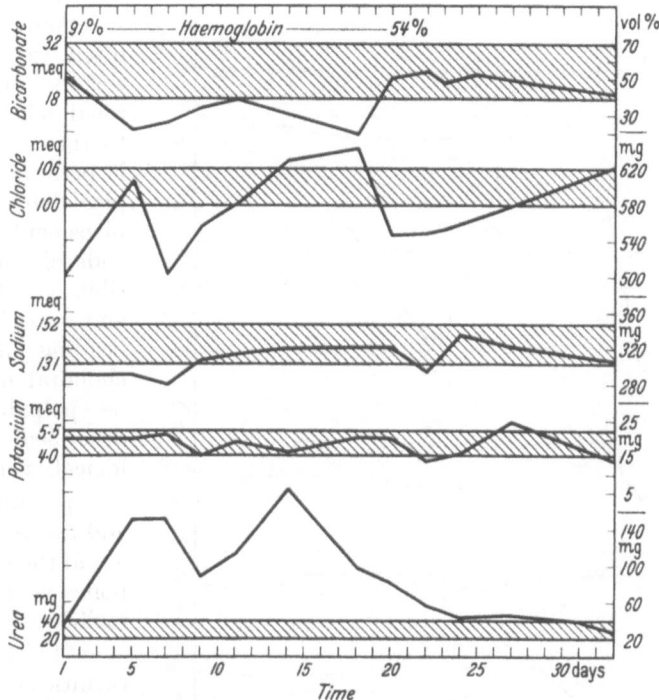

Fig. 133. Chart to show variations in the serum chemistry in a boy admitted at the age of 4 days, suffering from retention due to urethral valves. The hatched areas represent the limits of normality for the electrolytes and urea; the continuous lines represent the actual levels throughout the first 32 days of treatment. Marked acidosis with lowered sodium levels occurred during the first weeks

due to adrenal tumour, but one of my cases of lower urinary obstruction died of hypokaliaemia which appeared to result from excessive urinary losses, and milder chronic depletion has occurred in others.

Phosphate and sulphate are retained because of a low glomerular filtration rate, and are partly responsible for the acidosis. This rise in serum phosphate causes a corresponding depression in the total serum calcium, but because an acidosis is present at the same time, the ionized calcium remains near normal levels. Tetany will appear if the ionized calcium level falls, and although latent tetany is often detectable in late renal failure, actual tetanic spasms usually result from the ill-judged administration of alkalis. Although vomiting is common in these cases, it seldom results in alkalaemia since there is hypochlorhydria.

Occasionally the renal loss of electrolytes has proceeded rapidly but the child has only had water to drink: thus although the child may be dehydrated, the serum is hypo-electrolytaemic (Fig. 134). The great danger of this state lies in the fact that if more water or isotonic fluid is administered, the extra-cellular fluid is expanded but is hypotonic in relation to the intracellular fluid. Osmotic forces then drive water into the cells, and consequent cellular overhydration leads to convulsions, coma and death.

3. Bone changes — renal osteodystrophy

The recognition that retardation of growth in renal disease was accompanied by bone changes was first emphasized by BARBER, and later described by PARSONS, by DUKEN and others. In children the changes often resemble dietary rickets, and the term renal rickets was applied to them. Genu valgum is perhaps the most typical deformity, but displacement of the lower ends of the radius and tibia is also common, and a "rickety rosary", beading of the costochondral junctions may be palpable. PARSONS described three radiological varieties:

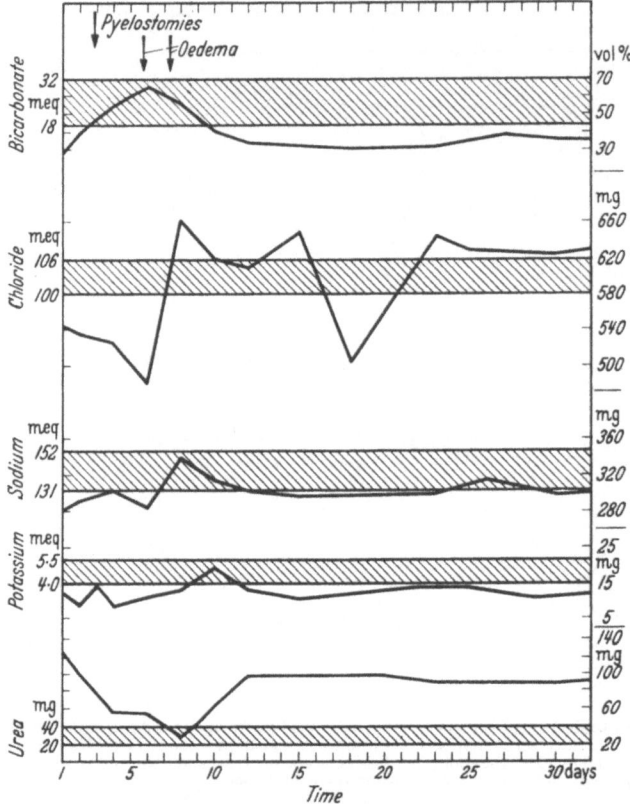

Fig. 134. Chart to show variations of the serum chemistry in a boy aged 20 months with chronic retention due to bladder neck obstruction. On admission all the electrolyte levels were depressed, although there was severe dehydration; water and electrolyte had been lost, largely into the bowel, and had been replaced only by water. The fall in blood urea at the end of the first week was associated with cerebral and pulmonary oedema, the later rise came with a considerable improvement in the clinical condition

a) Atrophic type: in addition to rachitic changes at the epiphyses, the bones as a whole were rarified.

b) Florid type: severe rachitic changes without alteration of the shaft.

c) "Woolly" type: entirely peculiar to this condition, the metaphyses were enlarged, and the distal end of the diaphysis honeycombed and woolly in appearance.

LANGMEAD and ORR, and subsequently many other writers, recognized the similarity of many of the changes to osteitis fibrosa resulting from hyperparathyroidism, and for a time it was supposed (ALBRIGHT and RIEFENSTEIN) that all the bone lesions were due to parathyroid dysfunction. Parathyroid hyperplasia is almost always found at post-mortem in long standing cases of renal failure, and DRESKIN and FOX were even able to demonstrate improvement in the bone state after removal of a hyperplastic parathyroid gland in the course of "biopsy". It was believed that phosphate retention led to a fall of serum calcium with consequent stimulation of the secretion of parathyroid hormone. This factor then resulted in mobilization of calcium from the bones, and the changes of osteitis fibrosa. However, on rare occasions normal phosphate values may be recorded in these cases, and histological studies do not confirm the hypothesis that osteitis fibrosa accounts for all cases (GILMOUR, FOLLIS). The possibility of a disorder of Vitamin D action was suggested by many observations: DUKEN, GRAHAM and OAKLEY, SHELDON and other writers recorded the apparent healing which could be obtained by the administration of very large doses of Vitamin D, and finally LIU and CHU demonstrated that these cases have an acquired insensiti-

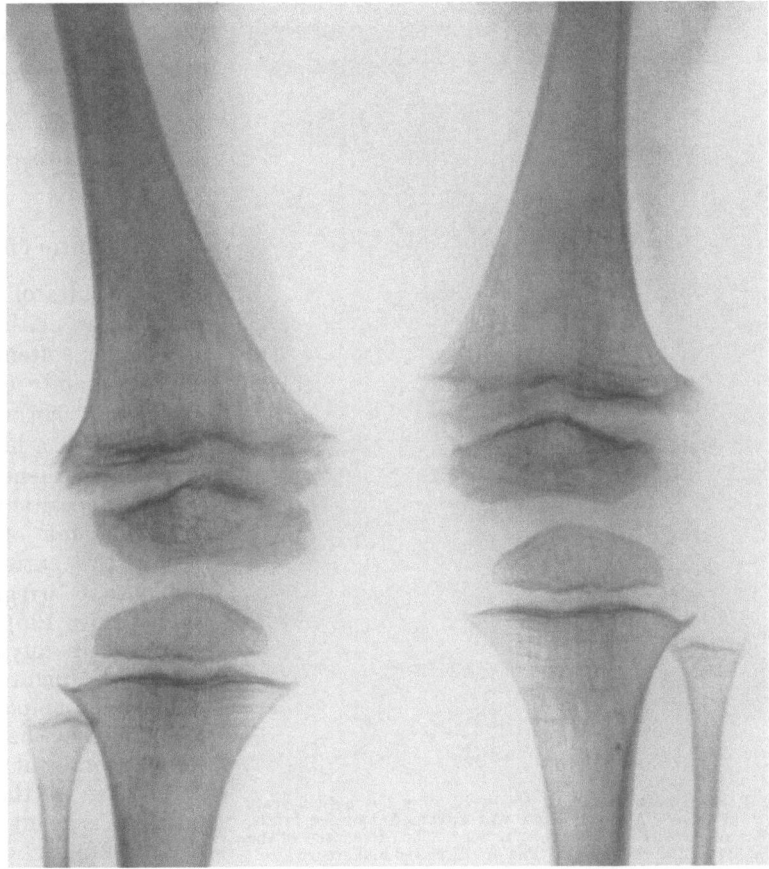

Fig. 135. Renal rickets of the "tubular" variety. X-ray of the knees of a boy aged 6 years with nephrocalcinosis, a normal blood urea, and a severe hyperchloraemic acidosis. He was first treated for multiple calculi in dilated ureters at the age of 3 years (Fig. 101) and the disorder of renal function only became evident later

vity to Vitamin D in normal doses, resulting in impaired absorption of calcium from the gut. The relationship between this defect and parathyroid hyperplasia is not fully explained.

In the cases with reduced glomerular filtration and raised blood urea it is doubtful whether the bone changes can be attributed to chronic acidosis which results in the mobilization of calcium. Correction of the acidosis alone has not resulted in any improvement in the bone disease and advanced changes may be demonstrable in children with little alteration of the serum bicarbonate level. Bone changes can occur, however, in cases with predominantely tubular lesions, having a normal blood urea but a severe hyperchloraemic acidosis ("tubular rickets"). This is most often seen in ALBRIGHT'S syndrome (p. 234), but may also complicate obstructive uropathies where the renal damage has been selective (Fig. 135). A case of this type in which acidosis is playing an important part in osteodystrophy may be recognized from the high level of the urinary calcium: this is characteristic of the tubular cases but is not found in the typical azotaemic disease.

Most contemporary writers agree that the bone lesions in renal disease are due in various degrees to hyperparathyroidism and to Vitamin D insensitivity with impaired absorption of the calcium. The radiological signs of these two disorders are distinguishable, though both may be present in the same child. The appearance are discussed by BRAILSFORD and by DENT and HODSON.

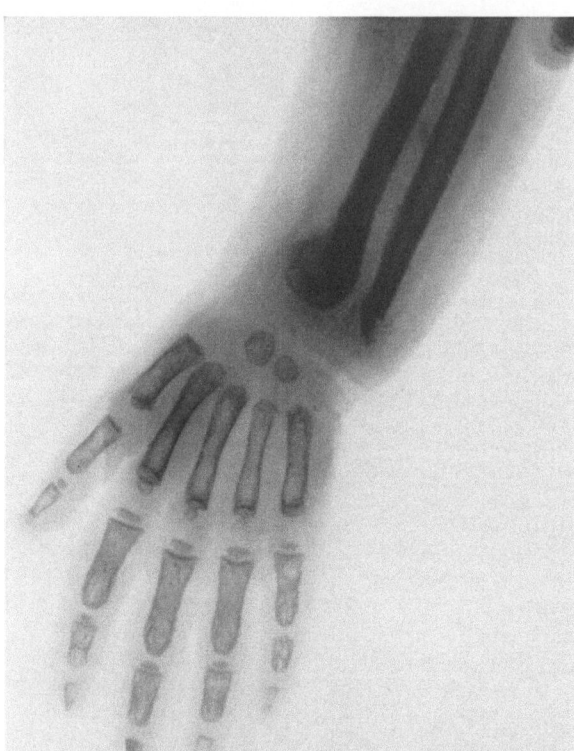

Fig. 136. Renal rickets. X-ray of the wrist of a boy aged 3 years with urethral valves. Although there was advanced hydronephrosis, no disorder of micturition had been noticed. The extremities of the diaphyses of the radius and ulna are displaced and eroded

a) Rachitic changes

The shafts of the long bones show neither osteoporosis nor softening, both compact and cancellous zones are normal. The metaphysis is a little deepened and widened owing to the deposition of the large amount of osteoid tissue; the extremity of diaphysis is irregular and woolly (Fig. 136), but the bone immediately behind it is normal. Slight displacement of the epiphysis may occur. The changes are more prominent at the knees than at the ankles, and there is no involvement of the skull.

b) Osteitis fibrosa changes

There is osteoporosis of the whole skeleton, and in advanced cases long bones consist of coarse cancellous bone only. Early changes are found in the cortical zone of the middle phalanges which shows sub-periosteal erosion (Fig. 137). The metaphysis is much thicker than normal, the extremity of the diaphysis is cupped, and has a "ground glass" structureless appearance. Bending of the shaft and gross displacement of the epiphysis may occur in this type.

Unfortunately there is still disagreement and confusion in regard to these radiological appearances: for instance the term "rotting stump" originated by TEALL has been applied to the rachitic change as well as to the osteitis fibrosa type. CRAWFORD et al. have further drawn attention to the existence of a third type of bone reaction — osteosclerosis. Hyperparathyroidism is not invariable in this type, and no explanation can be given for the appearance.

In the late stages of the osteitis fibrosa type, calcifications appear in the soft tissue. The media of the arteries of the limbs may be chiefly affected, or soft malleable masses of putty-like substance may be deposited in the subcutaneous tissues. Such calcification is particularly likely to complicate cases where large doses of Vitamin D have been administered. It may also be noted that ANDERSEN and SCHLESINGER have described arterial calcification in infants with renal failure and hyperparathyroidism without any bone change.

The serum chemistry in renal osteodystrophy has been indicated in the preceding section: the phosphate level is almost always raised (4—12 mg/100 ml), the calcium is normal or slightly depressed (6—10 mg/100 ml). The alkaline phosphate is increased (15 to 100 units). Uraemia and acidosis of some degree are invariable.

4. Management

Chronic renal failure due to loss of functioning renal tissue cannot be repaired but superimposed upon this loss there may be an element of circulatory failure, obstructive uropathy, or active pyelonephritis. Correction of these factors may restore chemical equilibrium and allow hypertrophy of surviving nephrons, so that a somewhat precarious life may be prolonged. Moreover even where no improvement in renal function can be obtained, biochemical treatment may allow considerable symptomatic relief.

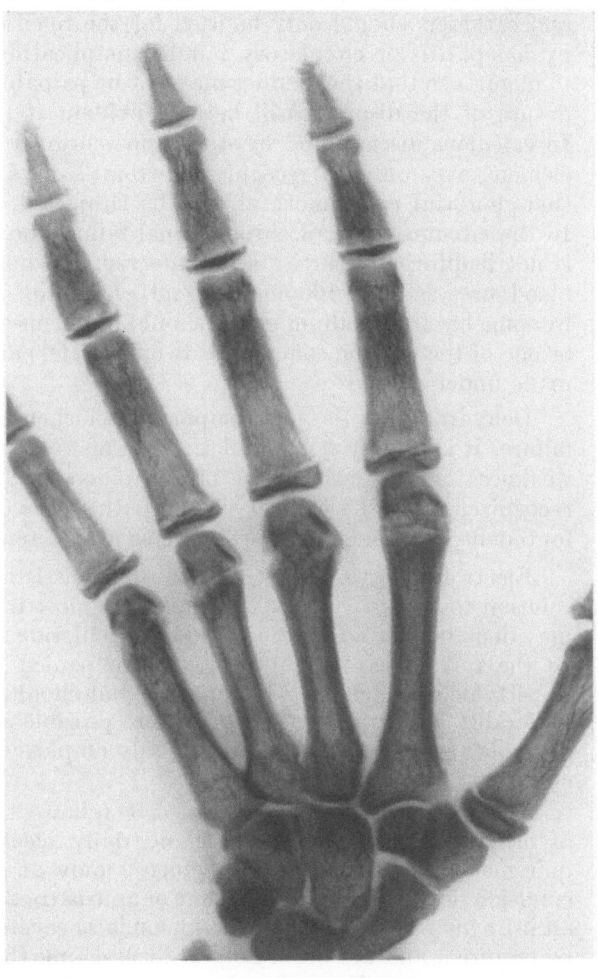

Fig. 137. Renal osteodystrophy. The phalanges of a girl aged 12 years with chronic pyelonephritis, and a blood urea which had persisted over 100 mgm/100 ml for 5 years, but was accompanied by only a mild acidosis. Films show the characteristic erosion of the terminal phalanx and the cortical spicules in the middle phalanx. Administration of Vitamin D in large doses resulting in great symptomatic improvement, and radiological healing of the bone lesion

The presence of a urinary obstruction can be recognized by the palpation of a distended bladder or enlarged kidneys: if retention has become acute, urgent drainage is required, but in chronic cases the urine is usually dribbling away and it may be preferable to spend some hours or even a day in resuscitation and control of infection, so that a planned operation may be performed. The type of operation required is discussed elsewhere in this volume, but in the presence

15*

of a very high blood urea and urinary infection, it is wiser to perform pyelostomies or nephrostomies as an emergency measure, rather than to spend time in investigating the site of obstruction. Suprapubic cystostomy is justifiable when the infant's condition permits no more than a "stab" under local anaesthetic; an indwelling urethral catheter may be employed in older children, or rarely in young girls, but in male infants the lumen is seldom adequate to allow free drainage and catheters should only be used for the relief of acute retention. Very severe pyelonephritis or circulatory failure complicating urinary obstruction may lead to oliguria so that the bladder may not be palpably distended, but the obstructive nature of the disorder will become evident if the general condition improves. In calculous disease, and in other upper urinary tract disorders, the obstructive element may only be recognisable from X-rays and retrograde pyelograms, so that doubtful cases must always be subjected to full urological investigation. In the circumstances of chronic renal failure, however, intravenous pyelography is not helpful, and carries a definite risk: it should not be performed when the blood urea is over 100 mgm/100 ml. Ureteric catheterization is also attended by some hazards; sodium iodide should not be used as a contrast medium (diodone or one of the organic compounds is much safer) and the injection should never be made under pressure.

Dehydration is the most important biochemical disturbance of chronic renal failure: it is usually a mixed deficiency of water and salt. Headaches, thirst and weakness are the complaints of the older children, but in infants it must be recognized from the clinical signs, apathy, loss of elasticity in the skin, sunken fontanelle, dry tongue, and sometimes a high temperature.

Electrolyte estimations are of great assistance in choosing the "repair" solution to be used: water is usually the most immediate necessity, but acidosis may demand lactate solution, and a low chloride may indicate the need for saline. In the rare cases of dehydration accompanied by low total electrolyte levels, hypertonic solutions may be required, but should be used with great caution and preferably by intragastric drip. Where possible all fluids should be administered by mouth, and a parenteral route only employed in the very weak or comatose children.

The progress of rehydration must be followed by daily weighing, measurement of urinary output, and at first by daily electrolyte estimations. Calorie requirements should be met by glucose only at first, or the glucose-peanut oil emulsion devised for the treatment of anuria (p. 220) which may be given through an intragastric tube. When the anaemia is severe, small blood transfusions may be required, and are often helpful in assisting the control of chronic urinary infection, but must be used with caution in the presence of high blood urea. Fresh rather than stored blood should be used, as potassium leaves the cells in the stored variety and transfusion may result in an abrupt rise of serum potassium which the damaged kidneys cannot correct.

A sudden rise of serum potassium associated with a rise of blood urea and a fall in chloride may be seen in some infants with chronic renal failure after operation, or at the onset of a generalized infection. It is a temporary phenomenon perhaps associated with increased protein catabolism, and may be corrected by the administration of insulin and glucose.

In long standing cases of renal failure the correction of acidosis carries the risk that because of lowered calcium levels, alkalis may precipitate tetany. Calcium gluconate should therefore be administered at the same time as a sodium citrate mixture.

It has been seen that the bone changes of renal osteodystrophy appear to result primarily from an acquired insensitivity to Vitamin D, and DENT has shown the extraordinary radiological and symptomatic improvement which may be obtained by very large doses of this substance. Moreover, the hypotonic state of the musculature and general weakness which are seen in infants without bone changes are also improved by the same treatment, and are probably due to the same deficiency. Either calciferol or dihydrotachysterol may be employed, and doses may vary between 0.5 mgm and 5.0 mgm daily: these quantities carry a considerable risk of toxic damage to the kidneys and of precipitating metastatic calcification, and must therefore be carefully controlled. Treatment should be started in a unit equipped for metabolic work, and the dose judged from the biochemical response; hypercalcaemia or a strongly positive calcium balance indicates overdosage. In spite of these difficulties satisfactory treatment can lead to healing of the bone lesions, both in the rachitic and the hyperparathyroid types, to restoration of muscle power and to a general well being. Temporary lowering of the blood urea may be seen but no real improvement in renal function is to be expected and ultimately the disease will prove fatal.

III. Renal vascular disorders

1. Bilateral cortical necrosis

Symmetrical cortical necrosis has been reported in a considerable number of infants and children during the past seven years, and although the paper of CAMPBELL and HENDERSON in 1949 was the first to draw attention to the condition in this age group, it is clearly not a very rare lesion. Infants during the first year are most likely to be affected, and in the literature more boys have been reported than girls (LELONG et al.). The etiology of the disease remains obscure, but a severe bacterial infection has been present in the majority of cases, and a toxic effect upon the renal vascular system is postulated. Most authors believe that the vascular shunt mechanism described by TRUETA and his co-workers has some relevance to the problem.

Pathologically the kidneys exhibit a series of small infarcts of the cortex, together with haemorrhagic patches: in severe cases the entire cortex is necrosed and pale yellow in colour, but a rim of intact tissue remains immediately under the capsule. The main blood vessels are patent, and the urinary passages normal. Histologically there appears to be vasostasis in the glomeruli with consequent ischaemic necrosis of the cortical tubules and interstitial tissue. Vascular lesions may also occur in the intestine.

There is no distinctive clinical picture and the diagnosis is very seldom reached before the autopsy. The child is usually, though by no means invariably, suffering from some severe infection, for instance gastro-enteritis, or suppurative arthritis, and the sudden onset of oliguria or anuria is noticed. A small quantity of albuminous urine with a few red cells may be withdrawn by catheter, but nothing more. There is little evidence of pain in the renal area, no oedema or rise of blood pressure. Vomiting and abdominal distension appear later, and as the general condition deteriorates, convulsions occur. The blood urea rises steadily and death usually occurs within 4—5 days of the onset of anuria, though careful treatment may prolong life a little (LELONG et al.).

ZUELZER et al., suggest that mild cases may occur, in which the recovery is possible, but they have not yet been diagnosed. Treatment is simply the management of acute renal failure (p. 219).

2. Venous thrombosis with haemorrhagic infarction

Renal venous thrombosis occurs most frequently in the neonatal period, and at this stage is accompanied by haemorrhagic infarction. The thrombosis usually begins during a period of dehydration associated with toxaemia and severe infections, particularly during gastro-enteritis; it may also complicate previous renal infections and occasionally it occurs in apparently healthy children (the primary type, SANDBLOM).

a) Pathology

The pathological appearance depends upon the extent and stage of the disease: the thrombosis appears to start in the small venous radicles, arcuate and inter-lobular veins, and to spread to the main vessels (MORISON), though a simultaneous

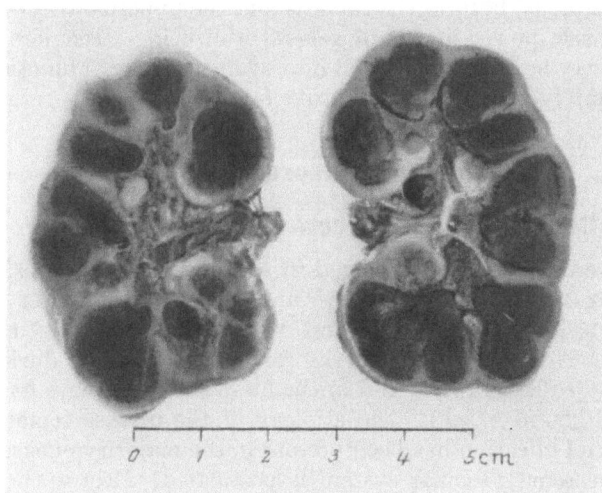

onset over a wide area probably occurs at times. The consequent infarction may be partial or complete, and in acute cases is haemorrhagic so that the kidney structure becomes completely disorganized. In fact it appears that in the most rapidly fatal cases there is extensive haemorrhagic infarction without thrombosis, so that perhaps haemorrhage and thrombosis both result from a common factor: ZUELZER et al. suggest sudden complete venous stasis due to dilatation. In less severe examples there is extensive coagulative necrosis and areas of liquefaction,

Fig. 138. Renal venous thrombosis with haemorrhagic infarction in the new-born. Nephrectomy specimen from a boy aged 3 days with haematuria and a hard enlarged right kidney. The thrombus extended into the inferior vena cava, but the opposite kidney was not involved. The infant died shortly after operation from shock

with haemorrhages chiefly in the medullary zone (Fig. 138). Where local infection precedes or follows infarction, abscess formation will occur. The disease may be bilateral from the onset, and in unilateral cases there is a risk of extension to the opposite kidney. A fatal outcome is to be expected when both kidneys are involved, though a recovery has been recorded by FALLON. Canalization of the thrombus may restore circulation, though atrophy of the kidney perhaps complicated by hypertension is likely. Unilateral cases may be cured by nephrectomy.

b) Clinical features

The clinical picture is variable; where the destructive process is rapid the infant dies soon after its admission to hospital and no diagnosis is made: the severity of the gastro-enteritis and toxaemia diverts attention from the urinary tract, so that no signs relevant to the kidney are observed.

A sudden enlargement of the kidney coinciding with a rapid deterioration of the general condition is characteristic. One or both kidneys may be palpable, they are very firm or even hard, and since the disease is occurring in the neonatal period, lobulated. There may be some evidence of pain in the renal area. The urine is often heavily blood stained for a time, but in extensive bilateral infarction no urine will be secreted. Except in the cases with antecedent infection, the urine passed will only contain a few white cells, with a considerable quantity of albumin.

Intravenous pyelography may be performed in some of the older infants whose general condition permits it: the affected kidney is non-functioning. On retrograde pyelograms, the renal pelvis may not fill at all, or there may be an extensive extravasation of dye throughout the necrotic kidney substance (CAMPBELL and MATTHEWS). Unless this picture is obtained, cases of infarction are very likely to be mistaken for renal tumour or polycystic disease, although the nature of the onset should suggest the correct diagnosis.

c) Treatment

In unilateral cases, where the opposite kidney is normal, urgent nephrectomy is the treatment of choice. The operation in best performed by the trans-abdominal approach so that the extent of thrombosis is the renal vein and inferior vena cava can be clearly visualized, and a thrombus removed from the latter if necessary. The kidney is often friable, and attached to surrounding structures so that tearing is very likely to occur. There is little perinephric fat at this stage to provide a clear plane of separation. Since CAMPBELL and MATTHEW's original case, a number of successful nephrectomies have been reported in unilateral disease.

In bilateral cases, heparin may be administered in the hope of preventing spread of the thrombosis, and the regime recommended for anuria should be adopted. The prognosis is almost but not entirely hopeless.

3. Venous obstruction with thrombosis of inferior vena cava

This form is rare, and more likely to affect older children. Inferior vena cava thrombosis alone will cause oedema of the lower limbs and dilatation of the veins on the abdominal wall: the onset of the thrombosis is seldom recognized, and its effects are insidious in their appearance. When the renal veins are partially occluded, there is often albuminuria and generalized oedema simulating nephrosis; hypertension may also be a feature (PERRY and TAYLOR). The diagnosis by venography is discussed by STEINER. No surgical treatment is advocated at present.

4. Arterial occlusion

Large emboli rarely lodge in the renal arteries but these may be occluded by emboli and thrombosis in the aorta. Most of the recorded cases have been neonates, and the source of the emboli has been the ductus arteriosus or the obliterating umbilical arteries. Death has resulted from anuria (ZUELZER et al., GROSS).

Small septic emboli in bacterial endocarditis produce pyaemic foci in the kidney (p. 150).

Chronic partial obliteration of the arteries causing hypertension is discussed on p. 212.

IV. Polyuria and the renal tubular disorders

The disorders which result in the production of excessively high volumes of urine are not for the most part amenable to surgical treatment, but brief mention of them must be made here as they often enter the differential diagnosis of cases with frequency of micturition and enuresis. Disorders of renal tubular function may also come to the urologist's attention because of pyuria and nephrocalcinosis with stone formation.

Physiological polyuria occurs during "water diuresis" or during "osmotic diuresis". The distal convoluted tubules, under the influence of the pituitary anti-diuretic hormone are responsible for varying the rate of excretion of water and water diuresis occurs when reabsorption ceases at this level, but since the quantity of excreted solute remains unchanged the urine is of low specific gravity. Diabetes insipidus, resulting from a pathological lack of the anti-diuretic hormone, produces a typical water diuresis. Osmotic diuresis occurs when there is an unusually heavy load of osmotically active solute to be excreted: water is retained within the tubules by the presence of this solute and the urine produced must therefore always be hypertonic compared with a plasma ultra-filtrate. Diabetes mellitus provides a classical example of an osmotic diuresis.

The polyuria of total renal failure is not easily explained: PLATT has suggested that because the nephrons are greatly reduced in number, the normal solute load in the functioning survivors produces an osmotic diuresis. However, it is characteristic of renal failure in the young that the urine produced even with a high blood urea is hyposthenuric, with a specific gravity of 1002—1006, well below that of a plasma ultrafiltrate, so that the osmotic process cannot be responsible. EARLEY ascribes this type of hyposthenuria in renal failure to a specific defect of the tubules, comparable to the lesion of "salt-losing nephritis".

From the diagnostic view point, polyuria due to chronic renal failure, or to diabetes mellitus is easily recognized from simple chemical tests: other diseases which may be responsible are briefly listed below.

1. Diabetes insipidus

Deficiency in the production of the anti-diuretic hormone by the posterior lobe of the pituitary results in a failure of reabsorption of water by the loop of Henle and distal convoluted tubule. Very large volumes of urine of low specific gravity (1001—1005) are therefore secreted, and in order to maintain hydration large volumes of fluid must be drunk. Restriction of fluid intake makes little difference to the volume of urine flow, and therefore results in their rapid loss of weight and collapse.

This disorder may be "idiopathic", a form which is usually hereditary (see WARKANY and MITCHELL, FANCONI). Males are affected slightly more often than females, and the first manifestations are usually noticed in the second year of life, they are probably overlooked earlier. Provided hydration is adequate there is no serious interference with health (though a good deal of inconvenience) and the disease is not incompatible with long life.

Diabetes insipidus may also be acquired following direct interference with the pituitary or with the hypothalamus due to fracture of the base of the skull, to tumours and xanthomatosis (Hand-Schuller-Christian syndrome), to encephalitis and syphilis.

In infants thirst is the most noticeable symptom, though it is apt to be mistaken for hunger. If fluids are denied severe dehydration will result. During the following years the child can regulate his own fluid intake, and thirst is easily recognized. Frequency and enuresis are other complaints and with the acquired diseases the onset of enuresis may be the first sign. Headache, irritability, constipation and in infants high fever are common signs of dehydration.

The bladder becomes very large to accomodate the increased volume of urine, and the ureters may show a moderate dilatation, which is reversible if the polyuria is controlled (Fig. 139). The blood urea and electrolyte values are normal except in states of acute dehydration. If fluid is with held for 24 hours, the urine volume continues at a high level, and the specific gravity does not rise above 1005—1007. The child becomes acutely miserable with a raging thirst, the body weight falls

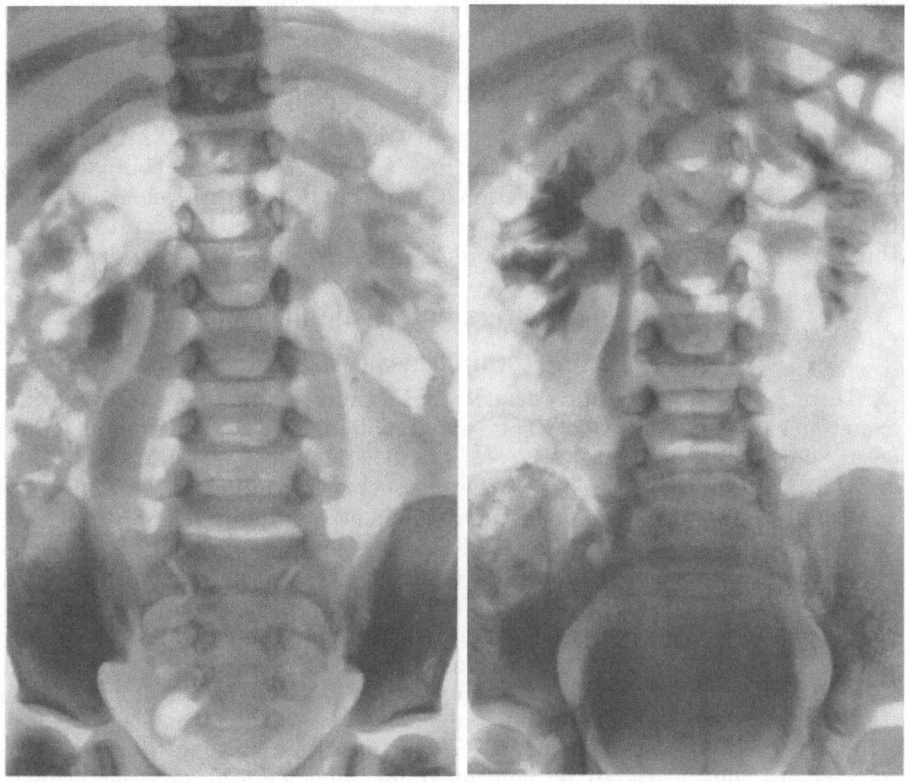

A   B

Fig. 139 A und B. Diabetes insipidus. Intravenous pyelograms in a girl aged 3 years. A During polyuria, showing marked hydroureter. B Under control by pituitrin injections, ureteric calibre much reduced

rapidly, and there may be a rise in blood urea and chlorides. The administration of pitressin (0.5 B.P. units per sq. meter of body surface) will cause a fall in the urine output and a rise in its specific gravity up to normal levels.

The failure to concentrate during dehydration and the rapid response to pitressin usually suffice for diagnosis, and the treatment consists in the therapeutic use of the hormone. Pitressin tannate in oil 0.2—1.0 ml per day by intramuscular injection is a suitable regime, or in some cases pitressin is adequately absorbed from a snuff (e.g. Disipidin) by the nasal mucosa. Control is less precise by the latter method, but in both cases the dosage must be worked out by cautious experiment. Overdose leads to vasopressor effects and abdominal pain.

2. Diabetes insipidus renalis

During the past 10 years it has been recognized that some cases of diabetes insipidus do not respond to pitressin; they are believed to suffer from an abnormality of the renal tubules, which are resistant to the effects of the hormone (KIRMAN et al., DANCIS et al.).

In one of its forms the disease is hereditary, it affects only boys but is transmitted by girls. Unless hydration is fully maintained, the condition is associated with severe mental deficiency. Signs of the disease appear during infancy, usually because of failure to gain, constipation, and episodes of dehydration with fever. Despite dehydration the urine is plentiful and of low specific gravity; the blood urea, sodium and chloride are raised. Good health may be maintained by the provision of large volumes of fluid.

3. Primary polydypsia

Some children suffering from psychological disturbances exhibit a primary polydypsia, and their urine volume and specific gravity is comparable with cases of diabetes insipidus. Restriction of fluid will be met with vehement protests, but the urinary concentration will rise to normal levels. Moderate degrees of thirst may be the result of local disorders of the mouth, such as thrush.

4. Hyperchloraemic renal acidosis

a) Infantile form (Lightwood's syndrome)

This is a temporary disorder of renal tubular function, resulting in the excretion of an alkaline urine, despite a metabolic acidosis. The onset of symptoms occurs most often between the age of 6 and 9 months: constipation, vomiting, anorexia, and failure to thrive are the common complaints. Thirst and polyuria are usually present, though not always commented upon by the parents. In some cases the infant is wasted, dehydrated and febrile. The urine is alkaline except in extreme dehydration and contains a slight excess of pus cells (5—10 per high power field): it is usually but not invariably sterile on culture. The plasma bicarbonate is less than 18 m Eq/litre despite the alkaline urine and the serum chloride is higher than 108 m Eq/litre. The blood urea may be slightly raised (40—80 mg/100 ml) but falls with rehydration. X-rays of the kidney show a stippled medullary calcification in only a few case, though nephrocalcinosis is a constant finding at post-mortem. Treatment with alkalising solutions restores good health, but needs to be continued for some months or even years: the prognosis is excellent provided the initial dehydration and acidosis are overcome. A modified Shohl's solution is suitable (sodium citrate 10 gm, citric acid 6 gm, water 100 ml), and initial doses should be of the order of 15 ml four times a day.

b) Adult form (Albright's syndrome)

The biochemical disturbance is very similar to the infantile form, but is not recoverable. It is probably a congenital disorder, and the symptoms first appear in later childhood or adolescence. Thirst and polyuria are prominent complaints, but it is often the passage of small stones and the discovery of extensive nephrocalcinosis which leads to the biochemical investigation. The state of chronic acidosis produces bone changes, similar to those found in rickets or osteomalacia in adults, but these cases differ from the ordinary renal rickets of azotaemic renal failure in that the blood urea is not seriously raised, and there are no signs of secondary hyperparathyroidism (p. 224). Control of the acidosis by alkalizing mixtures relieves the symptoms and together with Vitamin D leads to an improvement in the bone changes. The nephrocalcinosis remains unchanged except in so far as calcified particles enter the urinary tract and pass out in the form of calculi.

5. Lignac-Fanconi disease (De Toni's syndrome)

This title may be conveniently used to describe a group of disorders in which cystine storage, glycosuria, amino-aciduria and Vitamin D resistant rickets are found: there are many variations or perhaps more than one disease (BICKEL et al., McCUNE et al., LIGNAC, FANCONI). The disorder is congenital but its mechanism remains unexplained; there appears to be a renal tubular defect, but this would not account for the wide-spread deposition of cystine crystals throughout the body, and clearly some more generalized disorder of metabolism is present. Although cystine is one of the amino-acids lost in the urine, there appears to be no relation to the cystinuria which commonly results in stone formation (p. 165). Cystine storage may be found without the other features of the Fanconi syndrome, and may then have a better prognosis.

In more acute forms, failure to thrive, thirst and polyuria, anorexia and constipation are noted from the age of six months onwards. More chronic cases present in childhood with dwarfism and bone changes which are radiologically indistinguishable from Vitamin D deficiency rickets. The ultimate prognosis is bad and many of the children die before reaching puberty. Examination shows an undersized, often wasted and dehydrated child; the urine is usually alkaline, and contains albumin, glucose and a wide range of amino-acids, including cystine. A mild degree of pyuria may be present without infection. Biochemical investigation shows a metabolic acidosis, and in the early stages a normal blood urea and lowered phosphorus. Potassium deficiencies may occur, and in the terminal stages of the disease there is a retention of phosphate and urea. The presence of cystine storage may be recognized by the observation of cystine crystals in the cornea by slit lamp microscopy. Stone formation is unlikely to occur in the urinary tract, though microscopic cystine calculi have been found.

Treatment consists in the correction of acidosis, provision of adequate potassium and Vitamin D in large doses to heal the bone lesions.

6. Idiopathic hypercalcaemia

This recently recognized (LIGHTWOOD; FANCONI et. al.) but not uncommon disorder of infants may come to the attention of the urologist because of a raised blood urea. It appears to exist in a mild and in a severe form: in the former the infant presents with failure to thrive, thirst, constipation and hypotonia. Urine examination may show slight pyuria. The serum calcium is between 12—14 mgm/100 ml, and in some cases the blood urea may be up to 100 mgm/100 ml, often associated with hypertension. In the severe form there are multiple deformities, osteosclerosis, mental retardation, hypercholesterolaemia, with a characteristic facies (SCHLESINGER et al.).

The mild form of the disease, which is recoverable, may perhaps represent a hypersensitivity to Vitamin D, though some authors dispute this theory. Treatment consists in a low calcium diet, and the use of cortisone to reduce the blood calcium.

V. Haematuria and nephritis

1. General considerations

In a work of this nature, it is scarcely necessary to emphasize the importance of haematuria as a symptom of surgical disease of the urinary tract and it is unlikely that the urologist will be content with anything short of a full investigation. Nevertheless, because neoplasms are comparatively rare in childhood and are easily diagnosed, while nephritis and unexplained haematuria are common, the observation of blood in the urine has a different significance in the young and in the old. It becomes clear that although a thorough investigation is required in all unexplained cases, the urological procedures need not be repeated in the child as they might be in the adult; the anxiety generated by numerous visits to hospital and continued observation of urine specimens is liable to disturb the child's emotional equilibrium without benefiting his physical condition.

Faced with a case of supposed haematuria, it is first essential to confirm that the urinary discolouration is due to blood, and that the blood is mixed with the urine, not derived from some external source. The pigment of beetroot and certain synthetic dyes used in the manufacture of sweets may colour the urine red, but to the practised eye the tint is easily distinguishable from blood pigment and further investigation is unnecessary. Urates and porphyrins may render the urine brown, and are occasionally mistaken for blood pigments. Haemoglobinuria can only be distinguished from haematuria by microscopy, which must be undertaken as a routine in suspected cases.

External bleeding, which may lead to confusion, derives from the vagina or urethra. A meatal ulcer is a common source of haemorrhage in infancy, and since the napkin is stained with blood, the symptom is often described as haematuria. Clinical examination will at once reveal the nature of the lesion. Urethral bleeding, sometimes with slight discharge of pus, is seen in boys from time to time. It may be due to the introduction of foreign bodies, but I have seen several for which no explanation could be given — all have ultimately recovered. Uterine haemorrhage in the intersex cases with occult vagina may present as urethral haemorrhage.

2. Surgical causes of haematuria

Almost all the renal diseases described in this volume are capable of producing haematuria, and no attempt will be made to set out all possible causes.

The possibility of malignant disease is naturally uppermost in the urologist's mind and a high proportion of nephroblastomata (p. 180) present with haematuria as the first symptom; they are rapidly growing tumours, however, and are almost always large enough to be palpated; they are certainly large enough to produce an unmistakable pyelographic deformity. Vesical and prostatic neoplasms (p. 197) cause retention rather than haematuria, which comes only as a complication of infection. Calculi (p. 162) are a frequent cause of bleeding, which may precede any other symptom; in urinary infection of all types, haematuria is usually accompanied by frequency. Tuberculosis of the urinary tract (p. 156) is very rare, but must be borne in mind during investigation of these cases. Hydronephrosis and hydro-ureter occasionally cause haematuria even when uncomplicated. Renal vascular disorders are naturally associated with bleeding: venous thrombosis with haemorrhagic infarction (p. 230) is of importance to the surgeon because unilateral cases may be successfully treated by nephrectomy. Renal haemangiomata (p. 187) are exceptionally rare and should not be diagnosed without definite pyelographic evidence.

Trauma to the kidney, often the result of a blow in the loin, is an important cause of bleeding: so too are foreign bodies introduced into the bladder or reaching the ureters by perforating the duodenum.

3. Haemorrhagic diseases

Haematuria may occur as a manifestation of a bleeding tendency in any generalized disease which affects the blood vessels or the mechanism of coagulation.

In many of these it is relatively an unimportant symptom and other manifestations will leave little doubt as to the nature of the disorder. Thus in haemorrhagic disease of the new-born, and in the thrombocytopenia which accompanies septicaemia, bleeding may occur from the urinary tract as from other mucous surfaces; microscopic haematuria is a regular feature of infantile scurvy and of bacterial endocarditis. At times, however, haematuria may be the presenting sign of such conditions as haemophilia, leukaemia, aplastic anaemia or thrombocytopenic purpura, and a haemotological investigation is therefore required in every case where no obvious local cause is discernible. In the anaphylactoid purpuras, haematuria may accompany or precede the manifestations in skin, joints, or intestine, and the diagnosis of these conditions is essentially clinical, laboratory tests being of little assistance. In all these generalized diseases, cystoscopy will show a bloody ureteric efflux on both sides, an observation which may help in excluding a local surgical cause for bleeding.

4. Nephritis

Haematuria is a prominent symptom of acute glomerulonephritis (ELLIS type I), it may also occur in the chronic phase particularly if there is a complicating hypertension, but is rare in the nephrotic type (ELLIS type II). In acute cases the bleeding may be brisk but the urine is a brownish red and it is unusual for clots to be found. Every specimen passed is evenly blood-stained for a few days and microscopic haematuria continues for days or weeks after the urine has cleared to naked eye examination. In the typical case, haematuria follows three weeks after an acute upper respiratory infection, and is accompanied by peri-orbital oedema, albuminuria, oliguria, hypertension and a raised blood urea. Where all these signs are present little doubt need be felt as to the diagnosis, but many milder examples are seen and in some the bleeding is the only unequivocal sign. The great majority of all acute cases (about 85%) clear up altogether and have no further symptoms: a few suffer recurrent acute episodes following sore throats, and some enter a chronic phase with persistent microscopic haematuria and albuminuria, later developing hypertension and renal failure. A few die during the acute phase with hypertensive encephalopathy, cardiac failure or uraemia. Many authors (e.g. FISHBERG) separate as a distinct clinical entity "focal nephritis", in which the haematuria is co-incident with the respiratory infection, is of short duration and never leads to chronic nephritic changes. The pathological evidence for such a disease has never been satisfactory and PAYNE and ILLINGWORTH, reviewing a series of cases at Great Ormond Street, reached the conclusion that no difference in prognosis existed between cases in which haematuria coincided with or followed the infection; furthermore that haematuria unaccompanied by oedema or by nitrogen retention might sometimes be followed by the changes of chronic nephritis.

The presence of granular casts in the urine supports the diagnosis of glomerulonephritis. Albumin is usually excreted in greater quantities in nephritis than in surgical lesions, but here again there is no clear cut distinction. It will be seen therefore that the diagnosis of glomerulo-nephritis as a cause of haematuria is based upon a variety of observations, most of them clinical, and none pathognomonic: should gross haematuria persist, it will be wise to have an intravenous pyelogram to exclude a surgical lesion.

5. Medicational haematuria

Until the introduction of sulphonamides excreted in soluble form, these drugs were a potent cause of haematuria during the treatment of any infection in children: an overdose or a restricted fluid intake was frequently responsible. Haematuria was accompanied by oliguria and might precede anuria with acute tubular necrosis. Sulphonamide crystals and epithelial debris could be found in the urine. Many other drugs have produced toxic renal damage at times, with haematuria and oliguria.

6. Unexplained haematuria

However careful the investigations, in a considerable proportion of children with haematuria no firm diagnosis can be made. Where the bleeding has occurred on only one occasion, it causes little concern: often the label acute glomerulo-nephritis is applied to the case, although this is probably unjustifiable unless microscopic haematuria persists for some days.

In other children attacks of haematuria are persistent, but usually unaccompanied by any other symptom. In one group of these cases, the bleeding follows any violent exercise, and ceases immediately the child is put to bed. The blood is apparently derived from both kidneys in these cases, as has been observed on cystoscopy, but no local pyelographic lesions are detectable. This type of haematuria may persist for years, though the violence of the exercise required to produce it varies from time to time. Blood loss is not sufficient to render the child anaemic, and ultimately the symptom appears to cease spontaneously.

In some children, bouts of haematuria seem to have an allergic basis; in one of my cases they were associated with asthma. Haematuria has occurred after serum injection, and as a response to various ingested substances (including beer!). Oxaluria may cause a little bleeding.

The initial investigation of haematuria must be thorough and exhaustive; when doubt exists pyelograms may be repeated. Nevertheless, the prognosis of unexplained haematuria in children is good and more harm may be caused by repetition of diagnostic urological procedures than by loss of blood. Too often these children are referred from one hospital to another, and are subjected to the full routine at each. The parents anxiously inspect every specimen of urine and demand some active treatment. It need hardly be emphasized, however, that bleeding is almost always bilateral in these unexplained cases, and the observation of a unilateral bloody efflux on one or two occasions should not beguile the surgeon into the belief that a nephrectomy will cure the condition: unexplained haematuria from a solitary remaining kidney is even more productive of anxiety than haematuria from two kidneys.

N. The male genital tract

I. Congenital abnormalities of the penis

The common anomalies of penile development are those in which the urethra is primarily at fault, e.g. hypospadias, ectopia vesicae, which have already been discussed. There are, however, a number of rare deformities of the penis which present during childhood.

1. Micropenis

A penis of normal size may be so completely concealed by the suprapubic fat during the first year of life, that the child's parents become seriously, though unnecessarily, perturbed about its size. A true congenital "micropenis" is an uncommon finding but easily recognizable when the infant fat is lost (Fig. 140). It may occur without any other genital malformation and growth will then be observed at puberty, but a full size is never attained, and considerable difficulty may be encountered in coitus: I have observed the condition in three generations in one family, however, so that diminutive proportions do not constitute a complete bar to procreation. The small penis with hypospadias is discussed on p. 105.

The penis in hypogonadism may fail to grow at puberty, and therefore retain the childish proportions: in these circumstances, however, growth may be stimulated by the administration of appropriate hormones (see p. 289).

2. Congenital absence of the penis

The penis may be entirely absent although the testicles are fully descended into a bifid scrotum: the urethra then opens in the perineum or the rectum. Cases have been reported by CAMPBELL, RUKSTINAT and HASTERLIK, BERARDINELLI, DRURY and SHWARZELL, and STOLL. A case of mine is illustrated in Fig. 141: in

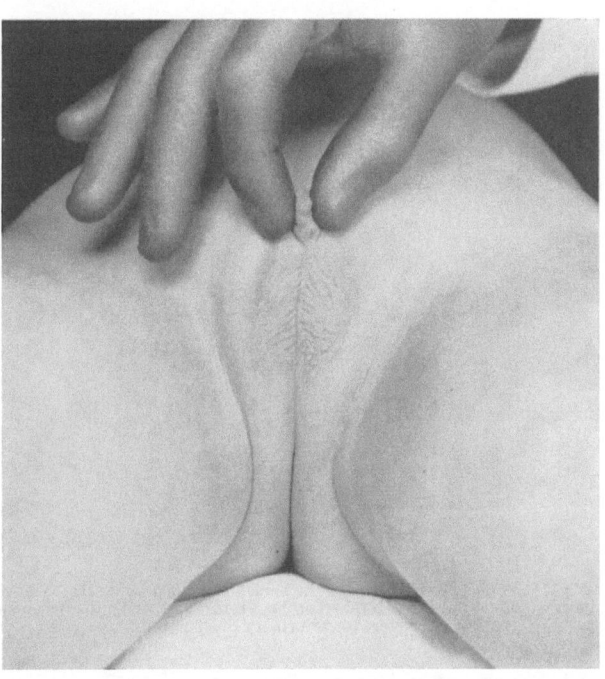

Fig. 140. Micropenis. The external genitalia of a boy aged 9 years: the penis is minute and the terminal urethra narrow. Both testicles were palpable and could be brought into the scrotum

this, as in other examples, minute corpora cavernosa could be palpated beneath the flat strip of skin separating the two halves of the scrotum. This deformity was associated with severe urethral stenosis, and bilateral hydronephrosis.

The methods of repair have been discussed by GILLIES.

3. Diphallus

Double penis is a rare condition, and frequently associated with other deformities. There may be a double bladder, each part drained through a separate urethra and penis, as in the child reported by NESBIT and BROMME, or one penis may serve a urinary and the other a genital function. One penis may possess no urethra (DONALD) or there may be an associated hypospadias; COCHRANE and SAUNDERS report a case with imperforate anus. In DAVIS' case there were three or four structures which may have represented penises. An association with ectopia vesicae is often reported, but a distinction must be made between the true double penis, and the separated halves which are common in epispadias. In the case reported by KIRSCH the pubic bones were widely separated, but there was no ectopia vesicae; a urethra in each penis led into a loculated bladder.

Treatment must depend upon the precise anatomy and no rules can be laid down.

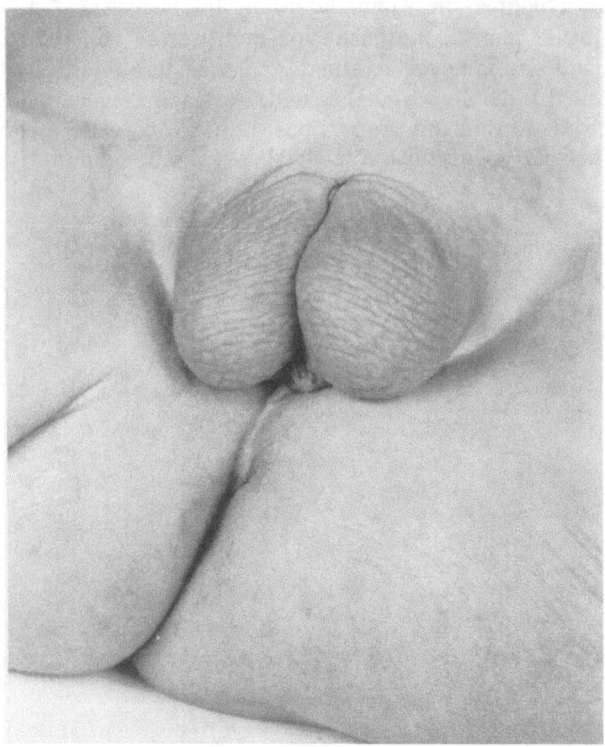

Fig. 141. Congenital absence of the penis. Boy aged 9 months. Testicles normally descended into bifid scrotum. Urethral meatus in the perineum. Severe lower urinary obstruction

Double clitoris may also occur and, in a girl treated by the author, was associated with intractable incontinence.

4. Pre-penile scrotum

In a case reported by CAMPBELL, the penis, containing a normal urethra, hung from the perineum behind the scrotum: no other abnormality was present, and by splitting the scrotum it was possible to restore a semblance of normality. In the examples recorded by FRANCIS and by HUFFMAN there were other fatal deformities, the urinary tract being absent in one. In FORSHALL and RICKHAM'S case an extreme degree of chordee with hypospadias brought the penis down to the perineum.

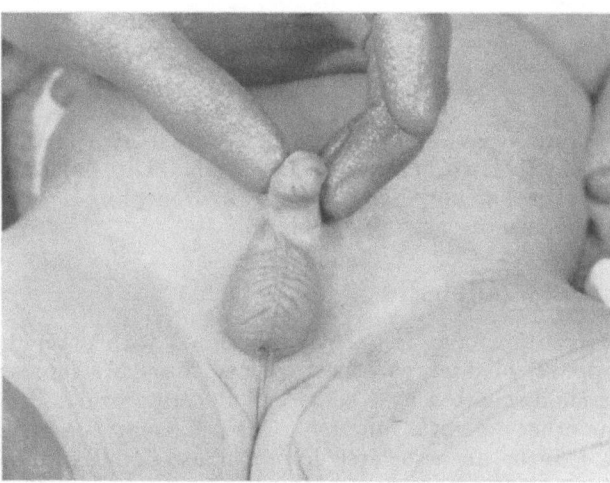

Fig. 142. Torsion of the penis. The genitalia of a boy aged 2 years. The penis exhibits a 90° twist to the left. the corpora cavernosa as well as the urethra being involved. There is also a coronal hypospadias with slight chordee

5. Torsion of the penis

In this deformity the penis appears to be rotated upon its long axis through 90—180°; the median raphe, urethra, and corpora cavernosa all taking part in the spiral. The deformity is probably not so rare as the sparsity of information in the literature would suggest, I have observed it on five occasions (Fig. 142), but other severe malformations are likely to be present, and no satisfactory treatment has been described. Simple torsion is not, however, a severe handicap, and does not preclude satisfactory sexual activity (SCHWART and FARR). The temptation to operate should be resisted.

6. Webbing of the penis

Although usually due to hypospadias or short urethra (p. 107) a state of chordee may be maintained by a web of skin fixing the penis down to the scrotum. The normal anatomy may be restored by a carefully planned plastic operation, though the local shortage of skin may be an embarrassment.

7. Cysts of the penile raphe

Partial canalization of the median raphe of the penis and scrotum may be seen, particularly in association with anal atresia. The simple formation of cysts in the preputial raphe of infants is recorded by OTTOW.

II. Phimosis and paraphimosis

1. The normal development

The preputial sac, the cavity separating the prepuce from the glans, is formed during foetal life by the splitting of a solid lamella of cells. This process is not always complete at birth, and congenital preputial adhesions are therefore present. Furthermore the prepuce of the new born infant is normally elongated and redundant; its orifice appears narrow, and this together with the adhesions may prevent retraction. In the normal course of development the redundancy is taken up, the orifice widens and the adhesions resolve during the first six to nine months of life, and retraction then becomes possible. Gentle stretching and separation of the adhesions with a probe may hasten this development and reassure the parents of the normality of the genitalia, but spontaneous freeing of the prepuce will occur in the vast majority of children.

2. Phimosis

Phimosis, stenosis of the preputial orifice, may be congenital or acquired. The congenital form is uncommon, and unless of extreme degree, is difficult to diagnose during the first months of life, when the prepuce is not normally retractile. The acquired form when seen in children usually results from the scarring following forcible stretching of the orifice, or from badly performed circumcision. Phimosis and, to a less extent, redundant prepuce may be responsible for the accumulation of smegma within the preputial sac, and consequent attacks of balano-posthitis. This form of inflammation, which commences within the preputial sac, must be distinguished from the effects of ammonia dermatitis, in which the external surface is primarily affected (see below). During the acute phase of balano-posthitis retraction of the foreskin may be impossible because of oedema, later it is sometimes accomplished without difficulty so that separation of adhesions and regular cleansing is all that is required to prevent recurrence. If, however, a tight phimosis is present circumcision should be performed.

Phimosis is on rare occasions responsible for urinary obstruction; the urine enters and distends the preputial sac with each act of micturition, only escaping in a slow dribble. The obstruction may be rendered more acute by inflammatory ulceration of the prepuce, and a sealing off of the orifice by scab formation: if in such cases the urine is infected, the infant may become seriously ill, and fatal results are on record (CAMPBELL) but circumcision is a sufficient cure for the majority. When ballooning of the prepuce occurs repeatedly over a long period, without acute obstruction, preputial calculi may be formed.

3. Paraphimosis

When the phimotic prepuce is forcibly drawn back behind the corona, and allowed to remain in the retracted position, oedema fluid rapidly accumulates in the loose tissues, and replacement is thereby prevented (paraphimosis). The swelling in the retracted prepuce may reach enormous proportions, and interference with the circulation may ultimately lead to skin necrosis. However, in small boys reduction can usually be achieved by firm pressure: if necessary the oedema can be lessened by the applications of a swab soaked in cocaine 10% with adrenaline (1 in 1,000) or by the injection of hyalase, and if all other measures fail the constriction ring can be released by incision. Circumcision should be performed after the tissue reaction has settled down.

4. Routine circumcision

The advisability of routine circumcision in infancy is a subject which has been hotly disputed by the medical profession, and for many years past the weekly medical journals of all countries have regularly published articles and letters, many of them written under the influence of powerful emotion, demanding on the one hand a wholesale removal of every foreskin, or on the other, a complete abandonment of the ancient operation. The disadvantages of circumcision are seen chiefly in childhood, its advantages in adult life, and as a result paediatricians are for the most part inflexibly opposed to it, while venerologists are keen advocates. Religious beliefs and traditions have an important bearing on the subject, and parents are themselves apt to hold strong views: men who have suffered from recurrent preputial inflammation, often in hot and dusty climates, not infrequently demand that their children should be spared that handicap even when the infant's prepuce appears normal, while in Scandinavian countries where circumcision is seldom performed, they may be reluctant to accept the operation despite a clear indication.

Routine circumcision in infancy undoubtedly protects the child against the complications of phimosis and balanitis, and protects the man against the considerably more unpleasent consequences of the same disorders after sexual life has begun. It gives a substantial measure of protection against the development of carcinoma of the penis, and removes much of the discomfort from such lesser disorders as penile herpes, penile warts and balanitis xerotica obliterans. It is true that most of the disadvantages inherent in the possession of a foreskin are seen in those men who are either unable or unwilling to retract it in order to maintain cleanliness, yet a few whose standard of hygiene is beyond criticism suffer from irritating recurrent attacks of preputial inflammation which ultimately result in scarring and phimosis.

The dangers of infantile circumcision result chiefly from poor operative technique and from meatal ulceration. The operation is often regarded as so simple that it can safely be left to the least skilled member of the surgical team, who has received no adequate instruction in its performance, and who, now that circumcision is losing its popularity, gets very little practice. Operative technique is discussed in another volume in this series, but the chief hazards may be mentioned here. Haemostasis may be inadequate because of an unwillingness to recognize the occasional need for ligatures in infancy. Too much skin may be removed so that the penis is pulled back against the abdominal wall; too little skin may be taken away in the frenal area leaving an untidy redundancy. Too much mucosa may be left so that the suture line, instead of being held back behind the glans, can slip forward, and with contraction will reconstitute a tight phimosis.

A deep suture may be placed in the frenal area which includes a portion of the urethral wall, and results in an obstinate fistula at the level of the coronal sulcus. These complications are commonly observed, and there are, of course, other rarer but more serious consequences of operative carelessness.

Meatal ulcer is discussed in a subsequent section: it results from exposure of the glans to the action of ammonia derived from the decomposition of urine entrapped within the napkins. It is a cause of much misery to small boys, but can be avoided by proper care.

In addition to the clinically apparent disadvantages of circumcision, it is sometimes claimed that the satisfaction derived from sexual intercourse is thereby diminished. No scientific observations upon this point have yet been published, but there does not appear to have been any serious falling off in the birth-rate of those races who always circumcise their infants.

These then are the advantages and disadvantages of routine circumcision; there can be no doubt as to its value in cases of phimosis, but unfortunately it is hard to be sure, in the infant whose prepuce is not normally retractile, whether phimosis is present or not. If operation is postponed until the age of one year, it will be found to be necessary in very few children, but performed at that age it is considerably more trouble to those who require it. The conclusion drawn from the facts presented will doubtless vary according to the prejudices of the reader: my view is that in Northern Europe routine circumcision of all infants is not justified on clinical grounds, but that periodic medical inspection with a view to early recognition of phimosis is desirable.

III. Skin lesions

Very few children pass through the first two years of their life without exhibiting, at some time, the signs of ammonia dermatitis or "napkin rash". The disorder usually appears after the first six months, and is apt to continue with remissions and relapses until urinary control is finally established. It is much more common in bottle fed than in breast fed babies, and its onset may be associated with the introduction of mixed feeding; periodic exacerbations (ammoniacal storms, HAMILTON and MIDDLETON) are common and are frequently attributed to teething.

The rash occurs on the prepuce, the scrotum, the inner aspects of the thighs, lower abdomen and buttocks, but spares the flexures. In its mildest degree, it is a bright red erythema; continuing, it causes the skin to be thickened and scaly, with the later appearance of vesicles. Secondary infection, usually seen in the older children with urinary incontinence, leads to the formation of many superficial ulcers. The appearance and distribution of the rash are so characteristic that diagnosis seldom presents any difficulty, but several other rashes appear in the napkin area. The buttocks may be excoriated in infants with loose stools, producing a septic peri-anal rash which may accompany, but is distinct from, ammonia dermatitis. Thrush napkin rashes affect the buttocks and genitalia, and have been found in young infants in association with maternal vaginal moniliasis. Thrush is characterised by dull red areas, and vesicles producing small ulcers surrounded by white collars of sodden epithelium. Intertrigo may be seen in the flexures, and in rare cases the napkin area may be affected by seborrhoeic dermatitis, and congenital syphilitic rashes.

The prepuce is often severely inflamed in cases of ammonia dermatitis, it is reddened, oedematous and elongated; in this state retraction is difficult and immediate circumcision is often advised by the unwary. Exposure of the glans to the effects of ammonia, however, leads to a more serious lesion, meatal ulcer, and circumcision should be avoided in these circumstances, for proper management will soon reduce the inflammation.

The role of ammonia in the production of the dermatitis was established by ZAHORSKY, by BRENNEMAN, and by COOKE. The last named showed that the ammonia was liberated from the urinary urea by bacterial action and identified a gram negative bacillus (B. ammoniagenes) commonly found in the infant's colon as the chief offender. There can be no doubt that the chemical action of the alkalis in the napkins can also lead to the breakdown of urea even where sterility is maintained.

The ammoniacal napkin must be in contact with the skin for some hours to produce the dermatitis, but the process is greatly accelerated when water-proof rubber or plastic pants are also used. By contrast, in warm climates, where little is worn outside the napkin, dermatitis is unlikely to be severe.

The cure of ammonia dermatitis is simple, but demands continuous care from the infant's mother. Napkins must be changed frequently and the child should not be left all night in the same sodden covering. The use of rubber pants should be confined to important social occasions, and they should not, on any account, be worn at night. In severe cases the napkin should not be wrapped around the child at all during sleep, but spread out beneath him. The napkins must be carefully washed and rinsed free of alkaline soaps before being dried. A talcum powder containing 5% of boric acid should be applied liberally to the genitalia, and to the interior of the napkin at each changing. These measures will relieve the vast majority of cases though if there is a superadded infection, the use of acriflavine (1 in 1000 aqueous solution) may be a valuable adjunct. During recent years, however, there has been a tendency to seek other methods of treatment, because of the supposed danger of boric acid poisoning following the liberal use of that substance on the inflamed surface (GOLDBLOOM and GOLDBLOOM). FISHER et al., also JOHNSON et al., have demonstrated, however, that the fatal cases followed the use of pure boric acid in place of a talcum powder containing only 5%, and that the usual powders are entirely harmless. Pure boric acid crystals have often been given to parents so that napkins can be soaked in a boric acid solution after washing: in view of the possible misuse of the crystals, this practice is inadvisable, and the efficacy of the 5% boric acid powder renders it unnecessary.

Other methods of treatment have included the use of barrier cream (e.g. Drapolene) and the soaking of napkins in antiseptics (e.g. Roccal) in order to prevent the bacterial decomposition of urea.

IV. Meatal ulcer and stenosis

Meatal ulcer is a very common affliction of boys from the age of 8 or 10 months onwards, until they achieve normal urinary control: it is the result of ammonia "burning" of the epithelium of the glans, and is therefore usually found in association with ammonia dermatitis affecting the scrotum and thighs. Only circumcised children are commonly affected by meatal ulcer, since only in them is the glans continually exposed: on rare occasions, a small raw ulcer is seen in an enuretic child with a long foreskin. The ulcer is a reddened area, 2—3 mm across, situated anywhere on the glans, but usually on the meatal margin: it is frequently covered by a grey, papery scab which also seals off the urinary meatus. The presence of the ulcer causes acute pain on micturition, and sometimes slight bleeding as the scab is torn away by the stream of urine; the pain or the fear of pain may be sufficient to cause retention in some children, though usually the urine will be passed soon after they have fallen asleep. While active ulceration is present, the meatus will be narrowed by the inflammatory swelling of its lips; later on, if the condition has been persistent there may be cicatrical stenosis leaving a narrow circular meatus surrounded by radiating scars. Some urologists have claimed that congenital meatal stenosis predisposes to ulcer formation (CAMPBELL, FREUD) and that meatotomy is curative. This view is not in accord-dance with my experience; simple measures are almost always sufficient to cure the ulcer, and meatotomy is scarcely ever required except in cases of very long standing (see also ABESHOUSE and BOGORAD).

The therapeutic measures are essentially those already described for ammonia dermatitis; in addition, a little boric ointment should be applied to the glans when the napkins are changed, and if there is severe pain preventing micturition, it can be relieved by soaking in a warm bath.

Congenital meatal stenosis, although not as common as the sequel to meatal ulceration, is an occasional cause of difficult micturition. The meatus instead of being a longitudinal slit is a circular "pin-hole". Treatment by dilatation is seldom adequate and a meatotomy should be performed. Meatal stenosis may complicate coronal hypospadias (p. 104).

V. Genital tract infections

1. Urethritis

The term posterior urethritis is sometimes applied to changes in the mucosa of the prostatic urethra (roughened and reddened areas with "hillocks" and polyp formation), which are occasionally found in children with sterile urine suffering from enuresis, frequency or slight dysuria. The significance of these lesions is discussed in Section F; the present section is only concerned with urethritis associated with urethral discharge.

Gonococcal urethritis in boys, though admittedly rarer than vulvo-vaginitis in girls, has been regarded by some writers (e.g. CAMPBELL) as relatively common disease, and BEILIN, writing from Chicago in 1931 reported that he had personally observed 91 cases of gonorrhoea in pre-pubertal boys. The infection is almost always acquired during a sexual encounter; sometimes a precocious boy will attempt intercourse with a girl his own age, while on other occasions the child may be "seduced" by an infected nursemaid in whose care he has been placed. At boarding schools for older children, epidemics of gonorrhoea are usually the result of homosexual practices, and are associated with proctitis as well as urethritis (WESTPHAL). The disease follows its usual course and, though complications are said to be uncommon, a gonococcal prostatic abscess has been recorded in a boy aged four years (FOX). With the declining incidence of gonorrhoea in general, urethritis due to this cause in boys has become very rare. Treatment should follow the customary lines.

Urethritis, together with inflammation of other mucous surfaces occurs in the STEVENS-JOHNSON syndrome: an acute febrile illness accompanied by severe erythema multiforme. It is self-limiting. Very rarely, urethritis complicates measles.

Abacterial urethritis is one of the manifestations of Reiter's syndrome, in which conjunctivitis and arthritis also occur. The syndrome is common in adults, but has only been reported on rare occasions in childhood: it may follow dysenteric infection with Shiga or Flexner organisms, or a venereal infection causing abacterial urethritis. The former is the common cause in childhood, though there may be a few signs of dysentery other than a raised titre of the corresponding antibodies (CORNER). The urethritis may cause only a slight discharge, but frequency and pyuria are common. The disease is fully described by HARKNESS; treatment with antibiotics is usually effective, though the arthritis may be persistent, and at times disabling. The use of cortisone in the treatment of joint lesions is discussed by HENCKEL.

Urethritis of a mild degree may follow the introduction of foreign bodies into the urethra during masturbation. In one of my cases the diagnosis was, at first, suspected as a result of the urethroscopic finding of a traumatized area on the floor of the urethral bulb. At other times, the foreign body is found in the bladder. An indwelling catheter is another possible cause of urethritis with resulting urethral stricture.

Sulphonamides, particularly sulphamerazine, occasionally irritate the urethral mucosa (HARKNESS) and have even been responsible for stricturing in a case observed by the author: sulphonamide obstruction to the urinary passages is partly the result of inflammation of the mucosa.

Urethritis and inflammation of the glans may be due to diphtheria, which has been reported on several occasions after ritual circumcision (BOROVSKY). A characteristic diphtheritic membrane is found, and the organisms are easily recovered from the lesion. Treatment with antiserum is effective.

Acquired genital syphilis is reported from time time in young boys (e.g. McKAY) and is responsible for typical chancre formation.

2. Prostatitis and prostatic abscess

The symptoms of acute non-suppurative prostatitis: frequency, dysuria, perineal pain, terminal haematuria and pyrexia are similar to those of cystitis, and estimates of the incidence of true prostatitis in boys vary greatly. The present writer has observed the condition, but believes it to be a rare phenomenon before puberty, while on the other hand CAMPBELL regards it as relatively common. There is a similar divergence of opinion in regard to chronic prostatitis with congestive inflammation but little evidence of bacterial invasion: CAMPBELL believes this to be a common result of habitual excessive masturbation, and a cause of sclerosis of the bladder neck which will produce urinary obstruction in adult life.

By contrast prostatic abscess is a disorder in which there can be little doubt as to the diagnosis, and all observers agree that it is rare, but can occur at a very early age. Gonorrhoea has been responsible for some cases (FOX) but in an infant of 1 month old, treated at the Hospital for Sick Children, there was a large staphylococcal abscess causing retention of urine, constipation, and bilateral epididymitis. The infection in this case was believed to have originated in umbilical sepsis, and to have been blood-borne. In another infant, however, there was a large infected haematoma, immediately lateral to, and behind the prostate gland, also causing acute retention of urine, and it is suggested that descending arteritis in the umbilical artery could be responsible for this extravasation of blood in the perivesical space. Both cases recovered with perineal drainage and chemotherapy.

3. Epididymitis

Acute epididymo-orchitis may complicate inflammatory disease of the lower urinary tract, particularly infections following surgical operation for urethral obstructions. In the pre-sulphonamide era it was also occasionally seen after simple urethral instrumentation.

Non-specific epididymitis may occur in older children in the absence of urinary infection, and though it is much less common than in adults, QVIST reported 12 cases between the ages of 3 months and 12 years which were all confirmed by exploration. So-called metastatic epididymitis, complicating distant infections has been recorded in neonates by GARROW and WERNE, and by LOMBARD. In one of my cases, acute epididymitis was the presenting symptom in a boy aged 2 years with an ectopic ureter which joined the vas deferens before entering the posterior urethra.

In the acute forms, and especially in inguinal testicles, epididymo-orchitis may be impossible to distinguish from torsion of the testis, though an accompanying urinary infection may lead to the correct diagnosis. In doubtful cases, exploration is fully justified, since no chance of correcting a torsion should be lost. In less acute disorders, the swelling of the epididymis is palpable behind a normal testis, and the clinical diagnosis presents no difficulty. Treatment consists in the administration of appropriate antibiotics, and if necessary drainage of an abscess cavity: epididymectomy should not be required now that powerful antibacterial agents are available.

Tuberculous epididymitis is discussed on p. 161.

4. Orchitis

Simple inflammatory lesions of the testis are very unusual: mumps orchitis is chiefly a disorder of adolescents and young adults, and seldom affects children. CONNOLLY, however, has recorded two cases in infancy where the diagnosis was made on serological grounds, though a known mumps contact was found in only one. Rarely the epididymis and cord are also involved during mumps orchitis. Subsequent testicular atrophy is likely, but not inevitable: local treatment is not commonly required, though oestrogens or if necessary incision of the tunica albuginea will relieve severe pain, and possibly preserve the spermatic tubules.

Orchitis as a complication of chicken-pox is described by ORMISTON.

Congenital syphilis is a rare cause of orchitis, and an exceptionally rare cause of symptoms (NABARRO). MENNINGER reported 12 post-mortem cases, in which bilateral testicular atrophy was found. Hydrocele has been attributed to syphilitic orchitis in some instances, but gumma formation is extremely uncommon.

VI. Urethral injuries, stricture and fistula

Injuries to the urethra and penis, although not uncommon in children, differ very little from those seen in adults, and for a full discussion the reader is referred to volume VII of this series.

1. Anterior urethral injuries

Injury of the penile urethra may be seen as a result of compression by rings or ligatures tied around the penis, often placed there during naive attempts to cure enuresis. In severe cases there may be gangrene of the entire distal penis, but more often the ligature can be released in time, leaving only some necrosis of the tissues beneath it. This necrosis can lead to the development of an obstinate stricture and to a fistula.

Rupture of the bulb of the urethra is most often due to falls astride sharp objects: the child is brought in with a perineal haematoma and some dysuria or retention. If a catheter can be passed, the rupture is incomplete and surgical repair is not required though, save in the most minor cases, a suprapubic diversion of urine during the period of healing is desirable. If the catheter is held up at the point of rupture, the severed ends should be exposed and sutured together. In cases when there is any tension on the suture line, it is wiser only to reconstitute the dorsal wall of the urethra, and allow the healing process to complete the channel.

2. Posterior urethral injuries

Rupture of the membranous urethra is seen in association with fractures of the pelvis: where there is a complete solution of continuity the apex of the prostate will be displaced upwards and usually forwards by the development of the haematoma, so that the severed ends become widely separated. Early operation is imperative, and in children it is often possible to visualize the site of the rupture through a retropubic approach; the proximal urethra may then be sutured down to the region of the perineal membrane, and healing allowed to take place over an indwelling catheter. Should direct exposure prove impossible a sound must first be manipulated across the gap, a process which is facilitated by passing an instrument down from the open bladder to meet another passed up through the urethra. Approximation of the severed ends may then be achieved by drawing a Foley catheter through the gap, inflating the balloon in the bladder, and applying light traction ($\frac{1}{2}$ lb) so that the prostate is held down in the pelvis. In young children the catheter should always be brought out through a perineal urethrostomy, so that the traction is applied in a straight line, and damage to the urethra at the peno-scrotal angle, where stricturing is likely to occur, is thus avoided.

3. Urethral stricture

Inadequate treatment of both forms of rupture is likely to be followed by the development of a urethral stricture, and trauma is in fact the most common cause of acquired stricture in childhood. Intermittent dilatation is not a suitable method of treatment in boys since the pain and the apprehension which precedes it often cause a serious emotional disturbance; every effort should therefore be made to produce a permanent cure by operative means. In the penile urethra the operation described by JOHANSON is the most suitable. The strictured part of the urethra is first laid open on to the surface and stitched to the skin, forming an artificial hypospadias. After the scar has become supple the urethra is reconstituted by the method described by DENIS BROWNE for congenital hypospadias, the strictured area being widened or replaced by the inclusion of the adjacent skin.

Some strictures of the bulb of the urethra may be repaired by a similar operation, though it will be necessary to turn flaps of perineal skin up to the urethra, as the latter cannot be brought to the surface. Short segment strictures may often be satisfactorily excised and sutured according to the method described by MARION.

Strictures of the membranous urethra (Fig. 143) are much more difficult to treat, because of the wide separation of the ends, and because the injury and subsequent fibrosis have often destroyed the external sphincter causing urinary incontinence. Nevertheless, if an adequate channel can be restored continence will ultimately be recovered. The strictured region is a good deal more accessible in the child than in the adult, and may be exposed simultaneously from the perineum, and from the retropubic space. The scar tissue should be excised and the severed ends of the urethra approximated by direct suture: with proper mobilization it will be found that this suture line often lies comfortably below the perineal membrane. The pull-through method of approximation described by BADENOCH may also be employed.

Instrumental trauma is another cause of urethral stricture in children as in adults, and the avoidance of this complication is the best evidence of urological skill. It need scarcely be stated here that catheters and bougies should be passed with the utmost gentleness, and that no attempt should be made to introduce a larger instrument than can be comfortably accommodated. The greatest

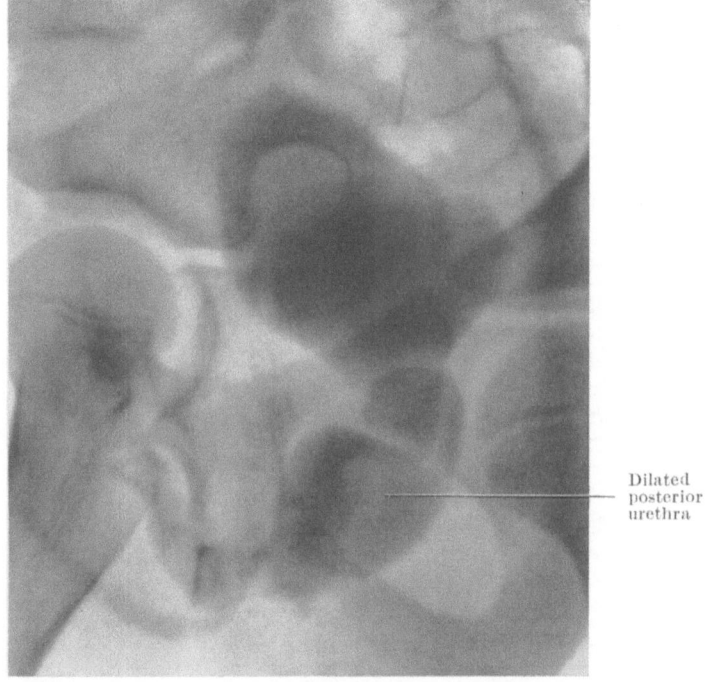

Dilated
posterior
urethra

Fig. 143. Traumatic stricture of the membranous urethra. Micturating cystogram in a boy aged 9 years. The posterior urethra is dilated, elongated and tortuous, having been pulled up from the site of the rupture. Fracture of the pubic bones

temptation to transgress the latter rule occurs during cystoscopy, but it should always be remembered that a perineal urethrostomy will permit a much less traumatic approach. Neither gum elastic nor red rubber indwelling urethral catheters should be employed; a soft latex rubber Foley catheter is best adapted for continuous drainage, but even this should be avoided if it is too tight in the urethra, and instead a supra-pubic cystostomy should be made. Urethritis complicating the use of an indwelling catheter is particularly destructive, and in one case referred to the author the urethral lumen was completely obliterated from the fossa navicularis to the bulb. The commonest site for stricture due to instrumentation, apart from the external meatus, is the region of the peno-scrotal angle; in these cases treatment by intermittent dilatation may be given a short trial, but if there is no improvement within the first six months, operative repair by the JOHANSON method should be undertaken.

Stricture due to infective urethritis is now almost unknown in children, but other acquired causes, such as the inflammatory reaction complicating sulphon-amide obstruction may be seen from time to time.

4. Urethral fistula

External urethral fistulae are most often a result of unsatisfactory repair of hypospadias, but may be traumatic in origin. A common type is the fistula at the level of the coronal sulcus (Fig. 144) resulting from a stitch, carelessly placed

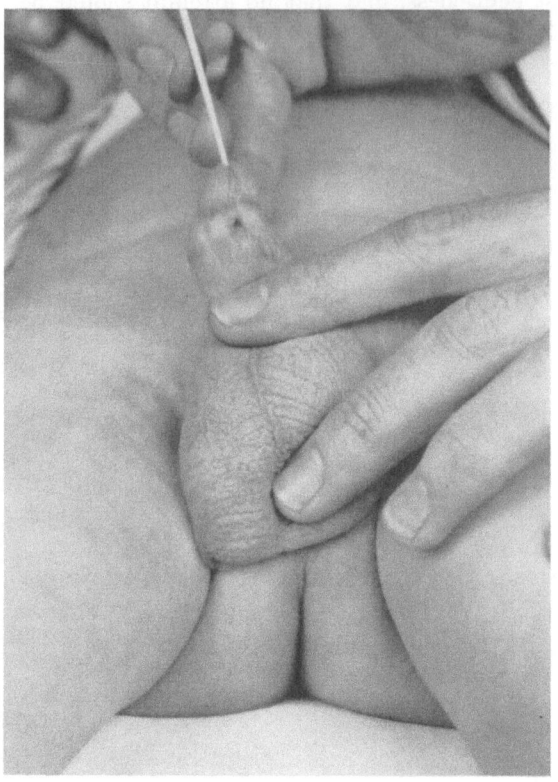

Fig. 144. Urethral fistula: the penis of a aged boy 2 ¹/₂ years showing a urethral fistula at the level of the coronal sulcus. Necrosis of the urethral wall had resulted from a deeply placed suture during circumcision

during circumcision, which includes the urethral wall and causes necrosis. All such fistulae should be carefully repaired after a full mobilization of the surrounding skin, and a diversion of urine by cystostomy or perineal urethrostomy is essential.

Congenital urethral fistulae are discussed on p. 108.

VII. Priapism

Spontaneous penile erections occur normally even in young infants, unassociated with masturbation, but perhaps stimulated by the mother's handling of the genitalia while bathing or changing napkins. Such erections are transitory, and relatively frequent.

True priapism, however, is very seldom observed in childhood. It may be associated with blood disorders, leukaemia (MACCIOTTA) or sickle-cell anaemia, and may indeed be the first evidence of disease. COWIE has recorded the case of a boy of 9 years in whom priapism resulted from the extension of a sarcoma of the prostate. Injury and haematoma of the perineum can produce a lasting priapism, as in the boy described by FRASER, in whom the use of anticoagulants lead to a satisfactory relief. For a full discussion of causes and treatment the reader is referred to vol. XI.

VIII. Undescended testicles

1. Embryology

Embryologically the testis is formed on the dorsal wall of the coelom, from the genital ridge which extends from the level of the diaphragm down to the sacral segments; in the course of early development the foetus elongates rapidly, while the testis by shrinkage at its cranial extremity, becomes a compact body lying a little above the inguinal region. It remains in this position until the 7th month of foetal life, after which descent into the scrotum occurs rapidly. The testis is preceded by a pouch of peritoneum, the processus vaginalis, which for a time remains in continuity with the general peritoneal cavity: after full descent the lumen of the processus is obliterated, and the tunica vaginalis, surrounding the testis is thus isolated. The mechanism of descent is still not clearly understood, though it seems likely to be connected in some way with the gubernaculum, a broad strand of condensed mesenchyme which first appears at 25 mm; it is attached above to the Wolffian duct near its junction with the gonad, and splays out below to reach the surface at the groin, scrotum and thigh. The gubernaculum grows rapidly until the 7th month and after that its rapid shrinkage is associated with the descent of the testis. It has often been pointed out that since it is only attached to the skin, its shortening can scarcely draw the testicle out of the abdomen, yet in shrinking it may create a passage down which the testicle may be pushed by abdominal pressure. The "milking" action of cremaster activity is also said to play a part. Endocrine secretions have clearly some influence over the process of descent, though the manner in which they act is obscure. The embryological findings are discussed by WELLS and by WYNDHAM.

2. Incidence

Descent is not always complete at birth. SCORER, examining 1,700 full term infants, found undescended testicles in 4%: in the majority of these full descent occurred within the first three months of post-natal life, leaving only 0.7% undescended at the end of the first year. The frequency with which spontaneous descent occurs after this age is hotly disputed: most surgeons with a long experience of the condition (e.g. BEVAN, CAMPBELL, GROSS) believe that such descent is rare, while other observers (e.g. SMITH) regard it as usual. The latter view ignores the distinction between the retracted and the true undescended testicle, and it is clear that the more careful the examiner, the less often will he observe late descent.

Estimates of the incidence of the disorder in children and adults vary considerably, and many of them are based on inadequate data. The retractile testicle is a frequent source of confusion, and unless therefore a careful and repeated examination of each child is undertaken the incidence of undescended organs will certainly be overestimated. Post-mortem statistics in children also overestimate the incidence of the anomaly in the general population since it is a common concomitant of other congenital abnormalities which may be responsible for death during the pre-pubertal period. Clinical data in adults usually relate to the examination of Army recruits, and will incline to underestimate since certain groups who are frequently affected by the disorder, such as the mental defectives, are apt to be excluded from the examination. CAMPBELL reports that undescended testicles were found in 292 instances in a post-mortem series of 10,712 boys (1 in 36), and in 107 cases in 22,606 adult males (1:211). SOUTHAM and COOPER, reviewing various previous estimates reached the conclusion that 1 in 200 adults was approximately the incidence, but most recent authors in America appear to regard 1 in 500 as a more likely figure.

3. Surgical anatomy

The best description of the anatomy of the undescended testicle is that given by BROWNE, and the following remarks are based upon his work. He points out that the testicle is a mobile organ, and that its position must be described in terms of its possible range of movement.

The normal testicle in the child may be confined to the scrotum, but most have a range of movement which extends from the bottom of the scrotal sac up to the fascial pouch which lies lateral to the external inguinal ring, deep to Scarpa's fascia and superficial to the external oblique aponeurosis. The testicle is drawn up from the scrotum under the influence of cremaster contractions, and slips into the superficial inguinal pouch because this is the line of least resistance when once the pubis is crossed. The normal testicle does not retract into the inguinal canal: it remains palpable only when placed on the superficial surface of the external oblique, while a testicle within the canal is scarcely ever palpable, and is abnormal in position. It should be noted that some American surgeons (e.g. GROSS and JEWETT) do not accept this latter statement: they believe that the normal retractile testicle enters the inguinal canal where it still remains palpable, although lying deep to the tense anterior wall. My own experience leads me to support BROWNE's view; wherever a testicle, palpable lateral to the external ring, has been explored it has been found to lie superficial to the external oblique.

The mobile normal testicle which ranges from the deep scrotum to the superficial inguinal pouch, BROWNE designates the "low retractile" type. Active retraction occurs readily when attempts are made to palpate the organ, often leading the inexperienced to suppose that descent has not occurred. The condition is usually, though not invariably, bilateral and in fat boys, in whom the scrotum remains small, and the retracted testicles are buried beneath a deep layer of adipose tissue, is often mistaken for bilateral abdominal cryptorchidism. Active retraction ceases to occur at or soon after puberty, and the scrotum enlarges at the same time: these phenomena undoubtedly account for the great majority of instances of so-called spontaneous late descent of the testicles. The pubertal change can also be brought about by the administration of gonadotropic hormones, though it should be clear that if a proper examination is made, and the true state of affairs discovered, no treatment is required.

BROWNE also describes as a variant of the normal the "high retractile" testicle, which has a range of movement extending from the superficial inguinal pouch to the upper part of the scrotum, but which cannot be coaxed to the bottom of the scrotal sac. He believes that all these testicles achieve the full scrotal position after puberty (or after gonadotropins) and that he has never seen this range of movement in an adult. Some doubt may be felt with regard to this latter observation, however, and this group constitutes the most difficult problem in diagnosis: as will be seen later, the author believes that treatment is necessary for some of these cases in which spontaneous descent cannot always be relied upon.

The true undescended testicles may be classified according to the lowest point of their range. The "emergent" testicle lies within the inguinal canal or emerges for a short distance from the external ring: its mobility is essentially dependent upon the presence of a hernial sac within which it moves. The sac may be narrow at its upper end so that the intestines cannot enter it, though often a little omentum is able to come down. Where the neck of the sac is wider and there is an evident clinical hernia, the fundus of the sac may become enlarged and extend below the testicle. The range of movement of this type of testicle will increase at puberty, but full spontaneous descent will not occur.

The "middle inguinal" testicle can enter the canal from above, but cannot leave it below; it is not palpable, though a hernial sac may emerge from the external inguinal ring and produce a palpable swelling. On rare occasions the external ring is found to be very small or absent, so that there is a simple mechanical bar to progress, but more often no evident cause for the failure can be demonstrated. The "entrant inguinal" is placed even higher, and is hardly distinguishable from the "abdominal" in which the testicle does not engage in the inguinal canal at all. Some of the abdominal testicles are found in pseudo-hermaphrodites and lie on a broad ligament adjacent to the uterus and Fallopian tubes: others have a short pedicle from the lateral pelvic wall, and others again lie entirely retroperitoneally, but they are seldom found more than a short distance above the internal inguinal ring. A hernial sac may or may not be present in association with an abdominal testis, the gubernaculum is poorly formed or absent.

In very rare cases the testicle may be high up on the posterior abdominal wall; WHITEHORN found it occupying the renal fossa in a case with congenital absence of the kidney; KAYS and COLEMAN found one high and one low testicle in a case of polyorchism.

The "inguinal ectopic" testis is one which lies in the superficial inguinal pouch, but which cannot be made to enter the scrotum. The limitation of its range is partly due to the closure of the normal channel of descent, and partly to the length of the spermatic cord. In the typical case there is no complete hernial sac, though there may be a short processus at the upper end of the inguinal canal, and the testicle cannot be pushed back into the canal. It remains easily palpable on the superficial aspect of the external oblique and usually produces a visible swelling there. The upper pole of the testis and epididymis (with appendix testis) is placed laterally. Gubernacular tissue is often found connecting the testicle to the scrotum, and the failure of descent cannot be attributed to the lack of this structure. The onset of puberty will not lead to any change in the position of the inguinal ectopic testicle. A variant of this type is the "emergent inguinal ectopic" in which a hernial sac is present and permits reduction into the canal. Rarer forms of testicular ectopia, in which a greater displacement has occurred, are discussed in a later section.

All forms may be unilateral or bilateral: GROSS and JEWETT recording a total of 1,222 cases note that right unilateral undescended testicles constituted 44%, left unilateral 30%, and bilateral 26%.

The undescended or ectopic testis differs from the normal, not only in its position, but also in its relation to the Wolffian duct derivatives. Gross abnormalities of the epididymis are often seen in the abdominal and emergent types, this organ being long and drawn out, and having only a tenuous connection with the testis itself. When there is a complete failure of union between the testis and epididymis, the latter is drawn down further towards the scrotum than the former, and at times a vas deferens will be found extending to the bottom

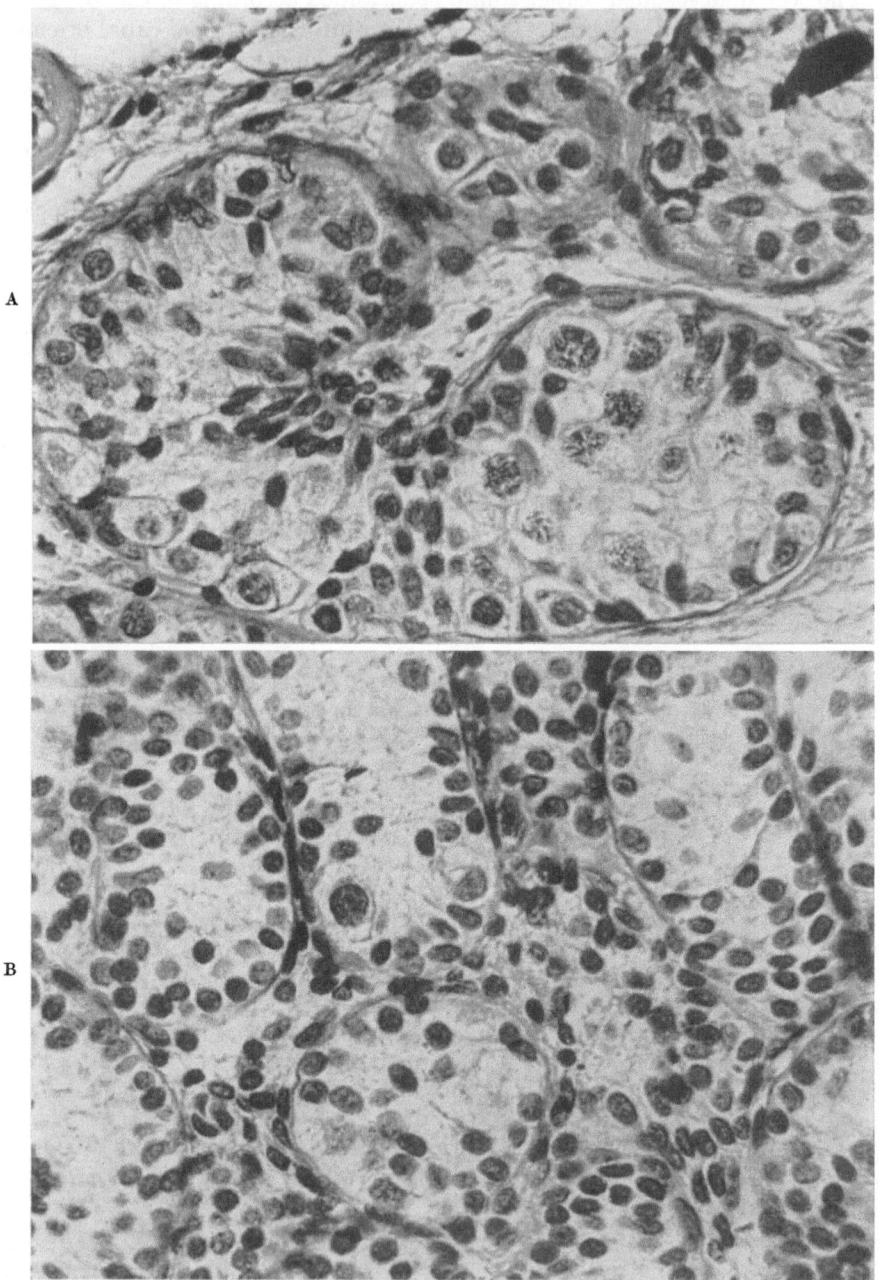

Fig. 145 A and B. Histology of the undescended testicle. Section from A the normal testis, B the undescended testis, both at the same magnification (× 300), from a boy aged 7 years. The undescended organ shows smaller tubules with little differentiation of spermatogonia

of the scrotum where it exhibits a swelling representing the epididymis, but the testis is completely absent. The undescended testicle is almost always smaller than its fellow, though it may be necessary to have them both exposed at operation to appreciate this fact.

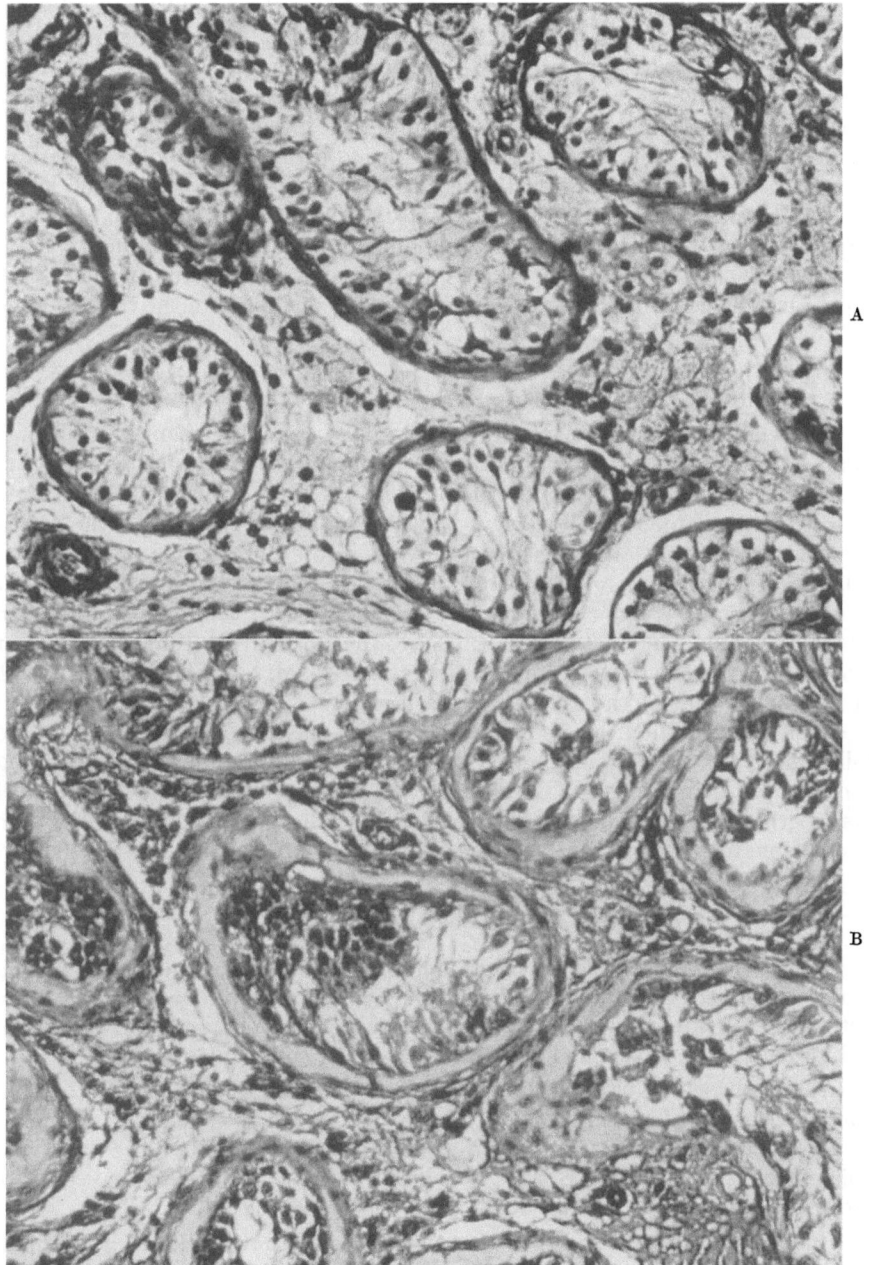

Fig. 146 A and B. Histology of the undescended testicle. A from a boy aged 11 years (× 125), B from an adult (× 125), showing sclerosis of the tubules

4. Histology

Until recent years it was believed that the undescended testis did not differ microscopically from the normal until puberty, but it is now clear that the divergence begins not later than the sixth year of life (Fig. 145). The normal spermatic tubules at this stage are slowly increasing their diameter, and becoming more tortuous; the cells lining them are developing more than one layer, and spermatogonia are beginning to appear. Studies by SNIFFEN, by ROBINSON and ENGLE, and subsequently by many other observers demonstrate that the undescended testicle, whatever its type or level, lags behind the normal in these developments. The lag becomes much more marked at puberty; interstitial cells appear and some of the tubules exhibit a trend towards normal differentiation, but others remain immature (even when the fourth decade is reached), and contain no germ cells or Sertoli cells. After some years all the tubules become sclerotic and shrunken (Fig. 146), but the interstitial cells remain numerous and prominent. Although, at times, the interstitial cells appear hyperplastic in the undescended testis, in most cases their prominence is due rather to the shrinkage of the tubular elements.

5. Function

The endocrine function of the undescended testis is essentially normal, and bilateral cryptorchids are not eunuchoid unless some other abnormality is present. This observation accords well with the continued development of the interstitial cells. Tubular function, however, is very seldom adequate for the production of spermatozoa, and although there may be rare exceptions to the rule (see REA) bilateral cryptorchids are infertile. It appears well established that the failure of spermatogenesis is to some extent correlated with the higher temperature to which the undescended testis is exposed, the normal scrotum with its variable length being a mechanism for keeping the testis at a temperature of a degree or two below that of the abdominal tissues. A testis which is artificially retained in the inguinal region, as for instance when it has become adherent to the scar following repair of inguinal hernia in infancy, will undergo the same changes as the naturally undescended organ. On the other hand, a structural inferiority may perhaps be an inherent characteristic of the undescended testicle, and be responsible for the failure of its migration (SOHVAL).

6. Cause

It has been indicated at the beginning of this section that the normal mechanism of descent is still not understood, and the causes of failure are not better known. Although FRAZER believed that a defect of the gubernaculum could be demonstrated in most cases, subsequent observers have not confirmed this view.

At operation, several mechanical factors may make it difficult to secure an adequate length of spermatic cord; the hernial sac is one such factor, and a tight medial pillar to the internal inguinal ring another, yet from the embryological point of view neither abnormality can be regarded as a sufficient cause: a patent processus has been present in all testicles at one stage.

Endocrine failure is often held responsible for the condition, and this hypothesis has given a scientific background to the treatment by hormones. Undescended testicles may certainly be found in association with definite endocrine disorders, yet in the majority the child is otherwise normal and the testicular disorder unilateral. Moreover, since the normal testicle is descended before or very shortly after birth, the endocrine failure must be foetal in origin, and the precocious inducement of pubertal changes by hormones cannot be regarded as comparable.

Except therefore in the cases of gross departure from the normal anatomy or physiology, the cause of undescent remains unexplained.

7. Complications

An inguinal hernia is much the most common concomitant of the undescended testicle. A complete funicular sac is found in 30 to 40%, but in many of these the neck is too narrow to allow the bowel to enter, and a hernia large enough to cause symptoms occurs only in a few cases. Incarceration and strangulation may complicate the picture, however, and demand urgent treatment.

Torsion is much more liable to occur in the undescended than in the normal testicle, and the periodic attacks of inguinal pain, of which some of the boys complain, are sometimes perhaps transient episodes of torsion. Torsion may also occur in the intra-abdominal testicle (KELLY and UHRICH).

The increased liability to malignancy is a topic which has received considerable attention in the literature: it has been stated that the undescended testicle is between 20 and 50 times more liable to the development of tumour than the normally placed organ. Evidence of this increased risk has been presented by GORDON TAYLOR and TILL, and by many other authors. ROBINSON and ENGLE are so convinced of the danger that they believe that all testicles which cannot be satisfactorily brought down to the scrotum at the age of six or seven years should be excised. On the other hand, malignant disease has been recorded several times (e.g. CHAUVIN, THOMAS) in testicles which have been successfully operated upon, and the suggestion has been made that the risk of malignancy is related to the inherent structure of the testicle, not simply to its position, which may indeed be a reflection of its structural inferiority. However, many surgeons (e.g. GROSS and JEWETT, CAMPBELL, H. E., CARROLL) consider that there are many statistical fallacies in the conclusions regarding the liability to malignancy, that the risk has been overestimated and that testicles which cannot be brought down may safely be left within the abdomen where their endocrine function may continue.

8. Clinical picture

Most undescended testicles cause no symptoms at all during childhood, and are discovered only on routine examination. A few boys complain of local pain, but often it is a generalized abdominal pain of intestinal origin which leads to the observation of the testicular condition. A hernia may cause discomfort, and on a few occasions will produce the acute symptoms associated with incarceration or strangulation.

The association of undescended testicles with endocrine disorders is well known, but its frequency is exaggerated; all too often the fat but well grown boy of 11 or 12 years is sent to hospital as a case of "Fröhlich's Syndrome" and is believed to have cryptorchidism, yet on examination he is found to have retractile testicles, and simple obesity. Puberty in these boys is often late, but with it the testicles cease to be actively retractile, the scrotum enlarges and often some of the adiposity is lost.

True hypogonadism may be seen when the testicles are hypoplastic as well as undescended, but it is comparatively rare. Male intersex cases and true hermaphrodites have testicles which are frequently misplaced, and any child in whom a unilateral or bilateral undescended testicle is found in association with hypospadias should be subjected to the careful investigations suggested on p. 287. Undescended testicles may accompany other severe deformities of the urogenital system, and are to be expected in cases of agenesis of the abdominal muscles. A familial incidence of unilateral undescended testicle is occasionally reported (WILES).

The clinical findings in the various forms of undescended testicles have been described under the heading of surgical anatomy. The importance of a careful examination can scarcely be overemphasized however; the child must be relaxed and at ease, the consulting room and the surgeon's hands must be warm. The examination should first be made with the child lying down, and the testicle should be coaxed downwards from the groin with the flat of the left hand, to be received between the fingers and thumb of the right. Subsequent examination in the erect position may help in the observation of accompanying hernia. If operation is advised a second careful review should be made when the child enters hospital, for it will occasionally be found on re-examination that a testicle, whose mobility was thought at first to be limited, can now be coaxed down to the scrotum, or that one which was completely impalpable has appeared at the external ring.

9. Management

There is as yet no unanimity among the medical profession concerning the management of undescended testicle, and much of the literature on the subject is confused by obvious inaccuracy of diagnosis, and by a regrettable lack of information regarding the late results of treatment.

The objects of treatment may be summarized as follows:

a) The presence of a testicle in the groin, and its absence from the scrotum are causes of slight physical and considerable psychological discomfort to the adult male, and for these reasons alone the correction of the misplacement is desirable. The exact age at which correction for this indication is undertaken is not of very great moment, but it must be before puberty if a shrunken testicle is to be avoided.

b) The untreated bilateral cryptorchid will almost certainly be sterile: the chances of fertility are definitely improved by securing descent. This consideration is not relevant to the unilateral case, whose chances of fertility are very unlikely to be increased by treatment. It is certain that in order to secure active spermatogenesis, the testicle must be in the scrotum before puberty, and the recent demonstration that histological divergence of the undescended from the normal begins in the sixth year may suggest that correction should be achieved before that age. We are, however, without accurate information as to whether a testicle, retarded because of its position, will "catch up" if replaced before puberty, or whether its structural deficiency is such that normal function can never be expected of it, at whatever age it reaches the scrotum. The earlier reports of fertility after correction of bilateral cryptorchidism (HANSEN) indicated that very little could be achieved by treatment, but GROSS and JEWETT record that 30 out of 38 of their cases became fertile after being treated by orchidopexy between the ages of 9 and 10 years. The advocates of earlier operation (e.g. HINMAN) have not been able to produce any comparable series as yet, though if the correction was as easily obtained at the earlier age, there would be little objection to their advice. This point is discussed later.

c) There may be a complication such as hernia or torsion which demands treatment. The age of the child is irrelevant to this consideration.

d) The undescended testicle may have an increased liability to malignant disease: as already stated the magnitude of this risk is variously assessed and regarded by many as negligible. The risk does not appear to be eliminated by replacement of the testicle in the scrotum, and if established as a serious factor, it must be regarded as an indication for orchidectomy. This conclusion is only acceptable, however, in unilateral cases and for testicles which cannot be brought to the scrotum, and even for these cases most surgeons to-day prefer to retain during childhood an abdominal testicle for its endocrine function, believing the risk of hypogonadism to be greater than the risk of malignancy. In operations after puberty and the establishment of secondary sex characteristics, preservation of the unilateral intra-abdominal testicle has little advantage.

From these considerations it may be concluded that all undescended testicles should be corrected before puberty, and where diagnosis has been accurate, nothing can be gained by awaiting the outcome of that event. The method of treatment, and the stage of childhood at which it should be applied, remain to be discussed.

The extravagant claims for endocrine therapy which were made in the earlier days of its use may now be largely discounted; there remains a small but important place for the use of hormones. The exhibition of gonadotropins such as Pregnyl, Folluitin, or Antuitrin S will produce a reaction mimicking the normal pubertal changes; testosterone should not be used as there is some danger that it will suppress normal testicular function.

It will be clear from the discussion of the surgical anatomy that gonadotropins will not cause descent in cases of inguinal ectopia, or in emergent testicles with hernial sacs, while in the low retractile type no treatment is required. In the high retractile group, however, there may be some doubt about the exact anatomy and about the outcome: in these cases, particularly where the condition is bilateral, a course of gonadotropin will settle the issue. Some of the testicles will descend to the bottom of the scrotum, and the surgeon may then rest assured that even if retraction takes place at the end of the course of treatment the changes of normal puberty will again set matters right. When there is no increase in the range of mobility, operation should be advised.

Pre-operative gonadotropins are advised by some surgeons on the grounds that they lengthen the cord structures and render the scrotal replacement easier. There cannot be any conclusive evidence for such an effect, however, and many operators, including the present author, remain unconvinced. Only in the case of bilateral impalpable testicle can hormones be usefully employed pre-operatively.

Hormone injections therefore assume a diagnostic rather than a therapeutic role, and are useful in only a small proportion. The author's practice is to give a course of Pregnyl, 500 units twice weekly for 8 weeks, but rather larger doses than this may be employed without danger. Some surgeons (e.g. HINMAN) use a much shorter course of a more concentrated drug, giving 1,000 units every other day for 2 weeks. Higher dosage for long periods will produce some undesirable side effects, including a very considerable enlargement of the penis, but these effects are transitory, and despite the many warnings which have been issued, no permanent harm has been reported.

Operative orchidopexy is required for all inguinal ectopic testicles, for emergent testicles, and for impalpable testicles. The operative technique is discussed in Vol. XIII and it may simply be remarked here that the method of freeing the cord, if necessary by extensive dissection, is much more important than the method of fixation. The hernial sac must be completely dissected off the cord, and excised; the testicular vessels must be freed from their attachment to the peritoneum above and lateral to the internal ring so that they can be swung in medially, and the posterior wall of the canal incised down to the epigastric vessels to allow the vas to shorten its course. After freeing, the majority of testicles can be brought easily to the scrotum, and require only to be kept there while healing occurs. GROSS uses a trans-scrotal stitch with elastic traction applied from the thigh;

the writer prefers DENIS BROWNE's method of slipping the testicle through a loop cut from the fascia covering pectineus and passing it on into the scrotum.

When the testicle cannot be brought fully down, it may be left immediately outside the inguinal ring, and a second operation attempted one or two years later. The secondary procedure is seldom easy, dissection of the adhesions is tedious and must be carried out with great care to avoid damage to the cord and vessels, but it will often be found that sufficient length can thereby be obtained, and a very satisfactory position secured. When it fails the testicle is likely to be in poor condition and may be removed.

When, at the first operation the cord is very short indeed and the testicle cannot be brought to the external ring, abdominal replacement should be performed in the child, orchidectomy in the adult.

Absence of the testicle is seen from time to time, and a very extensive dissection and search is not justifiable in childhood, but when no testicle is found in the inguinal canal, or in the nearby retro-peritoneal region, the peritoneum should be opened to see whether any Mullerian duct derivatives are present.

In unilateral cases, when the contralateral testicle is normal, and there is little risk of infertility, operation is best performed at the age of 9 or 10 years. An early intervention may be made when pain or the presence of a hernia demand it, but the tissues in the older child are tougher and make a satisfactory outcome more likely. This is particularly the case with the impalpable testicle, in which operative difficulties are frequent and may be formidable.

In bilateral cases, a somewhat earlier operation may be advised, but not before 5 years of age. The two sides may be treated at the same time only when length is easily obtained on the first, otherwise it is preferable to allow some months to elapse between the two procedures.

A small symptomless hernia need not indicate an early operation, and many may safely be watched until a suitable age is reached. Any suggestion of incarceration or strangulation will demand early attention.

Judged from the standpoint of clinical examination, the results of a carefully performed orchidopexy are satisfactory in about 90% of cases: accidents to the blood supply result in atrophy of some testicles, and the inherent structural inferiority accounts for other failures. Evidence as to the results in terms of fertility are difficult to obtain, and the results of GROSS and JEWETT have already been quoted.

IX. Other testicular anomalies

Although imperfect descent of the testicles is one of the most common problems of children's urology, other congenital testicular abnormalities are rare, and of interest to the clinician chiefly on account of their liability to be confused with simple failure of descent.

1. Anorchia and monorchia

In a small proportion of those cases in which no testicle is palpable on clinical examination none will be found at operation (COUNSELLOR et al.). From the operative standpoint complete absence of the testicle is difficult to establish since all the possible sites can hardly be adequately explored, but the diagnosis may be made with reasonable assurance when the vas deferens can be traced down into the scrotum where it ends in an expansion representing the epididymis yet no testicle can be found in the scrotum, the inguinal canal or the pelvis as exposed through an inguinal incision. Unilateral absence (monorchia) is commoner than complete anorchia (WILLIAMS and LEE); hypogonadism will occur only in the latter, and if it is diagnosed before the normal age of puberty replacement therapy is indicated.

2. Hypoplasia

The testicle is sometimes represented by a minute organ in the scrotum, no larger than a pea, though the histology during childhood may be normal. Cases are likely to be diagnosed only at operation for suspected abdominal testicles. Hormone replacement therapy is required in bilateral hypoplasia.

3. Polyorchism

A third testicle is a very exceptional finding, and usually presents as a tender swelling in the groin or upper scrotum, which is apt to be regarded as a hydrocele of the cord or an irreducible hernia (ANDERSON). The clinical finding is likely to lead to exploration and therefore to the correct diagnosis. A single vas commonly serves both organs, and must be preserved when the supernumerary member is removed.

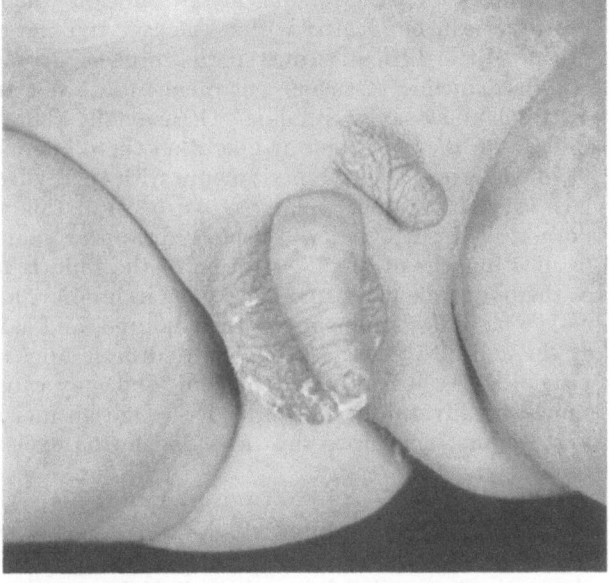

4. Rare forms of testicular ectopia

The form of maldescent known as inguinal ectopia has already been described: other forms of ectopia are rare, and can normally be diagnosed without difficulty.

a) Perineal ectopia. The testis passes downward from the external inguinal ring into the

Fig. 147. Ectopic scrotum. The external genitalia of an infant aged 2 months. Normal scrotal skin occurs only on the right side of the median raphe, but there is a separate pedicled scrotum in the region of the left pubic tubercle, which encloses a testicle

perineum (WAKELEY). In this situation it may cause some pain, particularly during such activities as riding a bicycle. It is easily palpable, but is apt to be overlooked unless a deliberate examination of the region is made.

b) Penile ectopia. The testis passes upwards and comes to lie at the root of the penis, or on the dorsum of the shaft (RASPALL).

c) Femoral ectopia. The testis takes up a position in the femoral triangle (BEETZ).

d) Transverse ectopia. Both testes pass out through the same inguinal canal and come to lie in the same half of the scrotum.

The first three forms are easily corrected, since the spermatic cord is of adequate length, and it is a simple matter to replace the testicle in the scrotum. Transverse ectopia may be associated with other abnormalities of the genital tract, including pseudohermaphroditism, and is seldom amenable to correction (HERTZLER).

An ectopic testicle occupying an ectopic scrotal pouch in the inguinal region is illustrated in Fig. 147.

X. Hydrocele

A collection of fluid within the tunica vaginalis is a common finding in infancy, but one that need cause little concern. The subject is reviewed by CAMP-BELL, by GROSS and by LANGER. As in adults, a secondary hydrocele may complicate epididymitis, orchitis or a traumatic lesion of the testicle, but the onset, pain, and associated signs will leave little doubt as to the nature of the disorder. Primary hydrocele in children is almost always accompanied by a congenital defect in the processus vaginalis, and the group may be sub-divided as follows:

1. Hydrocele of the tunica vaginalis

a) Irreducible

There is a cystic swelling in the scrotum which is brightly transilluminable, the testis can be located within the sac, and the cord is normal. The diagnosis presents little difficulty since spermatocele is virtually unknown in childhood, and other irreducible testicular enlargements do not transilluminate: a neoplasm is a harder and heavier swelling. Occasionally there is a palpable prolongation of the sac up the cord, and at operation there is almost always a definite processus vaginalis connecting the peritoneum with the hydrocele sac, even when its lumen has been obliterated. Bilateral hydrocele of this type is often seen in the new-born, and if untreated will usually disappear spontaneously during the first six or nine months of life. Aspiration of the fluid is not helpful, since the presence of the hydrocele causes no symptoms in infancy, and recurrence is the rule. The child's parents should simply be re-assured, and asked to bring him up for review at the end of a year. Irreducible hydrocele appearing after the end of the first year of life is likely to be persistent, and may cause some discomfort; operation should be advised and performed through an incision over the external inguinal ring, so that the processus vaginalis can be excised at the same time that the tunica is trimmed away.

b) Reducible

The usual signs of hydrocele are present, but the swelling can be reduced by digital pressure, or will disappear spontaneously in recumbency. Occasionally no change in size can be observed on clinical examination, but there is a clear history that the swelling is smaller when the child first gets out of bed, and enlarges towards the evening. There is evidently a patent processus vaginalis allowing the fluid to be displaced into the peritoneal cavity, though there need be no suggestion of ascites or any intra-abdominal disorder. Clinically, the fluid nature of the swelling is evident, so that hernia will not be suspected, though with a wide processus it is clear that hernia may follow in time, and the distinction is unimportant. Except in the neonatal period when spontaneous cure is likely, treatment should be operative, but need only comprise excision of the processus, and laying open of the tunica.

2. Hydrocele of the cord, or of the canal of Nuck

In these cases, the processus vaginalis has become obliterated at its upper and lower extremities, leaving an accumulation of fluid in the mid-portion. Clinically this presents as a tense cystic swelling in the inguinal region, painless and irreducible; transillumination is only possible when the cyst lies in the upper scrotum, for higher up the thickness of the overlying tissue obscures the effect. Differential diagnosis from incarcerated inguinal hernia may be difficult, but the absence of pain, and the length of history will usually be sufficient indication. In some cases, the hydrocele of the cord is elongated, and reaches down to the level of the testicle. In the majority, the cyst is found in infancy, and disappears spontaneously; operation may be required in later childhood.

3. Hydrocele with undescended testis

A collection of fluid may surround an "emergent" testicle (p. 253) or one entrapped within the inguinal canal. A patent processus vaginalis is usually present. Operation will be required for the testicular abnormality.

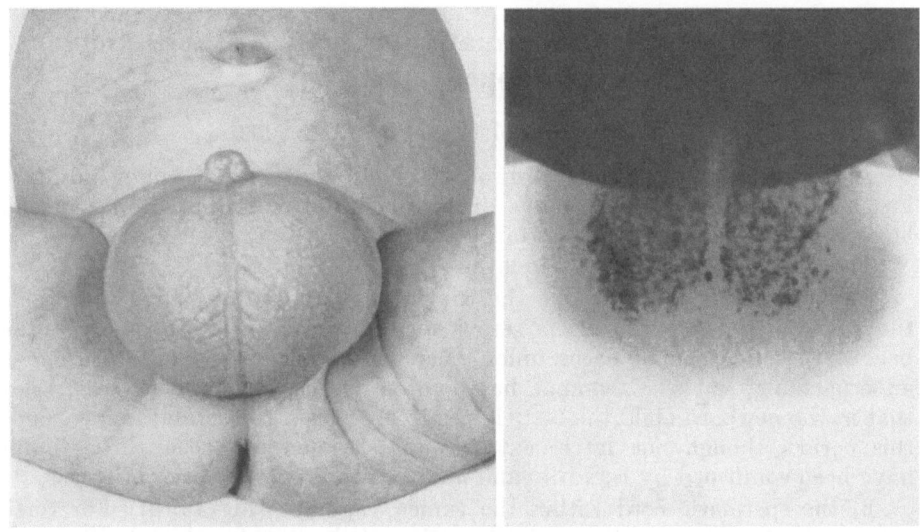

A   B

Fig. 148 A and B. Meconium hydrocele. A External genitalia; B X-ray of scrotum; boy aged 6 weeks with testicular swellings but in good general health. Calcified masses were seen in the X-ray of abdomen as well as in the scrotum and indicated healed meconium peritonitis. Masses of sticky meconium were removed from both hydrocele sacs with complete recovery. Mr. D. J. WATERSTON's case

4. Meconium hydrocele

The condition here described is very rare, and occurs as a complication of meconium peritonitis. A perforation of the bowel is assumed to have taken place during foetal life, releasing a quantity of meconium into the peritoneal cavity, where it sets up a sterile, chemical peritonitis. The bowel perforation heals, but the effects of the peritonitis and adhesions may cause obstruction. Calcification occurs in the masses of meconium, and these can therefore be visualized radiologically.

While the processus vaginalis is patent, the spilt meconium is free to enter it, and set up an inflammation around the testicle. After birth the infant may present with a considerable scrotal swelling, and both testicles are surrounded by partially calcified masses of meconium, as in WATERSTON's case illustrated in Fig. 148. Removal of the masses led to a satisfactory resolution of the inflammation.

XI. Varicocele

In the presence of large renal tumours, particularly on the left side, the veins of the pampiniform plexus may become tensely distended: the tumour obstructs the testicular veins by pressure rather than by invasion. This finding may be of

diagnostic importance, but it is easily distinguished from true varicocele formation, in which there is an easily compressed varicosity.

Varicocele, though normally a post-pubertal development is occasionally seen
in boys of 8 years and upwards, but it is seldom responsible for symptoms. CAMP-
BELL has emphasized that a renal abnormality may be found, and describes a
case with hydronephrosis due to vascular obstruction of the pelvi-ureteric junction,
with concomitant obstruction of the testicular veins. In the great majority,
however, no such abnormality is found, and treatment should follow the same
lines as for the disorder in adults. The present writer favours the high ligation
technique described by ROBB.

XII. Torsion of the spermatic cord and of the testicular appendages

1. Torsion of the spermatic cord

Although this is typically a disorder of adolescents and young adults, an
increasing number of reports have drawn attention to its importance in childhood, and particularly in the neonatal period.

The torsion can occur at three levels:

a) the spermatic cord above the tunica vaginalis, resulting in infarction of
the whole testicle as well as its serous membranes (Fig. 149a). Many authors
believe that this cannot occur unless there has been a previous rupture of the
gubernaculum, but as CAMPBELL has pointed out that it has long been known
that in the newborn child the testicle lies freely within the scrotal tissues, and at
this period, though not later, extra-vaginal torsion can occur. His findings
have been confirmed by LONGINO and MARTIN who report a series of 9 cases.

b) the spermatic cord within the tunica vaginalis (Fig. 149b). For torsion
to occur in this situation the tunica must invest the cord to a high level, and the
testicle and epididymis must be suspended by a comparatively long mesentery,
often hanging "like a clapper in a bell". This state of affairs is often bilateral, so
that if torsion has occurred on one side, it is likely that the predisposing factor
is present on the other side as well. MUSCHAT states that in this type the testicle
has not undergone its normal developmental inversion so that the appendix
testis is lying at the lower pole: he believes that early high investment of the cord
prevents this inversion, and leaves the testicle predisposed to torsion. Intravaginal torsion is apt to take place in the undescended testicle, though it may
be noted that a normally placed testicle is often pulled up to the groin during the
process of torsion.

c) the mesorchium between the epididymis and the testis (Fig. 149c). This
form is rare, and can only occur when the mesorchium is long.

The force causing the torsion is believed to be a spasm of the cremaster
muscle, though there is little proof of this. The onset occasionally follows a
sudden muscular effort or slight trauma, but may at other times occur at rest or
during sleep.

Clinically there is a severe spasmodic pain in the testicle and acute local tenderness. There may be nausea and vomiting, and sometimes collapse, but the
temperature is seldom raised and the bowels are unaffected. The pain subsides
after a few days, when the testicle is completely gangrenous. Spontaneous relief
may occur, however, with restoration of normal circulation and a history of
transitory attacks is not unusual: both testicles may be affected one after the
other.

On examination, the testicle is enlarged, firm or hard, and acutely tender. It is often drawn up to the groin, and some writers state that lifting it further tends to relieve the pain. After a time the overlying skin becomes oedematous and reddened, later it is slightly blue. Differential diagnosis must be made from strangulated inguinal hernia and from acute epididymo-orchitis: accompanying intestinal signs in the one case, and urinary disturbance in the other will usually be sufficient indication, but there should be no hesitation in advising immediate exploration.

The chances of preserving the testicle by untwisting it are small, unless the case is seen within the first few hours, though the degree of vascular obstruction must clearly vary from case to case. DE-MING and CLARKE believe that a deprivation of circulation lasting four hours is sufficient to render testicular gangrene and subsequent atrophy inevitable, yet they claim to have preserved the testis in 9 out of 20 cases. The treatment should be immediate operation, and reposition of the testicle if it is possible; if not orchidectomy should be performed. The replaced testicle should be stitched to the scrotal skin, and if there is any suspicion of contralateral involvement, the same operation should be performed on the opposite side. Some surgeons, who have been particularly impressed by the frequency of bilateral torsion, advise contralateral fixation in all cases.

Torsion in the new born presents a somewhat different problem, since pain is not a feature, and the only finding a hard, enlarged testicle. It is assumed that the onset has occurred before birth. A testicular tumour may sometimes be suspected, and in several cases hydrocele of the

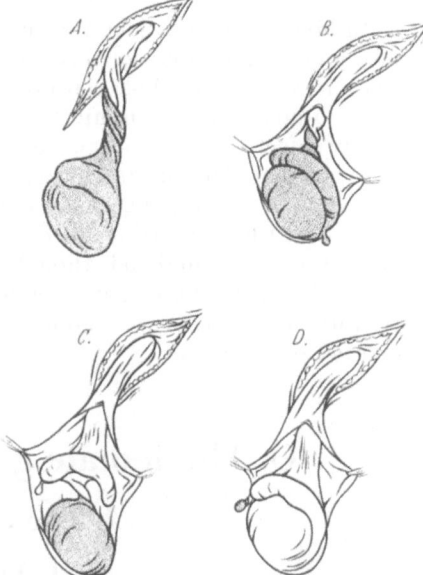

Fig. 149. Diagrams to show the varieties of torsion. *A* Extra-vaginal torsion of the spermatic cord. *B* Intravaginal torsion of the spermatic cord. *C* Torsion between testis and epididymis. *D* Torsion of appendix testis. The infarcted areas are stippled

opposite side has confused the diagnosis. It is likely that atrophy will ultimately follow, but little benefit will be derived from operation at the late stage at which the cases are seen. GLASER and WALLIS believe that surgery should be withheld altogether, while LONGINO and MARTIN replace even a blackened testicle within the scrotum, when it is found at operation, in the hope that some of the endocrine function at least will be preserved.

Infarction of the testicle without evident torsion is seen from time to time in infants: it can certainly complicate strangulated or incarcerated hernia (BENNETT-JONES, FUCHSIG) and may follow birth trauma in breech presentation (NOWA-KOWSKI) but in the new-born it is usually assumed that an intra-uterine torsion has occurred (RAVICH, RHYNE et al., FERNICOLA). Once again the condition is painless and little is gained by orchidectomy.

2. Torsion of the testicular appendages

Torsion of the testicular appendages is characteristically a disorder of children approaching the age of puberty. The subject has been fully reviewed by DIX, and good case reports have been added by HESLIN and ALLYN, and SEIDAL and YEAW. The appendix testis (hydatid of Morgagni) is most frequently affected (Fig. 149d), the appendix epididymis, the paradidymis and the organ of Giraldés less often. There is a sudden onset of acute pain and tenderness: the twisted hydatid can occasionally be felt as a separate nodule, but may be obscured by slight hydrocele or by oedema of the overlying skin. A severe case may be difficult to distinguish from torsion of the spermatic cord, but operation will reveal the true state of affairs, and the hydatid is easily removed.

XIII. Scrotal oedema and gangrene

In breech presentations the scrotum is particularly liable to become oedematous, and may in addition become severely traumatized. NIELSON et al. record a case in which the whole scrotal and penile skin became gangrenous as a result of the injury in these circumstances; the testicles were exposed, and the wound heavily infected, but spontaneous healing was ultimately complete.

Strangulated hernia and local infection in the groin may, in a debilitated infant, lead to a spreading gangrenous infection of the scrotal skin (LEVINSON), which in times past has proved fatal. Extravasation of urine and peri-urethral phlegmon are very rare in childhood, though they have been recorded by CAMPBELL: they may follow impaction of a calculus in the urethra, or complicate a congenital stricture. Spontaneous gangrene of the scrotum (Fournier's Gangrene) has been reported by ALDERS.

O. The female genital tract and urethra

I. The clitoris and labia

1. Ligated clitoris

The most important changes observed in the clitoris during childhood have an endocrine basis and are discussed in the following chapter. Traumatic lesions are seen, however, resulting from the tying of a hair or thread around the clitoris, which becomes reddened, oedematous and considerably enlarged. Since a clear history of the cause of the trouble is unlikely to be obtained, other origins for the enlargement may be suspected : one reported case was originally thought to be a paraphimosis (BROWN) and a similar lesion ascribed to riding a bicycle may perhaps be regarded with scepticism (WILLAN). Careful inspection under anaesthesia will reveal the presence of the ligature, and its removal may be all that is required: advanced necrosis may demand amputation.

An accumulation of smegma beneath the prepuce may cause irritation, cleansing only is needed, and circumcision has no place in the modern treatment.

2. Labial fusion

This is a common disorder of young girls which is too little known by the medical profession. The margins of the labia minora adhere to one another in the midline, and form an almost complete membrane closing the vulva save for a minute opening anteriorly (Fig. 150). The condition may certainly be present at birth, but in other instances it is acquired, and follows a mild vulvitis. The appearance is quite characteristic, and the adhesions can be separated with ease by the use of a probe: a normal hymen and vaginal orifice are then displayed to the great satisfaction of the parents, who have often anticipated, and have been told to expect, multiple operations for reconstruction of the absent vagina. Recurrence of adhesions may occur in cases of vulvitis, and the mother should be instructed to maintain strict cleanliness, and to apply a smear of vaseline to the labia after each bath.

3. Ammonia dermatitis

Ammonia dermatitis occurs as often in girls as in boys, though its effects are much less serious: the urinary meatus is protected, and the skin lesions are

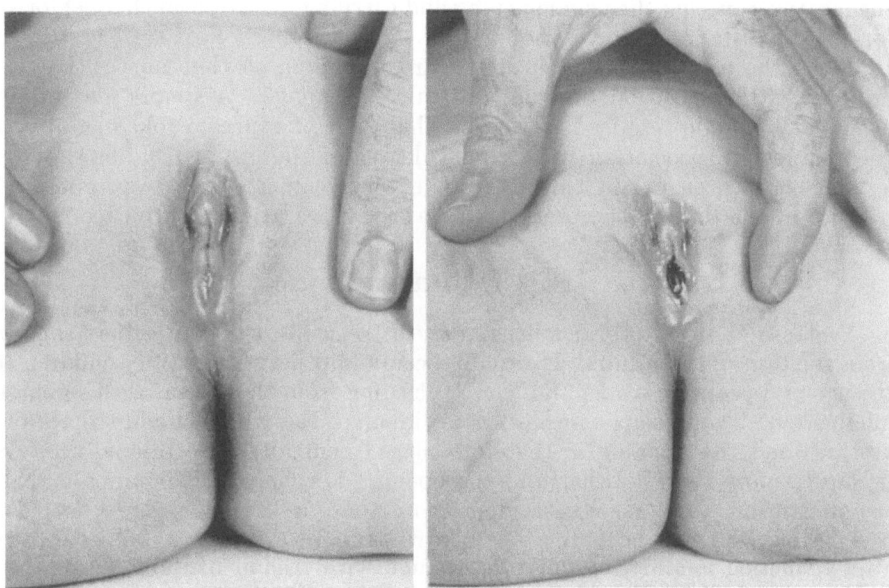

A   B

Fig. 150 A and B. Labial fusion. The external genitalia of a girl aged 3 years. A Showing adhesion of the edges of the labia minora. B After separation — normal vaginal introitus

confined to the labia minora, and thighs. In older children with urinary incontinence, more severe changes may be encountered, the vulval tissues becoming sodden, oedematous, and perhaps ulcerated.

4. Labial thickening

A leathery thickening of the labia results from habitual masturbation in some girls: it somewhat resembles the pubertal changes, but may be distinguished by the absence of other signs of precocity.

II. The external urinary meatus

1. Stenosis

Simple stenosis of the external urinary meatus may be seen from time to time in girls complaining of frequency and enuresis, though it is seldom a cause of serious urinary obstruction. The stenosis responds readily to instrumental dilatation, but the symptoms may take longer to disappear.

2. Hypospadias

Much more severe stenosis is seen in association with the deformity known as hypospadias of the female urethra, in which the meatus is placed above its normal situation on the anterior vaginal wall. With this deformity, chronic retention of urine may be encountered and the hidden opening of the urethra makes diagnosis difficult. Regular intermittent dilatation must be carried out over a prolonged period to ensure an adequate channel.

3. Covered meatus

In some otherwise normal girls, a fold of mucosa projects forward from behind the meatus, covering the usual opening and carrying the urethral channel forwards for a short distance towards the clitoris. At times this fold is sufficiently strong to divert the urinary stream in a forward direction, so that micturition in the ordinary sitting position becomes difficult to manage. A simple meatotomy is usually all that is required for cure. This type of mucosal fold has also been encountered in association with a mild degree of the epispadias deformity, and a very short urethra: in this case an extensive meatotomy was not advised because of the danger of upsetting the already precarious continence.

III. Urethral prolapse

Prolapse of the urethral mucosa may be seen in girls, and differs somewhat from the disorder in adults. It usually occurs in otherwise healthy children from the age of 3 years onwards, and causes bleeding from the vulva, with soreness on micturition. The prolapse in most cases involves the whole circumference of the urethra, and the opening is therefore placed centrally; exceptionally one wall prolapses more than another and the opening is then found in front or behind the protrusion. The mass is seldom more than 1—2 cm across, it is red and oedematous and can be reduced only with difficulty or not at all. Recurrence after reduction is almost invariable, though with rest in bed and sitz-baths the oedema may subside considerably and relieve all the symptoms. HIGGINS et al. have emphasized that conservative management may ultimately lead to spontaneous cure, but most authors have treated these cases by excision of the prolapsed portion of the urethra. This may be done by a circular incision with a diathermy knife on to a catheter, or the mass may be divided into two portions and ligatured. No stricture formation has been recorded after these operations.

In one case, now under my care, excision of a prolapse containing angiomatous tissue in a new born infant has left the child with a very short urethra and some stress incontinence of urine.

IV. Urethro-trigonitis

As in the case of the adult female, there is considerable difference of opinion among urologists as to the importance of minor changes in the urethral mucosa. Some authors (e.g. HODGES, ROEN and STEPT, SPENCE and MOORE, WINSBURY-WHITE) believe that in a high proportion of girls with frequency, dysuria, enuresis, and recurrent urinary infections, symptoms are due to urethritis although the urine may be sterile and free from deposit. The endoscopic findings in these cases include polyp formation at the bladder neck, granular areas and hillocks in the urethra and to a lesser extent on the trigone. It is claimed that very good results from instrumental dilatation are obtained in such cases.

The present writer believes that these changes are sometimes, though not frequently, important in cases of recurrent infection in the otherwise normal urinary tract, and has observed good results following instrumental dilatation of the urethra, but the significance of minor changes in cases where no infection has been present is more doubtful, and in enuresis the results of treatment of girls with "urethro-trigonitis" appear to be much the same as those with normal findings on urethroscopy.

V. Vulvo-vaginitis

The vaginal mucosa of the new born infant is comparable with that of the adult, being thick and stratified; the cells contain glycogen, the secretion is acid and Döderlein's bacilli are present. At this stage, vaginitis is unlikely to occur, though a slight white discharge may be seen as a result of the secretory activity of the cervical glands. As the influence of the maternal hormones recedes, the vaginal mucosa thins, until it is represented only by three or four layers of cells, and shows no keratinization of the superficial layers. The cells lose their glycogen content and the pH of the secretion increases to 7 or 8. This is the state of affairs before puberty, until which time the vagina presents little resistance to infection should any pathogenic organisms be introduced. Gonococcal vulvo-vaginitis was, in fact, a common and severe disease of childhood which could be acquired by simple non-venereal contact with clothing or towels used by infected individuals: fortunately the introduction of the antibiotics has so reduced the incidence of this infection that involvement of pre-pubertal girls is now very rarely seen. There remain, however, many cases of non-specific vaginitis of no great severity, but offering considerable resistance to treatment.

1. Gonococcal vulvo-vaginitis

The incidence and mode of infection differ considerably in various communities: thus in India MUKHERJEE reports that the age group 3—5 years was most commonly involved, and that cases were sporadic, the infection being transferred by infected parents or servants; while in Western countries epidemics in rather older children have accounted for most cases, infection being transferred from child to child in boarding schools and other institutions. In London in 1938, gonorrhoea accounted for 20 to 30% of all cases of vaginal discharge in children, whereas MUKHERJEE found gonococci in 54%.

The disease is characterized by a profuse, and irritating purulent discharge: there is marked dysuria and frequency, but other complications are uncommon. The vulva is acutely tender so that examination may be difficult; the urethral orifice is reddened and pouting, and in severe cases there may be some ulceration of the labia. The discharge should be washed away by a gentle stream of water, and a drop of pus taken with a pipette from within the vagina: microscopic examination of a smear and culture will confirm diagnosis.

Penicillin treatment is rapidly curative in the majority of cases and antibiotics will be successful in resistant infections. While the discharge is present, strict precautions must be taken against spread of infection to other children; clothes, towels etc., should be sterilized after use, baths and toilets should be carefully washed with disinfectant (see SCHAUFFLER).

2. Non-gonococcal vulvo-vaginitis

This category includes a variety of disorders, in some of which no definite infecting organism can be found. In a few cases a haemolytic Streptococcus, or a Staph. aureus produces an intense purulent discharge comparable with the gonococcal variety and as easily cured by chemotherapy. A retained foreign body will set up an acute inflammation with a discharge which is frequently blood-stained as well as purulent: it is seldom possible to obtain any history relevant to the introduction of the object for which the curiosity of the child or her companions is most frequently responsible. A careful search should be made in all cases. In many instances, the only organisms cultured from the discharge are diphtheroids, coliforms and other obvious contaminants: in these the discharge is often white rather than yellow and is comparatively scanty. This type of vulvo-vaginitis is frequently attributed to lack of hygiene and to general debility, and it is true that it is often found in children who are poorly cared for, who have deformities such as spastic diplegia which render cleansing difficult, or who are recovering from acute specific fevers. Periodic and self-terminating attacks of mild vulvo-vaginitis are also encountered in healthy girls, however, and are a source of great concern to parents with high standards of hygiene. SCHAUFFLER regards this type as the result of "hypoestrinism" and comparable to the senile vaginitis of the post-menopausal woman: there is no doubt that most of these cases recover at puberty. Trichomonas infection, and vaginal moniliasis are almost unknown in the pre-pubertal age group.

Where there is an acute onset and purulent discharge, bacteriological investigations and chemotherapy are clearly the immediate requirements, and internal examination may be deferred, but in less acute disorders a careful inspection of the vagina should be made. A urethroscope is a suitable instrument, which easily passes through the hymen of any normal child: some are quite tolerant of such procedures, but in most girls they are better conducted under anaesthesia. Removal of a foreign body, which may be quite small, will lead to immediate recovery.

In cases which resist systemic chemotherapy, and in which no foreign body is found, local hygiene and frequent baths are of the greatest importance, but little benefit is likely to be derived from douches or the introduction of chemotherapeutic agents in pellet form. Such intravaginal procedures should in fact be avoided in young girls if possible. Often the discharge is intermittent and so slight that the parents may simply be reassured that no serious infection is present, and that the disorder will clear spontaneously at puberty: when it is severe and troublesome oestrogens may be employed to bring about prematurely the pubertal changes in the vaginal mucosa. Stilboestrol, 0.5 mgm b.d., may be taken orally, or dienoestrol cream may be squeezed into the vagina from an ointment tube. Side effects, such as uterine bleeding and breast development may complicate oestrogen therapy if it is carried on for a long period.

VI. Urethral injuries and fistulae

Injury to the urethra of the female child is rare, but may result from falls astride sharp objects which penetrate the vagina from below, or very rarely from fractures of the pubis. In both cases, the formation of a urethro-vaginal fistula may follow, with or without, stricture formation in the distal urethra. At times the whole mid-portion of the urethra appears to be destroyed leaving only the external meatus below, and the bladder neck above opening directly into the vagina. Concomitant injury to the vagina and stenosis of the hymenal region may lead to a urinary hydrocolpos. The surgical repair of extensive urethro-vaginal fistulae is difficult, but exposure from below may be improved by a wide episiotomy, and closure of the defect in layers should be attempted.

VII. Hydrocolpos and haematocolpos

"Gynatresia", congenital vaginal obstruction, may produce symptoms at the two extremes of childhood: during the first weeks of life, and again at the onset of puberty.

In infants the obstruction is usually a tough membrane, considerably thicker than the normal hymen and often higher up the vagina. MAHONEY and CHAMBERLAIN believed that the commonly applied term "imperforate hymen" was incorrect, but the majority of cases have not been sufficiently carefully examined to determine the point. In my case, the membrane bulged down to the vulva from an attachment deeply within the vagina (Fig. 151).

Behind the obstruction there is an accumulation of white mucoid fluid, which causes an enormous distension of the vagina (hydrocolpos), and sometmes also a distension of the uterus (hydrometra). This fluid appears to be derived from the cervical glands which in utero and during the first week of life are actively secreting, being stimulated by the maternal hormones. The hydrocolpos displaces the bladder and frequently causes retention of urine, sometimes with upper urinary tract dilatation; the bowel is also obstructed, and in advanced cases there may

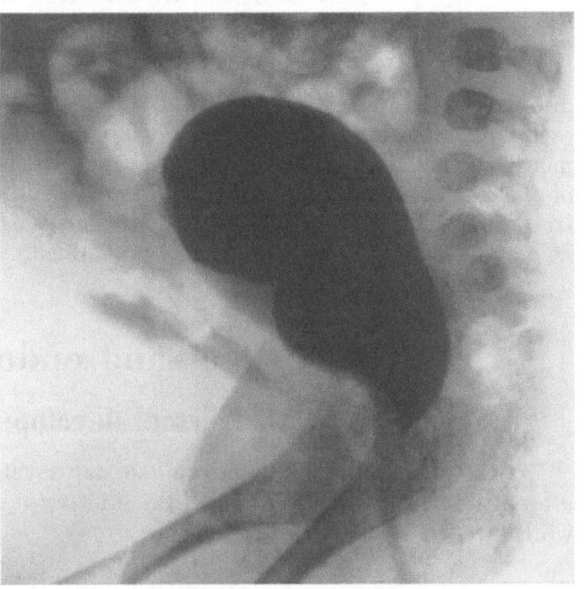

Fig. 151. Hydrocolpos. Colpogram in a premature female infant presenting with an abdominal tumour, due to the enormously distended vagina. Under anaesthetic an obstructing membrane was found some distance above the hymen, and this film was obtained after rupture of the membrane. A small amount of dye can be seen in the bladder, on the ventral aspect of the hydrocolpos

be a respiratory embarrassement, and oedema of the legs. The diagnosis is easily made, provided the vulva is carefully examined in all cases where a swelling is found arising from the pelvis.

Treatment should consist in simple ablation of the obstructing membrane. GROSS warns that where the bulging is extreme there may be some danger of injuring the urethra, and advises laparotomy, and drainage from above. In the majority, however, relief is rapidly obtained by simple incision and the only risk is that infection may be introduced.

Hydrocolpos may occasionally be seen in pubertal girls (MALIPHANT), but in the latter age group, haematocolpos due to the accumulation of menstrual fluid is the common finding. The child is brought up because of recurrent lower abdominal pain, and a blue bulging membrane is found at the vulva. Haematometra and haematosalpinx may complicate the haematocolpos, but provided adequate drainage is established and infection avoided, recovery is satisfactory and fertility is not threatened.

Hydrocolpos and hydrometra with septate vagina may be seen in association with anal atresia and urinary obstruction: these rare forms are discussed on p. 95.

Vaginal atresia may be acquired: trauma and infection can cause severe scarring and constriction of the outlet. Falls astride sharp objects may result in damage to the urethra as well, and producing a urethro-vaginal fistula with stricturing of the meatus. Urine was found dribbling through a minute opening in the posterior part of the scarred vulval orifice in one of my cases, and the vaginal cavity formed a large reservoir of infected urine. In this type of stenosis, simple dilatation of the vaginal constriction is inadequate, and a flap of skin should be turned in to enlarge the vulval opening.

VIII. Congenital absence of the vagina

Few symptoms appear during childhood in cases where the vagina is completely or partially absent, though on routine examination it may be found that only a dimple is present behind the urethral meatus. A uterus may be palpable on rectal examination in some, but it is usually rudimentary and incapable of menstruation. The anatomical findings, and the methods of plastic reconstruction of the vagina are described by McINDOE, and by BRYAN et al. Upper urinary tract abnormalities are frequently found in these cases: PHELAN et al. reported 26 examples in a series of 72 women examined.

P. Intersex states and endocrine disorders

I. Normal development

A brief discussion of the normal sexual development of the foetus and child is essential to the understanding of the intersex states and endocrine abnormalities which are the subject of this section.

1. The genetic basis

The genetic factors responsible for sexual development have been worked out in detail in insects and lower vertebrates in which experimental embryological methods are applicable. As far as can be judged from the simple histological observations, the conclusions reached are equally applicable to the mammals.

The genes concerned with female development are carried upon the X chromosome, and nuclei in the female possess an equal pair of these sex chromosomes (XX). The genes concerned with male developments are carried upon one of the autosomes (certainly in drosophila and probably in mammals); the male nuclei possess an unequal pair of sex chromosomes, one X chromosome, and one much smaller body, the Y chromosome. It appears that when the combination XX is present the female genes are strong enough to overcome the male autosomal genes, whereas with the combination XY the male factor dominates. During spermatogenesis and ovogenesis, a reduction division takes place so that the gamete possesses half the normal complement of autosomes, and only one sex chromosome: all ova must naturally have an X chromosome, whereas a sperm may have either an X or a Y. Fertilization of the ovum, and union of the gamete nuclei restores the full number of chromosomes and gives either an XY or an XX combination, a potential male or a potential female. This genetic combination determines the later development of the gonads, but once differentiation of the ovary or testis occurs, endocrine factors play an important part. During recent years it has been realised, largely as a result of the observation of BARR and his co-workers, that the ordinary somatic nuclei present a distinctive appearance in the two sexes. The phenomenon was first recognized in the nerve cells of the brain stem in the cat but the earliest cells used for routine examination were those in the skin. A small densely stained plano-convex body can be found lying immediately within the nuclear membrane in at least 70% of normal female cells, and in less than 5% of normal male cells. This body is believed to be connected with the XX combination of sex chromosomes, and is known as the sex chromatin (Barr) or chromocentre (Danon and Sachs). Similar chromatin masses have been identified in the mucosal cells derived from buccal or vaginal smears.

Davidson and Smith have described a distinctive appearance in the nuclei of the polymorph leucocytes. A rounded chromatin mass about 1 μ in diameter may be attached by a thread to some part of the nucleus, having something of the appearance of a drum stick. In some cells, the chromatin mass appears to be sessile and is much more difficult to identify. Typical drum sticks are found in 7—15% of normal female nuclei, none in normal male nuclei, though multiple nuclear tags may cause confusion to the inexperienced.

Either the epidermal or the polymorph method requires an experienced observer if it is to give reliable results, and there is little difference in their accuracy. Standard preparations of blood films are perhaps the more easily obtained.

This method of nuclear sexing has obviously provided a useful tool for research, and is of assistance in the diagnosis of the individual abnormalities. Its implications have yet to be fully worked out, and it is still too early to say to what extent abnormalities result from genetic factors affecting the sex chromosomes as opposed to later endocrine factors. Experimentally it has been possible (Chang and Witschi) to transform genetic male amphibians into functioning females so that the chromosomal factors are clearly not of paramount importance: similarly in the human Klinefelters's syndrome it has been observed that spermatogenesis may occur in genetic females (Bunge and Bradbury).

In gonadal agenesis (p. 287), the genetic sex of apparently female individuals is male, but in some it has been suggested that skin from different portions gives different results. Danon and Sachs suggest that these "mosaics" have an XO constitution, but most authors (e.g. Segal and Nelson) believe that the chromosome make-up is normal and that the anomaly lies in a failure of the germ cells.

In the pseudohermaphrodites there is little evidence to suggest any abnormality of the sex chromatin, with the doubtful exception of the intersex male with purely feminine genitalia (p. 283). Of the true hermaphrodites (Hinglais and Hinglais, Barr, Nelson) some are found to have the male, and some the female pattern of sex chromatin in the epithelial cells. In the case of Greene et al., there was a suggestion of an XXY formation, and Cathie has twice noted an incidence of 2—3% of drumsticks in the polymorph nuclei, a finding abnormal for either male or female. This variability in the true hermaphrodites limits the value of the test in the clinical diagnosis of intersex states, and it is still preferable to classify these conditions according to the histology of the gonad.

2. Endocrine factors

The embryonic gonad is indeterminate until the seventh week of foetal life, when medullary elements first show differentiation towards testicular tissue. The gonad destined to be an ovary does not differentiate until the tenth week when primordial follicles appear in the cortex. The subsequent development of the genital passages is dependent upon the presence of the gonad, and it has been shown experimentally in the rabbit (JOST) that if the gonad is destroyed, the female type of genitalia will appear whatever the genetic sex. A gonadal endocrine influence is therefore postulated, though its exact nature remains obscure, and there may be a more local effect since unilateral abnormalities may follow unilateral damage. Very little is in fact known about the normal endocrine influences operative during foetal life, and although many of the intersex abnormalities are attributed to such influences, few of these hypotheses can be proved.

The initiation of normal puberty is apparently due to changes in the hypothalamus, which acts upon the peripheral organs through the secretions of the anterior pituitary gland. Two pituitary gonadotropic hormones are known: one, the follicle stimulating hormone (F.S.H.) stimulates the development of Graafian follicles in the ovary, and the spermatic tubules in the testis. The other, the luteinizing hormone (L.H.) controls the corpora lutea and the interstitial cells of the testis. The gonads in their turn produce two hormones, which have an effect on the secondary sex organs, and also by a "feed-back" mechanism modify the pituitary activity. The ovarian hormones are oestrogen and progesterone, the testicular hormones, testosterone from the interstitial cells, and probably also "inhibin" from the tubules.

Gonadotropic hormone excretion, chiefly F.S.H., can be measured in the urine; it is normally almost undetectable in childhood, but rises sharply at puberty to the adult level (< 60 mouse units/24 hours). In the absence of a normal response from the testicle or ovary, an even greater rise will occur as in gonadal agenesis and some forms of male hypogonadism.

Oestrogens may be present in minimal amounts in young children of both sexes: in girls a slight rise commences at about the age of eight years, and then there is a rapid increase about three years later. Thereafter, with normal menstruation, there is a cyclical rise and fall, so that single estimations are of little value, and must always be considered in relation to the period. This same observation applies to cases of precocious puberty. Progesterone estimation has little place in paediatric work.

Testosterone, derived from the testicular interstitial cells, is excreted in the form of 17-ketosteroids, together with androgenic substances derived from the adrenal cortex, and despite numerous attempts at fractionation it is still not possible to identify the precise origin of urinary 17-ketosteroids.

The anterior pituitary also produces a hormone ACTH which stimulates the adrenal cortex, and the latter in turn secretes hydrocortisone which among other things regulates ACTH production. The adrenal cortex is responsible for many hormones, among them androgens and to a lesser extent oestrogens, disorders of which are discussed later in this section. Both adrenal and gonadal factors can produce abnormalities of sexual development in both pre-natal and post-natal life. In the prepubertal stage the measurement of the 24 hour output of 17-ketosteroids provides an adequate estimate of the androgenic activity of the adrenal cortex: the normal levels are set out in the table below. It will be seen that the excretion is very low during the first six years of life, it rises a little after this time and then more steeply at puberty in both sexes. It is believed that adrenal androgens are responsible for the growth of pubic hair in girls.

Normal excretion of 17-ketosteroids

Age		
0— 1 years	. . . . . .	0.25 ± 0.12 mgm/24 hours
1— 5 years	. . . . . .	0.78 ± 0.4 mgm/24 hours
6—10 years	. . . . . .	1.38 ± 0.64 mgm/24 hours
11—16 years	. . . . . .	4.96 ± 1.97 mgm/24 hours

(Ref.: PROUT, M., and A. H. SNAITH, awaiting publication)

Normal excretion of oestrogen in prepubertal girls

Age 0— 6 years . . . . . . nil
7—10 years . . . . . . less than 1.0 μgm/24 hours
11—12 years . . . . . . 2.9—4.1 μgm/24 hours
(Ref.: SNAITH, A. H., personal communication)

3. The anatomical growth changes

During the first two or three weeks after birth, the female genital organs exhibit the effects of stimulation by the maternal hormones. The uterus is congested and is almost twice the weight of that in an infant aged one year: the cervical glands are active and may produce a slight white discharge, and vaginal bleeding from the endometrium is said to occur in 1% of normal infants (TALBOT et al.). A slight enlargement of the breasts and the production of a few drops of milk may be observed in most infants of either sex. The labia and clitoris appear larger and more prominent in the new born partly because of the relative absence of subcutaneous fat in the surrounding area.

The ovaries in infancy are long and slender, having an almost ribbon-like appearance: they enlarge slowly until puberty, when they have attained the characteristic almond shape, but the surface is quite smooth, in contrast to the irregular pitted surface of the adult organ. After the age of 10 years a few follicles begin to develop sufficiently to produce some oestrogens.

The age of onset of puberty varies greatly from one individual to another, and from one race to another: it is also influenced by the nutritional state of the child. Puberty is a gradual process which takes some years to complete: breast enlargement is the first sign, and is followed by the appearance of pubic hair. Menstruation, irregular and often anovular at first, comes later, and axillary hair is the last development. Menstruation normally starts between 10 and $16^1/_2$ years of age, most often at 13 years.

In the normal male infant at birth, the penis and scrotum are large and lax; the testicles are easily palpated. During the subsequent months, subcutaneous fat accumulates so that the penis, which is growing slowly, appears to be relatively smaller, and may even become buried in pubic fat. The dartos muscle is active and the scrotum varies in size but is seldom as lax as in the neonate. The cremasteric activity results in readily retractile testicles, which when drawn up into the groin are difficult to feel in the surrounding fat.

During the earlier years of childhood, the baby fat may be lost, allowing the penis to be more evident, but actual growth of the external genitalia is very slow indeed. Normal puberty may occur at any age between 9 and 17 years, and the process may take as long as 3 years to complete. Externally the first change to be noted is an increase in the size of the testicles: subsequently androgen stimulation results in the enlargement of the penis, growth of pubic hair, deepening of the voice, and the appearance of acne on the face. The testicles now cease to be actively retractile, and remain in the scrotum.

Histologically the testicles of the normal infant at birth contain a high proportion of well differentiated interstitial cells, due it is believed to the stimulation by maternal gonadotropic hormones, and these cells disappear almost entirely during the first three weeks of post-natal life.

From the age of 3 weeks to 4 years the seminiferous tubules are small (66 μ) and straight, they are almost without a lumen, and the cells have a uniform character save for occasional large cells destined to be spermatogonia. During the next 6 years, changes are slow; the tubules become more tortuous, and very slightly larger, a lumen is clearly defined but only a single layer of cells is present

18*

around it. Rapid enlargement of the tubules occur at about the age of 10, and is followed by the appearance of interstitial cells. Differentiation within the tubules, and the maturation of spermatozoa may take 3—4 years to complete (CHARNEY et al.).

II. Female pseudohermaphroditism

In the female pseudohermaphrodite, the only gonadal tissue is ovarian and the external genitalia are partly or completely masculine in appearance. The majority of cases are hormonal in origin.

1. Congenital adreno-cortical hyperplasia

Following the pioneer work of LAWSON WILKINS this disorder is now recognized as a common affliction of both sexes, although more often diagnosed in the female in whom it produces an intersex state. At present it appears to account for a majority of infant admissions to hospital for diagnosis of sex. GRUMBACH has estimated that in Maryland one individual in 58,000 was affected, and with CHILDS has traced the family history of a large group of patients: they believe the disorder to be genetically determined, by a recessive autosomal gene, and find some evidence of a minor adrenal abnormality in healthy parents of their cases.

a) Anatomy

At birth, the female pseudohermaphrodite with adrenocortical hyperplasia has a moderately enlarged phallus, prominent and often slightly rugose labia, and a urogenital sinus opening in a hypospadiac position (Fig. 152). Often this opening corresponds to a perineal hypospadias, but occasionally it simulates the penile variety, and when the phallus is acutely kinked downward by chordee, the urethra may reach the coronal sulcus. BENTINCK et al. have recorded a case with a complete penile urethra, but more common is the perineal opening in which the vaginal orifice can just be visualized. The vagina, which is normally capacious, opens into the urethra through a small orifice at the level of the perineal membrane; the uterus, Fallopian tubes and ovaries are normal in size and position. Both adrenal glands are grossly hypertrophied; the origin of the hypertrophied cells cannot be identified precisely though they resemble somewhat the "foetal cortex".

b) Clinical progress

The virilizing effects of the adrenal activity continue unchecked after birth, and result in precocious somatic growth and sexual development upon male lines. The phallus becomes considerably enlarged, and frequent erections occur from the age of 3 of 4 years onwards; pubic hair appears during the first few years and quickly thickens. The skin is coarse and acne-form, the voice breaks early. Muscular development is advanced, and the centres of ossification appear early; during the first years these individuals are considerably bigger than their contempories but, in spite of the early spurt of growth, premature fusion of the epiphyses occurs and by adolescence they are short for their years, particularly in the limbs (Fig. 153). Menstruation very seldom occurs in untreated cases, though it is on record (EVERIDGE). Breast development is absent. The sexual inclinations of these children usually accord with the role in which they have been brought up (MONEY and HAMPSON), which in turn depends largely upon the anatomy of the vulva noted at birth: those raised as boys have often led an active sexual life after repair of hypospadias, and have made satisfactory though sterile husbands. There are some records of untreated cases voluntarily changing their role from female to male in early adult life (GENITIS and BRONSTEIN); there is no doubt that those brought up as girls, before the introduction of cortisone, passed very unsatisfactory lives and a behaviour disorder was not uncommon.

Apart from the virilizing effect of adrenal hyperplasia, many of these children suffer in early infancy from episodes of acute adrenal insufficiency, resembling Addisonian crises, and in the past they have often died from this condition undiagnosed. Vomiting is sometimes projectile, and mistaken for the effects of pyloric stenosis. Severe dehydration and collapse are the characteristic signs but hypotension is not a feature. These crises are apt to occur after operation or instrumentation, and this fact should be born in mind when a newborn is brought up for the diagnosis of sex. The liability to this type of imbalance lessens

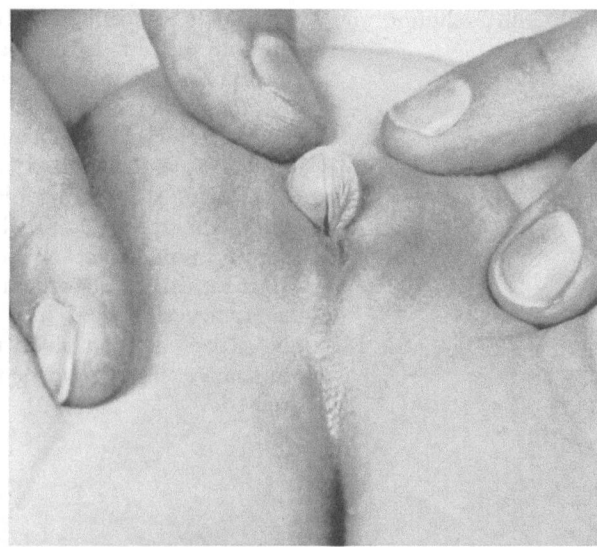

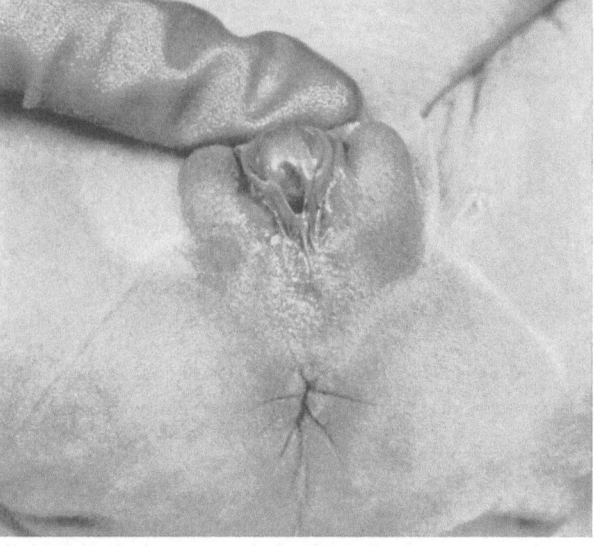

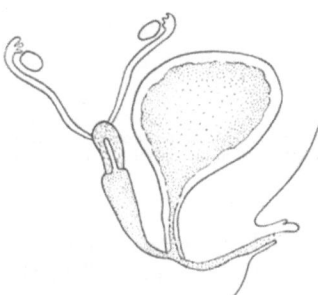

Fig. 152. Female pseudohermaphrodites with adrenal hyperplasia. The external genitalia of two infants brought up for determination of sex. Both suffered from severe electrolyte disturbances. The anatomical arrangement is shown in the inset diagram

in the later years of childhood, but until then a mild infection may sometimes be rapidly fatal.

Hypertension is a feature of some older children recorded by WILKINS, and may also be due to overtreatment with cortisone or related steroids. Urinary infection, perhaps due to an undrained vaginal reservoir has been seen in some.

c) Laboratory findings

The nuclear chromatin is invariably of the female pattern.

The 17-ketosteroid excretion is raised: in the newborn it is usually over 2 mgm/ 24 hour, and rises steadily during the first six or seven years of life, up to 20 to 40 mgm/24 hours, and even higher in adult life. In a few neonates, the 17-keto-steroid output is normal, and the figures should be checked again after three months in doubtful cases.

Pregnanetriol excretion is also raised along with the total ketosteroids (normal 0—1.8 mgm/24 hours, BON-GIOVANNI and EBERLEIN).

During the "Addisonian" crises there is a depression of serum sodium and chloride, and a marked rise of serum potassium, which not infrequently reaches 10 mEq/litre. Electrocardiographic changes may accompany this rise, but are not as marked as might be expected. The blood urea is also raised in the crises in some cases even after the dehydration has been corrected.

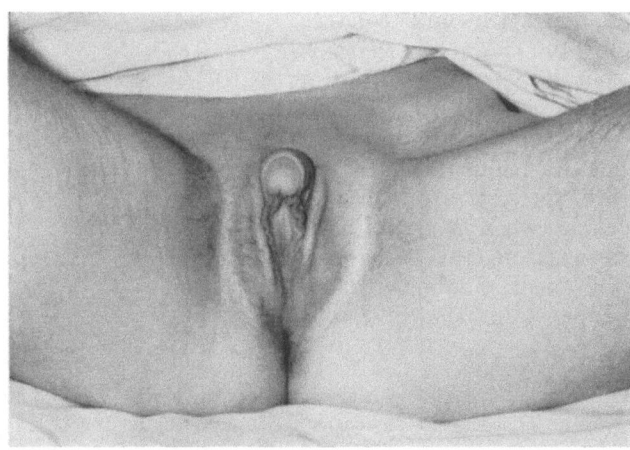

A   B

Fig. 153 A and B. Adrenal cortical hyperplasia causing pseudohermaphroditism in the female: appearance at 12 years after cortisone therapy commenced at the age of 9 years. Menstruation has started and breast development is normal, but the large phallus remains unchanged. The premature fusion of epiphyses has led to shortening of the limbs compared to the trunk

The effects of treatment in cases of adrenal hyperplasia have greatly aided the understanding of the fundamental disorder. Cortisone causes a rapid fall in the androgens, and clinically brings to a halt the virilizing process; started in infancy and continued over a long period it allows normal development to proceed, and appears to act as substitition therapy. It is postulated that the primary failure is an inability on the part of the adrenals to complete the synthesis of hydrocortisone, the process stops short at the formation of 17-hydroxyprogesterone which is excreted in the form of pregnanetriol. In the absence of circulating hydrocortisone which normally inhibits pituitary secretion, ACTH is produced in large amounts and leads to adrenal hypertrophy: this in turn raises the output of androgenic substances. Cortisone administration leads to a fall in the ACTH output, and therefore allows the adrenals to drop back to a more normal level of activity. This hypothesis explains most of the features of the disease, though some problems still remain: it might be anticipated that in the crises there would be a lowered output of aldosterone, but this has not in fact been observed.

d) Diagnosis

An infant with genitalia of equivocal sexuality and a raised 17-ketosteroid and pregnanetriol output is undoubtedly suffering from adrenal hyperplasia: the appearance of the external genitalia is mimicked both by other forms of male and female pseudohermaphroditism, and by true hermaphrodites, while a raised 17-ketosteroid output occurs in adrenal tumour. Hyperplasia cases presenting in childhood have almost always had the disorder since birth, whereas most tumours are post-natal developments. Pregnanetriol output is raised only in hyperplasia, and cortisone therapy reduces both this and total 17-ketosteroid output in hyperplasia but not in tumour.

An infant with severe hypospadias and unexplained vomiting is probably a female pseudohermaphrodite; the observation of female sex chromatin confirms this, and indicates the need for immediate investigation of the electrolytes and androgen excretion before anything further is attempted. Endoscopy will reveal an occult vagina and normal uterine cervix.

e) Management

Cases seen in infancy must be treated continuously with cortisone and, provided the dose is correctly judged, may achieve normal female development. Dosage must be worked out empirically, as in balancing a diabetic, and should be adjusted to keep the 17-ketosteroid output at a normal level. Young infants often require about 25 mgm a day by mouth as initial therapy, but this can sometimes be lowered for maintenance. WILKINS emphasizes that oral cortisone should be given in three or four daily doses, as its effect is short-lived, and believes that some failures to control these cases have resulted from infrequent administration. The dose will rise with increasing age, up to 50 mgm/day.

Cortisone therapy cannot of course reverse the anatomical abnormality, and when it is started late in childhood, will not cause loss of pubic hair or any change in the voice if this has broken. If the treatment is commenced after the bone age (not the chronological age) has reached 11 or 12 years, there is likely to be an immediate onset of menstruation and breast development (WILKINS). Late treatment cannot, of course, affect bone growth when epiphyseal fusion has already occurred, but when the child has been brought up as a girl there is no doubt at all that the feminization which it produces is of great value, and the appearance of the genitalia can be corrected by excision of the clitoris and opening up of the vaginal orifice.

When an infant has been regarded as a male, the parents should be advised to change the sexual role; when an older child has been brought up as a boy, and is already well adapted to the male role, it is better to with-hold cortisone, repair the hypospadias, and accept the stunting of growth processes, for a change of established sex is fraught with grave psychological dangers. HAMPSON suggests that it is unwise to change after the age of $2^{1}/_{2}$ years.

The infant with Addisonian crises requires very careful management: cortisone therapy must be supplemented by the administration of DOCA (1—2 mgm/day) and salt (about 5 gm/day). The exact dosage must be judged by the regular estimation of the serum electrolytes. Fluorohydrocortisone produces a more rapid response in electrolyte imbalance, given in a dose of

0.1—0.2 mgm/day: higher doses may lead to excessive sodium retention and hypertension (Cox) and it is seldom a suitable drug for maintenance.

Surgical excision of adrenal tissue, which was extensively practised before the introduction of cortisone (BROSTER) now has little place in therapy. Unilateral adrenalectomy does bring down the 17-ketosteroid output, though there is usually a later rise. In one of my cases, in which cortisone alone appeared to be inadequate, the operation did, however, seem to be of value.

2. Other forms of female pseudohermaphroditism

Rarely children whose genitalia resemble those of the previous group and have female sex chromatin, may be found to exhibit no signs of adrenal hyper-plasia. There is no exces-sive excretion of 17-keto-steroids or pregnanetriol, precocious development does not occur, the uterus and ovaries are normal, and at least some have ulti-mately commenced men-struation: after plastic sur-gery COTTE's case became pregnant. Usually no cause can be assigned for this abnormality, and the cases must be regarded as com-parable to, though much less common than, the male pseudohermaphrodites de-scribed in the next section. When the genital deformity is severe, great difficulty is encountered in diagnosis, and laparotomy with gona-dal biopsy is essential. PA-PADATOS and KLEIN record

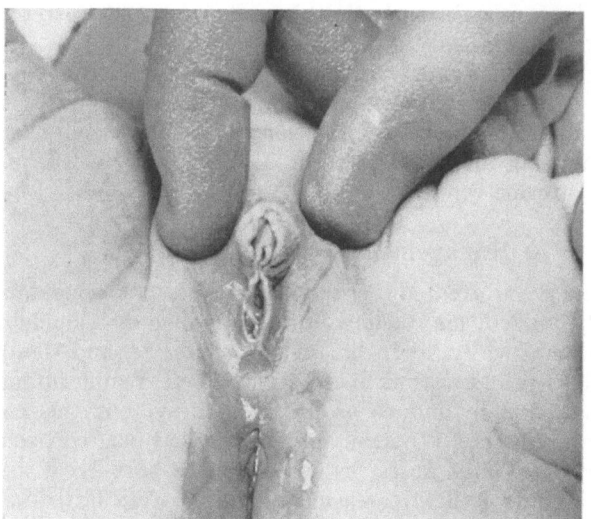

Fig. 154. Female pseudohermaphroditism. The external genitalia of a child aged 3 weeks, whose mother had received testosterone therapy starting at the twelfth week of pregnancy. The clitoris is grossly enlarged but the genitalia are otherwise normal. Sex chromatin of the female pattern. No excess of 17 ketosteroids in the urine

two cases in which renal failure, and a consequent electrolyte disturbance, led to the suspicion of adrenal deficiency, which was later disproved. In less severe cases an extrinsic hormonal influence may be detected: the enlargement of the clitoris, illustrated in Fig. 154, occurred in a child whose mother had received large doses of methyl testosterone from the 12th week of pregnancy in order to prevent abortion, and several other examples of this association of events are on record (HAYLES and NOLAN, ZANDER and MÜLLER). A similar appearance has been observed in the child born of a woman suffering from arrhenoblastoma (BRENTNALL). The follow-up of these infants is not on record, but there seems little reason to doubt that, apart from the anatomical deformity, development will be normally feminine.

In a different category are the female pseudohermaphrodites with genital passages of the arrangement shown in Fig. 155, and usually with urinary obstruction. A minute penis is present, with a terminal meatus, indistinguishable from the organ illustrated in Fig. 140, but testicles cannot be palpated. In a specimen of this type preserved in the museum of the Royal College of Surgeons,

London, the bladder was heavily trabeculated with two large diverticula (see WILLIAMS). A minute vaginal opening may be found in the perineum, and there may be some communication between the vagina and urethra (HOWARD and HINMAN, BROSTER). The sex chromatin is female, the uterus and ovaries normal. These cases are likely to have been reared as boys, yet satisfactory relief of urinary

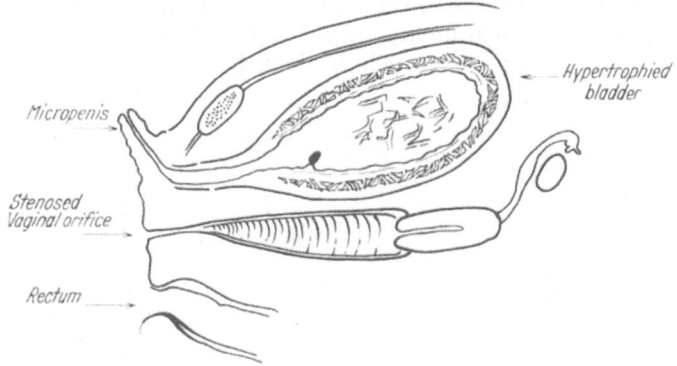

Fig. 155. Diagram to show the arrangement of the genital and urinary passages in the type of female pseudo-hermaphroditism with micropenis and urinary obstruction

obstruction may demand a perineal opening for the urethra, and a change of role may be desirable.

III. Male pseudohermaphroditism

The male pseudohermaphrodite has testicles, but incomplete masculine development of the external genitalia, often accompanied by Müllerian duct differentiation. There is no clear distinction between male pseudohermaphroditism and simple hypospadias of severe degree.

1. Male pseudohermaphrodites with external genitalia of equivocal sexuality

In this group there is a wide variation in anatomy, and though a familial incidence is sometimes recorded it is not common. A severe degree of hypospadias is always present, and this together with a small penis may be the only abnormality (Fig. 156): the testicles in such a case may be simply overlooked at birth, although they descend fully into the labio-scrotal folds. In other case, there is a development of the Müllerian duct system along female lines: a vagina may open into the urethra, or may be evident in the "vulva", it may be short and blind or of normal length, though it is seldom so capacious or so supple as in the female. It often leads up to a small and eccentric uterus. Both Fallopian tubes and vasa deferentia may be present, and the testicles may lie on the broad ligament, on the posterior abdominal wall, or in the inguinal region. Occasionally only one testicle can be found.

At birth the external genitalia are often indistinguishable from those of the female pseudohermaphrodite or the true hermaphrodite, and the diagnosis can only be made clinically when both testicles are definitely felt in the labio-scrotal folds. Growth proceeds normally throughout childhood, and male pubertal changes will occur at the usual age unless there is a severe degree of hypogonadism. Periodic uterine haemorrhage is not observed but intermittent and irregular bleeding is sometimes a feature: in one of my cases a male pseudo-hermaphrodite developed a severe haematocolpos shortly after birth.

The psychological orientation depends largely upon the diagnosis which is made at birth and the mode of upbringing: when the child is recognized as a male, development is normal; when he is put in the female category there are three possible effects. Most accept their role, but, being conscious of some anatomical and physiological abnormality, avoid any intimate contacts. A few develop a voracious sexual appetite which is denied satisfaction by their deformity. Others again, in later childhood or adolescence, have such a markedly masculine outlook that a change of role becomes inevitable.

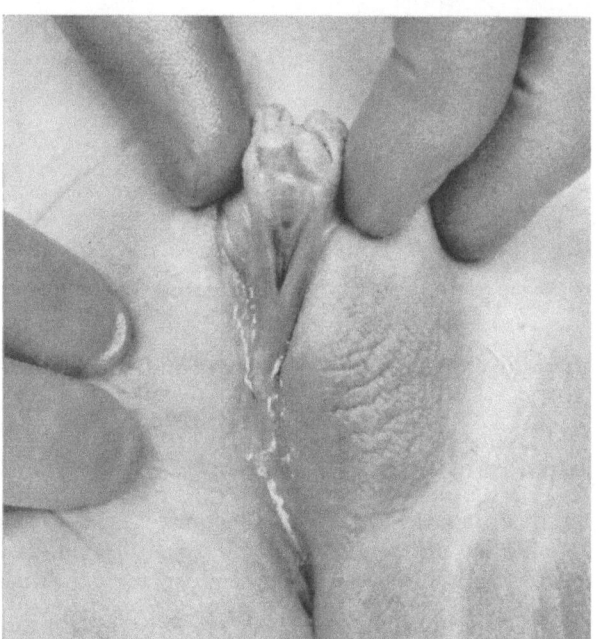

Fig. 156. Male pseudohermaphrodite. Child aged 2¹/₂ years with small penis, perineal hypospadias and no palpable gonads. Two testicles were present within the abdomen

A diagnosis of male pseudohermaphroditism can be made with certainty in a child with genitalia of equivocal sexuality, when both testicles are palpable, when urethroscopy shows a normal verumontanum, when the sex chromatin is male in pattern, and when the 17-ketosteroid excretion is normal. In the more complex cases the differential diagnosis from true hermaphroditism presents great difficulties, and if a vagina and uterus is present, it will be necessary to proceed to gonadal biopsy in order to establish the facts beyond doubt. In an infant with a large phallus, whose external appearance indicates that he is best suited for the male role, this confirmatory biopsy may be postponed until the time of the hypospadias repair, for even if ovarian tissue is found, it will need to be excised.

As in other varieties of pseudohermaphroditism the management will depend upon the circumstances in which the child is brought up. In a new born infant sent for diagnosis of sex, the male role is usually advisable unless the phallus is so minute that no adequate penis could be constructed. In a child recognized as male, plastic surgery is required, and at the same time that hypospadias repair is completed, it is wise to perform a hysterectomy and colpectomy. This prevents the accumulation of secretions in what amounts to a urethral diverticulum, and obviates the danger that later slight haemorrhage will raise once more doubts as to the sex of the individual. In a child raised as a girl it is difficult to lay down definite rules. For the adolescent who is well adapted to the female role, there should be no question of a change, and any child with a minute phallus is better left as a girl, since no satisfactory male sex life would be possible. Castration and oestrogen therapy are then advisable. A change is inevitable in a few cases, when the outlook and appearance of the genitalia are strongly masculine.

Some male pseudohermaphrodites have normal external genitalia except for an undescended testicle on one or both sides, yet operation reveals a well developed muscular uterus, perhaps with Fallopian tubes reaching down to the testicles (NILSON, KOZOLL, KEEN and DE VILLIERS). The only treatment required in these cases is hysterectomy combined with orchidopexy.

Pseudohermaphroditism is not infrequently found in infants with multiple congenital abnormalities, especially those involving the cloaca (p. 95).

2. Male pseudohermaphrodites with purely feminine external genitalia

These cases, which form a well defined group, have been variously classified under the heading of "Adenoma tubulare type" and "Testicular feminization" (MORRIS). Neither term is satisfactory, however, since the first describes an occasional and unimportant feature of the testicular histology, while the second makes an entirely unjustifiable assumption as to the nature of the disease. Affected individuals exhibit external genitalia of normally feminine appearance (Fig. 157) and the general bodily form is also of the female type. The vagina is short, however, and ends immediately above the hymen in a small mass of

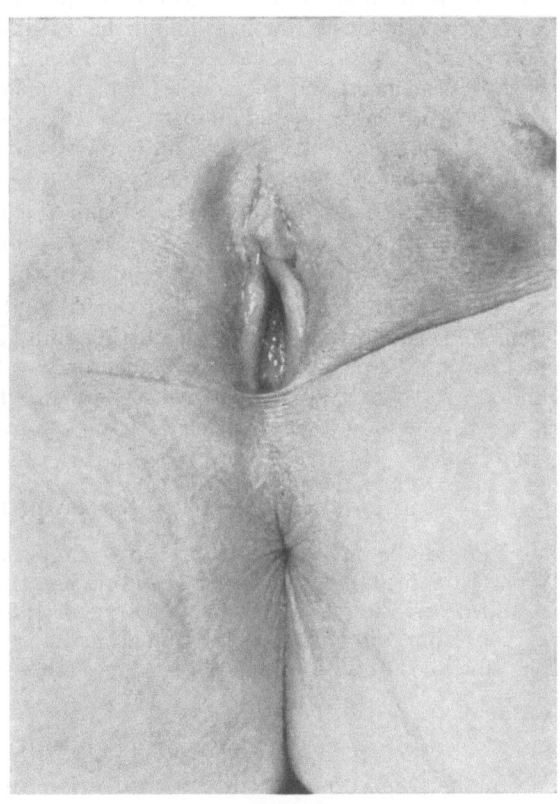

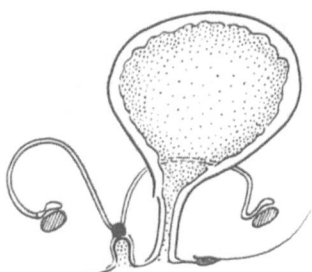

Fig. 157. Male pseudohermaphrodite with purely feminine external genitalia. Child age 1 year examined for a mass in the groin, which proved to be a testicle. Anatomy of the genital passages shown in the inset diagram

fibrous tissue, perhaps representing the uterus, from which spring vasa deferentia. Testicles, of normal appearance in childhood, lie just within the abdomen, in the inguinal canal, or the labio-scrotal folds. Growth is normal throughout childhood, and cases only present at this stage with suspected hernia. After puberty, the pubic and axillary hair is found to be scanty or absent; breast development occurs but is less than normal and there is amenorrhoea. The testicles undergo the characteristic changes seen in the undescended organs, and some show small tubular adenomata. The emotional orientation is female, and many of these individuals have entered marriage, though intercourse is unsatisfactory for physical reasons. A high familial incidence is recorded in this condition; in some families all the male offspring have been affected (MISHELL, SEGAL and NELSON).

The sex chromatin is usually reported as of the ordinary male pattern, though DANON and SACHS have maintained that examination of the epithelial cell nuclei suggests an XXY formation. They thus believe that the condition has a genetic basis, due perhaps to the presence of an XXX formation in the mother or of a failure of the normal reduction division in the maternal ova. Examination of the chromatin pattern in the polymorphs in my own cases by Dr. I. A. B. CATHIE does not appear to support this view. SEGAL and NELSON accept that the sex chromatin is of the XY pattern, and suggest that a maternal anti-testis factor may be at work during foetal life, preventing the normal development of the genital passages. The levels of hormone excretion are reported to be within the normal limits in most cases (STERN and VANDERVORT), despite the suggestion that the testicle might be responsible for an unusual output of oestrogen (MORRIS). HEALEY and GUY record a case dying at the age of 26 years with hypertension and considerable enlargement of both adrenals, while PRADER and GURTNER investigated an infant with this anatomy who died of an Addisonian crisis at the age of 6 weeks. The adrenals were hyperplastic but the output of 17-Ketosteroid was normal. These cases are exceptional but deserve attention.

Diagnosis in childhood is made from the observation of the gonads in the groin, the short vagina and the male sex chromatin. The last two facts will distinguish them from cases of prolapse of the ovaries into hernial sacs.

All these children are brought up as girls, and there is no indication for changing their sex. The testicles are often a little painful and are a source of embarrassment in later life: it is likely that orchidectomy will be undertaken sooner or later, and provided oestrogen therapy is commenced at puberty, there is little to be lost by removing these testicles early, before the child has any idea of their significance.

IV. True hermaphroditism

Individuals in this category are comparatively rare, yet the number of reported cases increases steadily, and no less than five have come under my care. A full description was given by YOUNG in 1937, based on the 20 cases reported at that time, and in spite of numerous subsequent papers very little addition has since been made to our knowledge of the condition.

1. Anatomy

In the true hermaphrodite both ovarian and testicular tissue is present, and at puberty there is evidence of both male and female development. The gonads may appear as typical ovaries or testicles, perhaps one on either side, perhaps both forms on the same side. In many cases an ovotestis is found, a body which is ovarian at one end and testicular at the other. The distinction between the two parts is usually evident to the naked eye, but in some the dual nature is only discovered on histological examination. In the mature ovaries there are Graafian follicles and corpora lutea, so that ova are probably released normally, but sometimes atrophic tissue is found containing only stromal elements. There is no known instance of pregnancy in a true hermaphrodite. In the testicles, spermatogenesis is occasionally complete and live spermatozoa in the ejaculate have been observed: paternity was presumed in GREENE and MATTHEWS case. Often, however, the testicle is retained within the abdomen and sclerotic.

The anatomy of the genital passages is extremely variable. A phallus of moderate size is the rule, and a urethra usually opens in a hypospadiac position (Fig. 158), but a complete penis with a terminal urethral meatus, or a female type of urethra opening into the vulva may also occur. A uterus is almost always present, though it is often eccentric or bicornuate. A vagina will certainly be found if it is sought; it may open into the urethra at or below the level of the verumontanum, it may open nor-mally in the vulva, or through a small meatus in the skin of the perineum.

A scrotum, complete or bifid is often found, and a testicle or ovotestis may descend fully into it, even though accompanied by a Fallopian tube. An ovary, however, exhibits no tendency to descend into the scrotum, and no true hermaphrodite is on record with two fully descended gonads.

The sex chromatin may be either of the male or female pattern (BARR), but anomalous results may be obtained in performing this in-vestigation. Hormone excretion studies have not produced any useful information.

2. Clinical features

Growth proceeds normally in childhood, but a confusion of signs appears in puberty. Breast deve-lopment reaches normal female proportions, and periodic uterine bleeding commences at 12—14 years of age: where the vagina opens into

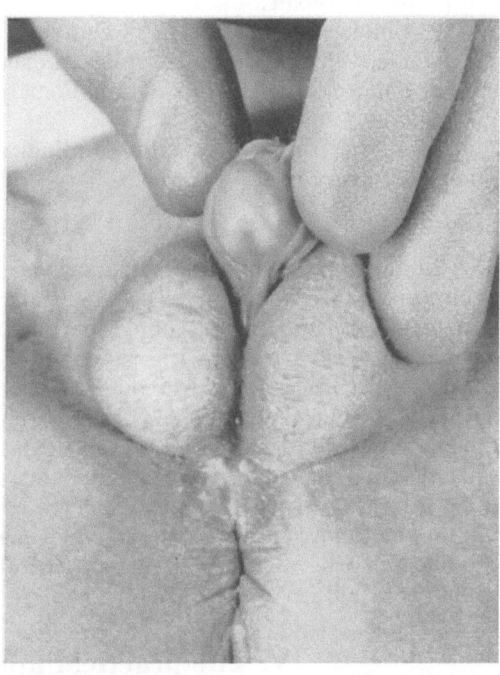

Fig. 158. True hermaphrodite. Child aged 2 months brought up for determination of sex. Sex chromatin estimation in the polymorphs give equivocal results. Endoscopy showed a well formed vagina and cervix. At laparotomy, the uterus and Fallopian tubes appeared normal: a well developed testicle was present on the right side, where there was an inguinal hernia; an atrophic ovary lay beneath the left tube

the urethra, this bleeding is often interpreted as haematuria. At the same time, the phallus enlarges, hair appears on the face, and the voice breaks. The psycho-logical orientation of the true hermaphrodite depends very largely upon the upbringing, and therefore follows the parents' initial decision as to the sex based upon the general form of the genitalia. The pubertal developments naturally lead to a serious emotional disturbance, though very few have been bivalent in their sexual relations. It is clearly desirable that the diagnosis should be made during childhood, so that removal of the gonad inappropriate to the sexual role will prevent these pubertal complications.

3. Diagnosis

The diagnosis can only be made with certainty from biopsy of both gonads, a procedure which usually involves laparotomy, but in view of the importance of surgical treatment before puberty there should be no hesitation in taking this step in doubtful cases. Paediatric surgery has now reached the stage where such an exploratory operation carries a risk very little greater than a simple endoscopy, and I am accustomed to advise laparotomy for diagnosis even in early infancy. The types of cases which require investigation are:

a) Children with genitalia of equivocal sexuality, in whom a vagina is found by simple examination or endoscopy, and whose sex chromatin pattern is male. When the genitalia are predominantly masculine, and it is certain the child must be reared as a boy, laparotomy may be postponed until the time of hypospadias repair.

b) Children with genitalia of equivocal sexuality whose sex chromatin pattern is female, yet who do not excrete an excess of 17-ketosteroids or pregnanetriol.

c) Children with micropenis and no palpable gonads, whether the sex chromatin is male or female.

In taking the biopsy a longitudinal strip should be removed from the full length of every gonad found.

4. Management

In an infant brought for diagnosis of sex, the choice of role will depend upon the appearance of the external genitalia: this is more often male than female. In an older child, there should be no attempt to change the role unless it is obviously at variance with the child's inclinations and appearance. In the "males", ovarian tissue should be excised and the uterus and tubes removed. Repair of hypospadias and, when practical, orchidopexy may follow. Late cases also require mastectomy. In the "females", orchidectomy, clitoridectomy and plastic enlargement of the vaginal orifice are indicated. As in all intersex states, it is essential that parents should have confidence that following treatment there is no longer any question of the child being half one thing or half the other: he or she must be allowed to live an entirely normal life in the chosen role, unhampered by any sense of deformity.

V. The practical approach to intersex

Deformities of the external genitalia which throw doubt upon the true sex of the child constitute an important problem confronting the paediatric urologist: cases are relatively common, and important decisions must be taken which affect the whole life and happiness of the child. In the past, and sometimes even more recently, great misery has been occasioned by indecision and inadequate diagnosis: parents who have been told to wait and see how the child develops are in a state of perpetual anxiety which is inevitably communicated to the child, and if a change of sexual role is advised they often find it necessary to give up all their friends and move to a part of the world where the family was previously unknown. Not only is such temporizing disastrous to the emotional balance of all concerned, but it is also apt to be inconclusive since the majority of cases the sexual orientation depends upon the upbringing and therefore upon the initial decision. Exceptions to this rule certainly occur, as has been noted in the previous discussion, and they reinforce the view that an accurate diagnosis must be made in infancy. It cannot of course be predicted with certainty that an infant correctly assigned to a male or female role will not ultimately develop homosexual tendencies, but an anatomically normal infant is in no better position from this viewpoint, and clinical histories leave little doubt that the emotional problems of the intersex cases are due chiefly to unresolved doubts and to a sense of deformity which could have been avoided by early diagnosis and treatment. Transvestists, individuals anatomically and physiologically normal in one sex, yet convinced that they should properly belong to the other, cannot be diagnosed in childhood and are outside the scope of this discussion.

Early and complete diagnosis is therefore essential, and obstetricians and paediatricians bear the primary responsibility. The preceding discussion makes it clear that the diagnostic problem is seldom a simple one, and even the most experienced observer would not be justified in making a pronouncement simply on the appearance of the external genitalia. Full investigation must therefore be undertaken before the infant is named or the birth registered. The following routine is suggested for the infant born with genitalia of equivocal sexuality.

1. Careful clinical examination should be made particularly with a view to determining the presence of gonads in the groin or labio-scrotal folds. If two testicles are definitely palpable, the problem is settled immediately.

2. A 24-hour specimen of urine should be collected for the estimation of the 17-ketosteroid output. Collection may be made on a metabolic bed, or by an indwelling urethral catheter: the latter is simpler and safe if sulphonamide cover is provided. A raised 17-ketosteroid level will place the infant in a category of female pseudohermphroditism with adrenal cortical hyperplasia, and further management may follow the lines of those suggested on p. 279.

3. The sex chromatin pattern should be assessed either from the leucocytes or epithelial cells, depending upon the experience of the pathologist available.

4. Provided there is no evidence of adrenal disorder, an endoscopic examination under anaesthetic should be made to determine the precise anatomy.

A child with male sex chromatin and a normal verumontanum may be placed in the male pseudohermaphrodite category. A child with female sex chromatin and no anatomical abnormality other than simple enlargement of the clitoris may be placed in the non-adrenal female pseudohermaphrodite group. A child who has a large phallus, prominent labio-scrotal folds with perhaps one gonad palpable, but has also a vagina evident externally or on urethroscopy, requires laparotomy and biopsy of gonads in order to settle the diagnosis.

Once the diagnosis has been reached and a decision made as to the management, the parents must be given to understand that the child is either a boy or a girl, who may perhaps require treatment or operation, but who must be treated as a normally sexed individual. The intersex factor should not be stressed, for popular journalism has led many parents to expect the most extraordinary behaviour from intersex cases. Where, as in the male pseudohermaphrodite with purely feminine external genitalia, it is inevitable that the gender role should be at variance with the nature of the gonad, only well balanced and intelligent parents should be informed of the true facts, otherwise the strain of bringing up as a girl a child known to have testicles may be too great. It may be sufficient simply to say that the girl has no womb and will not menstruate or bear children.

VI. Gonadal agenesis

Hypogonadism in the female is not a problem of childhood, and lies entirely outside the scope of this volume; there is, however, a syndrome in which individuals of apparently female sex exhibit a total gonadal agenesis, and this diagnosis has usually to be made during the early years of life.

Failure of gonadal development is found in association with a normally formed, though infantile uterus and Fallopian tubes; the gonads are represented by narrow ribbon like structures lying in the normal ovarian position, and showing on microscopy tissue resembling ovarian stroma with or without cells having some likeness to the Leydig cells of a normal testis. The affected children also manifest the signs of "Turner's Syndrome" having webbing of the neck and sometimes of the other joints, cubitus valgus, shortened fourth and fifth fingers, and generally stunted growth. The external genitalia are poorly developed, the nipples small and often inverted. coarctation of the aorta is a common complication, and renal abnormalities, particularly horse-shoe kidney may be found.

These features may all be noticed in childhood: in adult life the sexual infantilism, absence of menstruation and breast development are the chief complaints. The condition was originally regarded as ovarian agenesis, although coarctation of the aorta, which is a common complication, is a disorder affecting males much more frequently than females. Study of the chromosomal sex of theese patients (POLANI et al., GRUMBACH et al., RUSSELL et al.) has now established that sex chromatin is absent in the skin nuclei, and in the leucocytes, of the majority. SEGAL and NELSON find in a male chromatin pattern predominates over the female in a ratio of 5:1 over a large series. This finding implies that most subjects are denetic males, and that the failure of development of the gonad has allowed differentiation of the genitalia to occur along female lines. In this connection, the experimental work of JOST may be recalled; when the gonads were removed from embryo rabbits at any early stage, the subsequent development was invariably feminine, whatever their genetic sex. It appears that gonadal rather than ovarian agenesis is the better description of this condition, although some genetic females may suffer the same changes, which are usually ascribed to a primary failure of the germ cells.

It should be noted that although the webbing is characteristic of gonadal agenesis, it may also occur in females with normal genital function, and rarely in males.

The diagnosis may be made from the association of TURNER's syndrome with a male chromosomal sex, and laparotomy is not required; the only genital disorder which simulates it is male pseudohermaphroditism with purely feminine external genitalia (p. 283) but in the latter condition no true uterus is present, and the webbing syndrome does not occur.

Plastic surgery may be required for the correction of webbing. In adolescence, some feminization may be obtained from the administration of oestrogens.

VII. Hypogonadism in the male

Since the hormones derived from the testicles have little influence on postnatal development until after puberty, the serious effects of male hypogonadism are not evident until later adolescence or adult life. The causative lesions, however, are often congenital or have their origin during childhood; cryptorchidism and other congenital abnormalities are likely to come to notice during the early years, and although normal puberty may not be complete until 16 or 17 years, yet the abnormal developments associated with hypogonadism, such as gynaecomastia, frequently make their appearance from the age of 10 onwards. These early manifestations may enable effective treatment to be undertaken and for this reason a brief review of the hypogonad syndromes is included in this volume.

Many classifications of male hypogonadism have been published, and though the natural complexity of the problem has so far defied a simple analysis, the schemes devised by HELLER and NELSON, and by ALBERT et al., are the best known and most widely accepted. The former authors rely primarily upon the presence or absence of pituitary disease, and upon measurement of the excretion of gonadotropic hormones; the latter upon the histology of the testicle as seen in biopsy specimens. The two schemes have, however, a great deal in common.

1. Pituitary deficiency

The pituitary defect may be general or specific: where many functions fail during childhood, sexual infantilism is only one aspect of the complex problem of pituitary dwarfism. The individual remains child-like in all the bodily proportions, and growth is considerably retarded; obesity is seldom a feature though it may occur. Fröhlich's syndrome, usually resulting from a suprasellar tumour, is a form of generalized pituitary failure, but there has been a considerable misuse of the term; it is often applied to obese children, whose growth is more rapid than the normal although sexual development may be delayed (see BRUCH). It has been emphasized by BAUER that hypothalamic lesions, particularly those affecting the tubero-infundibular region may cause hypogonadism, but that other evidence of a neurological disorder will be found; for instance there may be diabetes insipidus, hyperthermia, or somnolence, as well as eye signs.

A specific failure of the gonadotropic function of the pituitary will lead to the so-called "idiopathic eunuchoidism". The testicles themselves are normal, but in the absence of stimulation retain the histological pattern of the child, with absence of Leydig-cells and immature tubules. The absence of androgens results in delayed closure of the epiphyses, and therefore in the typical elongated limbs of the "eunuchoid habitus". Clinically it will be noticed that the genitalia appear infantile, and there is little growth of pubic or facial hair. Some obesity is not uncommon, and a few adolescents show a considerable deposition of fat in the breast area giving the appearance of gynaecomastia. Gonadotropic hormones are absent from the urine of these eunuchs after the age of normal puberty and 17-ketosteroid excretion is very low. If facilities for hormone estimation are not available, the diagnosis of

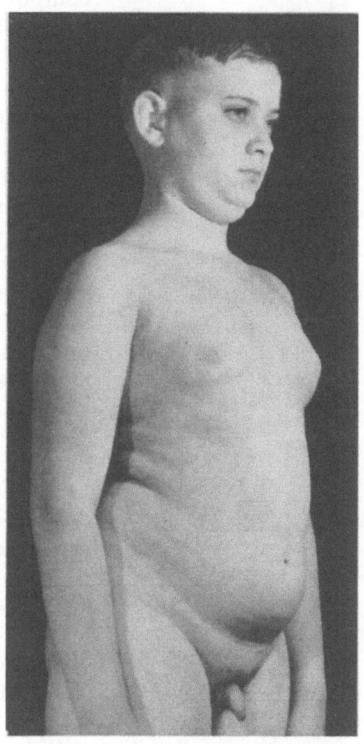

Fig. 159. Hypogonadism with congenital hypoplasia of testicles. Boy aged 13 with a small penis and excessive deposition of fat in the breast area, there is no true breast development. Scrotal exploration revealed two minute testicles

pituitary failure may be made from the effect of administration of gonadotropic hormones (e.g. Pregnyl, 500 units twice weekly for 6 to 8 weeks): testicular development and subsequently growth of the penis and pubic hair will be observed. This measure may be continued as treatment, and in some cases, the natural function may recover or at least be adequate to maintain masculinity. In other cases it may be wiser to change over to testosterone for maintenance since this drug can be given orally instead of by injection.

In a few instances it appears that the pituitary defect is confined to the excretion of luteinizing hormone (L.H.) which normally stimulates the interstitial cells. In these circumstances androgens are not produced in adequate amounts, and the eunuchoid appearance may result, yet the spermatic tubules are still capable of function and may produce spermatozoa (fertile eunuchs).

2. Testicular deficiency

Where pituitary function is normal, hypogonadism is due to a testicular failure, associated sometimes with an evident causative lesion (Fig. 159) such as congenital anorchia, cryptorchidism, orchitis or trauma, but also at times

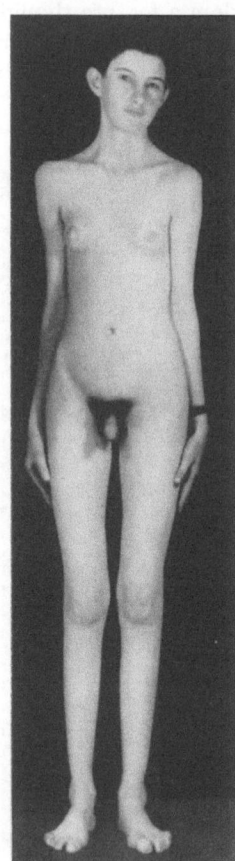

"idiopathic". The specific testicular disorders which may be encountered are discussed in Section N. Testicular biopsies will show lesions of both tubules and interstitial cells, but an endocrine disturbance is naturally only a complication when the lesions are bilateral. Once again the absence of androgens will lead to eunuchoid proportions and infantile genitalia, but the urinary excretion of gonadotropins will be comparatively high, and no improvement will result from the administration of Pregnyl or other gonadotropic substance. In this "surgical" group it is usually possible to start substitution therapy at approximately the normal age of puberty: at 13 years oral methyl testosterone may be started in doses of about 5 mgm a day, it should be increased very slowly, but large doses are seldom necessary or desirable. Subcutaneous implantation of 100 mgm tablets is an alternative method, but must be repeated every 3 to 6 months, and treatment may need to be continued indefinitely.

3. Klinefelter's syndrome

It has been customary to include the Klinefelter syndrome (KLINEFELTER, RIEFENSTEIN and ALBRIGHT) under the heading of hypogonadism, though recent work seems to indicate that the defect is more fundamental. In this syndrome a well marked gynaecomastia is a prominent feature, eunuchoid proportions are usual, but the penis is often normal in size and pubic hair plentiful (Fig. 160). The testes are small and firm, and on biopsy show sclerosis of the tubules and considerable overgrowth of the interstitial cells which are hyperplastic and clumped. Sperma-

Fig. 160. Hypogonadism of the Klinefelter type. Boy aged 15 years with four years history of enlargement of the breasts. Eunuchoid proportions. Penis well formed with pubic hair plentiful. Testicles small and firm: biopsy shows poorly formed spermatic tubules, and a large masses of Leydig cells. Androgenic excretion normal, gonadotropin excretion raised. Polymorphs show the female pattern of sex chromatin

togenesis is sometimes seen. Gonadotropic excretion reaches high levels, though despite the presence of so many interstitial cells the 17-ketosteroid output is low. Recently it has been demonstrated (PLUNKETT and BARR, JACKSON et al.) that these subjects have nuclei exhibiting the female sex chromatin in epithelial cell nuclei, although there is no suggestion of the presence of ovarian tissue. In the polymorph nuclei there was a low incidence of "drum sticks" but not a complete absence as in the normal male. The significance of this finding is far from clear, though it will undoubtedly simplify the problem of diagnosis, and it is now possible to distinguish "true" Klinefelter's syndrome with female sex chromatin and a congenital testicular anomaly, from "false" cases with male sex chromatin and post-pubertal peri-tubular sclerosis (SEGAL and NELSON). Treatment of the Klinefelter syndrome may often be confined to mastectomy, since androgenic stimulation has produced adequate development of the penis and pubic hair: fertility is unobtainable.

Gynaecomastia, it will be noted, may occur in some degree in many forms of hypogonadism, though there is seldom a development of true breast tissue. In the differential diagnosis true hermaphroditism (p. 284) should be kept in mind, since in this condition breast development is to be expected at puberty, while on very rare occasions a feminizing adrenal tumour (p. 194) may be responsible for the same manifestations.

4. Familial hypogonadism

Many rare conditions complicated by hypogonadism are described in the literature, perhaps the most well known being the LAWRENCE-MOON-BIEDL syndrome. This is a familial disorder characterized by mental defect, polydactylism, retinitis pigmentosa and obesity: fully developed cases will be diagnosed without difficulty (see ROTH) and treatment is not required. For a discussion of other forms of familial hypogonadism, the paper by SOHVAL and SOFFER should be consulted.

VIII. Sexual precocity

The term precocious puberty should be confined to those cases in which pubertal changes occur in their natural order, and which therefore result from a disorder of the hypothalamus. Iso-sexual precocity may also be due to an endocrine disorder which causes a development of secondary sex characteristics, but does not stimulate the normal evolution of the gonads. In the male, this distinction is easily made since testicular enlargement will be found in the true precocious puberty group, but not in other forms unless local tumour formation has occurred. Heterosexual precocity, usually virilism in girls, may also result from endocrine abnormalities; the stimulation of somatic growth parallels that found in iso-sexual precocity but the secondary sex characteristics are paradoxical.

In all forms of precocious puberty there is a general acceleration of bodily growth, and the children are advanced in their somatic as well as in their sexual development. The centres of ossification appear early, and a radiological estimation of the bone age provides a useful measurement. Epiphyseal fusion also occurs prematurely, so that the children who were much bigger than their contemporaries in the first few years appear stunted by the age of 11 or 12, the limb bones being short in relation to the trunk (Fig. 153). By contrast mental development is seldom advanced, and because it is difficult in conversation with these children to remember their chronological age, they often seem backward. Sexual interest is also surprisingly lacking, though behaviour disorders and even delinquency are common.

1. Constitutional precocious puberty

A precocious onset of puberty for which no cause can be found is more common in girls than in boys (Fig. 161). The evolution of pubertal changes is unusually rapid, but does not depart from the normal course: breast development is the first sign, pubic hair then appears, and menstruation follows. Often there is some white vaginal discharge before the bleeding starts. Precocious puberty may occur at any stage in childhood; JOLLY reviews the subject fully and finds that the earliest recorded onset of uterine bleeding was at six months, but in

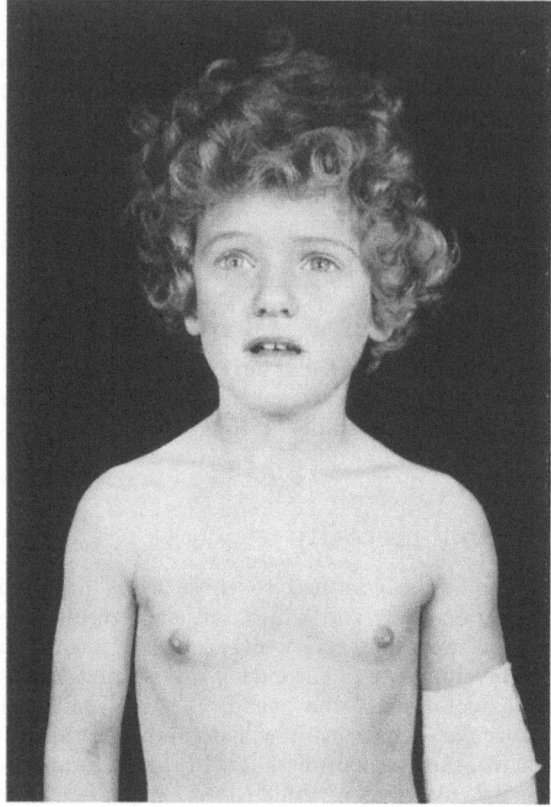

A

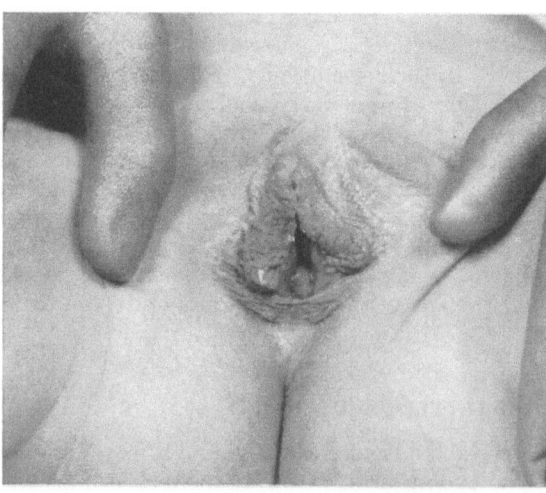

B

Fig. 161 A and B. Constitutional precocious puberty. Girl aged
7 years with vaginal bleeding, hypertrophy of the labia, breast
development and pigmentation of the nipples. No cause found

the majority regular menstruation does not begin until much later. Ovulation probably starts many months or years after menstruation, but the Peruvian child described by ESCOMEL gave birth to an infant at the age of 5 years and 8 months.

Oestrogen excretion in constitutional precocity is only slightly raised until a regular menstrual cycle is established when levels will reach those occuring at normal puberty. The prognosis is good provided the child can be steered through the psychological hazards of the abnormality: fertility is unimpaired, and as far as can be gathered from the scanty records, the menopause comes at a normal age, or is even somewhat delayed. The only permanent physical handicap is the short stature which results from the early fusion of epiphyses. No medical or surgical treatment should be given, but the parents must be advised in the handling of the emotional problems.

Apart from true precocious puberty isolated development of some of the secondary sexual characteristics may be seen in young girls without other evidence of disease. Thus breast hypertrophy may appear many years before the normal age, unaccompanied by any acceleration of somatic growth or by any changes in the genital organs. Alternatively pubic hair and labial hypertrophy may be the only signs of precocity. In both instances the prognosis is entirely favourable and normal development follows at the usual age.

In the rare male cases of constitutional precocity bilateral testicular enlargement precedes the other developments, and the 17-ketosteroid output shows only a slight rise.

2. Precocity due to hypothalamic lesions

Precocious puberty may result from cerebral lesions of various types: the lesions have in common an effect upon the posterior hypothalamus, and WEIN-BERGER and GRANT postulate that they remove an inhibitory influence which is normally exerted from this area upon the pituitary gland. They thus promote the secretion of gonadotropic hormones, and set in motion the changes of normal puberty.

A cerebral tumour arising in the hypothalamic region apart from causing precocity is likely to produce neurological signs fairly rapidly: particularly there is likely to be interference with the visual mechanisms. Most of the tumours are inoperable and though the rate of growth is variable, they are ultimately fatal. Precocity has also resulted from benign lesions such as hydrocephalus, tuberose sclerosis, tuberculous meningo-encephalitis and congenital defects: the various causes are reviewed by JOLLY and by WILKINS.

3. Albright's syndrome

Precocious puberty is a feature of Albright's syndrome, a disorder much more frequently recorded in girls than in boys. A recent review of the topic, with a list of earlier references is given by ARLIEN-SØBERG and IVERSEN. Bone changes (poly-ostotic fibrous dysplasia) are the most serious causes of disability in this syndrome, causing pain, limp and fractures. Radiologically there are cyst-like areas of lessened density in the long bones, and dense formations in some areas such as the base of the skull. The bone changes may be the only signs of the disease, and even in the absence of sexual manifestations skeletal precocity is always found when the disease is recognized in childhood (FALCONER and COPE). Patchy pigmentation of the skin is characteristic; the café-au-lait pigmented areas are not elevated, they are well defined, with very irregular edges, and occur predominantly on the side of the bone lesions. They appear between 4 months and two years of age. The sexual precocity appears to be of central origin, but the cause of the condition remains obscure. Menstruation has occurred as early as 8 weeks in some cases, though it may cease for a time later in childhood: normal fertility has been reported in at least one case.

4. Iso-sexual precocity in the male

Adrenal cortical hyperplasia, equivalent to the disorder found in the female pseudohermaphrodite, is the most common cause of precocious development in the male child, but the action of the hormone is upon the secondary sex characteristics, and therefore spermatogenesis will not occur. The biochemical abnormality is precisely as described on p. 278, the excretion of 17-ketosteroids and of pregnanetrol is raised, and Addisonian crises, with salt loss and hyper-kaliaemia, are common in infancy. The male disorder is not so often diagnosed as the female pseudohermaphroditism, since its manifestations are not so striking, but it has been undoubtedly responsible for many unexplained infant deaths in the past.

The external genitalia may not be noticeably enlarged at birth, and curiously enough a mild degree of hypospadias has been seen in some. During the first year, or sometimes later, there is the characteristic acceleration of somatic growth, development of pubic hair and enlargement of the penis. The testicles are usually small, being normal for the child's age, but a case is on record in which bilateral testicular enlargement resulted from infiltration of the testes by cells resembling those of the hyperplastic adrenal cortex (GARDNER et al.). In mild cases, the precocity causes the child no inconvenience, and the only permanent handicap is the short stature which results from the premature fusion of the epiphyses.

The treatment of early cases, particularly when there are Addisonian signs, is the administration of cortisone, as in female pseudohermaphroditism. This treatment should be continued until growth is complete, and may then cease. Mild cases seen later in childhood when the bone age is already advanced do not require cortisone.

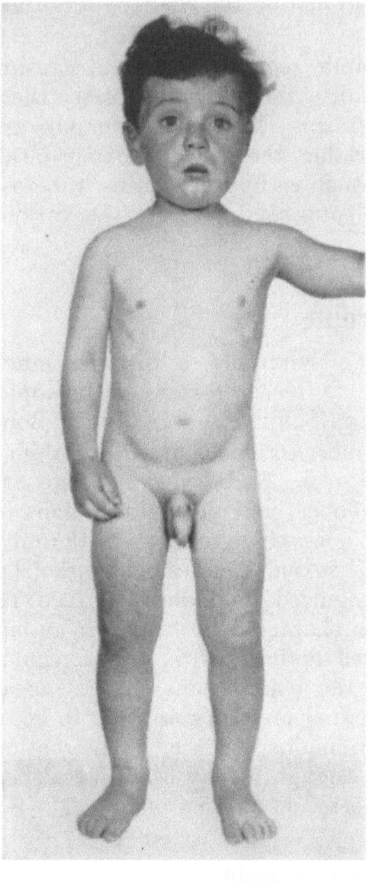

Adrenal cortical tumours (p. 192) (Fig. 162), cause a similar type of precocity; the 17-ketosteroid excretion is raised, but the pregnanetriol is normal since the disorder is not a failure of the normal synthesis of hydrocortisone. Cortisone treatment will not be followed by any consistent fall in the 17-ketosteroid output, as it is in hyperplasia. The penis is large, the testicles small. A mass may be palpable high in the loin, the renal shadow is displaced downwards in the pyelogram and air insufflation may outline the actual tumour.

Interstitial cell tumour of the testis (p. 204) causes sexual precocity: one testicle is enlarged by tumour, the other is small, though bilateral cases are on record. 17-ketosteroid excretion is raised, but the pregnanetriol is normal.

Androgenic stimulation has also been observed in a case of sacrococcygeal tumour (RHODEN).

Fig. 162. Adrenal cortical tumour. Boy aged 2 years with recent enlargement of the penis, growth of pubic hair, and acceleration of skeletal development. Mass palpable in the right upper quadrant of abdomen. Right adrenalectomy with subsequent regression of signs. The tumour was encapsulated but histologically malignant. No recurrence after 4 years

5. Iso-sexual precocity in the female

Ovarian tumours, and very rarely adrenal tumours may be responsible for a high level of oestrogen production, which causes iso-sexual precocity. The changes are not strictly comparable to true puberty since ovulation does not occur, but periodic uterine bleeding is common.

The granulosa cell tumour (p. 208) is the characteristic ovarian lesion though teratomata and carcinomata have the same effects on occasion. The reported tumours have always reached a considerable size before the signs of precocity have appeared, and bimanual pelvic examinations, particularly if carried out under anaesthesia, should therefore be adequate for diagnosis. Follicular cysts are sometimes found in the ovaries of precocious children, and it is difficult to decide whether these are the cause or the result of precocity: periods have sometimes ceased after unilateral oophorectomy (KIMMEL) but have often recommenced long before the normal age, and breast development may not regress at all. If therefore a small ovarian cyst is found at laparotomy it seems better to perform a biopsy rather than a radical excision.

Adrenal tumours (p. 195) very seldom produce simple iso-sexual precocity, and those which have caused a premature onset of menstruation have usually caused also virilism or signs of Cushing's syndrome. In all adrenal cases the 17-keto-steroid, as well as the oestrogen output, is raised.

Sexual precocity may result from the use of synthetic oestrogens: this has been seen during the course of treatment of various conditions (Jolly) but also when the child has had access to stilboestrol tablets prescribed for elderly relatives.

The approach to the problem of precocity in the female may be summarized as follows: apart from the routine clinical assessment, a bimanual pelvic examination under anaesthetic and a careful neurological investigation including if necessary air studies are important. The urinary output of 17-ketosteroids and of oestrogens should be estimated. If all these investigations are negative a constitutional precocity should be diagnosed and no medical or surgical treatment given.

6. Heterosexual precocity in the male

A stimulation of growth processes accompanied by gynaecomastia, and due to adrenal cortical tumour has been reported by Wilkins. Gynaecomastia may also result from interstitial cell tumour and gonadal stromal- cell tumour (androblastoma) of the testicle. It is seen at puberty in Klinefelter's syndrome and in true hermaphroditism.

7. Heterosexual precocity in the female

Adrenal cortical tumours are the usual cause of a post-natal onset of virilism in a girl: hyperplasia is very seldom responsible at this stage. The diagnosis of the tumours has already been discussed.

Arrhenoblastoma is exceptionally rare in children, but has been recorded by Flannery in a 13 year old girl.

References

A. Introduction

III. Investigation

Brockhaus, J.: Subkutane Pyelographie bei jungen Kindern mit Hilfe der Hyaluronidase und mit Anwendung des Tomographen. Fortschr. Röntgenstr. 77, 602 (1952). — Brodny, M. L., and S. A. Robins: Urethrocystography in the male child. J. Amer. med. Ass. 137, 1511 (1948). — Cammenos, A.: L'urographie intramusculaire chez le nourisson et enfant (hyaluronidase et diodone). J. Urol. méd. chir. 59, 505 (1953). — Campbell, M. F.: Miniature sound. J. Urol. (Baltimore) 60, 653 (1948). — Radiologic diagnosis of urinary tract tumours in infants and children. Radiology 54, 646 (1950). — Christiansen, H.: Some practical hints in the performance of urography in infants. Acta radiol. (Stockh.) 26, 46 (1945). — Cohen, R., and M. L. Blatt: Urine collector for female infants. Amer. J. Dis. Child. 60, 897 (1940). — Epstein, B. S.: Subcutaneous urography in infants. J. Amer. med. Ass. 164, 39 (1957). — Fainsinger, M. H.: Excretory urography in the young subject. Hyaluronidase and tomography as aids. S. Afr. med. J. 1950, 418. — Friese-Christiansen, A.: Urography on children after administration of the contrast substance by mouth. Acta radiol. (Stockh.) 27, 197 (1947). — Gladnikoff, H., u. E. Jacobsson: Hyaluronidase in the urographic examination of children. Acta paediat. (Uppsala) 42, 393 (1953). — Hackworth, L. E.: Urethrography in infants and children. J. Urol. (Baltimore) 60, 947 (1948). — Harder, E.: Micturition cysto-urethrogram in children. Radiography 21, 255 (1955). — Helmholz, H. F.: Simple procedure for catheterizing girls. Amer. J. Dis. Child. 82, 426 (1951). — Landelius, E.: Death following renal arteriography in a child. Acta chir. scand. 109, 469 (1955). — McCrea,

L. E.: New infant cystoscope. J. Urol. (Baltimore) **58**, 217 (1947). — Infant curved urethral sounds. J. Urol. (Baltimore) **59**, 330 (1948). — PONCHER, H. G., and J. C. RICEWASSER: Quantitative collection of urine from infants and young children. J. Pediat. **20**, 759 (1942). — SILVERMAN, F. N.: Urologic problems in pediatric X-ray diagnosis. Radiology **58**, 325 (1952). — SINGLETON, E. B., and G. H. HARRISON: Excretory pyelography in infants: technique for intravenous injection. Amer. J. Roentgenol. **75**, 896 (1956). — ST. MARTIN, E. C., J. H. CAMPBELL and C. M. PESQUIER: Cystography in children. J. Urol. (Baltimore) **75**, 151 (1956). — STEPHENS, F. D.: Urethral obstruction in childhood. The use of urethrography in diagnosis. Aust. N.Z. J. Surg. **25**, 89 (1955). — WYATT, G. M.: Excretory urography for children. Indications and methods. Radiology **36**, 664 (1941).

IV. Management of surgical cases

ANDERSON, S. M.: Controlled hypotension with arfonad in paediatric surgery. Brit. med. J. **1955**II, 103. — CAMPBELL, M. F.: Caudal anaesthesia in children. J. Urol. (Baltimore) **30**, 245 (1933). — GROSS, R. E.: Surgery of childhood. Philadelphia: W. B. Saunders Company 1953. — MARTIN, S. J., and T. M. FELNEY: Anaesthesia in pediatric urology. J. Amer. med. Ass. **148**, 180 (1952). — ÖRSTEN, P., u. A. MATTSSON: Hospitalisation symptoms in children. Acta paediat. (Uppsala) **44**, 79 (1955). — RICKHAM, P. P.: The surgery of premature infants. Arch. Dis. Child. (awaiting publication). — VAUGHAN, G. F.: Children in Hospital. Lancet **1957**I, 1117.

V. Fluid balance

BARNETT, H. L.: Kidney function in young infants. Pediatrics **5**, 171 (1950). — BARNETT, H. L., and F. SERENI: Kidney function tests in infants and children. Pediat. Clin. N. Amer. **2**, 191 (1955). — BLAND, J. H.: The clinical use of fluid and electrolyte. Philadelphia: W. B. Saunders Company 1952. — CAMERON, G., and R. CHAMBERS: Direct evidence of function in kidney of an early human foetus. Amer. J. Physiol. **123**, 482 (1938). — DALY, H., L. J. WELLS and G. EVANS: Experimental evidence of secretion of urine by the foetal kidney. Proc. Soc. exp. Biol. (N.Y.) **64**, 78 (1947). — GROSS, R. E.: Surgery of Childhood. Philadelphia: W. B. Saunders Company 1953. — GRUENWALD, P., and H. POPPER: Physiology of the renal glomerulus in early postnatal life. J. Urol. (Baltimore) **43**, 452 (1940). — McCANCE, R. A., N. J. NAYLOR and E. M. WIDDOWSON: The response of infants to a large dose of water. Arch. Dis. Childh. **29**, 104 (1954). — McCANCE, R. A., and E. M. WIDDOWSON: Renal function before birth. Proc. roy. Soc. B **141**, 488 (1954). — New thoughts on renal function in the early days of life. Brit. med. Bull. **13**, 3 (1957). — McNAIR SCOTT, T., and W. W. PAYNE: In: Diseases of Children, editor A. MONCRIEFF and P. R. EVANS, 5. edit. London: Arnold & Co. 1953. — POTTER, E. L., and T. THIERSTEIN: Glomerular development in the kidney as an index of foetal maturity. J. Pediat. **22**, 695 (1943). — RICKHAM, P. P.: The metabolic response to neonatal surgery. Cambridge, Massachusetts: Harvard University Press 1957. — TAUSCH, M.: Der Fetalharn. Arch. Gynäk. **162**, 217 (1936). — VESTERDAL, J.: Renal excretion of water and osmotically active substances in young infants. Helv. paediat. Acta **10**, 167 (1955). — WELLS, L. J., and E. T. BELL: Functioning of the foetal kidney as reflected by stillborn infants with hydroureter and hydronephrosis. Arch. Path. (Chicago) **42**, 274 (1946).

B. Congenital abnormalities of the upper urinary tract

I. Renal agenesis

BOUND, J. P.: Two cases of congenital absence of the kidney in the same family. Brit. med. J. **1943**, ii, 747. — BRAUM, O., u. H. GROSS: Zur Kenntnis der eigenartigen mit Nierenfehlbildungen kombinierten Gesichtsveränderungen (Dysplasia renofacialis). Virchows Arch. path. Anat. **329**, 433 (1956). — CAMPBELL, M. F.: Clinical paediatric urology. Philadelphia and London: W. B. Saunders Company 1951. — GUNTER, J. U., and F. S. OSER: Ante-mortem diagnosis of bilateral renal agenesis. N. C. med. J. **9**, 307 (1948). — GUTIERREZ, R.: Surgical aspects of renal agenesis. Arch. Surg. (Chicago) **27**, 686 (1933). — NATION, E. F.: Renal agenesis; a study of 30 cases. Surg. Gynec. Obstet. **79**, 175 (1944). — POTTER, E. L.: Bilateral renal agenesis. J. Pediat. **29**, 68 (1946). — Facial characteristics of infants with bilateral renal agenesis. Amer. J. Obstet. Gynec. **51**, 885 (1946). — SELBY, G. W., and A. H. PARMELEE: Bilateral renal agenesis and oligohydramnios. J. Pediat. **48**, 70 (1956).

II. Renal hypoplasia

BAGENSTOSS, A. H.: Congenital anomalies of the kidney. Med. Clin. N. Amer. **35**, 987 (1951). — BELL, E. T.: Renal diseases. London: Kimpton & Co. 1950. — BLACKLOCK, J.W.S.: Renal aplasia in an infant. J. Path. Bact. **37**, 502 (1933). — COLLINS, D. C.: Congenital renal aplasia. Ann. Surg. **95**, 715 (1932). — EINECKE, F.: Zur Pathogenese der Schrumpf-niere im Kindesalter. Mschr. Kinderheilk. **42**, 130 (1929). — EKSTROM, T.: Renal hypoplasia. Acta chir. scand. Suppl. **203** (1955). — HUTCHISON, R., and A. A. MONCRIEFF: Primary Hypertension in a Child. Brit. J. Child. Dis. **27**, 201 (1930). — LIGHTWOOD, R.: Specimens and clinical history of a case of renal aplasia with adrenal cortical hyperplasia. Proc. roy. Soc. Med. **27**, 400 (1934). — MACKENZIE, D. W., and A. B. HAWTHORNE: Unilateral renal aplasia. Surg. Gynec. Obstet. **46**, 42 (1928). — MARSHALL, A. G.: Persistence of foetal structures in pyelonephritic kidneys. Brit. J. Surg. **41**, 38 (1953). — MULLER, H. P.: Über doppelseitige Aplasie der Nieren beim Neugeborenen. Zbl. Gynäk. **57**, 1055 (1933).

III. Cystic disease

BANSILLON et GUICHARD: Reins polykystiques bilateraux chez un nouveau-né. (Étude anatomo-clinique.) Bull. Soc. Obstét. Gynéc. Paris **22**, 415 (1933). — BELL, E. T.: Cystic disease of the kidneys. Amer. J. Path. **11**, 373 (1935). — BEESON, H. G.: Polycystic disease in a premature infant. J. Urol. (Baltimore) **30**, 285 (1933). — BIALESTOCK, D.: Morphogenesis of renal cysts in the stillborn. J. Path. Bact. **7**, 51 (1956). — BOCIAN, J. J., and M. LIANG: Rare case of polycystic disease of the kidneys. Amer. J. Dis. Child. **89**, 615—617 (1955). — BOURLAND, J. W.: Polycystic disease of the kidneys causing dystocia. Urol. cutan. Rev. **50**, 669 (1946). — BURRELL, N. L.: Multilocular cyst of the kidney. J. Urol. (Baltimore) **43**, 656 (1940). — CADERAS, J., et J. M. BERT: Hematome perirénal spontane bilateral avec maladie polykystique des reins chez un nouveau-né mort en hyperthermie au cinquieme jour. Arch. Soc. Sci. méd. Montpellier **20**, 34 (1939). — CAMPBELL, M.: Clinical pediatric urology. London and Philadelphia: W. B. Saunders Company 1951. — CHALKLEY, T. S., and L. E. SUTTON: Infected solitary cyst of kidney in a child. J. Urol. (Baltimore) **50**, 414 (1943). — CHAUVIN, M. E.: Un cas de rein polykystique partiel. J. Urol. méd. chir. **52**, 210 (1944/45). — CHRISTE-SON, W. W.: Simple renal cysts in the new born. Report of two cases. J. Urol. (Baltimore) **72**, 1137 (1954). — FERGUSSON, J. D.: Observations on familial polycystic disease of the kidneys. Proc. roy. Soc. Med. **42**, 806 (1949). — FÈVRE, M., et T. VAN HOA: Reins poly-kystiques chez l'enfant. Presse méd. **1945**, 106. — FRAZIER, T. H.: Multilocular cysts of the kidney. J. Urol. (Baltimore) **65**, 351 (1951). — GONNET, BANSILLON, MENEAULT and BUCHER: Dystocie grave par reins polykstiques avec éclatement du dome vaginal. Bull. Soc. Obstét. Gynéc. Paris **26**, 774 (1937). — GREEN, C.: Bilateral hypoplastic kidneys. Amer. J. Dis. Child. **24**, 1 (1922). — HART, L. B., W. BECKLEY, E. J. DOBOS and R. P. FORBES: Congenital cystic dilatation of a single kidney calyx. J. Pediat. **16**, 206 (1940). — HIGGINS, T. T., D. I. WILLIAMS and D. F. E. NASH: Urology of childhood. London: Butterworth & Co. 1951. — HINKEL, C. L., and L. C. SANTINI: Polycystic Disease of the kidney in Infants. Amer. J. Roentgenol. **76**, 153 (1956). — HOWZE, C. P., and J. H. HILL: Unilateral multiple cysts of the kidney. J. Urol. (Baltimore) **61**, 187 (1949). — KORNBLUM, K., and J. A. RITTER: Retroperitoneal cyst with agenesis of the kidney. Radiology **32**, 416 (1939). — KRETSCHMER, H. L.: Renal rickets and polycystic disease of the kidney. J. Urol. (Baltimore) **59**, 773 (1948). — LAMBERT, P. P.: Polycystic disease of the kidney. Arch. Path. (Chicago) **44**, 34 (1947). — LIENHARDT, E., J. BOUCOMENTS et H. GUIBERT: Rein polykystiques congenitaux a kystes miliaires. Ann. Méd. **45**, 71 (1939). — LIGHTWOOD, R., and G. H. LOOTS: Three cases of familial congenital cystic disease of kidney and liver. Proc. roy. Soc. Med. **25**, 1230 (1932). — LORENZ, G.: Cystennieren mit weiteren mesodermalen Mißbildungen. Z. Urol. **48**, 653 (1955). — LYNCH, K. D., and R. F. THOMPSON: Unilateral multicystic kidney in an infant. J. Urol. (Baltimore) **38**, 58 (1937). — MOORE, T.: Unilateral cystic kidneys. Brit. J. Urol. **29**, 3 (1957). — NORRIS, R. F., and L. HERMAN: Pathogenesis of polycystic kidneys: reconstruction of cystic elements in 4 cases. J. Urol. (Baltimore) **46**, 147 (1941). — PARNELL, J. L., and I. KESSEL: Congenital polycystic disease of the kidneys in infancy. S. Afr. med. J. **1953**, 344. — PARROTT, R. H., L. G. JOSEPH and R. R. NESBIT: Left ventricular hyper-trophy in infantile polycystic kidney disease. J. Amer. med. Ass. **147**, 648 (1951). — POTTER, E. L.: Pathology of the foetus and the newborn. Chicago: Yearbook Publ. 1952. — RALL, J. E., and H. M. ODELL: Congenital polycystic disease of the kidney. Review of literature and data in 207 cases. Amer. J. med. Sci. **218**, 399 (1949). — RAVITCH, M. M., and M. C. SANDFORD: Unilateral multicystic kidney in infants. Pediatrics **4**, 769 (1949). — Roos, A.: Polycystic kidney: report of a case studied by reconstruction. Amer. J. Dis. Child. **61**, 116 (1941). — SCHWARTZ, J.: Unusual unilateral multicystic kidney in infant. J. Urol. (Baltimore) **35**, 259 (1936). — SMITH, C. H., and J. B. GRAHAM: Congenital medullary cysts of the kidneys with severe refractory anaemia. Amer. J. Dis. Child. **69**, 369 (1945). — SORRELL, E.: Rein polykystique chez un enfant de deux mois. Bull. Soc. nat. Chir. Paris **61**, 290 (1935). — SPENCE, H. M.: Congenital unilateral multicystic kidney: an entity to be distinguished from polycystic kidney disease and other cystic disorders.

J. Urol. (Baltimore) **74**, 693 (1955). — TOULSON, W. H., and J. A. WAGNER: Congenital encapsulated multilocular serous cast of the kidney associated with hypertension: occurrence in a 19 months old infant. Report of the case. Bull. Sch. Med. Maryland **26**, 177 (1942). — VAIL, A. S., and T. P. STONE: Congenital hypertrophy of the neck of the bladder with bilateral hydro-ureter. Hydronephrosis and polycystic kidney. Arch. Path. (Chicago) **43**, 427 (1947). — WAKELEY, C. P. G.: Cystic kidney in an infant. Proc. roy. Soc. Med. **23**, 547 (1929/30). — WEERD, J. H. DE, and H. B. SIMON: Simple renal cysts in children. J. Urol. (Baltimore) **75**, 912 (1956). — WEINBERG, S. R., W. T. O'CONNOR and F. L. SENGER: Unilateral multicystic renal disease of the newborn. Amer. J. Dis. Child. **92**, 576 (1956). — WEYRAUCH, H. M., and A. E. FLEMING: Congenital hydrocalycosis. J. Urol. (Baltimore) **63**, 582 (1950).

IV. Malrotated, fused and ectopic kidneys

ANSON, B. J., J. W. PICK and E. W. CAULDWELL: Anatomy of commoner renal anomalies: ectopic and horse-shoe kidneys. J. Urol. (Baltimore) **47**, 112 (1942). — BOISSONNAT, P.: Rein en L a trois uretères (l'un d'eux termine en ureterocele) associé a avec une fistule trigonovaginale chez une fillette de 14 jours. Intervention plastique creant un rein droit et un rein gauche independants. J. Urol. méd. chir. **61**, 408 (1955). — BOYLSTON, G. A., and B. J. ANSON: Pelvic kidney and renal vessels in a newborn child. J. Urol. (Baltimore) **40**, 502 (1938). — CARLETON, A.: Crossed ectopia of the kidney. J. Anat. (Lond.) **71**, 292 (1937). — CHAUVIN, E., et H. F. CHAUVIN: Les hematuries dans le rein en fer a cheval. J. Urol. méd. chir. **60**, 172 (1954). — GAMMELGAARD, A.: Horseshoe kidney in a child of 16 months elucidated aortographically. Acta chir. scand. **107**, 163 (1954). — GUTIERREZ, R.: Clinical management of horseshoe kidney. Amer. J. Surg. **15**, 132 (1932). — HANLEY, H. G.: Horse-shoe and supernumerary kidney. A triple kidney with a horse-shoe component. Brit. J. Surg. **30**, 165 (1942). — HANLEY, H. G., and W. A. STEEL: The solitary ectopic kidney (with reports of 2 further cases). Brit. J. Surg. **34**, 402 (1947). — KEUSENHOFF, W.: Gekreuzte Nierendystopie. Z. Urol. **49**, 114 (1956). — LOWSLEY, O. S.: Surgery of horse-shoe kidney. J. Urol. (Baltimore) **67**, 565 (1952). — THOMPSON, G. J., and J. M. PACE: Ectopic kidney, a review of 97 cases. Surg. Gynec. Obstet. **64**, 935 (1937). — WALTERS, W., and J. B. PRIESTLEY: Horse-shoe kidney, a review of 68 surgical cases. J. Urol. (Baltimore) **28**, 271 (1932).

V. Hydronephrosis

ANDERSON, J. C.: Abnormal function on the upper urinary tract. Proc. roy. Soc. Med. **44**, 925 (1951). — Modern trends in urology, editor E. W. RICHES. London: Butterworth & Co. 1954. — CAMPBELL, M. F.: Vascular obstruction of the ureter in children. J. Urol. (Baltimore) **36**, 366 (1936). — Hydronephrosis in infants and children. J. Urol. (Baltimore) **65**, 734 (1951). — COVINGTON, T., and W. REESER: Hydronephrosis associated with overhydration. J. Urol. (Baltimore) **63**, 438 (1950). — CULP, O. S., and J. R. WINTERRINGER: Surgical treatment of the horse-shoe kidney: comparison of results after various types of operation. J. Urol. (Baltimore) **73**, 747 (1955). — DAVIS, D. M.: Ureteral obstruction. Brit. J. Urol. **19**, 71 (1947). — FISTER, G. M., and E. H. SMITH: Aberrant renal vessels in children. J. Urol. (Baltimore) **26**, 175 (1931). — FOLEY, F. E. B.: Plastic operation for stricture at the uretero-pelvic function. J. Urol. (Baltimore) **38**, 643 (1937). — GERARD, L., et J. W. SAMSON: Double hydronéphrose congénitale méconnue chez un enfant. J. Urol. méd. chir. **47**, 25 (1939). — GRAUHAN: Über Wachstum und Form der Hydronephrosen. Arch. klin. Chir. **180**, 517 (1934). — HAGENBACH, E.: Seven cases of hydronephrosis in children. Schweiz. med. Wschr. **1940**, 226. — HESS, E., and B. W. WRIGHT: Pyelocystomosis, report of two cases. J. Amer. med. Ass. **127**, 267 (1945). — HESSE, F.: Zur kongenitalen Hydronephrose, zugleich ein pathologisch-anatomischer Beitrag. Kinderärztl. Prax. **23**, 395 (1955). — JEWETT, H. J.: Accessory renal vessels. Surg. Gynec. Obstet. **68**, 666 (1939). — KRETSCHMER, H. L.: Hydronephrosis in infancy and childhood. Surg. Gynec. Obstet. **64**, 634 (1937). — McCREA, E. F. W.: Large hydronephrosis in an infant. Brit. J. Urol. **2**, 154 (1930). — MURNAGHAN, G. F.: Awaiting publication. — NIXON, H. H.: Hydronephrosis in children, a clinical study of 78 cases. Brit. J. Surg. **40**, 601 (1953). — ÖSTLING, K.: The genesis of hydronephrosis. Acta chir. scand. Suppl. **72** (1942). — PIEPENBORN, J.: Ein Beitrag zur Frage der Hydronephrose bei Neugeborenen. Z. urol. Chir. **26**, 384 (1929). — RAFFLE, R. B.: Familial hydronephrosis. Brit. med. J. **1955** I, 580. — SCHNEIDER, H.: Operative Entfernung einer Sackniere bei einem Säugling. Dtsch. Z. Chir. **237**, 115 (1932). — SWENSON, O., and D. MARCHANT: Uretero-pelvic obstruction in infants and children. J. Urol. (Baltimore) **73**, 945 (1955). — WHITE, R. R., and G. M. WYATT: Surgical importance of aberrant renal vessels in infants and children. Amer. J. Surg. **58**, 48 (1942).

VI. Congenital ureteric stricture, hypoplasia and valves

HAMILTON., J. L.: Hypoplasia of the ureter with renal agenesis. J. Urol. (Baltimore) **56**, 530 (1946). — LANGSTON, W C.: Congenital absence of one kidney, report of a case showing aplasia of the secreting portions of uriniferous tubules. J. Urol. (Baltimore) **29**, 355 (1933). — MACKENZIE, D. W., and M. I. SENG: Obliteration of a ureter in an anomalous kidney with hydronephrosis. Trans. Amer. Ass. gen.-urin. Surg. **30**, 347 (1937). — MERIKALLIO, P.: Ein kongenitaler Hydronephros als Ursache für Dystokie. Acta obstet. gynec. scand. **25**, Suppl. 2, 99 (1945). — ROBERTS, R. R.: Complete valve of the ureter: congenital urethral valves. J. Urol. (Baltimore) **76**, 62 (1956). — SIMON, H. B., O. S. CULP and E. M. PARKHILL: Congenital ureteral valves. Report of 2 cases. J. Urol. (Baltimore) **74**, 336 (1955). — THIEMANN, A.: Beitrag zur Lehre von der angeborenen Hydronephrose und der poly-cystischen Mißbildung der Niere. Z. urol. Chir. **36**, 433 (1933).

VII. Duplications of the ureter

BURSTEIN, H. J.: Double kidney with Y shaped ureter and ureteral calculus in an infant. Urologic. Rev. **42**, 575 (1938). — CAMPBELL, M. F.: Hemipyonephrosis in infants and children. Treatment by heminephrectomy. Amer. J. Surg. **21**, 85 (1933). — CARLSON, H. E.: Super-numerary kidney: a summary of 51 reported cases. J. Urol. (Baltimore) **64**, 224 (1950). — CULP, O. S.: Ureteral diverticulum: classification and report of a case. J. Urol. (Balti-more) **58**, 309 (1947). — FEYDER, S., and C. L. DEMING: Congenital hydronephrosis in the lower half of a double kidney. Report of a case. New Engl. J. Med. **226**, 220 (1942). — FRANCK, A.: Uretère trifide et epispadias chez une fillette de dix ans. J. Urol. méd. chir. **35**, 255 (1933). — GLEIZE-RAMBAL, L., J. PROVANSAL, H. BARTHÉLEMY and E. HENRY: Volumi-neuse formation kystique d'origine renale chez un enfant de trois ans et demi. J. Radiol. Élec-trol. **34**, 400 (1953). — GOYANNA, R., and L. F. GREENE: Pathologic and anomalous conditions associated with duplications of the renal pelvis and ureter. J. Urol. (Baltimore) **54**, 1 (1945). — GRAVES, F. T.: Anatomy of the intra-renal Arteries. Brit. J. Surg. **42**, 132 (1955). — GUTIERREZ, R.: Double kidney as a source of impaired dynamism. Its surgical treatment by heminephrectomy. Amer. J. Surg. **65**, 256 (1944). — HARRIS, A.: Ureteral anomalies with special reference to partial duplication with one branch ending blindly. J. Urol. (Baltimore) **38**, 442 (1937). — KRETSCHMER, H. L.: Duplication of the ureters at their distal ends, one pair ending blindly: so-called diverticula of the ureters. J. Urol. (Baltimore) **30**, 61 (1933). — NATION, E. F.: Duplication of the kidney and ureter. A statistical study of 230 new cases. J. Urol. (Baltimore) **51**, 456 (1944). — PAPIN, E.: Sur un cas de basinnet bifurqué avec stenose du grand calices inferieur, anastomoses des deux grands calices. Bull. Soc. nat. Chir. Paris **58**, 686 (1932). — PHOKITIS, P.: L'uretère bifide caudal. J. Urol. méd. chir. **60**, 45 (1954). — RICHARDSON, E. H.: Diverticulum of the ureter. J. Urol. (Baltimore) **47**, 535 (1942). — RIHMER, B. v.: Von einem durch Gabelung des linken Ureters und Ein-mündung eines Zweiges in die Vagina verursachten Harnträufeln bei einem 17jährigen Mädchen. Z. urol. Chir. **29**, 55 (1930). — RUBIN, J. S.: Supernumerary kidney with aberrant ureter terminating externally. J. Urol. (Baltimore) **60**, 405 (1948). — SMITH, I.: Triplicate ureter. Brit. J. Surg. **34**, 183 (1946). — SPENCE, H. M.: Nephro-ureterectomy and hemi-nephro-ureterectomy in infancy and childhood. J. Urol. (Baltimore) **71**, 171 (1954). — STEPHENS, F. D.: Abnormalities. Double ureter in the child. Aust. N.Z. J. Surg. **26**, 81 (1956).

VIII. Ectopic ureter

ALLDRED, A. J., and T. T. HIGGINS: The ectopic ureter in childhood. Brit. J. Surg. **38**, 460 (1951). — BURFORD, C. F., J. E. GLENN and F. H. BURFORD: Ureteral ectopia. J. Urol. (Baltimore) **62**, 211 (1949). — CAMPBELL, M. F.: Ectopic ureteral orifice: a report of 17 cases in children. Surg. Gynec. Obstet. **64**, 22 (1937). — DEUTICKE, P. v.: Über ektope Harn-leitermündungen. Z. Urol. **46**, 533 (1953). — ERICSON, N. D.: Ectopic ureterocele in infants and children. Acta chir. scand. Suppl. **197** (1954). — HEPLER, A. B.: Bilateral pelvic and ureteral duplication with uterine ectopic ureter. J. Urol. (Baltimore) **57**, 94 (1947). — HRYNTSCHAK, T.: Ektope Uretermündung und Pyonephrose bei einem sechsmonatigen Säugling. Wien. klin. Wschr. **1930**, 169. — IDBOHRM, H., u. S. SJOSTEDT: Ectopic ureter not causing incontinence until adult life. Double kidney with hydronephrosis, diagnosed by renal angiography. Acta obstet. gynec. scand. **33**, 457 (1954). — LANGLEY, G. F.: Urinary incontinence due to ectopic ureter. Brit. J. Surg. **36**, 391 (1949). — MEADE, H. S.: Congenital absence of right kidney with cystic formation of lower end of ureter. Irish J. med. Sci. **1948**, 176. — MERTZ, H. O., J. W. HENDRICKS and R. A. GARRETT: Cystic uretero-vesical protrusion. Trans. Amer. Ass. gen.-urin. Surg. **40**, 180 (1948). — MOORE, T.: Ectopic openings of the ureter. Brit. J. Urol. **24**, 3 (1952). — MOORE, T. D.: Ureteral ectopia. J.

Urol. (Baltimore) **60**, 50 (1948). — OTTOW, B.: Relation between vaginal cysts and double ureters. Zbl. Gynäk. **62**, 1484 (1941). — POLITZER, G.: Die dystopische Mündung des Ureters und ihre formale Genese. Frankfurt. Z. Path. **64**, 324 (1953). — SANDMANN, H.: Der extravesikal mündende Ureter, eine seltene Mißbildung. Kinderärztl. Prax. **21**, 454 (1953). — SARGENT, J. C., and R. IRWIN: Ureteral ectopia: report of a case in infancy. J. Urol. (Baltimore) **24**, 645 (1930). — SMITH, G. G.: Empyema of the ureter associated with aplasia of the kidney. Trans. Amer. Ass. gen.-urin. Surg. **27**, 321 (1934). — TROLLE, D.: Ectopic hypoplastic kidney-ureter system opening into cystically dilated Gartner's duct n a 17 year old woman. Acta obstet. gynec. scand. **32**, 335 (1953). — VAZQUEZ, V. A., y M. VARELA: Desembocadura ectopia de un ureter supernumerario. Arch. esp. Urol. **9**, 301 (1954). — WEHRBEIN, H. L.: Double kidney, double ureter and bilocular bladder in a child. J. Urol. (Baltimore) **43**, 804 (1940). — WESSON, M. B.: Incontinence of vesical and renal origin (relaxed urethra and a vaginal ectopic ureter). J. Urol. (Baltimore) **32**, 141 (1934). — WILLIAMS, D. INNES: The ectopic ureter; diagnostic problems. Brit. J. Urol. **26**, 253 (1954). — WILLMARTH, C. L.: Ectopic ureteral orifice within an urethral diverticulum. J. Urol. (Baltimore) **59**, 47 (1948).

IX. Ureteroceles

BERNHEIM, M., J. A. ROUX, C. MOURIQUAND et M. LEVY: Dilatation kystique de l'extremité inférieure de l'uretère. Pédiatrie **10**, 554 (1955). — BINKS, J. B., and R. K. DEBENHAM: Ureterocele in childhood. Brit. J. Urol. **27**, 121 (1955). — BOISSONNAT, P.: L'urétérocèle de l'enfant. Rev. Chir. (Paris) **74**, 73 (1955). — CENDRON, J.: Sur six cas d'urétérocèle. Arch. franç. Pédiat. **13**, 20 (1956). — GREENFIELD, M.: True prolapse of the ureter, case report and review of the literature. J. Urol. (Baltimore) **75**, 223 (1956). — GROSS, R. E., and H. W. CLATWORTHY: Ureterocele in infancy and childhood. Pediatrics **5**, 68 (1950). — GUMMESS, G. H., D. A. CHARNOCK, H. I. RIDDELL and C. M. STEWART: Ureteroceles in children. J. Urol. (Baltimore) **74**, 331 (1955). — GUTIERREZ, R.: Ureterocele. Surg. Gynec. Obstet. **68**, 611 (1939). — KRETSCHMER, H. L., and W. G. HIBBS: Study of the vesical end of the ureter in hydronephrosis: report of 15 cases. Trans. Amer. Ass. gen.-urin. Surg. **25**, 341 (1932). — THOMAS, J. M. R.: Ureterocele prolapsed through the urethra in a child. Brit. J. Urol. **14**, 24 (1942).

X. Retrocaval ureter

CAMPOS, FREIRE, G. DE: Uretère rétro-cave et rein hypoplasique. J. d'Urol. **59**, 868 (1953). — MARCEL, J. E.: Grosse hydronephrose par uretère rétrocave. Arch. franç. Pédiatr. **10**, 274 (1953). — PARKS, R. E., and W. E. CHASE: Retrocaval ureter. Report of 2 cases diagnosed pre-operatively in childhood. Amer. J. Dis. Childr. **82**, 442 (1951). — SCHEARER, T. P.: Retrocaval ureter. J. of Urol. **62**, 159 (1949).

C. Hydro-ureter and mega-ureter

I. Normal ureteric funktion

BEGG, R. C.: Physiological variations in pyelograms commonly interpreted as pathological. Brit. J. Urol. **18**, 176 (1946). — BOZLER, E.: Electrical stimulation and conduction of excitation in smooth muscle. Amer. J. Physiol. **122**, 614 (1938). — GRUBER, M.: Autonomic innervation of the genito-urinary system. Physiol. Rev. **13**, 497 (1933). — LAPIDES, J.: The physiology of the intact human ureter. J. Urol. (Baltimore) **59**, 501 (1948). — MURNAGHAN, G. F.: The Experimental Investigation of the Dynamics of the Normal and Dilated Ureter. Brit. J. Urol. **29**, 403 (1957). — PIEPER, A.: Beitrag zur Nervenversorgung des Ureters. Z. Urol. **44**, 17 (1951). — SCHNEIDER, W.: The musculature of the upper urinary tract. Z. Anat. Entwickl.-Gesch. **109**, 187 (1938). — STEWART, C.: On the mechanism of the ureterovesical function. Quart. J. exp. Physiol. **27**, 193 (1937). — WHARTON, L. R.: The innervation of the ureter. J. Urol. (Baltimore) **28**, 639 (1933).

II. Radiography and other investigations

BAKER, R.: Ureteral electromyography in congenital megaloureter. Amer. J. Dis. Child. **87**, 7 (1954). — EDWARDS, D.: Cine radiology in congenital bladder neck obstruction and megaureters. Brit. J. Urol. **29**, 410 1957. — HANLEY, H. G.: The electro-ureterogram. Brit. J. Urol. **25**, 358 (1953). — JONA, J. L.: The kidney pelvis. Surg. Gynec. Obstet. **59**, 713 (1934). — SWENSON, O.: Congenital defects in the pelvic parasympathetic system. Arch. Dis. Childh. **30**, 1 (1955). — TRATTNER, H. R.: Graphic record of function of the human ureter. J. Urol. (Baltimore) **28**, 1 (1933).

III. Vesico-ureteric reflux

AUER, J., and L. D. SEAGER: Experimental local bladder edema causing urine reflux into ureter. J. exp. Med. **66**, 741 (1937). — BARKSDALE, E. H., and W. W. BAKER: The effect of denervation of the lower ureter upon the incidence of ureteral reflux in the dog. J. Urol. (Baltimore) **24**, 263 (1930). — GIBSON H. M.: Ureteral reflux in the normal child. J. Urol. (Baltimore) **62**, 40 (1949). — GRAVES, R. C., and L. M. DAVIDOFF: Studies on the ureter and bladder with especial reference to regurgitation of the vesical contents. Trans. Amer. Ass. gen.-urin. Surg. **16**, 25 (1923). — GREY, D. N., P. FLYNN and W. E. GOODWIN: Experimental methods of ureteroneocystostomy: experiences with the ureteral intussusception to produce a nipple or valve. J. Urol. (Baltimore) **77**, 154 (1957). — HUTCH, J. A.: Vesico-ureteral reflux in paraplegics. J. Urol. (Baltimore) **68**, 457 (1952). — HUTCH, J. A., R. G. BUNGE and R. H. FLOCKS: Vesico-ureteral reflux in children. J. Urol. (Baltimore) **74**, 607 (1955). — IANNACCONE, G., u. P. E. PANZIRONI: Ureteral reflux in normal infants. Acta radiol. (Stockh.) **44**, 451 (1955). — PRATHER, G. C.: Vesico-ureteral reflux. J. Urol. (Baltimore) **52**, 437 (1944). — VERMOOTEN, V., and C. H. NEUSWANGER: Effects on the upper urinary tract of incompetent uretero-vesical valve. J. Urol. (Baltimore) **32**, 330 (1934).

IV. Hydro-ureter in bladder disorders

BOPPE, M., et J. E. MARCEL: Coexistence chez un enfant de 8 ans d'une maladie du col vésical et de mega-uretères bilatéraux. Operations multiples. Guérison functionelle. Bull. Soc. Pédiatr. Paris **36**, 36 (1938). — HINMAN, I.: Obstructive hydro-ureteral angularity, with hydronephrosis in children: Surgical treatment. Arch. Surg. (Chicago) **18**, 21 (1929). — WILLIAMS, D. I.: Discussion on the chronically dilated ureter. Proc. roy. Soc. Med. **45**, 840 (1952).

V. Hydro-ureter in other reno-ureteral abnormalities

BERRY, J. V.: Bilateral torsion of the ureter. J. Urol. (Baltimore) **40**, 378 (1938). — CAMPBELL, M. F.: Congenital bilateral uretero-vesical stricture in infants and children. J. Urol. (Baltimore) **26**, 529 (1931). — Ureteral obstruction in children. J. Urol. (Baltimore) **41**, 660 (1939). — GREENE, L. F., J. T. PRIESTLEY, H. B. SIMON and R. H. HEMPSTEAD: Obstruction of the lower third of the ureter by anomalous blood vessels. J. Urol. (Baltimore) **71**, 544 (1954). — MURNAGHAN, G. F.: The Normal and Dilated Ureter. Brit. J. Urol. **29**, 403 (1957). — POOLE-WILSON, D. S.: Discussion on the chronically dilated ureter. Proc. roy. Soc. Med. **45**, 835 (1952). — PRATHER, G. C.: Ectopic testis as a cause of ureteral dilatation. New Engl. J. Med. **212**, 413 (1935). — WITHYCOMBE, J. F. R.: A case of trifid ureter and segmental hydro-ureter. Brit. J. Surg. **38**, 113 (1950/51).

VI. Infections

HEYMAN, W., and J. F. MARTIN: Bilateral megalo-ureter in a child: return to normal with control of infection. J. Pediat. **35**, 618 (1949). — MARCEL, J. E.: Le syndrome mége-vessie reflux cysto-pyélique. Presse méd. **1952**, 1793. — WILLIAMS, D. I.: The chronically dilated ureter. Ann. roy. Coll. Surg. Engl. **14**, 107 (1954).

VII. The mega-ureter-megacystis syndrom

BISCHOFF, P.: Brit. J. Urol. **29**, 416 (1957). — EDWARDS, D.: Cine-radiology in congenital bladder neck obstruction and mega-ureter. Brit. J. Urol. **29**, 410 (1957) — EISENSTAEDT, J. S.: Primary congenital megalo-ureters. Arch. Surg. (Chicago) **13**, 64 (1926). — GREVILLIUS, A.: Über einen Fall von Megaloureter bilateralis eines 5jährigen Mädchens. Acta chir. scand. **85**, 317 (1941). — GROGLER, F.: Über zwei Fälle von Megalureter. Z. urol. Chir. **34**, 55 (1932). — IRVIN, G. E., and J. E. KRAUS: Congenital megaloureter and hydro-ureter: pathogenesis and classification. Arch. Path. (Chicago) **45**, 752 (1948). — LEIBOVITZ, S.: Personal communication 1957. — LEIBOVITZ, S., and B. O'DONNELL: Cystometry in the mega-ureter-megacystis Syndrom. Brit. J. Urol. **29**, 399 (1957). — LEPOUTRE, C.: Dilatation de l'arbre urinaire et reflux vésico-urétéral d'origine congenitale. J. Urol. méd. chir. **33**, 560 (1932). — MARION, G.: Traité d'urologie, 4. edit. Paris: Masson & Cie. 1941. — ROUX, M., et A. CAILLET: A propos d'un cas de méga-uretère amélioré par la splanchnicectomie. J. Urol. méd. chir. **52**, 247 (1944/45). — SARGENT, J. C.: Bilateral uretero-nephrosis associated with congenital gaping ureteral orifices. J. Urol. (Baltimore) **16**, 23 (1926). — SCHMUTTE: Ein Fall von kongenitalem Megaloureter. Z. Urol. **21**, 608 (1927). — STEPHENS, F. D., R. A. JOSKE and R. T. SIMMONS: Mega-ureter with vesico-ureteric reflux in twins. Aust. N. Z. J. Surg.

24, 192 (1955). — STEPHENS, F. D.: Megaureter. Aust. N. Z. J. Surg. **23**, 197 (1954). — SWENSON, O., and J. H. FISHER: Relation of megacolon and megaloureter. New Engl. J. Med. **253**, 1147 (1955). — New techniques in the diagnosis and treatment of megaloureters. Pediatrics **18**, 304 (1956). — SWENSON, O., H. E. MacMAHON, W. E. JACQUES and J. S. CAMPBELL: New concept of the etiology of megaloureter. New Engl. J. Med. **246**, 41 (1952). — WILLIAMS, D. I.: The chronically dilated ureter. Ann. roy. Coll. Surg. Engl. **14**, 107 (1954). — WYLLIE, G. G.: Treatment of Hirschsprung's disease by Swenson's operation. Lancet **1957**, i, 850.

VIII. Simple mega-ureter

CAMPBELL, E. W.: Megalo-ureter. J. Urol. (Baltimore) **60**, 31 (1948). — CARLSON, H. E.: The intrapsoas transplant of megalo-ureter. J. Urol. (Baltimore) **72**, 171 (1954). — EVERIDGE, J.: Valvular obstruction of ureter. Proc. roy. Soc. Med. **25**, 1683 (1932). — GLOOR, H. U.: On the causes of megalo-ureters. Schweiz. med. Wschr. **1939**, 1080. — HEPLER, A. B.: Non-obstructive dilatations of upper urinary tract in children. J. Amer. med. Ass. **109**, 1602 (1937). — LAURET, G., et A. VIGNERON: Les malformations congénitales de la fonction uretèro-vésicale chez l'enfant. J. Urol. méd. chir. **61**, 15 (1955). — LEWIS, E. L., and R. W. CLETSOWAY: Megaloureter. J. Urol. (Baltimore) **75**, 643 (1956). — MacMYN, D. J.: On dilatation of the ureters and hydronphrosis in childhood. Brit. J. Urol. **1**, 152 (1929). — MURNAGHAN, G. F.: The Normal and Dilated Ureter. Brit. J. Urol. **21**, 403 (1957). — NESBIT, R. M., and J. F. R. WITYCOMHBE: Problem of primary megalo-ureter. J. Urol. (Baltimore) **72**, 162 (1954). — ORMOND, J. K.: Megalo-ureter and related conditions in children: report of 6 cases. J. Urol. (Baltimore) **70**, 171 (1953). — ORMOND, J. K., and R. W. OSBORNE: Plastic surgery of the ureter in children. J. Urol. (Baltimore) **67**, 860 (1952). — PUHL, H.: Die primäre Dilatation des Harnleiters. Z. Urol. **28**, 328 (1934). — SCARDINO, P. L.: Management of ureteral obstruction in children. J. med. Ass. Ga. **40**, 164 (1951). — SWENSON, O., J. H. FISHER and J. CENDRON: Megaloureter: investigation as to the cause and report on the results of newer forms of treatment. Surgery **40**, 223 (1956). — VERMOOTEN, V.: New etiology for certain types of the dilated ureters in children. J. Urol. (Baltimore) **41**, 455 (1939).

D. Congenital abnormalities of the lower urinary tract

I. Urachal abnormalities

BEGG, R. C.: The urachus. Surg. Gynec. Obstet. **45**, 165 (1927). — The urachus, its anatomy, histology and development. J. Anat. (Lond.) **64**, 170 (1929/30). — CAMPBELL, M. F.: Clinical paediatric urology. Philadelphia: W. B. Saunders Company 1951. — CHERRY, J. W.: Patent urachus. J. Urol. (Baltimore) **63**, 693 (1950). — DREYFUSS, M. L., and M. M. FLIESS: Patent Urachus with stone formation. J. Urol. (Baltimore) **46**, 77 (1941). — DUCLOUX, H., et S. BLONDIN: L'Ouraque et les fistules urinaires de l'ombilic. Rev. Chir. (Paris) **70**, 45 (1932). — HERBST, W. P.: Patient urachus. Sth. med. J. (Bgham, Ala.) **30**, 711 (1937). — LADD, W. E., and R. E. GROSS: Abdominal surgery of infancy and childhood. Philadelphia: W. B. Saunders Company 1941. — TRIMINGHAM, H. L., and J. R. McDONALD: Congenital anomalies in the region of the umbilicus. Surg. Gynec. Obstet. **80**, 152 (1945).

II. Rare bladder malformations

BOISSONNAT, P.: Vessie double (Vesica duplex) avec uretre unique chez un garcon de 4 ans. Operation plastique. Excellent resultat anatomique et fonctionnel. J. Urol. méd. chir. **59**, 883 (1953). — BOISSONNAT, P., et P. BOUTEAU: Volumineux kyste du trigone chez un garcon de 3 ans. J. Urol. méd. chir. **60**, 688 (1954). — BURNS, E., H. CUMMINS and J. HYMAN: Incomplete reduplication of the bladder with congenital solitary kidney. J. Urol. (Baltimore) **57**, 257 (1947). — CAMPBELL, M. F.: Clinical paediatric urology. Philadelphia: W. B. Saunders Company 1951. — CHWALLE, R.: Congenital hour glass bladder. Z. urol. Chir. **230**, 200 (1927). — IGNATESCU, M., H. SLOBOZIANU et E. ATHANASIU-VERGU: Absence de la vessie et abouchement des uretères dans l'uterus chez deux jumelles. J. Urol. méd. chir. **45**, 51 (1938). — KESSELBERG, C. O.: Über fehlerhafte Ausmündung eines Müllerschen Ganges in die Blase bei regelrechter Entwicklung des zweiten Müllerschen Ganges, der Blase und des Endarmes. (Bericht über zwei Beobachtungen.) Virchows Arch. path. Anat. **288**, 269 (1933). — KOHLER, H. H.: Septal bladder, with multiple genitourinary anomalies and uraemia. J. Urol. (Baltimore) **44**, 63 (1940). — KOOK, H., B. KAMBI and H. B. HERMANN: Trigonal curtain obstruction in a female child. J. Urol. (Baltimore) **73**, 1026 (1955). — LAUGHLIN, V. C., G. H. DERIAN and P. F. BOYD: Incomplete frontal septum of bladder complicated by congenital urethral valves and complete reduplication of upper left urinary tract. J. Urol. (Baltimore) **68**, 289 (1952). —

LEARMONTH, J. R., and K. H. WATKINS: Rare type of valvular obstruction of the neck of the bladder. Brit. J. Surg. **22**, 879 (1935). — LEPOUTRE, C.: Sur un cas d'absence congénitale de la vessie (persistance du cloaque). J. Urol. méd. chir. **48**, 334 (1939/40). — MEYER, R.: Zwei Fälle von Mißbildung der Harnblase bei Feten. Zbl. Gynäk. **56**, 1090 (1932). — MICHON, L., BOYET et CAMMENOS: Kyste du trigone chez une fillette de 3 ans. J. Urol. méd. chir. **59**, 529 (1953). — MILLER, H. L.: Agenesis of the urinary bladder and urethra. J. Urol. (Baltimore) **59**, 1156 (1948). — NESBIT, R. M., and W. BROMME: Double penis and double bladder. Amer. J. Roentgenol. **30**, 497 (1933). — OCKERBLAD, N. F., and H. E. CARLSON: Congenital hour-glass bladder. Surgery **8**, 665 (1940). — POOLE-WILSON, D. S.: Congenital valvular obstruction of the neck of the bladder. Brit. J. Urol. **15**, 11 (1943). — RAVITCH, M. M., and W. W. SCOTT: Duplication of the entire colon, bladder and urethra. Surgery **34**, 843 (1953). — ROLLER, C. S.: Intra-vesical external os uteri. A case of congenital absence of the vagina with external os of menstruating uterus opening into the bladder just below and internal to the right ureteral orifice. Urol. cutan. Rev. **38**, 730 (1934). — SWINNEY, J.: Case of congenital vesico vaginal fistula. Brit. J. Urol. **23**, 64 (1951). — WEBER, F. P., and M. SCHOLTZ: Congenital vesico-vaginal fistula with imperforate hymen; hydrops foetalis and erythroblastosis; polydactyly. Brit. J. Child. Dis. **36**, 131 (1939). — ZELLERMAYER, J., and H. E. CARLSON: Congenital hour-glass bladder. J. Urol. (Baltimore) **51**, 24 (1944).

III. Vesical diverticula

BADENOCH, A. W.: Congenital obstruction at the bladder neck. Ann. roy. Coll. Surg. Engl. **4**, 295 (1949). — BETHUNE, C. W., C. HAYDEN and M. WARWICK: So-called triple bladder. Report of a case of congenital diverticula. Urol. cutan Rev. **50**, 726 (1946). — CAULK, J. R.: The ureter as a possible origin of certain diverticula, the bladder. J. Urol. (Baltimore) **21**, 23 (1929). — CHWALLE, R.: Progress of formation of cystic dilatations of vesical end of ureter and of diverticula at ureteral ostium. Urol. cutan. Rev. **31**, 499 (1927). — ENGLISCH, J.: Über angeborene Verschließungen und Verengerungen der männlichen Harnröhre. Arch. Kinderheilk. **2**, 85 (1880/81). — HYMAN, A.: Diverticula of the bladder in children. J. Urol. (Baltimore) **9**, 431 (1923). — KRETSCHMER, H. L.: Diverticulum of the bladder in infancy and childhood. Amer. J. Dis. Child. **48**, 842 (1934).

IV. Bladder neck obstruction and urethral fibro-elastosis

ANDREASSEN, M.: Vesical neck obstruction in children. Acta chir. scand. **105**, 398 (1953). BADENOCH, A. W.: Congenital obstruction at the bladder neck. Ann. roy. Coll. Surg. Engl. **4**, 295 (1949). — BODIAN, M.: Congenital bladder neck obstruction. Brit. J. Urol. **29**, 393 (1957). — BOPPE, M., et J. E. MARCEL: Hypertrophie congenitale du col vesical operée et guerie chez un enfant de 7 ans. Bull. Soc. Pédiatr. Paris **31**, 315 (1933). — Les maladies du col vesical chez le nourrisson et l'enfant. Bull. méd. (Paris) **62**, 275 (1948). — BURNS, E., A. M. PRATT and R. G. HENDON: Management of bladder neck obstruction in children. J. Amer. med. Ass. **157**, 570 (1955). — CAMPBELL, M. F.: Submucous fibrosis of the bladder outlet in infancy and childhood. J. Amer. med. Ass. **94**, 1373 (1930). — EMMETT, J. L., and H. F. HELMHOLZ: Transurethral resection of the vesical neck in infants and children. J. Urol. (Baltimore) **60**, 463 (1948). — EMMETT, J. L., and H. B. SIMON: Transurethral resection in infants and children for congenital obstruction of the vesical neck and myelodysplasia. J. Urol. (Baltimore) **76**, 595 (1956). — GRANT, O.: Obstructions at the vesical neck in children. J. Urol. (Baltimore) **40**, 114 (1938). — LIEGE, R., et H. MARION: La maladie du col vesical chez l'enfant. Bull. Soc. Pédiatr. Paris **35**, 693 (1937). — MARION, G.: Traite d'urologie, 4. edit. Paris: Masson & Cie. 1940. — McDONALD, H. P., W. E. UPCHURCH and C. E. STURDEVANT: Vesical neck obstructions in children. J. Urol. (Baltimore) **70**, 94 (1953). — MILLER, A.: Cysto-urethroscopy of enuretic children. Proc. roy. Soc. Med. **49**, 895 (1956). — MITCHELL, J. P., and G. S. ANDREWS: Clinical aspects and pathology of bladder neck obstruction. Proc. roy. Soc. Med. **46**, 549 (1953). — RINKER, J. R.: Transurethral resection of the bladder neck in the treatment of congenital abnormalities in children. Sth. med. J. (Bgham, Ala.) **44**, 382 (1951). — STEPHENS, F. D.: Urethral obstruction in childhood. Aust. N.Z. J. Surg. **25**, 89 (1955). — THOMPSON, H. T.: Obstruction of the vesical neck in children. N. Y. St. J. Med. **56**, 361 (1956). — VAIL, A., and T. P. STONE: Congenital hypertrophy of the neck of the bladder. Arch. Path. (Chicago) **43**, 427 (1947). — YOUNG, B. W.: Retropubic approach to vesical neck obstruction in children. Surg. Gynec. Obstet. **96**, 150 (1953).

V. Urethral obstructions

ADDISON, O. L.: Congenital valvular obstruction of the urethra. Arch. Dis. Childh. **4**, 255 (1929). — ANGEN, G., u. E. KARLMARK: Zur Klinik und pathologischen Anatomie der angeborenen Urethralappen. Acta paediat. (Uppsala) 13, 20 (1932). — BALDRIDGE, R. R.: Case of congenital hypertrophy of the verumontanum. New Engl. J. Med. 213, 46 (1935). — BOISSONNAT, P.: Retrecissements congenitaux de l'urètre. J. d'Urol. 61, 399 (1955). — BOISSONNAT, P., et P. BOUTEAU: Valvule de l'urètre anterieur. J. d'Urol. 60, 949 (1954). — BRINKMAN, W., u. E. BONTKE: Harnverhaltung beim Neugeborenen. Z. Urol. 50, 21 (1957). — BROWN, H. S.: Congenital obstructions of the urethra — report of two cases. J. of Urol. 23, 275 (1930). — BUGBEE, H. G., and M. WALLSTEIN: Retention of urine due to congenital hypertrophy of the verumontanum. J. of Urol. 10, 477 (1923). — BUSCH, K. R.: Kongenitale Harnrohrenstenosen. Z. urol. Chir. 44, 460 (1939). — CAMPBELL, M. F.: Clinical Padiatric Urology. Philadelphia: W. B. Saunders Company 1951. — CHADWICK, R. T., and S. P. MEADOWS: Congenital obstruction of the posterior urethra. Brit. med. J. 1930, i, 443. — COUNSELLER, V. S., and J. G. MENVILLE: Congenital valves of the posterior urethra. J. Urol. (Baltimore) 34, 268 (1935). — CROWELL, W. M., and R. H. ANDERSON: Congenital urethral stricture. Clin. Proc. Child. Hosp. Wash. 6, 68 (1950). — DOURMASHKIN, R. L.: Complete urethral occlusion in living new-born. J. Urol. (Baltimore) 50, 747 (1943). — EHRLICH, A.: Congenital stenosis of prostatic urethra. Amer. J. Dis. Child. 91, 625 (1956). — EMMETT, J. L.: Obstruction of the vesical neck of a male infant produced by hypertrophy of the verumontanum. Proc. Mayo Clin. 15, 364 (1940). — FAGERSTROM, D. P.: Congenital obstruction of the lower urinary tract in the male. J. Urol. (Baltimore) 37, 166 (1937). — HASEN, H. B., and Y. S. SONG: Congenital valvular obstruction of the posterior urethra in two brothers. J. Pediat. 47, 207 (1955). — JORUP, S., u. S. R. KJELLBERG: Congenital valvular formations in the urethra. Acta radiol. (Stockh.) 30, 197 (1948). — KRUGER, R.: Über vesica gigantea. Z. urol. Chir. 32, 330 (1931). — LOWSLEY, O. S., and J. J. KIRWIN: A clinical and pathological study of congenital obstructions of the urethra. J. Urol. (Baltimore) 31, 497 (1934). — MARQUARDT, C., and A. FREDERICK: Congenital imperforate urinary meatus. Surgery 47, 78 (1943). — MAY, F.: Ein Fall von kongenitalem Verschluß der Urethra membranacea. Z. Urol. 42, 245 (1949). — MENEGAUX, G., et M. BOIDOT: Des obliterations congenitales du meat et de la portion balanique de l'urètre (hypospadias escepté). J. Chir. Paris 43, 641 (1934). — MUSCHAT, M.: Occlusion of urethral meatus. Amer. J. Dis. Child. 67, 275 (1944). — NESBIT, R. M., R. L. THIRLBY and F. P. RAPER: Diagnosis and treatment of congenital urethral valves. J. Mich. med. Soc. 50, 1244 (1951). — PILCHER jr., F., and H. W. PRICE: Congenital hypertrophy of the verumontanum. J. Amer. med. Ass. 115, 2072 (1940). — RAPER, F. P.: The recognition and treatment of congenital urethral valves. Brit. J. Urol. 25, 130 (1953). — TORP, K. H.: Congenital valvular formation of the posterior urethra. Acta paediat. (Uppsala) 43, 192 (1954). — TSENG, H. C.: Congenital diaphragm and fistula of penile urethra. J. Urol. (Baltimore) 65, 590 (1951). — WILLIAMS, D. I.: Congenital valves in the posterior urethra. Brit. med. J. 1954, i, 623. — YOUNG, H. H., and R. W. MCKAY: Congenital valvular obstruction of the prostatic urethra. Surg. Gynec. Obstet. 48, 509 (1929).

VI. Urethral diverticula and duplications

BOISSONNAT, P.: Absence congenitale des corps caverneux de l'urètre posterieur et du col vesical chez un nouveau-né. J. Urol. méd. chir. 60, 69 (1954). — Cinq cas de canaux accessoires, suivis d'un essai de classification anatomique de ces conduits surnumeraires. J. Urol. méd. chir. 60, 954 (1954). — BROWN, J. J. M.: Lesions of the anterior urethra in infancy and childhood. Proc. roy. Soc. Med. 49, 891 (1956). — CAMPBELL, M. F.: Clinical pediatric urology. Philadelphia: W. B. Saunders Company 1951. — COUVELAIRE, R.: A rare form of reduplication of the urethra in a child of six months. J. Urol. méd. chir. 53, 308 (1944/45). — FORSHALL, I., and P. P. RICKHAM: A case of congenital diverticulum of the anterior urethra in a male infant. Brit. J. Urol. 25, 142 (1953). — GEIRINGER, D., and M. O. ZUCKER: Diverticulum of the anterior urethra in a male child. Amer. J. Surg. 44, 463 (1939). — GROSS, R. E., and A. H. BILL: Concealed diverticulum of the male urethra as a cause of urinary obstruction. Pediatrics 1, 44 (1948). — GROSS, R. E., and T. C. MOORE: Duplication of the urethra: report of 2 cases and summary of the literature. Arch. Surg. (Chicago) 60, 749 (1950). — HIGGINS, T. T., D. I. WILLIAMS and D. F. E. NASH: The urology of childhood. London: Butterworth & Co. 1951. HOWELL, C., E. T. LISANSKY and E. SCOTT: Congenital cyst of the urethra in a 3 weeks old male infant causing pyonephrosis and death. A case report. Bull. Sch. Med. Maryland 26, 241 (1942). — JOHNSON, C. M.: Diverticula and cyst of female urethra. J. Urol. (Baltimore) 39, 506 (1938). — LANDES, R. R., and C. L. RANSOM: Müllerian duct cysts. J. Urol. (Baltimore) 61, 1089 (1949). — LIBAN, E.: Rare malformation of urethra as a cause of congenital obstruction of the lower urinary tract. Amer. J. Dis. Child. 84, 340 (1952). — LOWSLEY, O. S.: Accessary urethra. Report of two cases with a review of the literature. N.Y. St. J. Med. 39, 1022 (1939). — McKENNA, C. M., and J. H. KIEFER: Congenital enlargement of the prostatic utricle with inclusion of the ejaculatory ducts and seminal vesicles. Trans. Amer. Ass. gen.-urin. Surg. 32, 305 (1939). — McKENZIE, D. W.: In discussion re McKENNA and KIEFER's case. Trans. Amer. Ass. gen.-urin. Surg. **32**, 317 (1939). — MILLS, W. G. Q.: Chronic retention in boys caused by diverticula in the anterior urethra. Brit. J. Urol. **27**, 292 (1955). — NESBITT, T. E.: Congenital megalo-urethra. J. Urol. (Baltimore) **73**, 839 (1955). — NICOLA, R. R. DE, and R. C. McCARTNEY: Urethral duplication in a female child treated with sclerosing solution. J. Urol. (Baltimore) **61**, 1065 (1949). — RINKER, J. R.: Accessory urethra in a boy. J. Urol. (Baltimore) **50**, 331 (1943). — TERNOVSKY, S.: Congenital diverticulum of the urethra. Urol. cutan. Rev. **1930**, 578. — WRENN, E. L., and A. J. MICHIE: Complete duplications of the male urethra. Ann. Surg. **145**, 119 (1957).

VII. Malformations associated with absence of abdominal muscles

BORD, R. A. DE: Congenital deficiency of abdominal musculature. Ann. Surg. **142**, 863 (1955). — DAUT, D. R., J. L. EMMETT and R. L. J. KENNEDY: Congenital absence of abdominal muscles with urological complications: report of a patient successfully treated. Proc. Mayo Clin. **22**, 8 (1947). — EAGLE, J., and G. S. BARRETT: Congenital deficiency of abdominal musculature associated genito-urinary abnormalities. Pediatrics **6**, 721 (1950). — GREENE, L. F., J. L. EMMETT and O. S. CULP: Congenital absence of abdominal muscles with urologic complications: a further report. Proc. Mayo Clin. **27**, 325 (1952). — HENLEY, W. L., and A. HYMAN: Absent abdominal muscles. Genito-urinary anomalies and deficiency in the pelvic autonomic system. Amer. J. Dis. Child. **86**, 795 (1953). — HOWARD, P. J.: Congenital absence of the abdominal muscles and genito-urinary malformation. Amer. J. Dis. Child. **60**, 669 (1940). — JAMESON, S. G., and J. O. COOPER: Agenesis of abdominal musculature with ectopic ureteral orifice and congenital absence of opposite kidney and ureter. J. Pediat. **47**, 489 (1955). — MAUERMAYER, W.: Über kongenitale Mißbildungen an den Harnorganen, vergesellschaftet mit fehlender Bauchdeckenmuskulatur. Z. Kinderheilk. **75**, 671 (1955). — SILVERMAN, F. N., and N. HUANG: Congenital absence of the abdominal muscles, associated with malformations of genito-urinary and alimentary tracts. Amer. J. Dis. Child. **80**, 91 (1950).

VIII. Malformations associated with anal atresia

ANDERS, H. E.: Über Kloakenmißbildungen. Virchows Arch. path. Anat. **229**, 531 (1921). BUYS, R. DE, and H. CUMMINS: Persistent cloacae and other anomalies in a female infant. Amer. J. Dis. Child. **41**, 871 (1931). — CAMPBELL, M. F.: Urethrorectal fistula. J. Urol. (Baltimore) **76**, 411 (1956). — FITZPATRICK, L. J., and R. B. HILLSMAN: Congenital rectovesical anastomosis. Amer. J. Dis. Child. **47**, 593 (1934). — GERCKEN, F., u. R. KNEPPER: Fetale Riesenblase und kongenitale Pseudolebercirrhose mit eklamptischen Nekrosen und Ascites. Zbl. Gynäk. **61**, 710 (1937). — KRÜGER, R.: Über Vesica gigantea. Z. urol. Chir. **32**, 330 (1931). LADD, W. E., and R. E. GROSS: Congenital malformations of anus and rectum. Amer. J. Surg. **23**, 167 (1934). — LOWSLEY, O. S.: Persistent cloaca in the female. Report of 2 cases corrected by operation. J. Urol. (Baltimore) **59**, 692 (1948). — LYNCH, K. M., and A. J. JERVEY: Dystocia due to ascites in foetus with persistent cloaca. Surg. Gynec. Obstet. **22**, 618 (1916). MAJOR, S. G.: Persistence of the cloaca. Min. Med. **12**, 96 (1929). — MILLER, F.: Zur Kenntnis der Kloakenmißbildungen. Frankf. Z. Path. **54**, 378 (1940). — NORDENFELT, O.: Two cases of cloacal formation with congenital hydroureter and hydrocolpos. Acta obstet. gynec. scand. **5**, 1 (1926). — PARIN, B.: Atresia ani urethralis. Arch. klin. Chir. **166**, 386 (1931). — SPENCE, H. M.: Anomalies and complications of the urogenital tract associated with congenital imperforate anus. J. Urol. (Baltimore) **71**, 453 (1954). — STEWART, R. L., and J. A. ROSS: Congenital rectourinary fistula. Brit. J. Urol. **23**, 129 (1951). — THUNIG, L. A.: Atresia ani urethralis: report of a case. Arch. Surg. (Chicago) **38**, 501 (1939). — WATSON, P. C., and D. I. WILLIAMS: The urological complications of excision of the rectum. Brit. J. Surg. **60**, 19 (1952). WILLIAMS, D. I., and H. H. NIXON: Agenesis of the sacrum. Surg. Gynec. Obstet. **105**, 84 (1957). — YOUNG, H. H.: Imperforate anus; bowel opening into urethra, hypospadias: a presentation of a new plastic method. J. Amer. med. Ass. **107**, 1448 (1936).

IX. Ectopia vesicae and epispadias

BOEMINGHAUS, H.: Zur Behandlung der Blasenexstrophies mittels Blasen-Mastdarm-Anastomose. Chirurg **27**, 167 (1956). — BOYCE, W. H., and S. A. VEST: A new concept concerning the treatment of exstrophy of the bladder. J. Urol. (Baltimore) **67**, 503 (1952). — BRAKELEY, E.: Extrophy of the bladder, complicated by other congenital anomalies. Amer. J. Dis. Child. **43**, 931 (1932). — CAMPBELL, M.: Epispadias: a report of 15 cases. J. Urol. (Baltimore) **67**, 988 (1952). — DAVIES, D. V.: Ectopia vesicae. Brit. J. Urol. **14**, 1 (1942). — DAVIS, D. M.: Epispadias in females and its surgical treatment. J. Urol. (Baltimore) **20**, 673 (1928). — DEES, J. E.: Congenital epispadias with incontinence. J. Urol. (Baltimore) **62**, 513

(1949). — GARRETT, R. A., and J. H. O. MERTZ: Follow-up studies of bladder exstrophy with ureterosigmoidostomy. J. Urol. (Baltimore) 71, 299 (1954). — GAUDIN, H. J., and H. CABOT: Partial exstrophy of the bladder, embryological consideration: report of a case. Proc. Mayo Clin. 13, 216 (1938). — GODARD, H.: Epispadias total. Traitement de l'incontinence par transposition pre-rectale de la vessie. J. d'Urol. 53, 467 (1946). — GOODWIN, W. E., and P. B. HUDSON: Exstrophy of the bladder treated by rectal transplantation of the divided trigone. Surg. Gynec. Obstet. 93, 331 (1951). — GREY-TURNER, G.: The treatment of congenital defects of the bladder and urethra by implantation of the ureter with the bowel, 17 personal cases. Brit. J. Surg. 17, 114 (1929). — GRUBER, G. B.: Über Ektopie der Harnblase. Dtsch. Z. Chir. 227, 337 (1930). — HALL, E. G., A. E. McCANDLESS and P. P. RICKHAM: Vesicointestinal fissure with diphallus. Brit. J. Urol. 25, 219 (1953). — HARVARD, B. M., and G. J. THOMPSON: Congenital exstrophy of the urinary bladder: late results of treatment by Coffey-Mayo method of uretero-intestinal anastomosis. J. Urol. (Baltimore) 65, 223 (1951). — HEJT-MANCIK, J. H., W. B. KING and M. A. MAGID: Pseudo-exstrophy of the bladder. J. Urol. (Baltimore) 72, 829 (1954). — HEPBURN, T. N.: Repair of exstrophy of the bladder. J. Urol. (Baltimore) 65, 389 (1951). — HIGGINS, C. C.: Exstrophy of the bladder: review of 70 cases. J. Urol. (Baltimore) 63, 852 (1950). — KINDLER, K.: Beitrag zur Methodik der Harnleiter-Darmverbindungen, insbesondere für die Behandlung der Blasenexstrophie nebst klinischen Ergebnissen. Beitr. klin. Chir. 177, 489 (1948). — LATTIMER, J. K., A. L. DEAN, C. H. FUREY and L. BALLANTYNE: Reconstruction of the urinary bladder in children with exstrophy. N.Y. St. J. Med. 57, 746 (1957). — LUHMANN, K.: Über Blasenekstrophie und ihre chirurgische Behandlung. Beitr. klin. Chir. 165, 221 (1937). — MAKKAS, M.: Zur Behandlung der Blasenektopie. Beitr. klin. Chir. 163, 554 (1936). — MARION, G.: De la constitution d'un urètre continent chez la femme et de son emploi dans l'exstrophie vesicale. J. Urol. méd. chir. 37, 393 (1934). — MAYER, A.: Bemerkungen zur operativen Behandlung der Ektopia vesicae. Zbl. Gynäk. 73, 551 (1951). — MAYO, C. H.: Exstrophy of the bladder. Contributions to medical and biolocal research, p. 1095. New York: Paul B. Hoeber 1919. — McFARLAND, J.: Exstrophy of the bladder with imperforate anus, absence of the greater part of the small and large intestines, continuity of the duodenum with the colon, absence of the left testis, epididymis and cord, and enormous hydroureter. Amer. J. Path. 14, 509 (1938). — McINTOSH, J. F., and G. WORLEY jr.: Adenocarcinoma arising in exstrophy of the bladder: report of 2 cases and a review of the literature. J. Urol. (Baltimore) 73, 820 (1955). — MERCIER, O.: Personal technique for the cure of epispadias in a woman. Brit. J. Urol. 6, 313 (1934). — MICHON, L.: Conservative operations for exstrophy of the bladder, with particular reference to urinary continence. Brit. J. Urol. 20, 167 (1948). — PATTEN, B. M., and A. BARRY: Genesis of exstrophy of the bladder and epispadias. Amer. J. Anat. 90, 35 (1952). — PETERSSON, G.: Treatment of extroversion of the bladder with coexisting anal incompetence. Acta chir. scand. 102, 338 (1952). — POWELL, T. O.: Surgery on the exstrophied bladder: preliminary report. J. Urol. (Baltimore) 74, 67 (1955). — RUSSELL, K. F.: Case of complicated exstrophy of the bladder presenting many unusual features. Brit. J. Urol. 11, 31 (1939). — SANDERUD, A.: Exstrophy of the bladder: a follow-up examination of 17 cases. Acta chir. scand. 106, 117 (1953). — STRONG, G. H.: Repair of large abdominal defects following cystectomy for congenital vesical exstrophy: a new technique. J. Urol. (Baltimore) 64, 743 (1950). — SWEETSER, T. H.: Exstrophy of the urinary bladder. Further study of treatment by plastic surgery. Arch. Surg. (Chicago) 68, 525 (1954). — SWEETSER, T. H., T. C. CHISHOLM, W. H. THOMPSON, E. B. BERGLUND, S. P. WESOLOWSKI and T. H. SWEETSER jr.: Exstrophy of the urinary bladder, its treatment by plastic surgery. J. of Urol. 75, 448 (1956). — SWEETSER, T. H., T. C. CHISHOLM and W. H. THOMPSON: Exstrophy of the urinary bladder. Discussion of anatomical and surgical principles applicable to its repair, with preliminary report of a case. Minn. Med. 35, 654 (1952). — THOMPSON, A. R.: Vesical extroversion with control of micturition. Brit. med. J. 1937, ii, 3. — WYBURN, G. M.: Development of the infra-umbilical position of the abdominal wall with remarks on the aetiology of ectopia vesicae. J. Arat. (Lond.) 71, 201 (1937). — WILHELMI, O. J.: Exstrophy of the bladder with pyelographic follow-up. J. Urol. (Baltimore) 59, 1108 (1948). — WILLIAMS, D. I., and H. R. JOLLY: Long term results of transplantation of the ureters for ectopia vesicae. Gt. Ormond Str. J. 1952, No 3, 9. — YOUNG, H. H.: Exstrophy of the bladder: the first case in which a normal bladder and urinary control have been obtained by plastic operations. Surg. Gynec. Obstet. 74, 729 (1942).

X. Hypospadias and allied disorders

BARCAT, J. R.: Les formes antérieures de l'hypospadias. Sem. Hôp. Paris 23, 896 (1947). — BHANDARI, S. L.: Case of hypospadias with double urethral channel. Indian med. Gaz. 65, 444 (1931). — BROWNE, D.: Hypospadias. Postgrad. med. J. 25, 367 (1949). — BUCKNALL, R. T. H.: A new operation for penile hypospadias. Lancet 1907, ii, 887. — CAMPBELL, M. F.: Clinical Pediatric Urology. Philadelphia: W. B. Saunders Company 1951. — CECIL, A. B.:

Repair of hypospadias and urethral fistula. J. Urol. (Baltimore) **56**, 237 (1946). — Fèvre, M.: Généralitiés sur le traitement de l'hypospadias. Sem. Hôp. Paris **23**, 893 (1947). — Fogh-Andersen, P.: Hypospadias: 34 completed cases operated according to Denis Browne. Acta chir. scand. **105**, 414 (1953). — Howard, E. S.: Hypospadias with enlargement of the prostatic utricle. Surg. Gynec. Obstet. **86**, 307 (1948). — McKenna, C. M., and J. H. Kiefer: Unusual anomaly of the urogenital tract associated with hypospadias. Urol. cutan. Rev. **47**, 14 (1943). Nesbit, R. M.: Surgical treatment of congenital chordee without hypospadias. J. Urol. (Baltimore) **72**, 1178 (1954). — Nové-Josserand, G.: Traitement de l'hypospadias, nouvelle méthode. Lyon méd. **85**, 198 (1897). — Oberniedermayr, A.: Erfahrungen mit der Operation der Hypospadie nach Denis-Browne. Arch. klin. Chir. **282**, 936 (1955). — Ombrédanne, L.: Hypospadias penien chez l'enfant. Bull. Soc. nat. Chir. Paris **37**, 1076 (1911). — Pfeiffer, K. M.: Die Resultate der Hypospadie-Operation nach Ombrédanne. Ann. paediat. (Basel) **185**, 61 (1955). — Smith, D. R.: Hypospadias: its anatomic and therapeutic considerations. J. int. Coll. Surg. **24**, 64 (1955). — Young, F., and J. A. Benjamin: Repair of hypospadias with free inlay graft. Surg. Gynec. Obstet. **86**, 439 (1948).

E. Lower urinary tract obstruction

Bakker, N. J.: Over chronische urineretentie bij kinderen. Maandschr. Kindergeneesk. **24**, 1 (1956). — Bandler, C. G., and A. H. Milbert: Obstructive uropathies in children. J. Mt Sinai Hosp. **4**, 690 (1938). — Boissonnat, P.: L'absence de miction chez le nouveau-né. Rev. Prat. (Paris) **1955**, 1213. — Brown, R. K., and E. C. Brown: Sacrococcygeal teratoma with urinary retention. Arch. Surg. (Chicago) **60**, 535 (1950). — Burns, E., and P. Shashy: Problems in the management of bladder neck obstruction in children. Ohio St. med. J. **53**, 170 (1957). — Campbell, M. F.: Traumatic cord bladder in a premature infant; successful treatment by indwelling catheter. J. Urol. (Baltimore) **52**, 564 (1944). — Edgecombe, K.: Dystocia due to idopathic dilatation of the foetal urinary tract. J. Obstet. Gynaec. Brit. Emp. **37**, 832 (1930). — Ericsson, N. O., J. Winberg u. R. Zetterstrom: Renal function in infantile obstructive uropathy. Acta paediat. (Uppsala) **44**, 444 (1955). — Frontz, W. A.: Congenital urinary obstruction in male children, with reports of cases presenting unusual anomalies. J. Urol. (Baltimore) **27**, 489 (1932). — Goldberger, E.: Ein Fall von Kongenital-Erweiterung der fetalen Harnblase als Geburtshindernis. Mschr. Geburtsh. Gynäk. **81**, 253 (1929). — Hearn, J. B.: Urinary obstruction in a male infant. Brit. J. Radiol. **27**, 248 (1954). — Hoffman, W. L.: Retention of urine in a child due to an appendix abscess. Lancet **1932**, i, 778. — Hutch, J. A.: Pathological study of ureterovesical junctions of two stillborn infants with complete urethral atresia. J. Urol. (Baltimore) **74**, 795 (1955). — Jewett, H. J.: Diagnosis and management of urinary tract obstructions in children. Surg. Clin. N. Amer. **32**, 1371 (1952). — Ladd, W. E., and R. E. Gross: Abdominal surgery of infancy and childhood. Philadelphia and London: W. B. Saunders Company 1941. — Last, R. J.: Chronic urethral obstruction in children. Brit. med. J. **1949**, i, 179. — Lord, J. M.: Foetal ascites. Arch. Dis. Childh. **28**, 398 (1953). — McCahey, J. F.: Urinary bladder obstruction in children. J. int. Coll. Surg. **12**, 170 (1949). — Mitchell, J. M.: Retention of urine caused by faecal inpaction. Brit. med. J. **1929**, ii, 1198. — Morris, D. G.: Intraabdominal hydatid cyst causing renal failure. Brit. J. Surg. **40**, 402 (1953). — Nash, D. F. E.: Retention of urine in childhood. Med. Press. **229**, 569 (1953). — Nesbit, R. M., and W. C. Baum: Diagnosis and surgical management of obstructive uropathy in childhood. Amer. J. Dis. Child. **88**, 239 (1954). — Parrott, R. H.: Congenital urethral valve with apparent ascites. Clin. Proc. Child. Hosp. (Wash.) **7**, 309 (1951). — Pugh, R. C. B.: Personal communication. 1956. — Savage, J. E.: Dystocia due to dilatation of the foetal urinary bladder. Amer. J. Obstet. Gynec. **29**, 276 (1935). — Shaw, R. E., and H. J. Marriott: Origin of amniotic fluid and the bearing on this problem of foetal urethral atresia. J. Obstet. Gynaec. **56**, 1004 (1949). — Thompson, G. J.: Urinary obstruction of the vesical neck and posterior urethra of congenital origin. J. Urol. (Baltimore) **47**, 591 (1942). — Woodruff, S. R., and J. A. Begner: Sacroccygeal teratoma in an infant of five months causing acute urinary obstruction. J. of Urol. (Baltimore) **54**, 177 (1945). — Young, B. W., W. L. Anderson and G. G. King: Radiographic estimation of residual urine in children. J. of Urol. (Baltimore) **75**, 263 (1956).

F. Enuresis

Abernethy, A. C., and E. M. Tomlin: Treatment of enuresis in female children. J. Urol. (Baltimore) **72**, 1163 (1954). — Addis, R. S.: Statistical study of nocturnal enuresis. Arch. Dis. Childh. **10**, 169 (1935). — Anderson, F. N.: Psychiatric aspects of enuresis. Amer. J. Dis. Child. **40** (I), (II), 591 (1930). — Batty, R. J.: Enuresis. London: Staples Press 1948. — Behrle, F. C., M. T. Elkin and P. C. Laybourne: Evalution of a conditioning device in

the treatment of nocturnal enuresis. Pediatrics 17, 849 (1956). — BEVERLY, B. I.: Incontinence in children. J. Pediat. 2, 718 (1933). — BLOMFIELD, J. M., and J. W. B. DOUGLAS:
Bedwetting: prevalence among children aged 4 to 7 years. Lancet 1956, i, 850. — BONINE, M.: La
chirurgia della vesica nelf enuresi notturna. Nocturnal enuresis. Urologia Venezia 15, 87 (1948). —
BOSS, M.: Nocturnal enuresis. An example of the necessity of medical psychohygiene. Schweiz.
med. Wschr. 1945, 293. — BRODNY, M. L., and S. A. ROBINS: Enuresis: the use of cystoure-
thrography in diagnosis. J. Amer. med. Ass. 126, 1000 (1944). — CAMPBELL, M. F.: Clinical
pediatric urology. Philadelphia: W. B. Saunders Company 1951. — CIOFFARI, M. S., and
H. G. CLARK: Treatment of enuresis in children by means of chorionic gonadotropin. Arch.
Pediat. 64, 61 (1947). — CROSBY, N. D.: Essential enuresis: successful treatment based on
physiological concepts. Med. J. Aust. 1950, II 533. — FISHER, O. D., and W. I. FORSYTHE:
Micturating cystography in the investigation of Enuresis. Arch. Dis. Child 29, 451 (1954). —
FRARY, L. G.: Enuresis: a genetic study. Amer. J. Dis. Child. 49, 557 (1935). — GAYET. R.:
L'incontinence d'urine dite essentielle de la jeune fille. Son traitement par le resserrement du
sphincter vésical ou operation de MARION. Lyon méd. 161, 285 (1938). — GEPPERT, T.V.: Management of nocturnal enuresis by conditioned response. Automatic electric alarm. J. Amer. med.
Ass. 152, 381 (1953). — HEYMANN, K.: Enuresis in der Struktur des schwierigen Kindes. Ann.
paediat. (Basel) 158, 166 (1942). — HIGHAM, A. R. C.: Approach to the problem of simple
enuresis. Proc. roy. Soc. Med. 46, 849 (1953). — HUBBLE, D.: Enuresis. Brit. med. J. 1950, II
1108. — JOHNSON, S. H., and W. C. PRICE: Hypertrophy of the colliculus seminalis in childhood
a study of eighteen cases. Amer. J. Dis. Child. 78, 892 (1949). — KARLIN, I. W.: Incidence of
spina bifida occulta in children with and without enuresis. Amer. J. Dis. Child. 49, 125 (1935). —
KLACKENBERG, G.: Primary enuresis. Acta pediat. (Uppsala) 44, 513 (1955). — KUGELMASS,
I. N.: Androgenic arrest of familial enuresis. A study in 75 children. N. Y. St. J. Med.
47, 1369 (1947). — LANGE et MURET: Enuresis. Results obtained from PERRIN's operation.
J. Urol. méd. chir. 53, 479 (1946/47). — LESNÉ, E., J. A. LIEVRE et J. A. MMME. LIEVRE: Ra-
chischisis et incontinence nocturne d'urine. Bull. Soc. Pédiatr. Paris 32, 613 (1934). — LEWIS,
J. M., and J. OSTROFF: Psychic enuresis in normal children; an experimental study. Amer. J.
Dis. Child. 43, 1490 (1932). — MARSON, F. G. W.: Posterior pituitary snuff treatment of nocturnal enuresis. Brit. med. J. 1955, i, 1194. — McFADDEN, G. D. F.: Anatomical abnormalities
found in the urinary tract of enuretics, their significance and surgical treatment. Proc. roy.
Soc. Med. 48, 1121 (1955). — MICHAELS, J. J., and S. E. GOODMAN: Incidence of enuresis
and age of cessation in 1,00 neuro-psychiatric patients, with a discussion of. the relationship
between enuresis and delinquency. Amer. J. Orthopsychiat. 9, 59 (1939). — MOWRER,
O. H., and W. M. MOWRER: Enuresis, a method of its study and treatment. Amer. J. Orthopsychiat. 8, 436 (1938). — NASH, D. F. E.: Development of micturition control with special
reference to enuresis. Ann. roy. Coll. Surg. Engl. 5, 318 (1949). — POTTER, C. T.: Enuresis in
children. Practitioner 145, 33 (1940). — POULTON, E. M., and S. HINDEN: Classification of
enuresis. Arch. Dis. Childh. 28, 392 (1953). — ROSENSON, W., and R. LISWOOD: Sodium
chloride in the treatment of nocturnal enuresis in children. J. Pediat. 9, 751 (1936). —
SCHACHTER, M.: Contribution à l'étude des rapports de l'énuresie infantile avec les crises
commitiales. Ann. paediat. (Basel) 159, 19 (1942). — SCHLUTZ, F. W., and C. E. ANDERSON:
Endocrine treatment of enuresis. J. clin. Endocr. 3, 405 (1943). — SIENKIEWIEZ, E. M.:
Angeborene Minderwertigkeit der Prostata. Z. Urol. 31, 400 (1937). — SITKERY, J.: Untersuchungen über die Pathologie der sogenannten Enuresis nocturna. Z. Urol. 33, 409 (1939). —
STALKER, H., and D. BAND: Persistent enuresis, a psychosomatic study. J. ment. Sci. 92,
324 (1946). — STOCKWELL, L., and C. K. SMITH: Enuresis, a study of causes, type and thero-
peutic results. Amer. J. Dis. Child. 59, 1013 (1940). — SWEET, C.: Enuresis. A psychological
problem. J. Amer. med. Ass. 132, 279 (1946). — TAYLOR, J. A., and W. H. BERRY: Congenital absence of urinary sphincter with operative cure. J. Urol. (Baltimore) 70, 203 (1953). —
VULLIAMY, D.: Day and night output of urine in enuresis. Arch. Dis. Childh. 31, 439 (1956). —
WEXBERG, E.: Enuresis in neglected children. Amer. J. Dis. Child. 59, 490 (1940). — WINNICOT,
D. W.: Enuresis. Proc. roy. Soc. Med. 23, 255 (1929/30). — WINSBURY-WHITE, H. P.: A
study of 310 cases of enuresis treated by urethral dilatation. Brit. J. Urol. 13, 149 (1941).

G. Neurogenic bladder

CAMERON, A. H.: The spinal cord lesion in spina bifida cystica. Lancet 1956, ii, 176. —
CAMPBELL, M. E.: Incontinence clamp. J. Urol. (Baltimore) 64, 821 (1950. — CARR, T. L.: The
orthopaedic aspects of 100 cases of spina bifida. Postgrad. med. J. 32, 201 (1956). — CLARKE,
B. G.: Clinical study of the motor paralytic bladder in poliomyelitis. J. Urol. (Baltimore) 76,
66 (1956). CREEVY, C. D.: Treatment of paradoxical incontinence of urine associated with
spina bifida. J. of Pediat. 12, 747 (1938). — EMMETT, J. L., and H. F. HELMHOLZ: Transurethral resection of the vesical neck in infants and children. J. Urol. (Baltimore) 60, 463
(1948). — FISTER, G. M.: Fibrosis and submucous calcification of the vesical neck. J. Amer.

med. Ass. **118**, 604 (1942). — GODARD: Lumbo-sacral spina bifida with tumours and incontinence of urine treated by Goebell-Stoeckell operation. Bull. Soc. franç. Urol. **1937**, 92. — INGRAHAM, F. D., and H. SWAN: Spina bifida and cranium bifida: Survey of 546 cases. New Engl. J. Med. **228**, 559 (1943). — JENSEN jr., O. J., H. E. EGGERS, A. H. BILL and D. R. DILLARD: Urinary and fecal incontinence due to congenital abnormalities in children. Management by transplantation of ureters to an isolated ileostomy. J. Urol. (Baltimore) **73**, 322 (1955). — KARLIN, I. W.: Incidence of spina bifida occulta in children with and withour enuresis. Amer. Dis. Child. **49**, 125 (1935). — LAWSON, R. B., and F. K. GARVEY: Paralysis of the bladder in poliomyelitis. J. Amer. med. Ass. **135**, 93 (1947). — LORENZ, G.: Beitrag zum Problem der Myelodysplasie in der Urologie. Z. Urol. **47**, 611 (1954). — McCARROL, H. R.: Spina bifida urinary incontinence. Surg. Gynec. Obstet. **64**, 721 (1937). — MERTZ, H. O.: Relation of spina bifida occulta to neuromuscular dysfunction of the urinary tract, with a review of 6 cases operated by laminectomy. J. Urol. (Baltimore) **29**, 521 (1933). — MERTZ, H. O., and L. A. SMITH: Posterior spinal fusion defects and nerve dysfunction of the urinary tract. J. Urol. (Baltimore) **24**, 41 (1930). — NASH, D. F. E.: Ileal loop bladder in congenital spinal palsy. Brit. J. Urol. **28**, 387 (1956). — PICKRELL, K., N. GEORGIADE, H. CRAWFORD, C. MAGUIRE and A. BOOWE: Gracilis muscle transplant for correction of urinary incontinence in male children. Ann. Surg. **143**, 764 (1956). — PRINCE, C. L., and P. L. SCARDINO: Nonsurgical management of congenital neurogenic vesical dysfunction. J. Urol. (Baltimore) **69**, 520 (1953). — SMITH, C. K., and L. P. ENGEL: Neurogenic vesical dysfunction in children. J. Urol. (Baltimore) **28**, 675 (1932). — SWENSON, O., J. H. FISHER and J. CENDRON: Treatment of cord bladder incontinence in children. Ann. Surg. **144**, 421 (1956). — THIERMANN, E.: Ureterpenis. Z. Urol. **47**, 118 (1954). — THOMPSON, G. J., and C. E. JACOBSON jr.: Neurogenic vesical dysfunction due to spina bifida and myelodysplasia. Treatment by transurethral resection of the vesical neck. Amer. J. Surg. **61**, 224 (1943).

H. Non-tuberculous urinary infections

ABESHOUSE, B. S., and D. E. BOGORAD: Perinephric abscess and diseases of the vertebrae and spinal cord. Urol. cutan. Rev. **39**, 295 (1935). — ABT, I. A.: Diagnosis and treatment of urogenital infection in childhood. Illinois med. J. **66**, 521 (1934). — ANTELL, L.: Perinephritic abscess in children. Arch. Pediat. **49**, 743 (1932). — BLAIR, D. M., F. G. LOVERIDGE, C. V. MESSER and W. F. ROSS: Urinary schistosomiasis treated with miracil D. Lancet **1949**, i, 344. — BOURNE, N. W.: A case of urinary fistula complicating osteomyelitis of the pelvis. J. Urol. (Baltimore) **24**, 531 (1930). — BROOMBERG, A.: Localized pneumococcal peritonitis with rupture through the bladder. S. Afr. med. J. **12**, 18 (1938). — BRUNN, H., and G. K. RHODES: Acute haematogenous (metastatic) perinephric abscess. J. Amer. med. Ass. **94**, 618 (1930). — CAMPBELL, M. F.: Renal carbuncle in infancy. J. Amer. med. Ass. **98**, 1729 (1932). — Acute urinary infections in infants and children. N. Y. St. J. Med. **48**, 2397 (1948). — Clinical paediatric urology. Philadelphia: W. B. Saunders Company 1951. — CHOWN, B.: Pyelitis in infancy, a pathological study. Arch. Dis. Childh. **2**, 97 (1927). — CLAIREAUX, A. E., and M. G. PEARSON: Chronic nephritis in a new-born infant. Arch. Dis. Childh. **30**, 366 (1955). — CRAIG, W. S.: Urinary disorders occurring in the neonatal period. Arch. Dis. Childh. **10**, 337 (1935). — EISENSTAEDT, J. S.: Paranephritic abscess in childhood. J. Amer. med. Ass. **92**, 48 (1929). — FAHR, T.: Über pyelonephritische Schrumpfniere und hypogenetische Nephritis. Virchows Arch. path. Anat. **301**, 140 (1938). — GERLOCZY, F., K. SCHMIDT u. M. SCHOLZ: Beiträge zur Frage der Moniliasis im Säuglingsalter. Ann. paediatr. (Basel) **187**, 119 (1956). — GRIFFIN, M. A.:: Pyelonephritis in infancy and childhood: its bacterilogy and pathology. Arch. Dis. Childh. **9**, 105 (1934). — HAGE, W.: Pathologisch-anatomische Statistik der Pyelonephritis und pyelonephritischen Schrumpfniere. Z. urol. Chir. **44**, 172 (1938). — HELMHOLZ, H. F.: Diagnosis and treatment of infections of the urinary tract in childhood. Minn. Med. **15**, 703 (1932). — Is pyelitis of pregnancy a recrudescence of an infection in childhood? Proc. Mayo Clin. **18**, 33 (1943). — Acute infections of the urinary tract. In BRENNEMAN, Practice of pediatrics. Hagerstown, Maryland: W. F. Prior Company 1948. — Infection of the renal parenchyma from the pelvis of the kidney. Amer. J. Dis. Child. **54**, 1 (1937). — HEPLER, A. B., and C. F. EIKENBARY: Spontaneous perforation of the bladder, secondary to osteomyelitis of the pelvis. Amer. J. Surg. **22**, 113 (1953). — HUTCHISON, W. R. S., and J. V. S. A. DAVIES: Renal carbuncle treated by Penicillin. Brit. J. Urol. **19**, 229 (1947). — JUNGHANS, H.: Ein Fall von Myiasis der Harnwege. Z. Urol. **33**, 302 (1939). — KENNEDY, R. L. J.: Pathologic changes in pyelitis of children interpreted on the basis of experimental lesions. J. Urol. (Baltimore) **27**, 371 (1932). — KIMMELSTIEL, P., and C. WILSON: Inflammatory lesions in the glomeruli in pyelonephritis. Amer. J. Path. **12**, 99 (1936). — KLEIN, M.: Schrumpfnieren im Kindesalter. Frankfurt Z. Path. **41**, 317 (1931). — KRETSCHMER, H. L., and W. G. HIBBS: Actinomycosis of the kidney in infancy. J. Urol. (Baltimore) **36**, 123 (1936). — LEOPOLD, J. S., and E. GLASS: Case of perinephritic abscess in a child $2^1/_2$ years duration, associated with marked anaemia. Arch. Pediat. **49**, 346 (1932). — MALLURY, G. K., A. R. CRANE and J. E. EDWARDS: Pathology of acute and healed experimental pyelonephritis. Arch. Path. (Chicago) **30**, 330 (1940). — MARSHALL, A. G.: Persistence of foetal structures in pyelonephritic kidneys. Brit. J. Surg. **41**, 38 (1953). — MASTERS, P. L.: Urinary changes in infections of the urinary tract in childhood. Guy's Hosp. Rep. **102**, 76 (1953). — MAYO, H., and G. H. BURNELL: Carbuncle of the kidney. Aust. N.Z. J. Surg. **2**, 205 (1932). — McDONALD, H P., W. E. UPCHURCH and C. E. STURDEVANT: Interstitial cystitis in children. J. Urol. (Baltimore) **70**, 890 (1953). — MORRISON, J. E.: Malakoplakia of the bladder. J. Path. (Chicago) **56**, 67 (1944). — NAVASQUEZ, DE: Chronic pyelonephritis. Proc. roy. Soc. Med. **47**, 630 (1954). — NOEGGERATH, C.: Entstehung und Behandlung der kindlichen Pyurien oder Cysto-pyelitiden. Mschr. Kinderheilk. **56**, 4 (1933). — PORTER, K. A., and H. M. GILES: A pathological study of five cases of pyelonephritis in the new-born. Arch. Dis. Childh. **31**, 303 (1956). — PUTSCHAR, W.: Pyelitis, pyelonephritis and pyonephrose. In Handbuch der speziellen patholo-gischen Anatomie und Histologie, Bd. 6, Teil 2, S. 333. Berlin: Springer 1934. — SABADINI, L.: Retro-vesical cysts. Lyon chir. **43**, 179 (1948). — SANES, S., and G. D. DOROSHOW: Cystitis emphysematosa. J. Urol. (Baltimore) **32**, 278 (1934). — SAREWITZ, A. B.: Treatment of genito-urinary moniliasis with orally administered nystatin. Ann. intern. Med. **42**, 1187 (1955). — SCHWARZ, L.: Weitere Beiträge zur Kenntnis der Anatomischen Nierenveränderungen der Neugeborenen. Virchows Arch. path. Anat. **267**, 654 (1928). — SEMPLE, J. E.: Perinephric abscess. Brit. J. Urol. **11**, 1 (1939). — STANSFIELD, J. M.: Chronic pyelo-nephritis in children. Proc. roy. Soc. Med. **47**, 631 (1954). — STANSFIELD, J. M., and J. K. G. WEBB: Observations on pyuria in children. Arch. Dis. Childh. **28**, 386 (1953). — SPENCE, H. M., and L. W. JOHNSTON: Renal carbuncle. Ann. Surg. **109**, 99 (1939). — SWAN, H.: Perinephric abscess in infants and children. Amer. J. Surg. **61**, 3 (1943). — WEISS, S., and F. PARKER jr.: Pyelonephritis. Medicine (Baltimore) **18**, 221 (1939). — WHARTON, L. R., L. A. GRAY and H. G. GUILD: Late effects of acute pyelitis in girls. J. Amer. med. Ass. **109**, 1597 (1937). — WILLE-BAUMKAUFF, H.: Aktinomykose der Niere. Z. Urol. **43**, 240 (1950). — WILSON, J. R., and O. M. SCHLOSS: Pathology of so-called "acute pyelitis" in infants. Amer. J. Dis. Child. **38**, 227 (1929). — WINSBURY-WHITE, H. P.: The spread of infection from the uterine cervix to the urinary tract, and the ascent of infection from the lower urinary tract to the kidneys. Brit. J. Urol. **5**, 249 (1933). — WOODRUFF, A. W.: Paediatrics for the practitioner. Suppl. Editor W. GAISFORD and R. LIGHTWOOD. London: Butterworth & Company 1956. — WOODRUFF, J. D., and H. S. EVERETT: Prognosis in childhood urinary tract infections in girls. Amer. J. Obstet. Gynec. **68**, 798 (1954). — ZAPP, E.: Die Calicopapillitis als Sonder-form der kindlichen Harnwegsinfektion. Arch. Kinderheilk. **153**, 141 (1956).

I. Urogenital tuberculosis

ADDISON, O. L.: Tuberculosis of the kidney in childhood. Brit. Med. J. **1935**, ii, 565. — AUERBACH, O.: Tuberculosis in children. Amer. J. Dis. Child. **75**, 555 (1948). — BEKKER-MAN, A.: De la tuberculose rénale chez l'infant. J. Urol. med. chir. **31**, 236 (1931). — BELL, J. G. Y.: Urinary tuberculosis in children. J. Urol. (Baltimore) **61**, 671 (1949). — BODART et CORRET: Tuberculose orchi-epididymaire et prostatic chez le jeune enfant. Rev. méd. Nancy **65**, 605 (1937). — CAMPBELL, M. F.: Renal tuberculosis in juveniles. Amer. J. Dis. Child. **45**, 555 (1933). — ELLIS, R. W. B., and D. LEVI: Tuberculous epididymitis in a boy aged 9. Proc. roy. Soc. Med. **31**, 118 (1937). — FALCI, E.: La tuberculose rénale de l'enfant comparé a celle de l'adulte. J. Urol. méd. chir. **25**, 30 (1925). — GARIBALDI, B., et G. GAMBETTA: La tuberculose du testicule dans l'enfance. Acta urol. belg. **24**, 31 (1956). — HAWTHORNE, A. B., and M. SIMINOVITCH: Renal tuberculosis in children. Canad. med. Ass. J. **60**, 276 (1949). — KEARNS, W. M., and S. M. TURKELTAUB: Renal tuberculosis in children. Wis. med. J. **31**, 834 (1932). — LATTIMER, J. K.: Kidney tuberculosis in children. Pediat. Clin. N. Amer. **2**, 793 (1955). — MAIO, G. DI: Renal tuberculosis in children. Urologia Venezia **15**, 262 (1948). — MATHÉ, C. P.: Renal tuberculosis in the child. Arch. Mal. Reins **10**, 517 (1936). — MEDLAR, E. M.: Case of renal infection in pulmonary tuberculosis. Amer. J. Path. **2**, 401 (1926). — NOBÉCOURT: La tuberculose des reins chez les enfants. J. Prat. (Paris) **49**, 81 (1935). — ROSS, J. C.: The management of tuberculous bacilluria. Proc. roy. Soc. Med. **46**, 434 (1953). — SWOBODA, W., u. E. LIESS: Zur Symptomatologie der kindlichen Nierentuberkulose. Kinderärztl. Prax. **21**, 241 (1953). — WATTENBERG, C. A., M. ABRAMS, H. K. LEWIS and J. LEWIS: Bilateral epididymal tuberculosis in an infant. Pediat. **43**, 443 (1953).

J. Calculous disease

ALBRIGHT, F., and E. C. RIEFENSTEIN: Parathyroid glands and metabolic bone disease. London: Ballière, Tindall & Cox 1948. — ANDERSON, W. A. D.: Renal calcification in infancy and childhood. J. Pediat. **14**, 375 (1939). — APONTE, G. E., and T. R. FETTER: Familial idiopathic oxalate nephrocalcinosis. Amer. J. clin. Path. **24**, 1363 (1954). — ARCHER, H. E., A. E. DORMER, E. F. SCOWEN and R. W. E. WATTS: Primary hyperoxaluria. Lancet **1957**, ii, 320. — BAZLIEL, I. R.: Urethral diverticulum in the scrotum with calculi. Indian med. Gaz. **83**, 231 (1948). — BEGG, R. C.: Urethral calculus in the female, case occuring in a 5 year old child. Urol. cutan. Rev. **38**, 50 (1934). — BERMAN, L. S.: Twenty-second case of xanthine urinary calculus. J. Urol. (Baltimore) **61**, 420 (1948). — BICKEL, C.: Infantilism and bilateral calculi associated with a parathyroid adenoma in a boy 13 years old: spontaneous disappearance of infantilism and urinary calculi following extirpation of the adenoma. Helv. med. Acta **12**, 276 (1945). — BILGER, F., et G. GREINER: Calcul du bassinet chez un enfant de cinq ans developpée autour d'une barrette ingeree vraisemblement trois ans auparavant. Guerison apres nephrectomie. J. Urol. méd. chir. **55**, 259 (1949). — BLAINE, E. S.: An unusual foreign object in the kidney. Radiology **12**, 207 (1929). — BODIAN, M.: Personal communication. — BORMAN, M. C.: Bone suppuration and renal calculi in children. Amer. J. Dis. Child. **40**, 804 (1930). — BRATTSTROM, E.: An unusual case of foreign body in the kidney. Acta chir. scand. **62**, 56 (1927). — BROSCH, W.: Extraktion eines bohnengroßen Harnleitersteines mit der Zeiß-schlinge bei einem 2¹/₂jährigen Kind, rechtsseitige Restniere. Medizinische **1956**, 228. — BROWN, D. A.: Renal and ureteric calculi in childhood. J. Urol. (Baltimore) **18**, 285 (1927). — BROWN, R. K., and E. C. BROWN: Urinary stones. A study of their etiology in small children in Syria. Surgery **9**, 415 (1941). — BRUN, R. G.: Quelques reflexion sur la lithiase vésicale chez les enfants indigenes de tunisie d'apres 217 observations. Bull. Soc. nat. Chir. Paris **59**, 159 (1933). — Deux observations de complications rares chez deux fillettes indigenes atteintes de lithiase vesicale. Bull. Soc. nat. Chir. Paris **59**, 162 (1933). — Le signe de la main. Sa valeur clinique et pratique, sa frequence dans la lithiase vesicale de l'enfant. Presse méd. **1934**, 1139. — BUGBEE, H. G., and M. WALLSTEIN: Surgical pathology of the urinary tract in infants. J. Amer. med. Ass. **83**, 1857 (1924). — BUTT, A. J.: Ureteral calculi in children. J. Fla. med. Ass. **35**, 696 (1949). — CAMPBELL, M. F.: Urinary calculi in infancy and childhood. J. Amer. med. Ass. **94**, 1753 (1930). — CAPON, N. B., and C. WELLS: Foreign body in the kidney. Arch. Dis. Childh. **13**, 85 (1938). — CHAUVIN, E.: Pyonephrose lithiasique chez un enfant de onze ans nephrectomie, Guerison. J. Urol. méd. chir. **35**, 421 (1933). — CLARKE, H.: Report of a case of bilateral renal calculi in a child with normal kidneys. Brit. J. Urol. **24**, 56 (1952). — DAVIS, J. S., W. G. KLINGBERG and R. E. STOWELL: Nephrolithiasis and nephrocalcinosis with calcium oxalate crystals in kidneys and bones. J. Pediat. **36**, 323 (1950). — DEHERRIPON: Lithiase rénale chez un nourrisson de trois mois. Bull. Soc. Pédiatr. Paris **25**, 460 (1927). — DELL'ADAMI, G., and G. BORELLI: Una rara, e forde non ancora descritta, malformazione delle piramidi e dei fornici renali. Arch. ital. Urol. **28**, 386 (1955). — DENT, C. E., and G. G. ROSE: Amino-acid metabolism in cystinuria. Abstracts of communications 1. Internat. Congr. of Biochemistry, Cambridge 1950. — DENT, C. E., and G. R. PHILPOT: Xanthine: an inborn error of metabolism. Lancet **1954**, i, 182. — DENT, C. E., and B. SENIOR: Studies on the treatment of cystinuria. Brit. J. Urol. **27**, 317 (1955). — DIETRICH, E. A.: Harnsteine im Kindesalter. Arch. Kinderheilk. **101**, 26 (1934). — DUGAN, W. C.: Quoted by WINSBURY-WHITE. Kentucky med. J. **9**, 522 (1911). — ECKSTEIN, H. B.: Treatment of phosphate renal calculi with "Aludrox". Great Ormond Street J. **1954**, 117. — FREUND, G.: Über einen großen Blasenstein bei einem Kinde. Med. Klin. **1934**, 1334. — GOLDBERG, L. K.: Vesical calculi in infancy. Case report of vesical calculi in a 9 months old male infant. Arch. Pediat. **51**, 271 (1941). — GRAM, H. C.: The heredity of oxalic urinary calculi. Acta med. scand. **78**, 268 (1932). — GUTIERREZ, R.: Calculous pyonephrosis in a boy 13 years of age, complicated with vesico-uretero-renal reflux, cured by nephro-ureterectomy. Urol. cutan. Rev. **45**, 117 (1941). — HAMM, F. C.: Urinary lithiasis in infancy and early childhood. With report of a case occurring in an infant of 12 months. Amer. J. Surg. **49**, 368 (1940). — HARRIS, H., and F. L. WARREN: Quantitative studies on the urinary cystine in patients with cystine stone formation and in their relatives. Ann. Eugen. (Lond.) **18**, 125 (1953). — HERBST, W. P.: Appendectomy for a non-shadow casting ureteral calculus in a child. J. Amer. med. Ass. **94**, 338 (1930). — HRYNTSCHAK, T.: Horseshoe kidney with calculus in a child. Z. Urol. **22**, 823 (1928). — ISRAELS, S., H. MUTH and I. ZEAVIN: Nephrolithiasis with renal tubular failure. Amer. J. Dis. Child. **78**, 389 (1949). — JACKSON, J. W.: Nephrolithiasis in children. Arch. Dis. Childh. **16**, 55 (1941). — JOLY, F. S.: Stone and calculous disease of the urinary organs. London: Heinemann 1929. — KRETSCHMER, H. L.: Xanthine calculi: report of a case and review of the literature. J. Urol. (Baltimore) **38**, 183 (1937). — LECERCLE, M.: Vesical calculi in children. Rev. méd. franç. **11**, 605 (1930). — LETT, H.: On urinary calculus, with special reference to stone in the bladder. Brit. J. Urol. **8**, 205 (1936). — LEWIS, H. B.: The occurrence of cystinuria in healthy young men and women. Ann. intern. Med. **6**, 183 (1932). — LHIZ, A.: Le rein en éponge. J. Urol. méd. chir. **60**, 575 (1954). — LIGHTWOOD, R., W. W. PAYNE and J. A. BLACK: Infantile renal acidosis. Pediatrics **12**, 628 (1953). — MARTIN, A., et P. AIMÉ: Calcul vesical chez l'enfant. Bull. Soc. Pédiatr. Paris **32**, 350 (1934). — MAWSON, E. E.: Consideration of some possible factors concerned in the development of urolithiasis. Lpool med.-chir. J. **40**, 99 (1932). — McCarrison, R.: The causation of stone in India. Brit. med. J. **1931**, i, 1009. — McKay, H. W., and H. H. Baird: Giant ureteral stone in three year old child. Sth. med. J. (Bgham, Ala.) **40**, 891 (1947). — Mertz, H. O., and C. J. Lewis: Clinical study of urinary calculi in children. Urol. cutan. Rev. **38**, 56 (1934). — Mukherjee, M.: Vesical calculus in a child. Indian J. Pediat. **1**, 229 (1934). — Mulloy, M.: An unusual case of calcium oxalate deposits in the kidney of a young infant, $4^{1}/_{2}$ months. J. Pediat. **39**, 251 (1951). — Myers, W. A. A.: Urolithiasis in childhood. Arch. Dis. Childh. **32**, 48 (1957). — Naylor, J. M.: Case of hypothyroidism with nephrocalcinosis. Arch. Dis. Childh. **30**, 165 (1955). — Neustein, H. B., S. S. Stevenson and I. Krainer: Oxalosis with renal calcinosis due to calcium oxalate. J. Pediat. **47**, 624 (1955). — Newns, G. H., and J. A. Black: Case of calcium oxalate nephrocalcinosis. Great Ormond Street. J. **1953**, No 5, 40. — Noble, T. P.: Vesical calculus in Siam. Brit. J. Urol. **3**, 14 (1931). — Passmore, R.: Observations on the epidemiology of stone in Thailand. Lancet **1953**, i, 638. — Phillips, R. N.: Primary diffuse parathyroid hyperplasia in an infant on 4 months. Pediatrics **2**, 428 (1948). — Pitts, H. H. J. W. Schulte, and D. R. Smith: Nephrocalcinosis in a father and three children. J. Urol. (Baltimore) **73**, 208 (1955). — Prien, E. L., and B. S. Walker: Salicylamide and acetyl salicylic acid in recurrent urolithiasis. J. Amer. med. Ass. **160**, 355 (1956). — Pugh, R. J.: Primary hyperplasia of the parathyroids in a boy of 8 years. Proc. roy. Soc. Med. **39**, 694 (1945). — Rautenberg, A.: Urinary calculi in children. Z. urol. Chir. **37**, 111 (1933). — Reyes, A. I., and W. Fletcher: Cystolithiasis in children. J. Philipp. Islands med. Ass. **24**, 165 (1948). — Rutledge, R. C., W. G. Klingberg and M. L. Heideman: Nephrocalcinosis and pseudomonas aeruginosa pyelonephritis. J. Pediat. **35**, 88 (1949). — Schlesinger, B. E., N. R. Butler and J. A. Black: Severe type of infantile hypercalcaemia. Brit. med. J. **1956**, i, 127. — Schönlebe, J.: Beitrag zu den Prostatasteinen im Kindesalter. Z. Urol. **49**, 236 (1956). — Shoer, E., and A. C. Carter: Aluminium gels in the management of renal phosphatic calculi. J. Amer. med. Ass. **144**, 1549 (1950). — Smith, C. C. W.: On urinary lithiasis in childhood. Acta chir. scand. (I) **90**, 1 (1944); (II) **90**, 179 (1944). — Stevenson, F. H.: The prevention and control of decubitus stone formation. Proc. roy. Soc. Med. **48**, 835 (1955). — Sukhavanam, B.: Case of extravasation of urine due to a calculus in a child of 6 years. Indian med. Gaz. **69**, 450 (1934). — Szenthe, L.: Ein Fall von beiderseitigem Steinverschluß der Nieren im Kindesalter. Z. Chir. **66**, 190 (1939). — Thomas, J. M. R.: Vesical calculus in Norfolk. Brit. J. Urol. **21**, 20 (1949). — Thompson, J. O.: Urinary calculus at the Canton Hospital, China. Surg. Gynec. Obst. **32**, 44 (1921). — Tudor, R. B.: Stones in the urinary bladder in children. Diagnosis and treatment in 7 cases. Amer, J. Dis. Child. **65**, 591 (1943). — Vermooten, V.: Congenital cystic dilatation of the renal collecting tubules. A new disease entity. Yale J. Biol. Med. **23**, 450 (1951). — Vyas, K. G.: Urinary lithiasis. Indian J. Child. Hlth **5**, 64 (1956). — Waller, J. I., and F. Adney: Vesical calculi in young female children. Amer. J. Dis. Child. **79**, 684 (1950). — Winsbury-White, H. P.: Stone in the urinary tract, 2. edit. London: Butterworth & Co. 1954.

K. Neoplastic disease

I. Neoplasms in infancy and childhood

Bodian, M., and L. L. R. White: Neoplastic diseases in childhood. Great. Ormond Street. J. **1952**, No 4, 105. — *Metropolitan Life Insurance Co.:* Cancer among children. Statistics Bull. **30**, 1 (1949). — Stewart, A., J. Webb, D. Giles and D. Hewitt: Malignant disease in childhood and diagnostic irradiation in utero. Lancet **1956**, ii, 447. — Wells, H. J.: Occurrence and significance of congenital malignant neoplasms. Arch. of Path. **30**, 535 (1940).

II. The kidney

Adams, P. S., and H. B. Hunt: Differential diagnosis of Wilms' tumour assisted by intramuscular urography. J. Urol. (Baltimore) **42**, 689 (1939). — Barr, J. R., and J. W. Schulte: Bilateral Wilms' tumor: a case report. West. J. Surg. **58**, 567 (1950). — Beattie, J. W.: Hypernephroma in a 7 year old white girl. J. Urol. (Baltimore) **72**, 625 (1954). — Bernheim, M.: La forme occlusive de l'embryome de Wilms' chez le nouveau-né. Nourrisson **44**, 1 (1956). — Bertoye, P., G. Bertrand et B. Muller: Sur un cas d'epithelioma du rein chez l'enfant. Rev. franç. Pédiatr. **15**, 193 (1939). — Bixler, L. C., K. W. Stenstrom and C. D. Creevy: Malignant tumour of the kidney. Radiology **42**, 329 (1944). — Bjorklund, S. I.: Hemihypertrophy and Wilms' tumour. Acta paediat. (Uppsula) **44**, 287 (1955). — Blum, E., et L. Fruhling: Les tumeurs malignes du rein chez l'enfant. Considerations histopathologiques, cliniques et therapeutiques. Pédiatrie **8**, 797 (1953). — Bodian, M., and L. L. R.

WHITE: British Empire Cancer Campaign Reports for 1951 and 1955. — BRADLEY, J. E., and M. E. DRAKE: The effect of pre-operative roentgen-ray therapy on arterial hypertension in embryoma (kidney). J. Pediat. 35, 710 (1949). — BRADLEY, J. E., and M. C. PINCOFFS: Association of adeno-myosarcoma of the kidney (Wilms' tumor) with arterial hypertension. Ann. intern. Med. 11, 1613 (1938). — BRUN, H. I. LE, H. S. KELLETT and C. L. O. MACALISTER: Renal hamartoma. Brit. J. Urol. 27, 394 (1955). — CAMPBELL, M. F.: Clinical pediatric urology. Philadelphia: W. B. Saunders Company 1951. — Bilateral embryonal adeno-myosarcoma of the kidney (Wilms' tumor). J. Urol. (Baltimore) 59, 567 (1948). — CLINTON-THOMAS, C. L., and T. M. ROBINSON: Adenocarcinoma of the kidney in childhood. Brit. J. Urol. 28, 132 (1956). — CONSTANCE, T. L.: Bilateral rhabdomyoma of the kidney. J. Path. (Chicago) 59, 495 (1947). — COX, P. J. M., and J. M. SMELLIE: Case of nephroblastoma (Wilms' tumor) with severe hypertension. Great. Ormond Street. J. 1955/56, 112. — CURRIE, J. A.: Hypernephroma in a child of 5 years. S. Afr. med. J. 29, 730 (1955). — DEAN, A. L.: Wilms' tumor. N. Y. St. J. Med. 45, 1213 (1945). — DICKEY, L. B., and L. R. CHANDLER: Embryoma of kidney (Wilms' tumor) in children. Pediatrics 4, 197 (1949). — FALKINBURG, R. W. LE, M. N. KAY and E. A. SAYER: Recurrence of nephroblastoma (Wilms' tumor) 8 years after nephrectomy. J. Amer. med. Ass. 155, 1228 (1954). — FEENEY, M. J., R. B. MULLENIX, R. J. PRENTISS and J. M. WHISENAND: Clinical experiences with Wilms' tumors. J. Urol. (Baltimore) 74, 301 (1955). — FERRIS, D. O., and J. B. BEARE: Wilms' tumor: report of a case with unusual postoperative metastasis. Proc. Mayo Clin. 22, 94 (1947). — FITZGERALD, W. L., and H. C. HARDIN jr.: Bilateral WILMS' tumor in a Wilms' tumor family: case report. J. Urol. (Baltimore) 73, 468 (1955). — FOSTER, D. G.: Large benign renal tumours: a review of the literature and report of a case in childhood. J. Urol. (Baltimore) 76, 231 (1956). — GARRETT, R. A., and H. O. MERTZ: Wilms' tumor in children. J. Urol. (Baltimore) 70, 694 (1953). — GOWDEY, J. F, and E. B. D. NEUHAUSER: Roentgen diagnosis of diffuse leukemic infiltration of the kidneys in children. Amer. J. Roentgenol. 60, 13 (1948). — GROSS, R. E., and E. B. D. NEUHAUSER: Treatment of mixed tumours of the kidney in childhood. Pediatrics 6, 843 (1950). — GROSSMAN, B. J.: Radiation nephritis. J. Pediat. 47, 424 (1955). — HARVEY, R. M.: Wilms' tumor: evaluation of treatment methods. Radiology 54, 689 (1950). — HERTEL, E.: Beitrag zu den Hamartomen der Niere. Zbl. Chir. 80, 1752 (1955). — HIGGINS, T. T.: Malignant disease in childhood. Glasg. med. J. 36, 428 (1955). — HIGGINS, T. T., D. I. WILLIAMS and D. F. E. NASH: The Urology of childhood. London: Butterworth & Co. 1951. — HUGUENIN, R., et R. GERARD-MARCHANT: Diagnosis and treatment of malignant tumours in children. Presse méd. 1953, 909. — JOHNSON III, S. M., and M. MARSHALL jr.: Primary kidney tumours of childhood. J. Urol. (Baltimore) 74, 707 (1955). — JOSEPHS, C.: Embryoma of the kidneys with symptoms at birth. Arch. Dis. Childh. 24, 312 (1949). — KERR, H. D., and R. E. FLYNN: Role of irradiation in the treatment of Wilms' tumor in children. Amer. J. Roentgenol. 75, 971 (1956). — KRETSCHMER, H. L.: Malignant tumors of the kidney in children. J. Urol. (Baltimore) 39, 250 (1938). — Fibroblastoma of the kidney. Surg. Gynec. Obstet. 54, 524 (1932). — LADD, W. E.: Embryoma of the kidney (Wilms' tumor). Ann. Surg. 108, 885 (1938). — MASLOW, L. A.: Wilms' tumor: report of 3 cases and a possible fourth one in the same family. J. Urol. (Baltimore) 43, 75 (1940). — LANGHOF, J.: Über ein großes Hamartom der Niere. Z. Urol. 48, 321 (1955). — McCURDY, G. A.: Renal neoplasms in childhood. J. Path. Bact. 39, 623 (1934). — McGINN, E. J., and J. M. WICKHAM: Wilms' tumor in a horseshoe kidney. J. Urol. (Baltimore) 56, 520 (1946). — McLEAN, E. H., and T. MATTHEWS: Haemangioma of the kidney. West. J. Surg. 50, 47 (1942). — MILLICHAP, J. G.: Diffuse bilateral renal lymphosarcomatosis. Great. Ormond Street. J. 1952, No 3, 76. — MOOLTEN, S. E.: Hamartial nature of the tuberous sclerosis complex and its bearing on the tumour problem: report of a case with tumour, anomaly of the kidney and adenoma sebaceum. Arch. intern. Med. 69, 589 (1942). — MOONS, K. M., and M. K. RUCH: Hypertension in a 7 year old girl with Wilms' tumor relieved by nephrectomy. J. Amer. med. Ass. 115, 1097 (1940). — NESBIT, R. M., and F. M. ADAMS: Wilms' tumor: a review of 16 cases. J. Pediat. 29, 295 (1946). — NICHOLSON, G. W.: An embryonic tumour of the kidney in a foetus. J. Path. Bact. 34, 711 (1931). — ORMOS, J., u. A. JAKOBOVITS: Über das Nephroblastom (Wilms' Tumor) des Erwachsenenalters, mit besonderer Rücksicht auf die Bildung von Metastasen in den Genitalien. Virchows Arch. path. Anat. 327, 391 (1955). — PETERSON, C. A., and R. P. JOHNSON: Bilateral embryoma of the kidney: patient alive and well three years after treatment. Radiology 67, 99 (1956). — PRATT-THOMAS, H. A.: Tuberous sclerosis with congenital tumours of heart and kidney. Amer. J. Path. 23, 189 (1947). — PRIESTLEY, J. T., and A. C. BRODERS: Wilms' tumor. J. Urol. (Baltimore) 33, 544 (1935). — RICKHAM, P. P.: Bilateral Wilms' tumor. Brit. J. Surg. 44, 492 (1957). — RITTER, J. A., and E. S. SCOTT: Embryoma of contralateral kidney 10 years following nephrectomy for Wilms' tumor. J. Pediat. 34, 753 (1949). — ROBERTS, O. W.: Malignant papilloma of the left kidney in a boy. Lancet 1928, ii, 67. — ROSE, D. K., and C. A. WATTENBERG: Wilms' tumor in the isthmus of a horseshoe kidney. Urol. cutan. Rev. 49, 365 (1945). — RUSCHE, C.: Treatment of Wilms' tumor.

J. Urol. (Baltimore) **65**, 950 (1951). — Sansone, G., e C. Zunin: Considerazioni su 12 casi di tumori renali osservati nell'ultimo biennio nella Clinica Pediatricia di Genova. Minerva pediat. (Torino) **5**, 594 (1953). — Sauer, H. R.: Wilms' tumors. N.Y. St. J. Med. **48**, 497 (1948). — Schlapik, D.: Papillary carcinoma of the kidney in childhood. Urol. cutan. Rev. **47**, 283 (1943). — Scott, L. S.: Bilateral Wilms' tumor. Brit. J. Surg. **42**, 513 (1955). — Wilms' tumour: its treatment and prognosis. Brit. med. J. **1956**, i, 200. — Silver, H. K.: Wilms' tumor (embryoma of the kidney). J. Pediat. **31**, 643 (1947). — Smith, W. G., and A. W. Williams: Irradiation nephritis. Lancet **1955**, ii, 175. — Swan, Jocelyn R. H., and H. Balme: Angioma of the kidney: report of a case with an analysis of 26 previously reported cases. Brit. J. Surg. **23**, 282 (1935). — Tanner, C. H.: Intraperitoneal rupture of a Wilms' tumor. Brit. med. J. **1943**, ii, 714. — Thomas, G.: Papillary carcinoma of the renal pelvis in a child of $3^1/_3$ years. Surg. Clin. N. Amer. **3**, 1255 (1933). — Vuori, E. E.: Tumours of the kidney in children. Acta chir. scand. (Stockh.) **95**, 555 (1947). — Watkins, J. P.: Wilms' tumor with ureteral metastasis extending into the bladder. J. Urol. (Baltimore) **77**, 593 (1957). — Whitehouse, W. N., and I. Lampe: Osseus damage in irradiation of renal tumours in infancy and childhood. Amer. J. Roentgenol. **70**, 721 (1953). — Williams, I. G., T. T. Higgins and M. Bodian: British practice in radiothermy. London: Butterworth & Co. 1955. — Wilms, M.: Die Mischgeschwülste der Niere. Leipzig: Arthur Georgi 1899. — Zangemeister, W.: Untersuchungen über Altersverteilung, Häufigkeit und Morphologie der Nierenfibrome. Beitr. path. Anat. **97**, 142 (1936). — Zuckerman, C., D. Kershner, B. Laytner and D. Kerschel: Leiomyoma of the kidney. Ann. Surg. **126**, 220 (1947).

III. The adrenal gland and retroperitoneal space

Aird, I., and P. Helman: Bilateral anterior transabdominal adrenalectomy. Brit. med· J. **1955**, ii, 708. — Arnheim, E. E.: Combined pelvic and retro-peritoneal teratomas in infancy and childhood. Pediatrics **10**, 198 (1952). — Retroperitoneal tumours in infancy and childhood. Pediatrics **8**, 309 (1951). — Blacklock, J. W. S.: Neurogenic tumours of the sympathetic nervous system in children. J. Path. Bact. **39**, 27 (1934). — Bodian, M., and L. L. R. White: Neuroblastoma. Brit. Empire Cancer Campaign. 32. Report, p. 195, 1954; 34. Report, p. 213, 1956. — Cahill, G. F., and H. Aranow: Pheochromocytoma: diagnosis and treatment. Ann. intern. Med. **31**, 389 (1949). — Cahill, G. F., and J. N. Robinson: Androgenic symptom tumours of the adrenal cortex in children. A report of four cases. J. Urol. (Baltimore) **61**, 680 (1949). — Cushing, H., and S. B. Wolbach: Transformation of a malignant paravertebral sympatheticoblastoma into a benign ganglioneuroma. Amer. J. Path. **3**, 203 (1927). — Emery, J. L., and R. B. Zachary: Haematoma of the adrenal gland in the newborn. Brit. med. J. **1952**, ii, 857. — Euler, U. S. v., u. S. Hellner: The estimation of catechol amines. Acta physiol. scand. **22**, 161 (1951). — Farber, J. E., F. J. Gustina and V. A. Postoloff: Cushing's syndrome in children: review of the literature and report of a case. Amer. J. Dis. Child. **65**, 593 (1943). — Garrett, R. A.: Adrenal cortical carcinoma in children. J. Urol. (Baltimore) **66**, 477 (1951). — Glasser, S. T., C. Moran and A. J. Capute: Lumbar retroperitoneal ganglioneuroma. N. Y. St. J. Med. **50**, 717 (1950). — Goldenberg, M., and H. Aranow: Diagnosis of pheochromocytoma by the adrenergic blocking action of benzodioxane. J. Amer. med. Ass. **143**, 1139 (1950). — Guin, G. H., and E. F. Gilbert: Cushings' syndrome in children associated with adrenal cortical carcinoma. Amer. J. Dis. Child. **92**, 297 (1956). — Harrison, F. G., H. L. Warres and J. A. Fust: Neuroblastoma involving the urinary tract. J. Urol. (Baltimore) **63**, 598 (1950). — Heinecker, P., L. W. O'Neal and L. V. Ackerman: Functioning and non-functioning adrenal cortical tumours. Surg. Gynec. Obstet. **105**, 21 (1957). — Helps, E. P. W., K. C. Robinson and E. J. Ross: Phentolamine in the diagnosis and. management of pheochromocytoma. Lancet **1955**, ii, 267. — Higgins, T. T., D. I. Williams and D. F. E. Nash: The urology of childhood. London: Butterworth & Co. 1951. — Holl, G.: Two cases of suprarenal tumours with disturbance of internal secretion. Dtsch. Z. Chir. **226**, 277 (1930). — Holten, C., and V. P. Petersen: Malignant hypertension with increased secretion of aldosterone and depletion of potassium. Lancet **1956**, ii, 918. — Jolly, H. R.: Sexual precocity. Springfield, Ill.: Ch. C. Thomas 1955. — Kepler, E. J., W. Walters and R. K. Dixon: Menstruation in a child nineteen months as a result of tumour of the left adrenal cortex: successful surgical management. Proc. Mayo Clin. **13**, 362 (1938). — Kiefer, J. H., and I. P. Bronstein: Adrenal cortical tumours. J. Urol. (Baltimore) **62**, 639 (1949). — Kretschmer, H. L.: Retroperitoneal lipo-fibro-sarcoma in a child. J. Urol. (Baltimore) **43**, 61 (1940). — Ladd, W. E., and R. E. Gross: Abdominal surgery of infancy and childhood. Philadelphia: W. B. Saunders Company 1941. — Larson, L. M.: Lumbar retroperitoneal ganglioneuroma: review of literature and report of a case. Minn. Med. **30**, 969 (1947). — Mandeville, F. B.: Calcification in sympathoblastoma (neuroblastoma). Radiology **53**, 403 (1949). — Patterson, J.: Diagnosis of adrenal tumours. Lancet **1947**, ii, 580. — Robinson, M. J., and

A. WILLIAMS: Clinical and pathological details of 2 cases of pheochromocytoma in childhood. Arch. Dis. Childh. **31**, 69 (1956). — ROTH, G. M., and W. F. KVALE: A tentative test for pheochromocytoma. Amer. J. med. Sci. **210**, 653 (1945). — SNYDER, C. H., and L. J. RUTLEDGE: Pheochromocytoma — localization by aortography. Pediatrics **15**, 312 (1955). — SNYDER, C. H., and E. H. VICK: Hypertension in children caused by pheochromocytoma. Amer. J. Dis. Child. **73**, 581 (1947). — STOUT, A. P.: Ganglioneuroma of the sympathetic nervous system. Surg. Gynec. Obstet. **84**, 101 (1947). — TALBOT, N. B., E. H. SOBEL, J. W. McARTHUR and J. D. CRAWFORD: Functional endocrinology from birth through adolescence. Cambridge, Massachusetts: Harvard University Press 1952. — WILKINS, L.: Feminizing and virilizing adrenal tumours. Classification of adrenal disorders. J. clin. Endocr. **8**, 111 (1948). — The suppression of androgen secretion by cortisone in a case of congenital adrenal hyperplasia. Bull. Johns Hopk. Hosp. **86**, 249 (1950). — WILLIAMS, D. I.: Calcification in adrenal haemorrhage. Great. Ormond Street. J. **1955/56**, No 10, 100. — WITTENBORG, M. H.: Roentgen therapy in neuroblastoma. Radiology **54**, 679 (1950). — WYATT, G. M., and S. FARBER: Neuroblastoma sympatheticum: roentgenological appearances and radiation treatment. Amer. J. Roentgenol. **46**, 485 (1941).

IV. The bladder

BALLENGER, E. G., O. F. ELDER and H. P. McDONALD: Case of cavernous hemangioma of the bladder. Amer. J. Surg. **17**, 409 (1932). — CAMPBELL, M. F.: Clinical paediatric urology. Philadelphia: W. B. Saunders Company 1951. — CHALKLEY, T. S., and J. W. BRUCE: Neurofibromatosis of the bladder in a 9 year old boy. J. Pediat. **20**, 632 (1942). — FEGETTER, S. Y.: Sarcoma of the bladder. Brit. J. Surg. **25**, 382 (1937/38). — GANEM, E. J., and L. B. AINSWORTH: Benign neoplasms of the bladder in children. J. Urol. (Baltimore) **73**, 1032 (1955). — HENRY, G. W.: Sarcoma of the urinary bladder in children, with a review of the literature. Amer. J. Roentgenol. **62**, 843 (1949). — HIGGINS, T. T.: Rhabdo-myosarcoma of the bladder. Brit. J. Urol. **24**, 158 (1952). — HIGGINS, T. T., D. I. WILLIAMS and D. F. E. NASH: Urology of childhood. London: Butterworth & Co. 1951. — HUNT, R. W.: Rhabdo-myosarcoma in the lower urinary tract. N.Y. St. J. Med. **43**, 513 (1943). — KASS, J. H.: Neurofibromatosis of the bladder. Amer. J. Dis. Child. **44**, 1040 (1932). — KHOURY, E. M., and F. D. SPEER: Rhabdo-myosarcoma of the urinary bladder. A clinico-pathological case report with a review of the literature including a tabulation of rhabdo-myosarcoma of the prostate. J. Urol. (Baltimore) **51**, 505 (1944). — KRETSCHMER, H. L.: Rhabdo-myosarcoma of the bladder. Report of a case and review of the literature. Arch. Path. **44**, 350 (1947). — LANGE, G.: Lebensbedrohliche Blutung bei einem Myom der Harnblase. Z. Urol. **49**, 108 (1956). — LAZARUS, J. A., and A. A. ROSENTHAL: Myxosarcoma of the bladder. J. Urol. (Baltimore) **37**, 695 (1932). — LOWRY, E. C., W. A. SOANES and K. A. FORBES: Carcinoma of the bladder in children: case report. J. Urol. (Baltimore) **73**, 307 (1955). — MacALPINE, J. B.: Two cases of haemangioma of the bladder. Brit. J. Surg. **28**, 205 (1930). — MARSHALL, V. F.: Pelvic exenteration for polypoid myosarcoma (sarcoma botryoides) of the urinary bladder of an infant. Cancer (Philad.) **9**, 620 (1956). — MEADE, H.: Myxomatous tumour of the bladder simulating stone in the bladder, in a child of 5 years. Brit. J. Urol. **15**, 10 (1943). — MOSTOFI, F. K., and W. H. MORSE: Polypoid rhabdo-myosarcoma (sarcoma botryoides) of the bladder in children. J. Urol. (Baltimore) **67**, 681 (1952). — PEZZOLI, A.: Il rabdomiosarcoma della vesica urinaria. Contribution casistico e rivista della letteratura. Arch. ital. Urol. **26**, 229 (1953). — PITTS, H. H.: Neurofibromatosis of the urinary bladder in a 7 year old boy. Urol. cutan. Rev. **53**, 623 (1949). — RANSOM, H. K.: Sarcoma of the urachus. Amer. J. Surg. **22**, 187 (1933). — RATHBUN, N. P.: Primary bladder tumour in infancy and young children. Surg. Gynec. Obstet. **64**, 914 (1937). — RIDLON, G. R.: Benign bladder tumour in a 2 years 9 months child. J. of Urol. **41**, 173 (1939). — SHAW, R. E.: Sarcoma of the urachus. Brit. J. Surg. **37**, 95 (1949). — SLOTKIN, E. A., and R. D. DAVIS: Rhabdo-myosarcoma of the bladder. N.Y. State J. Med. **54**, 2837 (1954). — WHITE, E. W.: Very rare bladder tumour in a child. J. Urol. (Baltimore) **26**, 253 (1931). — WHITE, L. L. R.: Embryonic sarcoma of the urogenital sinus. M. D. Thesis, University of Wales 1955.

V. The prostate and urethra

GMELIN, L.: Neoplasma der Prostata im jungen Kindesalter. Kinderärztl. Prax. **16**, 76 (1948). — HESS, E.: Sarcoma of prostate. J. of Urol. **40**, 629 (1938). — HOLMES, R. J., and M. M. COPLAN: Sarcoma of the prostatic area in an infant of four months. J. of Urol. **24**, 539 (1930). — LOWSLEY, O. S., and F. N. KIMBALL: Sarcoma of prostae: with a review of the literature. Brit. J. Urol. **6**, 328 (1934). — MERTZ, H. O., R. D. HOWELL and R. C HAMMOND: Sarcoma of prostate in children with report of a case of rhabdomyosarcoma in a 4 year old boy. J. of Urol. **64**, 681 (1950). — TRUC, GUILLAUME et BAUMEL: Fibro-myxosarcome prostatique chez un enfant de 4 ans. J. d'Urol. **61**, 882 (1955). — Tzovaru, S., et C. Vasilescu: Primitives leiomyoxosarcom der Prostata bei einem Kind mit diffuser Infiltration der ganzen Blasenwand. Frankf. Z. Path. **52**, 41 (1938). — Wallgren, G. R.: Sarcoma of the prostate in children. Acta chir. scand. (Stockh.) **108**, 205 (1954).

VI. The penis and scrotum

Ferguson, G.: Cystic lymphangioma: an uncommon type of scrotal swelling. Brit. J. Urol. **26**, 264 (1954). — Helland, N. J., and J. B. Miale: Cystic lymphangioma of the scrotum. J. of Urol. **69**, 708 (1953). — Kini, M. G.: Cancer of the penis in a child of 2 years. Indian Med. Gaz. **79**, 66 (1944). — Mahoney, M. T.: Cavernous hemangioma of the scrotal septum. J. of Pediatr. **49**, 744 (1956). — Matthews D. N.: Personal communication. — Winslow, N.: Cavernous haemangioma of the scrotum: report of a case. Arch. of Surg. **19**, 829 (1929). — Zschau, H.: Angeborene Elephantiasis penis et scroti. Dtsch. Z. Chir. **245**, 312 (1935).

VII. The epididymis and spermatic cord

Burros, H. M., and P. P. Maycock: Adenomatoid tumours of the epididymis: report of a case in a newborn. J. Urol. (Baltimore) **63**, 712 (1950). — Culp, O. S.: Adrenal heterotopia: a survey of the literature and report of a case. J. Urol. (Baltimore) **41**, 303 (1939). — Guekdjian, S. A.: Lymphangioma of the groin and scrotum. J. int. Coll. Surg. **24**, 159 (1955). — Hirsch, E. F.: Rhabdo-myosarcoma of the spermatic cord (funiculus spermaticus). Amer. J. Cancer **20**, 398 (1934). — Sundarasivarao, D.: The Müllerian vestiges and benign epithelial tumours of the epididymis. J. Path. Bact. **66**, 417 (1953). — Thompson, G. J.: Tumours of the spermatic cord, epididymis and testicular tunics. Surg. Gynec. Obstet. **62**, 712 (1936).

VIII. The testicle

Blunden, K. E., S. Russi and R. C. Bunts: Interstitial cell hyperplasia or adenoma. J. Urol. (Baltimore) **70**, 759 (1953). — Bodian, M., and L. L. R. White: Testicular tumours. Brit. Empire Cancer Campaign, 30th Report, p. 172, 1952. — Culp, D. A., R. G. Frazier and J. J. Butler: Sertoli cell tumours in an infant. J. Urol. (Baltimore) **76**, 162 (1956). — Dean, A. L.: Cancer of the genito-urinary organs in children. In: Cancer in childhood, editor H. W. Dargeon. St. Louis: C. V. Mosby Comp. 1940. — Doyle, G. B.: Embryonal carcinoma of the testis in an infant. Brit. J. Urol. **27**, 287 (1955). — Gordon-Taylor, G., and N. R. Wyndham: On malignant tumours of the testicle. Brit. J. Surg. **35**, 6 (1947). — Gross, E.: Surgery of childhood. Philadelphia: W. B. Saunders Company 1953. — Guilleminet, M., et P. Fourrier: Evolution actuelle du traitement des tumeurs malignes du testicule chez l'enfant et l'adolescent. Lyon chir. **44**, 57 (1949). — Huffman, L. F.: Feminizing testicular tumours in a 6 year old boy. J. Urol. (Baltimore) **45**, 692 (1944). — Jolly, H. R.: Sexual precocity. Springfield, Ill.: Ch. C. Thomas 1955. — Julien, R.: Étude des tumeurs de testicule chez l'enfant. Thèse Paris 1925. — Jungck, E. C., A. M. Thrash, A. P. Ohlmacher, A. M. Knight and L. Y. Dyrenforth: Sexual precocity due to interstitial cell tumour of the testis. J. clin. Endocr. **17**, 291 (1957). — Magner, D., J. S. Campbell and F. W. Wigglesworth: Testicular adenocarcinoma with clear cells, occurring in infancy. Cancer (Philad.) **9**, 165 (1956). — Matassarin, F. W.: Embryonal adenocarcinoma of the testicle in an infant: case report. J. Urol. (Baltimore) **52**, 575 (1944). — Meltzer, A., and B. Bloom: Malignant testicular neoplasm in infancy: report of a case with six years survival. New Engl. J. Med. **237**, 513 (1947). — Newns, G. H.: Precocious sexual development due to an interstitial-cell tumour of the testis. Brit. J. Surg. **39**, 379 (1952). — Pfarschner, W.: Maligne Hodentumoren im Säuglings- und Kindesalter. Zbl. Chir. **77**, 1093 (1952). — Pomer, F. A., R. E. Stiles and J. H. Graham: Interstitial cell-tumour of the testis in children. Report of a case and review of the literature. New Engl. J. Med. **250**, 233 (1954). — Rezek, P., and H. C. Hardin jr.: Bilateral interstitial cell-tumour of the testicle: report of a case observed for 14 years. J. Urol. (Baltimore) **74**, 628 (1955). — Rosenthal, A. A.: Haemangioma of the testis in an infant. J. Urol. (Baltimore) **55**, 542 (1946). — Rusche, C.: Twelve cases of testicular tumours occurring during infancy and childhood. J. Pediat. **40**, 193 (1952). — Sacrez, R., Y. Le Gal, G. Kurtzemann and R. Korn: A propos d'un cas de dysembryonne du testicule chez un nourrisson de dix mois. Arch. franç. Pédiat. **13**, 97 (1956). — Schmid, R.: Zur Klinik der malignen Testikeltumoren im Säuglings- und Kindesalter. Arch. Kinderheilk. **152**, 71 (1956). — Schmidt, G. W., u. E. Tonutti: Pseudopubertas praecox und unvollständige Pubertas praecox bei einem Leydig-Zell-Tumor des Hodens. Helv. paediat. Acta **11**, 436 (1956). — Thamdrup, E.: Macrogenitosomia caused by interstitial cell-tumour of the testis. A case of a 7½ year old boy. Acta paediat. (Uppsala) **42**, 369 (1953). — Thompson, J. R.: Infantile teratoma testis. Brit. J. Surg. **42**, 437 (1955).

IX. The ovary

COSTIN, M. E., and R. I. S. KENNEDY: Ovarian tumours in infants and in children. Amer. J. Dis. Child. **76**, 127 (1948). — FLANNERY, W. E.: Arrhenoblastoma before puberty. Amer. J. Obstet. Gynec. **60**, 923 (1950). — GORDON, V. H., and H. N. MARVIN: Theca-cell tumour of ovary in child of 1 year. J. Pediatr. **39**, 133 (1951). — HARRIS, R. H.: Carcinomatous ovarian teratoma with premature puberty and precocious somatic development. Surg. Gynec. Obstet. **41**, 191 (1925). — KIMMEL, G. C.: Sexual precocity and accelerated growth in a child with follicular cyst of the ovary. J. Pediat. **30**, 686 (1947). — MANDEVILLE, F. B., P. F. SAHYOUN and L. E. SUTTON jr.: Dysgerminoma of the ovary in a 4 year old girl with metastases clinically simulating Wilms' tumor and adrenal neuroblastoma. J. Pediat. **34**, 70 (1949). — RINYIK, R.: Granulosa cell tumour in a case of precocious puberty. Acta obstet. gynec. scand. **32**, 222 (1953). — TAYLOR, S.: Torsion of the ovary in childhood. Arch. Dis. Childh. **27**, 368 (1952). — ZEMKE, E. E., and W. E. HERRELL: Bilateral granulosa cell tumours: successful removal from a child of 14 weeks of age. Amer. J. Obstet. Gynec. **41**, 704 (1941).

X. The vagina and uterus

BODIAN, M., and L. L. R. WHITE: Carcinoma of vagina and cervix. Brit. Empire Cancer Campaign, 31. Report, p. 172, 1953. — LOCKHART, H.: Cancer of the uterus in childhood. Amer. J. Obstet. Gynec. **30**, 76 (1935). — McFARLAND, J.: Dysontogenetic mixed tumours of urogenital region. Surg. Obstet. Gynec. **61**, 42 (1935). — POLLACK, R. S., and H. C. TAYLOR: Carcinoma of the cervix during the first two decades of life. Amer. J. Obstet. Gynec. **53**, 135 (1947). — SHACKMAN, R.: Sarcoma Botryoides of the genital tract in female children. Brit. J. Surg. **38**, 26 (1950). — ULFELDER, H., and S. H. QUAN: Sarcoma botryoides vaginae. Complete excision of the tumours in an infant by combined abdominal and perineal approach. Surg. Clin. N. Amer. **27**, 1240 (1947).

L. Hypertension

BERNHEIM, M., J. CIBERT, J. LANTERNIER, R. FRANCOIS et Y. FOUILLET: Hypertension arterielle infantile et hypoplasie renale congenitale. Rev. Lyon Méd. **2**, 131 (1953). — BOTHE, A. E.: Pyelonephritis in children and adults with hypertension. J. Urol. (Baltimore) **42**, 969 (1939). — BRADLEY, J. E., and M. C. PINCOFFS: Association of adeno-myosarcoma of the kidney (Wilms' tumour) with arterial hypertension. Ann. intern. Med. **11**, 1613 (1938). — BUTLER, A. M.: Chronic pyelonephritis and arterial hypertension. J. clin. Invest. **16**, 889 (1937). — COURT, D.: Malignant hypertension in childhood. Arch. Dis. Childh. **16**, 132 (1941). — ENGELSON, G., U. ISING u. S. WIDELL: Hypertension associated with adrenal tumour in an infant. Nord. Med. **56**, 1030 (1956). — FLOYER, M. A.: The role of the kidney in experimental hypertension. Brit. med. Bull. **13**, 29 (1957). — GRIFFITHS, A. L.: Hypertension of renal origin in childhood. Arch. Dis. Childh. **25**, 81 (1950). — HAGGERTY, R. J., M. W. MARONEY and A. S. NADAS: Essential hypertension in infancy and childhood. Amer. J. Dis. Child. **92**, 536 (1956). — HIGGINS, T. T., D. I. WILLIAMS and D. F. E. NASH: The urology of childhood. London: Butterworth & Co. 1951. — HILLEBRAND, H. J.: Einseitige Nierenerkrankungen und Hochdruck. Z. Urol. **49**, 65 (1956). — HOCK, E. F., and E. M. JONES: Aneurysm of the renal artery, causing hypertension. Amer. J. Dis. Child. **89**, 606 (1955). — HOWARD, T. L., R. P. FORBES and W. R. LIPSCOMB: Aneurysm of the left renal artery in a child of 5 years old with persistent hypertension. J. Urol. (Baltimore) **44**, 808 (1940). — HUTCHISON, R., and A. A. MONCRIEFF: Case of primary hypertension in a child. Brit. J. Child. Dis. **27**, 201 (1930). — ISAACSON, C., and S. WAYBOURNE: Malignant hypertension in a child due to unilateral kindey disease. Arch. Dis. Childh. **32**, 106 (1957). — KENNEDY, R. L. J., N. W. BARKER and W. WALTERS: Malignant hypertension: cure following nephrectomy. Follow up of report of the case of a child. Amer. J. Dis. Child. **69**, 160 (1945). — KILLIAN, S. T., and J. K. CALVIN: Renal hypertension in children. Clinico pathologic studies. Amer. J. Dis. Child. **62**, 1242 (1941). — KOBAYASHI, O., and S. SAKAGUCHI: Unilateral renal hypertension in a girl cured by nephrectomy. J. Pediat. **48**, 57 (1956). — LEADBETTER, W. F., and C. E. BURKLAND: Hypertension in unilateral renal disease. J. Urol. (Baltimore) **39**, 611 (1935). — MATZNER, R.: Ein Beitrag zum Problem des renalen Hochdrucks. Mschr. Kinderheilk. **101**, 479 (1953). — MORISON, J. E.: Pyelonephritis, malignant hypertension and ulceration of small intestine in a child. Arch. Dis. Childh. **20**, 90 (1945). — MOVIN, R., A. SØEBORG OHLSEN u. A. M. PEDERSON: Arterial hypertension - nephrectomy. Acta med. scand. **119**, 439 (1944). — ØSTER, J.: Arterial hypertension in a child cured by nephrectomy. Acta med. scand. **128**, 42 (1947). — PAGE, I. H.: Production of persistent arterial hypertension by cellophane perinephritis. J. Amer. med. Ass. **113**, 2046 (1939). — PERRY, C. B., and A. L. TAYLOR: Hypertension following thrombosis of the renal veins. J. Path. Bact.

51, 369 (1940). — PICKERING, G. W., A. D. WRIGHT and R. H. HEPTINSTALL: The reversibility of malignant hypertension. Lancet **1952,** ii, 952. — POUTASSE, E. F., A. W. HUMPHRIES, L.J. McCORMACK and A. C. CORCORAN: Bilateral stenosis of renal arteries and hypertension. J. Amer. med. Ass. **161,** 419 (1956). — REINHOLD, J. D. J.: Blood pressure determinations in the arms and legs of normal infants by the flush method. Arch. Dis. Childh. **30,** 127 (1955). — SEELEMAN, K., u. G. LINNEKOGEL: Über den Hochdruck im Kindesalter bei einseitiger Nierenerkrankung. Z. Kinderheilk. **70,** 568 (1952). — SNYDER, C. H., R. B. BOST and R. V. PLATOU: Hypertension in infancy with anomalous renal artery. Pediatrics **15,** 88 (1955). — SOBEL, I. P.: So-called essential hypertension in childhood. Amer. J. Dis. Child. **61,** 280 (1941). — TAUSSIG, H. B., and D. B. REMSEN: Essential hypertension in a boy of two years of age. Bull. Johns Hopk. Hosp. **57,** 183 (1935). — VERGER, P.: Hypertension arterielle maligne et hypoplasie renale unilaterale chez l'enfant. A propos d'un nouveau cas: resultats de la nephrectomie. Pédiatrie 8, 693 (1953). — WEISS, S., and F. PARKER jr.: Pyelonephritis: its relation to vascular lesions and to arterial hypertension. Medicine (Baltimore) **18,** 221 (1939). — WILSON, C., and D. G. ABRAHAMS: Treatment of hypertension in primary renal disease. Brit. med. Bull. **13,** 39 (1957). — WILSON, C., and F. B. BYROM: Renal changes in malignant hypertension. Lancet **1939,** i, 136. — ZUELZER, W. W., S. CHARLES, R. KURNETZ, W. A. NEWTON and R. FALLON: Circulatory diseases of the kidneys in infancy and childhood. Amer. J. Dis. Childr. **81,** 1 (1951).

M. Renal failure and allied disorders

I. Acute renal failure

BARTHÉLEMY: 200 cas d'anurie traités par infiltration anésthesique du pédicule rénal. J. Urol. méd. chir. **54,** 63 (1948). — BULL, G. M., A. M. JOEKES and K. G. LOWE: Conservative treatment of anuric uraemia. Lancet **1949,** ii, 229. — CAMPBELL, M.F.: Clinical pediatric urology. Philadelphia:·W. B. Saunders Company 1951. — CARRÉ, I. J., and J. R. SQUIRE: Anuria ascribed to acute tubular necrosis in infancy and early childhood. Arch. Dis. Childh. **31,** 512 (1956). — DARMADY, E. M., and F. STRANACK: Microdissection of the nephron in disease. Brit. med. Bull. **13,** 21 (1957). — DUVERGEY, H., P.VERGER et P. DUPUY: Anurie chez un enfant de 16 mois. Calculs de cystine pure au niveau des voies urinaires superieures des deux cotés. J. Urol. méd. chir. **57,** 88 (1951). — JONSSON, B.: Lower nephron nephrosis in asphyxia neonatorum. Acta paediat. (Uppsala) **40,** 401 (1951). — KAPLAN, S. A., and S. J. FOMON: Function recovery pattern in acute renal failure following ingestion of mercuric chloride. Amer. J. Dis. Child. **85,** 633 (1953). — MacDONALD, W. B., and M. J. ROBINSON: Use of a cation exchange resin in the management of anuria in childhood. Aust. Ann. Med. **3,** 123 (1954). — MATEER, F. M., L. GREENMAN and T. S. DANOWSKI: Hemodialysis of the uremic child. Amer. J. Dis. Child. **89,** 645 (1955). — McCANCE, R. A., and E. M. WIDDOWSON: Protein catabolism and renal function in the first 2 days of life in premature infants and multiple births. Arch. Dis. Childh. **30,** 405 (1955). — OLIVER, J., M. MACDOWELL and A. TRACY: The pathogenesis of acute renal failure associated with traumatic and toxic injury. J. clin. Invest. **30,** 1305 (1951). PETERSILGE, C. L.: Prolonged anuria following single injection of bismuth preparation; possible response to therapy with BAL. J. Pediat. **31,** 580 (1947). — PRATT, E. L.: Treatment of anuria. Amer. J. Dis. Child. **76,** 14 (1948). — RIDDELL, H. I.: Lower nephron syndrome in children. J. Urol. (Baltimore) **65,** 513 (1951). — RUBIN, M. I.: In W. E. NELSON, Textbook of paediatrics, 6. edit. Philadelphia: W. B. Saunders Company 1954. — SCHWARTZ, R., E. J. TOMSOVIC and I. L. SCHWARTZ: Hyperpotassemia and body water distribution in an anuric child. Pediatrics **7,** 516 (1951). — SWAN, H., and H. H. GORDON: Peritoneal lavage in the treatment of anuria in children. Pediatrics **4,** 586 (1949). — TZANCK, A., et DAUSSETT: L'exsanguino-transfusion dans les anuries. Bull. Soc. méd. Hôp. Paris **64,** 563 (1948). — WARD, O. C.: Treatment of acute uraemia in childhood. J. Irish med. Ass. **35,** 277 (1954). — WILSON, C. L., and C. B. BILLINGSLEY: Anuria for 96 hours in a 2 year old infant following sulfapyridine. J. Amer. med. Ass. **117,** 285 (1941).

II. Chronic renal Failure

ALBRIGHT, F., and E. C. RIEFENSTEIN: The parathyroid glands and metabolic bone disease. Baltimore: Williams & Wilkins Company 1948. — ANDERSEN, D. H., and E. R. SCHLESINGER: Renal hyperparathyroidism with calcification of the arteries in infancy. Amer. J. Dis. Child. **63,** 102 (1942). — BARBER, H.: Renal dwarfism. Guy's Hosp. Rep. **76,** 307 (1926). — BRAILSFORD, J. F.: The radiology of bones and joints, 5. edit. London: J. G. A. Churchill 1953. — CRAWFORD, T., C. E. DENT, P. LUCAS, N. H. MARTIN and J. R. NASSIM: Osteosclerosis associated with chronic renal failure. Lancet **1954,** ii, 981. — DEBRÉ, R. G., et LAURET H. BOISSIERE: L'hyperazotemie dans les malformations des voies urinaires chez les enfants. Sem. Hôp. Paris **25**, 371 (1949). — DENT, C. E.: Rickets and osteomalacia from renal tubular defects. J. Bone Jt Surg. B **34**, 266 (1952). — Azotaemic renal osteodystrophy. Lancet **1957**, i, 253. — DENT, C. E., and C. J. HODSON: Radiological changes associated with certain metabolic bone diseases. Brit. J. Radiol. **27**, 605 (1954). — DRESKIN, E. A., and T. A. FOX: Adult renal osteitis fibrosa with metastatic calcification and hyperplasia of one parathyroid gland. Arch. Intern. Med. **86**, 533 (1950). — DUKEN, J.: Beitrag zur Kenntnis der malacischen Erkrankungen des kindlichen Skelettsystems. Z. Kinderheilk. **46**, 137 (1928). — ELLIS, A., and H. EVANS: Renal dwarfism, a report of 20 cases with special reference to its association with certain dilatations of the urinary tract. Quart. J. Med. **26**, 231 (1933). — FOLLIS, R. H.: Renal rickets and osteitis fibrosa in children and adolescents. Bull. Johns Hopk. Hosp. **87**, 593 (1950). — GILMOUR, J. R.: The parathyroid glands and skeleton in renal disease. London 1947. — GRAHAM, G., and W. G. OAKLEY: Treatment of renal rickets. Arch. Dis. Childh. **13**, 1 (1938). — HOTTINGER, A.: Über "renalen Zwergwuchs" im Kleinkindesalter. Schweiz. med. Wschr. **1937**, 977. — KLUGE, E.: Neue Beiträge zur Kenntnis des renalen Zwergwuchses und der renalen Rachitis. Virchows Arch. path. Anat. **298**, 406 (1938). — LANGMEAD, F. S., and J. W. ORR: Renal rickets associated with parathyroid hyperplasia. Arch. Dis. Childh. **8**, 265 (1933). — LIU, S. H., and H. I. CHU: Studies of calcium and phosphorus metabolism with special reference to pathogenesis and effects of dihydrotachysterol and iron. Medicine (Baltimore) **22**, 103 (1943). — PARSONS, L. G.: The bone changes occurring in renal and coeliac infantilism and their relationship to rickets: renal rickets. Arch. Dis. Childh. **2**, 1 (1927). — PRICE, N. L., and T. B. DAVIE: Renal rickets. Brit. J. Surg. **24**, 548 (1937). — RULE, C., and A. GROLLMAN: Osteo-nephropathy: a clinical consideration of "renal rickets". Ann. intern. Med. **20**, 63 (1944). — SHELDON, W.: Healing of renal rickets. Arch. Dis. Childh. **18**, 194 (1943). — SINCLAIR, K.: Studies in a case of "renal rickets". Arch. Dis. Childh. **31**, 140 (1956). — SMYTH, F. S., and L. GOLDMAN: Renal rickets with metastatic calcification and parathyroid dysfunction. Amer. J. Dis. Child. **48**, 596 (1934). — STANBURY, S. W.: Azotaemic renal osteodystrophy. Brit. med. Bull. **13**, 57 (1957). — TEALL, C. G.: A radiological study of bone changes in renal infantilism. Brit. J. Radiol. **1**, 49 (1928). — THORN, G. W., G. E. KOEPF and M. CLINTON: Renal failure simulating adrenocortical insufficiency. New Engl. J. Med. **231**, 76 (1944).

III. Renal vascular disorders

CAMPBELL, A. C. P., and J. L. HENDERSON: Symmetrical cortical necrosis of the kidneys in infancy and childhood. Arch. Dis. Childh. **24**, 269 (1949). — CAMPBELL, M. F., and W. F. MATTHEWS: Renal thrombosis in infancy. Report of 2 cases in male infants urologically examined and cured by nephrectomy at 13 and 33 days of age. J. Pediat. **20**, 604 (1942). — CLARK, C. D., and J. D. PICKUP: Haemorrhagic infarction of the kidney treated by nephrectomy. Arch. Dis. Childh. **28**, 302 (1953). — DODD, K., R. J. JOHANSMANN and S. RAPOPORT: Thrombosis of the vena cava and hepatic veins in a patient with nephrosis. Amer. J. Dis. Child. **76**, 316 (1948). — FALLON, M. L.: Renal venous thrombosis in the new born. Arch. Dis. Child. **24**, 125 (1949). — FOURNIER, A., and A. PAULI: Les infarctus renaux par thrombose des veines renales chez le nouveau-né et le nourrisson. Nourrisson **43**, 229 (1955). — FREUND, J., u. G. BICK: Über hämorrhagische Niereninfarkte im Kindesalter. Z. Kinderheilk. **67** 23 (1949). — GROSS, R. E.: Arterial embolism and thrombosis in infancy. Amer. J. Dis. Child. **70**, 61 (1945). — HEPLER, A. B.: Thrombosis of the renal veins. J. Urol. (Baltimore) **31**, 527 (1934). — KOBERNICK, S. D., J. R. MOORE and F. W. WIGGLESWORTH: Thrombosis of the renal veins with massive haemorrhagic infarction of the kidneys in childhood. Report of 4 cases. Amer. J. Path. **27**, 435 (1951). — LELONG, M., R. JOSEPH, J. BERTRAND, LE TAW VINH, CHR. NEZELOFF, G. MATHÉ, J. C. JOB and M. ROIDOT: La nécrose corticale symetrique des reins chez le nourrisson et l'enfant. Arch. franç. Pédiat. **12**, 793 (1955). — MILLS, W. G. Q., and T. K. OWEN: Renal thrombosis complicating pink disease. Cured by nephrectomy. Arch. Dis. Childh. **28**, 300 (1953). — MORISON, J. E.: Renal venous thrombosis and infarction in the new-born. Arch. Dis. Childh. **24**, 129 (1945). — PERRY, C. B., and A. L. TAYLOR: Hypertension following thrombosis of the renal veins. J. Path. Bact. **51**, 369 (1940). — SANDBLOM, P.: Renal thrombosis with infarction in the new-born. Two different forms. Acta paediat. (Uppsala) **35**, 160 (1945). — SMITH, B. A.: Renal vein thrombosis in the new-born. J. Urol. (Baltimore) **73**, 765 (1955). — STEINER, R. E.: Venography in relation to the kidney. Brit. med. Bull. **13**, 61 (1957). — TRAGGIS, D. G., and M. M. ELLISON: Unilateral renal vein thrombosis. J. Pediat. **48**, 229 (1956). — TRUETA, J., A. E. BARCLAY, P. M. DANIEL, K. J. FRANKLIN and P. M. PRICHARD: Studies in the renal circulation. Springfield, Ill.: Ch. C. Thomas 1947. — WAHLE jr., G. H., and E. E. MUIRHEAD: Bilateral renal cortical necrosis in a child associated with an incompatible blood transfusion. Tex. St. J. Med. **49**, 770 (1953). — ZUELZER, W. W., S. CHARLES, R. KURNETZ, W. A. NEWTON and R. FALLON: Circulatory diseases of the kidneys in infancy and childhood. Amer. J. Dis. Childr. **81**, 1 (1951).

IV. Polyuria and the renal tubular disorders

ALBRIGHT, F., C. H. BURNETT, W. PARSONS and E. C. RIEFENSTEIN: Osteomalacia and late rickets. Medicine (Baltimore) 25, 399 (1946). — BICKEL, H., H. S. BAAR, R. ASTLEY, M. A. DOUGLAS, E. FINCH, H. HARRIS, C. C. HARVEY, E. M. HICKMANS, M. G. PHILPOTT, W. C. SMALLWOOD, J. M. SMELLIE u. C. G. TEALL: Acta paediat. (Uppsala) 42, Suppl. 90 (1953). — CARTER, C., and M. SIMPKISS: The carrier state in nephrogenic diabetes insipidus. Lancet 1956, ii, 1069. — CHUNG, R. C. H., and L. K. MANTELL: Urographic changes in diabetes insipidus. J. Amer. med. Ass. 150, 1307 (1952). — DANCIS, J., J. R. BIRMINGHAM and S. LESLIE: Congenital diabetes insipidus resistant to treatment with pitressin. Amer. J. Dis. Child. 75, 316 (1948). — EARLEY, L. E.: Extreme polyuria in obstructive uropathy. Report of a case of "water-losing nephritis" in an infant with a discussion of polyuria. New Engl. J. Med. 255, 600 (1956). — FANCONI, G.: Zur Differentialdiagnose des Diabetes insipidius. Helv. paediat. Acta 11, 506 (1956). — FANCONI, G., P. GIRARDET, B. SCHLE-SINGER, W. BUTLER and J. A. BLACK: Chronische Hypercalcämie, kombiniert mit Osteo-sklerose, Hyperazotämie, Minderwuchs und kongenitalen Mißbildungen. Helv. paediat. Acta 7, 314 (1952). — JAMES, J. A.: Renal tubular disease with nephrocalcinosis. Report of 2 unusual cases. Amer. J. Dis. Child. 91, 601 (1956). — JEUNE, M., et A. CHARRAT: L'acidose rénale idiopathique du nourrisson. Pédiatrie II, 205 (1956). — KIRMAN, B. H., J. A. BLACK, R. H. WILKINSON and P. R. EVANS: Familial pitressin-resistant diabetes insipidus with mental defect. Arch. Dis. Childh. 31, 59 (1956). — LIGHTWOOD, R.: Hypercalcaemia. Proc. roy. Soc. Med. 45, 401 (1952). — LIGHTWOOD, R., W. W. PAYNE and J. A. BLACK: Infantile renal acidosis. Pediatrics 12, 628 (1953). — LIGNAC, G. O. E.: Syndrome consisting of affec-tions of the kidney, stunted growth, rickets and disturbed cystine metabolism. Amer. J. med. Sci. 208, 542 (1938). — McCUNE, D. J., H. H. MASON and H. T. CLARKE: Intractable hypophosphatemic rickets with renal glycosuria and acidosis (the Fanconi syndrome): report of a case in which increased urinary organic acids were detected and identified, with review of the literature. Amer. J. Dis. Child. 65, 81 (1943). — PLATT, R.: Structural and functional adaptation in renal failure. Brit. med. J. 1952, i, 1313, 1372. — SCHLESINGER, B. E., N. R. BUTLER and J. A. BLACK: Severe type of infantile hypercalcaemia. Lancet 1956, i, 127. — SCHREINER, G. E., L. H. SMITH and L. H. KYLE: Renal hyperchloraemic acidosis: familial occurrence of Nephrocalcinosis with hyperchloraemia and low serum bicarbonate. Amer. J. Med. 15, 122 (1953). — STICKLER, G. B., and A. B. HAYLES: Chronic renal tubular insuffi-ciency in infants and children. Amer. J. Dis. Child. 93, 140 (1957). — VEST, M., and G. STALDER: Zum Pitressintest im Kindesalter. Ann. paediat. (Basel) 186, 36 (1956). — WAR-KANY, J., and A. B. MITCHELL: Diabetes insipidus in Children. Amer. J. Dis. Child. 57, 603 (1939).

V. Haematuria and nephritis

BOISSONNAT, P.: Les hematuries de l'enfant. Rev. Prat. (Paris). 1955, 65. — CAMPBELL, J. L.: Hereditary haemorrhagic telangiectasia as a cause of haematuria. J. Urol. (Baltimore) 62, 80 (1949). — ELLIS, A.: The classification of nephritis. Lancet 1942, i, 34, 72. — FINK, A. J., A. A. STEIN and W. GARLICK: Haematuria following minimal trauma. A sign of congenital uropathy. Amer. J. Dis. Child. 92, 157 (1956). — FISHBERG, A. M.: Hypertension and nephritis. Philadelphia: Lea a. Febiger 1939. — FRÄNKEL, W. K.: Hämaturie beim Kind. Kinderärztl. Prax. 3, 259 (1932). — GAHLEMANN, C.: Essentielle Hämaturie im Kindesalter. Mschr. Kinderheilk. 74, 45 (1938). — GARDNER jr., K. D.: "Athletic pseudonephritis" alteration of urine sediment by athletic competition. J. Amer. med. Ass. 161, 1613 (1956). — GLASER, J., and J. EPSTEIN: Winckel's disease. Amer. J. Dis. Child. 60, 1375 (1940). — JOCHIMS, J.: Differentialdiagnose der Hämaturie im Kindesalter. Kinderärztl. Prax. 24, 409 (1956). — OCHSENIUS, K.: Alimentäre Hämaturie im Kindesalter. Mschr. Kinderheilk. 53, 220 (1932). — PAYNE, W. W., and R. S. ILLINGWORTH: Acute nephritis in childhood with special reference to the diagnosis of focal nephritis. Quart. J. Med. 9, 37 (1940). — RHODES, J.: Haematuria after use of tetanus antitoxin; report of a case. J. Urol. (Baltimore) 38, 410 (1937). — WEDGWOOD, R. J. P., and M. H. KLAUS: Anaphylactoid purpura. Pediatrics 16, 196 (1955). — WYLLIE, G. G.: Haematuria in children. Proc. roy. Soc. Med. 48, 1113 (1955).

N. The male genital tract

I. Congenital abnormalities of the penis

BERARDINELLI, W., J. MATTOSO, D. DE ALBUQUERQUE and J. G. CORDEIRO: Aplasia of the penis. Presse méd. 1953, 432. — BOCKAY, J. v.: Über Diphallie. Jb. Kinder-heilk. 127, 127 (1930). — BROUSSARD, E. R.: Uncomplicated congenital torsion of the penis. J. Pediat. 46, 456 (1955). — CAMPBELL, M. F.: Clinical pediatric urology. Philadelphia and London: W. B. Saunders Company 1951. — COCHRANE, W. J., and R. L. SAUNDERS: Rare anomaly of the penis associated with imperforate anus. J. Urol. (Baltimore) **47**, 810 (1947). — DAVIS, D. M.: Cases of double, triple, or quadruple penis associated with dermoid of the perineum. Trans. Amer. Ass. gen.-urin. Surg. **40**, 112 (1948). — DONALD, C.: A case of human diphallus. J. Anat. (Lond.) **64**, 523 (1930). — DRURY, R. B., and H. H. SHWARZELL: Congenital absence of penis. Arch. Surg. (Chicago) **30**, 236 (1935). — FORSHALL, I., and P. P. RICKHAM: Transposition of the penis and scrotum. Brit. J. Urol. **28**, 250 (1956). — FRANCIS, C. C.: Case of prepenial scrotum (marsupial type of genitalia) associated with absence of urinary system. Anat. Rec. **76**, 303 (1940). — GILLIES, H.: Congenital absence of the penis. Brit. J. plast. Surg. **1**, 8 (1948). — HUFFMAN, L. F.: Case of prepenile scrotum. J. Urol. (Baltimore) **65**, 141 (1951). — KIRSCH, E.: Totale Diphallie. Z. Urol. **48**, 711 (1955). — LANE, V.: Pre-penile scrotum. Irish J. med. Sci. **1956**, 283. — NESBIT, R. M., and W. BROMME: Double penis and double bladder. Amer. J. Roentgenol. **30**, 497 (1933). — OTTOW, B.: Cyst of the preputial raphe. Z. urol. Chir. **30**, 50 (1930). — RUKSTINAT, G. J., and R. J. HASTERLIK: Congenital absence of the penis. Arch. Path. (Chicago) **27**, 984 (1939). — SCHWART, J. W., and J. L. FARR: Congenital torsion of the penis. J. Urol. (Baltimore) **78**, 425 (1957). — STOLL, H. G.: Angeborener Penismangel. Z. Urol. **47**, 360 (1954).

II. Phimosis etc.

CAMPBELL, M. F.: Clinical paediatric urology. Philadelphia: W. B. Saunders Company 1951. — GAIRDNER, D.: Fate of the foreskin: a study of circumcision. Brit. med. J. **1949**, ii, 1433.

III. Ammoniacal dermatitis

BOUND, J. P.: Thrush napkin rashes. Brit. med. J. **1956**, i, 782. — BRENNEMAN, J.: Ulceration of the meatus. In: Practice of paediatrics, vol. 4. Hagerstown, Ma.: W. F. Prior & Co. 1942. — COOKE, J. V.: The etiology and treatment of ammonia dermatitis of the gluteal region of infants. Amer. J. Dis. Child. **22**, 481 (1921). — FISHER, R. S., H. C. FREIMUTH, K. A. O'CONNOR and V. JOHNS: Boron absorption of borated talc. J. Amer. med. Ass. **157**, 503 (1955). — GOLDBLOOM, R. B., and A. GOLDBLOOM: Boric acid poisoning. J. Pediat. **43**, 631 (1953). — HAMILTON, A. J. C., and D. S. MIDDLETON: Phimosis and dysuria in infancy. Lancet **1927**, ii, 639. — JOHNSTONE, D. E., N. BASILA and J. GLASER: A study on boric acid absorption in infants from the use of baby powders. J. Pediat. **46**, 160 (1955). — ZAHORSKY, J.: The ammoniacal diaper in infants and young children. Amer. J. Dis. Child. **10**, 436 (1915).

IV. Meatal ulcer and stenosis

ABESHOUSE, B. S., and D. E. BOGORAD: Ulceration of the external urethral orifice in male children. Urol. cutan. Rev. **42**, 748 (1938). — CAMPBELL, M. F.: Stenosis of the external urethral meatus. J. Urol. (Baltimore) **50**, 740 (1943). — FREUD, P.: Ulcerated urethral meatus in male children. J. Pediat. **31**, 131 (1947). — FRITZSCHE, F.: Kongenitale Meatusstenose. (Stenose des orificium urethrae externum.) Chirurg **28**, 56 (1957). — KAPLAN, J. H., and W. M. TASEM: Stenosis of the urethral meatus in boys. Surgical correction. Calif. med. **79**, 231 (1953). — McNULTY, P. H.: Complete retention of urine in infancy — a common cause. Urol. cutan. Rev. **50**, 144 (1946).

V. Genital tract infections

BEILIN, L. M.: Gonorrheal urethritis in male children: with some observations on their sexual impulses. J. Urol. (Baltimore) **25**, 69 (1931). — BOROVSKY, M. P.: Diphtheria of the penis. J. Amer. med. Ass. **104**, 1399 (1935). — CAMPBELL, M. F.: Gonococcal prostatic abscess in infancy. J. Urol. (Baltimore) **22**, 445 (1929). — Clinical paediatric urology. Philadelphia: W. B. Saunders Company 1951. — CONNOLLY, N. K.: Mumps orchitis without parotitis in infants. Lancet **1953**, i, 69. — CORNER, B. D.: Reiter's syndrome in children. Arch. Dis. Childh. **25**, 398 (1950). — FLORMAN, A. L., and H. M. GOLDSTEIN: Arthritis, conjunctivitis and urethritis (so-called Reiter's syndrome) in a four-year-old boy. J. Pediat. **33**, 172 (1948). — FOX, C. P.: Gonorrheal prostatic abscess in 4 year old boy. J. Amer. med. Ass. **103**, 748 (1934). — GARROW, I., and J. WERNE: Metastatic epididymitis with a report of occurrence in an infant during acute respiratory infection. Urol. cutan. Rev. **51**, 3 (1947). — HARKNESS, H. H.: Nongonococcal urethritis. Edinburgh: E. & S. Livingstone 1950. — HENCKEL, H.: Das Reitersche Syndrom bei Kindern und seine Therapie. Z. Kinderheilk. **74**, 303 (1954). — LOMBARD, P.: Orchi-épididymites des nouveau-nés. Bull. Soc. nat. Chir. Paris **55**, 1201 (1929). — McKAY,

H.: Acquired genital syphilis in young male children. Arch. Pediat. **47, 467** (1930). — MENNINGER, W. C.: Congenital syphilis of the testicle. Amer. J. Syph. **12, 221** (1928). — MURRAY, J. D.: Stevens Johnson syndrome. Lancet **1947**, i, 328. — NABARRO, D.: Congenital syphilis. London: Ed. Arnold 1954. — ORMISTON, G.: Orchitis as a complication of chicken-pox. Brit. med. J. **1953**, i, 1203. — QVIST, O.: Swelling of the scrotum in infants and children, and non-specific epididymitis. Acta chir. scand. **110, 417** (1956). — STEVENS, A. M., and F. C. JOHNSON: A new eruptive fever associated with stomatitis and ophthalmia. Amer. J. Dis. Child. **24, 526** (1922). — SZENKIER, D.: Ein Prostataabsceß bei einem zweieinhalbjährigen Knaben. Z. Urol. **23, 119** (1929). — WESTPHAL, R. S.: Report of outbreak of gonorrhea at boy's school. N.Y. State med. J. **44, 493** (1944).

VI. Injuries and strictures

BADENOCH, A. W.: A pull-through operation for impassable traumatic stricture of the urethra. Brit. J. Urol. **22, 404** (1950). — BROWNE, D.: Hypospadias. Postgrad. med. J. **25, 367** (1949). — JOHANSON, B.: Reconstruction of the male urethra in strictures. Modern trends in urology. London: Butterworth & Co. 1953. — MARION, J.: Traité d'urologie, 4. edit. Paris: Masson & Cie. 1940. — PETKOVIC, S.: Verletzungen der Harnröhre bei Kindern. Z. Urol. **47, 737** (1954).

VII. Priapism

CONN, J. H., and L. KANNER: Spontaneous erections in early childhood. J. Pediat. **16, 337** (1940). — COWIE, D. M.: Case of priapism resulting from rapidly growing myxosarcoma. Amer. J. Dis. Child. **20, 211** (1920). — FRASER, W. J.: A case of priapism. Brit. Med. J. **1955**, ii, 419. — MACCIOTTA, G.: Priapismo rivelatore di una mielosi leucemica in un bambino di 10 anni. Pediatria (Napoli) **42, 1093** (1934).

VIII. Undescended testicles

ALNOR, P., u. H. HARTIG: Das funktionelle Ergebnis nach Kryptochismusoperationen. Chirurg **25, 294** (1954). — BEVAN, A. D.: Operation for undescended testis. Ann. Surg. **90, 847** (1929). — BISHOP, P. M. F.: Studies in clinical endocrinology. Management of the undescended testicle. Guy's Hosp. Rep. **94, 12** (1945). — BLECHSCHMIDT, E.: Wachstums-faktoren des Descensus testis. Z. Anat. Entwickl.-Gesch. **118, 175** (1955). — BOLL, Z.: Zum Problem; Retentio Testium. Z. Urol. **49, 582** (1956). — BREGADSE, I. L.: Der eingeklemmte Hoden im Leistenkanal als Komplikation des Kryptorchismus. Z. urol. Chir. **36, 301** (1933). — BROWN, D.: Anatomical points in operation for undescended testicle. Lancet **1933**, i, 460. — Diagnosis of undescended testicles. Brit. med. J. **1938**, ii, 168. — CAMPBELL, H. E.: Incidence of malignant growth of the undescended testicle: a critical and statistical study. Arch. Surg. (Chicago) **44, 353** (1942). — CARROLL, W. A.: Malignancy in cryptorchism. J. Urol. (Baltimore) **61, 396** (1949). — CHARNEY, C. W., A. S. CONSTON and D. R. MERANZE: Development of the testis: a histologic study from birth to maturity with some notes on abnormal variations. Fertil. a. Steril. **3, 461** (1952). — CHAUVIN, E.: Séminome développé sur un ancien testicule ectopique abaissé par le procédé d'Ombrédanne. Bull Soc. franç. Urol. **1938**, 196. — COOPER, E. R. A.: Histology of the retained testis in the human subject at different ages, and its comparison with the scrotal testis. J. Anat. (Lond.) **64, 5** (1929). — DAHL-IVERSEN, E., u. A. BERTELSEN: Du traitement de la rétention du testicule. Acta chir. scand. **87, 513** (1942). — DEMING, C. L.: Evaluation of hormonal therapy in cryptorchidism. J. Urol. (Baltimore) **68, 354** (1952). — DRAKE, C. B.: Spontaneous late descent of the testis. J. Amer. med. Ass. **102, 759** (1934). — FRAZER, J.: The surgery of childhood. London: Ed. Arnold 1926. — GORDON-TAYLOR, G., and A. S. TILL: On malignant disease of the testicle, with special reference to neoplasms of the undescended organ. Brit. J. Urol. **10, 1** (1938). — GREWE, H. E., and D. FRANKE: Zur Behandlung des Leistenhodens. Zbl. Chir. **78, 1781** (1953). — GROSS, R. E., and T. C. JEWETT jr.: Surgical experiences from 1,222 operations for undescended testis. J. Amer. med. Ass. **160, 634** (1956). — GRUENWALD, P.: Structure of the testis in infancy and in childhood, with a discussion of the so-called under-developed testis. Arch. Path. (Chicago) **42, 35** (1946). — HANSEN, T. S.: Fertility in operatively treated and untreated cryptorchism. Acta chir. scand. **94, 117** (1946). — HINMAN jr., F.: Implications of testicular cytology in the treatment of cryptorchidism. Amer. J. Surg. **90, 381** (1955). — KAFKA, V.: A contribution to hormonal treatment of incomplete descent of the testis. Schweiz. med. Wschr. **1946**, 561. — KAYS and F. P. COLEMAN: Duplication of the left undescended testicle: report of case. J. Urol. (Baltimore) **75, 815** (1956). — KELLY, C. M., and G. E. UHRICH: Infarction of intraperitoneal undescended testicle. Amer. J. Surg. **83, 233** (1952). — MIMPRISS, T. W.: The treatment of retention of the testis. Lancet **1938**, i, 533. — Cryptorchidism. Brit. J. Urol. **24, 23** (1952). — MOSZKOWICZ, L.: Über falschen und echten Kryptorchismus. Arch. klin. Chir. **192**, 209 (1938). — REA, C. E.: Functional capacity of the undescended testis. Arch. Surg. (Chicago) **38**, 1054 (1939). — Fertility in cryptorchids. Minn. Med. **34**, 216 (1951). — ROBINSON, J. N., and E. T. ENGLE: Some observations on the cryptorchid testis. J. Urol. (Baltimore) **71**, 726 (1954). — Cryptorchism. Pathogenesis and treatment. Pediat. Clin. N. Amer. **2**, 729 (1955). — SCORER, C. G.: Descent of the testicle in the first year of life. Brit. J. Urol. **27**, 374 (1955). — Incidence of incomplete descent of the testicle at birth. Arch. Dis. Childh. **31**, 198 (1956). — SMITH, R. E.: Observations on the descent of the testicles with special reference to spontaneous descent at puberty. Arch. Dis. Childh. **14**, 1 (1939). — SNIFFEN R. C.: Histology of the normal and abnormal testis at puberty. Ann. N. Y. Acad. Sci. **55**, 609 (1952). — SNYDER, W. H., and L. CHAFFIN: Surgical management of undescended testicles. J. Amer. med. Ass. **157**, 129 (1955). — SOHVAL, A. R.: Testicular dysgenesis as an etiological factor in cryptorchidism. J. Urol. (Baltimore) **72**, 693 (1954). — SOUTHAM, A. H., and E. R. A. COOPER: Retained testis in childhood. Lancet **1927**, i, 805. — STÄHLI, W.: Zur Behandlung des Kryptorchismus. Schweiz. med. Wschr. **1947**, 1119. — THOMAS, D. W.: Malignant transformation following orchidocleisis. Brit. J. Urol. **23**, 260 (1951). — WELLS, L. J.: Descent of the testis: anatomical and hormonal considerations. Surgery **14**, 436 (1943). — WHITEHORN, C. A.: Complete unilateral Wolffian duct agenesis with homolateral cryptorchidism. J. Urol. (Baltimore) **72**, 685 (1954). — WILES, P.: Family tree, showing hereditary undescended right testicle and associated deformities. Proc. roy. Soc. Med. **28**, 157 (1934). — WYNDHAM, N. R.: Descent of testicle. J. Anat. (Lond.) **77**, 179 (1943).

IX. Other testicular anomalies

AMELAR, R. D.: Anorchism without eunuchoidism. J. Urol. (Baltimore) **76**, 174 (1956). — ANDERSON, P. ST. G.: Case of polyorchidism. Lancet **1953**, i, 826. — BADENOCH, A. W.: Failure of urogenital union. Surg. Gynec. Obstet **82**, 471 (1946). — BEETZ, F.: Zur Ätiologie der Ectopia testis. Z. Chir. **66**, 1322 (1939). — BOGGON, R. H.: Polyorchidism. Brit. J. Surg. **20**, 630 (1933). — COUNSELLER, V., and M. A. WALKER: Congenital absence of testes (anorchia). Ann. Surg **98**, 104 (1933). — COUNSELLER, V. S., D. R. NICHOLS and H. L. SMITH: Congenital absence of testis: a report of 7 cases of monorchidism. J. Urol. (Baltimore) **44**, 237 (1940). — GOLJI, H.: Polyorchidism: a case report. J. Urol. (Baltimore) **74**, 207 (1955). — GORRO, A. P.: Testicule ectopique perineal. J. d'Urol. **48**, 114 (1939). — HERTZLER, A. E.: Transverse ectopia of the testicle. Surg. Gynec. Obstet **23**, 597 (1916). — LAZARUS, J. A., and M. S. MARKS: Anomalies associated with undescended testis: complete separation of a partly descended epididymis and vas deferens, and an abdominal testis. J. Urol. (Baltimore) **57**, 567 (1947). — RANSON, F. T.: Case of polyorchidism. Brit. med. J. **2**, 137 (1949). — RASPALL, G.: Anomalies congénitales génito-urinaires rares. J. Urol- méd. chir- **55**, 265 (1949). — WAKELEY, J. C. N.: Perineal testis. Lancet **1953**, i, 1025. — WENGER, W.: Über perineale Hodendystopie beim Neugeborenen. Zentralblatt f. Gynäk. **57**, 2077 (1933). — WILLIAMS, B. L., and J. LEE: Monorchia. Brit. J. Urol. **28**, 95 (1956).

X. Hydrocele

CAMPBELL, M. F.: Hydrocele of the tunica vaginalis: a study of 502 cases. Surg. Gynec. Obstet **45**, 192 (1927). — FRIES, J. W., and B. S. TALBOT: Scrotal calcification due to meconium peritonitis. J. Urol. (Baltimore) **73**, 1059 (1955). — GROSS, R. E.: Surgery in childhood. Philadelphia: W. B. Saunders Company 1953. — LANGER, M.: Über die Hernie und Hydrocele des Kindesalters. Arch. klin. Chir. **181**, 418 (1934). — Low, H., G. COOPER and L. COSBY: Meconium peritonitis. Surgery **26**, 223 (1949).

XI. Varicocele

CAMPBELL, M. F.: Variocele due to anomalous renal vessel: an instance in a 13 year old boy. J. Urol. (Baltimore) **52**, 502 (1944). — ROBB, W. A. T.: Operative treatment of varicocele. Brit. med. J. **1955**, ii, 355.

XII. Torsion of the spermatic cord and testicular appendages

ALLEN, P. D., and T. H. ANDREWS: Torsion of the spermatic cord in infancy. Amer. J. Dis. Child. **59**, 136 (1940). — BENNETT-JONES, M. J.: Strangulation of the testicle by hernia in infancy. Liverpool Med.-Chir. J. **45**, 121 (1937). — BIORN, C. L., and J. H. DAVIS: Torsion of the spermatic cord in the new-born. J. Amer. med. Ass. **145**, 1236 (1951). — BROSTER, L. R., and R. COYTE: Torsion of the appendix of the testis (hydatid of Morgagni). Brit. med. J. **1929**, i, 145. — CAMPBELL, M. F.: Torsion of the spermatic cord in the newborn infant. J. Pediat **33**, 323 (1948). — DEMING, C. L., and B. G. CLARKE: Torsion of the spermatic cord. J. Amer. med. Ass. **152**, 521 (1953). — Dix, V. W.: On torsion of the appendages of the testis and epididymis. Brit. J. Urol. **3**, 245 (1931). — Fernicola, A. R.: Idiopathic haemorrhagic infarction of the testicle in the newborn. J. Urol. (Baltimore) **72**, 230 (1954). — Idiopathic septic gangrene of the testicle in the newborn. Amer. J. Surg. **93**, 466 (1957). — Fuchsig, P.: Bruchreposition als Ursache eines beiderseitigen Hodeninfarktes bei einem Säugling. Öst. Z. Kinderheilk. **1**, 308 (1948). — Glaser, S., and H. R. E. Wallis: Torsion or spontaneous haemorrhagic infarction of testicle in newborn infant. Brit. med. J. **1954**. ii, 88. — Heslin, J. E., and R. E. Allyn: Torsion of the appendix testis. Urol. cutan, Rev. **47**, 210 (1943). — Koehler, H. D., and R. P. Koehler: Volvulus of the spermatic cord, caused by an embryonal anomaly. J. Int. Coll. Surg. **26**, 53 (1956). — Longino, L. A., and L. W. Martin: Torsion of the spermatic cord in the newborn infant. New Engl. J. Med. **253**, 695 (1955). — Muschat, M.: Pathological anatomy of testicular torsion. Surg. Gynec. Obstet. **54**, 758 (1932). — Nowakowski, H.: Bilateral testicular atrophy as a result of scrotal hematoma in the newborn. Acta endocr. **18**, 501 (1955). — Ravich, R. H.: Haemorrhagic infarction of the testicle in the newborn. J. Urol. (Baltimore) **57**, 875 (1947). — Rhyne, J. L., F. A. Mantz and J. F. Patton: Haemorrhagic infarction of the testis in newborn. Relationship to testicular torsion. Amer. J. Dis. Child. **89**, 240 (1955). — Rosenblaat, M. S., and W. H. Bueermann: Strangulated hernia with acute haemorrhagic infarction of testicle in infants. Northw. Med. **38**, 18 (1939). — Seidal, R. F., and R. C. Yeaw: Torsion of the appendix testis and appendix epidimymis: a report of 8 cases. J. Urol. (Baltimore) **63**, 714 (1950). — Trillat, A.: Un cas de torsion du testicule en position normale chez un nouveau né de trois jours. Castration. Guérison. Nourrisson **28**, 32 (1940).

XIII. Scrotal oedema and gangrene

Alders, N.: Scrotal gangrene in a new-born baby. Arch. Dis. Childh. **29**, 160 (1954). — Campbell, M. F.: Periurethral phlegmon (urinary extravasation). Surg. Gynec. Obstet. **48**, 382 (1929). — Levinson, A.: Scrotal gangrene in infants and children. Amer. J. Dis. Child. **41**, 1123 (1931). Nielson, H. K., D. O. Ferris and G. B. Logan: Injury of the penis scrotum and buttocks of the newborn resulting in gangrene. Amer. J. Dis. Child. **75**, 85 (1948).

O. The female genital tract and urethra

I. Clitoris and labia

Brown, K. S. McA.: Paraphimosis of the clitoris. Brit. med. J. **1929**, ii, 146. — Willan, R. J.: Paraphimosis of clitoris. Brit. med. J. **1928**, ii, 1130.

II. External urinary meatus

Campbell, M. F.: Clinical pediatric urology. Philadelphia: W. B. Saunders Company 1951. — Stevens, W. E.: Congenital obstructions of the female urethra. J. Amer. med. Ass. **106**, 89 (1936).

III. Urethral prolapse

Abrams, M., and H. K. Lewis: Prolapse of the urethra in young girls. J. Urol. (Baltimore) **72**, 222 (1954). — Barns, H. H. F.: Prolapse of the urethra in young girls. Brit. med. J. **1953**, ii, 765. — Hepburn, I. N.: Prolapse of the urethra in female children. Surg. Gynec. Obstet. **44**, 400 (1927). — Higgins, T. T., D. I. Williams and D. F. E. Nash: Urology of childhood. London: Butterworth & Co. 1951. — Moffet, J. D., and R. Banks: Prolapse of the urethra in young girls. J. Amer. med. Ass. **146**, 1288 (1951). — Moir, J. C.: Prolapse of urethra in a child of 6 years. Proc. roy. Soc. Med. **37**, 436 (1943).

IV. Urethro-trigonitis

Hodges, C. V.: Chronic urethritis in girls. J. Amer. med. Ass. **149**, 753 (1952). — Roen, P. R., and R. R. Stept: Urethritis in girls. Amer. J. Dis. Child. **72**, 529 (1946). — Spence, H. M., and H. Moore: Female urethra in childhood. Tex. St. J. Med. **35**, 234 (1939/40). — Winsbury-White, H. P.: Textbook of genito-urinary surgery. Edinburgh: Livingstone 1949.

V. Vulgo-vaginitis

Boisvert, P. L., and D. N. Walcher: Hemolytic streptococcal vaginitis in children. Pediatrics **2**, 24 (1948). — Clauberg, K. W.: Zur Bakteriologie der pseudogonorrhoischen Vulvovaginitiden beim Kinde. Dtsch. med. Wschr. **1930**, 524. — Mukherjee, C.: Gonococcal vulvo-vaginitis in infants and children: a study of 240 cases. Arch. Dis. Childh. **25**, 262 (1950). — *Report of Committee to Medical Officer of Health, County of London:* Vulvo-vaginitis in children. Brit. med. J. **1938**, i, 961. — SCHAUFFLER, G. C.: Pediatric gynaecology. Chicago: Year Book Publ. 1953.

VII. Hydrocolpos

ALTHOFF, F.: Ein ungewöhnlicher Fall von Serokolpos und Serometra bei Atresia hymenalis. Zbl. Gynäk. **65**, 1398 (1941). — ANTELL, L.: Hydrocolpos in infancy and childhood. Pediatrics **10**, 306 (1952). — BLOXSOM, A., and N. POWELL: Urinary retention due to hematocolpometra. Report of 2 cases, one with spontaneous recovery. Pediatrics **2**, 567 (1948). — FÈVRE, M.: L'hydrocolpos et l'hydro-pyocolpos. Arch. franç. Pédiat. **13**, 569 (1956). — GROSS, R. E.: Surgery of childhood. Philadelphia: W. B. Saunders Company 1953. — KERESZTURI, C.: Imperforate hymen causing hydrocolpos, hydro-ureter and hydronephrosis and pyuria. Amer. J. Dis. Child. **59**, 1290 (1940). — MAHONEY, P. J., and J. W. CHAMBERLAIN: Hydrocolpos in infancy. J. Pediat. **17**, 772 (1940). — MALIPHANT, R. G.: Gynatresia. Brit. med. J. **1948**, ii, 555. — MORRIS, P.: Hydrometrocolpos in infancy. A cause of urinary retention, intestinal obstruction and oedema of the lower extremities. Amer. J. med. Sci. **210**, 751 (1945). — TOMPKINS, P.: The treatment of imperforate hymen with hematocolpos: a review of 113 cases in the literature and a report of 5 additional cases. J. Amer. med. Ass. **113**, 913 (1939).

VIII. Absent vagina

BRYAN, A. L., J. A. NIGRO and V. S. COUNSELLER: One hundred cases of congenital absence of vagina. Surg. Gynec. Obstet. **88**, 79 (1949). — McINDOE, A.: The treatment of congenital absence and obliterative conditions of the vagina. Brit. J. plast. Surg. **2**, 254 (1950). — PHELAN, J. T., V. S. COUNSELLER and L. F. GREENE: Deformities of the urinary tract with congenital absence of the vagina. Surg. Gynec. Obstet. **97**, 1 (1953). — THOMSON, G. R.: Complete congenital absence of the vagina associated with bilateral herniae of uterus, tubes and ovaries. Brit. J. Surg. **36**, 98 1948).

P. Intersex states and endocrine disorders

I. Normal development

BARR, M. L.: In modern trends in obstetrics and gynaecology, 2. Ser. Editor K. BOWES. London: Butterworth & Co. 1955. — BUNGE, R. G., and J. T. BRADBURY: Genetic sex: chromative test versus gonadal histology. J. clin. Endocr. **16**, 1117 (1956). — CATHIE, I. A. B.: Personal communication. — CHANG, C. Y., and E. WITSCHI: Breeding of sex-reversed males of Xenopus laevis Daudin. Proc. Soc. exp. Biol. (N. Y.) **89**, 150 (1955). — CHARNEY, C. W., A. S. CONSTON and D. R. MERANZE: Testicular developmental histology. Ann. N. Y. Acad. Sci. **55**, 597 (1952). — DANON, M., and L. SACHS: Sex chromosomes and human sexual development. Lancet **1957**, ii, 20. — DAVIDSON, W. M., and D. R. SMITH: A morphological sex difference in polymorphonuclear leucocytes. Brit. med. J. **1954**, ii, 6. — GREENE, R., D. N. MATTHEWS, P. E. HUGHESDON and A. HOWARD: A case of true hemaphroditism. Brit. J. Surg. **40**, 263, (1953); **41**, 548 (1954). — HINGLAIS, H., et M. HINGLAIS: Le diagnostic chromosomique du sexe chez l'adulte. Presse méd. **1955**, 337. — JOST, A.: Recherches sur le controlle hormonal de l'organogenèse sexuelle du lapin et remarques sur certaines malformations de l'appareil génital humain. Gynéc. et Obstétr. **49**, 44 (1950). — LENNOX, B.: Nuclear sexing: a review incorporating some personal observations. Scot. med. J. **1**, 97 (1955). — MOORE, C. R.: Sex endocrines in development and prepubertal life. J. clin. Endocr. **4**, 135 (1944). — MOORE, K. L., and M. L. BARR: Nuclear morphology, according to sex, in human tissues. Acta anat. (Basel) **21**, 197 (1954). — Smears from oral mucosa in the detection of chromosomal sex. Lancet **1955**, ii, 57. — NATHANSON, I. T., L. E. TOWNE and J. C. AUB: Normal excretion of sex hormones in childhood. Endocrinology **28**, 851 (1941). — NELSON, W. O.: Sex differences in human nuclei. Acta endocr. (Kbh.) **23**, 227 (1956). — SCHONFELD, W. A.: Primary and secondary sexual characteristics. Study of their development in males from birth through maturity with biometric study of penis and testes. Amer. J. Dis. Child. **65**, 535 (1943). — SEGAL, S. J., and W. D. NELSON: Developmental aspects of human hermaphroditism: the significance of sex chromatin patterns. J. clin. Endocr. **17**, 676 (1957). — TALBOT, N. B., E. H. SOBEL, J. W. McARTHUR and J. D. CRAWFORD: Functional endocrinology from birth through adolescence. Cambridge, Massachusetts: Harvard University Press 1952. — WILKINS, L.: The diagnosis and treatment of endocrine disorders in childhood and adolescence. Springfield, Ill.: Ch. C. Thomas 1950.

II. Female pseudohermaphroditism

BENTINCK, R. C., H. LISSER and W. A. REILLY: Female pseudohermaphrodism with penile urethra masquerading as precocious puberty and crytorchidism. J. clin. Endocr. 16, 412 (1956). — BONGIOVANNI, A. M., and W. R. EBERLEIN: Certain aspects of steroid metabolism in the adreno-genital syndrome, in "Adrenal Function in Infants and Children". Editor L. I. GARDNER. New York: Grune & Stratton 1956. — BRENTNALL, C. P.: A case of arrhenoblastoma complicating pregnancy. J. Obstet. Gynaec. Brit. Enp. 52, 235 (1945). — BROSTER, L. R.: Form of intersexuality. Brit. med. J. 1956, i, 149. — BROSTER, L. R., J. PATTERSON and B. CAMBER: Adrenal pseudohermaphroditism. Brit. med. J. 1953, ii, 288. — CHILDS, B., M. M. GRUMBACH and J. J. VAN WYK: Virilizing adrenal hyperplasia: Genetic and hormonal study. J. clin. Invest. 35, 213 (1956). — COTTE, G.: Plastic operations for sexual ambignity. J. Mt Sinai Hosp. 14, 170 (1947). — COX, P.: Personal communication 1957. — EVERIDGE, J.: Case of pseudohermaphroditism and adrenalism. Proc. roy. Soc. Med. 38, 649 (1945). — GENITIS, V. E., and I. P. BRONSTEIN: Pregnandiol excretion in female pseudohermaphroditism. J. Amer. med. Ass. 119, 704 (1942). — GOLDBERG, M. B.: Experience with long term cortisone therapy in congenital adrenocortical hyperplasia. J. clin. Endocr. 14, 389 (1954). GREENE, R. R., and A. C. IVY: Experimental production of intersexuality in rats. Science 86, 200 (1937). — HAMPSON, J. G.: Hermaphroditic genital appearance, rearing and eroticism in hyperadrenocorticism. Bull. Johns Hopk. Hosp. 96, 265 (1955). — HAYLES, A. B., and R. B. NOLAN: Female pseudohermaphroditism: report of case in an infant born of a mother receiving methyltestosterone during pregnancy. Proc. Mayo Clin. 32, 41 (1957). — HOWARD, F. S., and F. HINMAN: Female pseudohermaphroditism with supplementary phallic urethra, report of 2 case. J. Urol. (Baltimore) 65, 439 (1951). — NEIMANN, N., M. PIERSON and G. LASCOMBES: Le pseudo-hermaphrodisme par hyperplasie congenitale des surrenales. I. Forme avec manifestations addisoniennes. II. Forme purement genitale. Arch. franç. Pédiat. 13, 596 (1956). — OWEN, J. A., F. L. ENGEL and T. B. WESTER: 9-α-Fluorohydrocortisone-induced hypertension in an infant with adrenogenitalism. J. clin. Endocr. 17, 272 (1957). — PAPADATOS, C., and R. KLEIN: Nonadrenal female pseudohermaphrodism. Report of 2 patients simulating mixed adrenal disease. J. Pediat. 45, 662 (1954). — PRADER, A.: Der Genitalbefund beim Pseudohermaphroditismus femininus des kongenitalen adrenogenitalen Syndroms. Morphologie, Häufigkeit, Entwicklung und Vererbung der verschiedenen Genitalformen. Helv. paediat. Acta 9, 231 (1954). — SWYER, G. I. M.: Male pseudohermaphroditism, a hitherto undescribed form. Brit. med. J. 1955, ii, 709. — WILKINS, L.: In: Adrenal function in infants and children. Editor L. I. GARDNER. New York: Grune & Stratton 1956. — WILKINS, L., M. M. GRUMBACK, J. J. VAN WYK, T. H. SHEPARD and C. PAPADATOS: Hermaphroditism: classification, diagnosis, selection of sex and treatment. Pediatrics 16, 287 (1955). — WILLIAMS, D. I.: The diagnosis of intersex. Brit. med. J. 1952, i, 1262. — WOLFF, S.: Female pseudohermaphroditism with adrenocortical failure in identical twins. Arch. Dis. Childh. 29, 132 (1954). — ZANDER, J., u. H. A. MÜLLER: Über die Methylandrostendiolbehandlung während einer Schwangerschaft. Geburtsh. u. Frauenheilk. 13, 216 (1953).

III. Male pseudohermaphroditism

CATHIE, I. A. B.: Personal communication. — DANON, M., and L. SACHS: Sex chromoomes and human sexual development. Lancet 1957, ii, 20. — FINESINGER, J. E., J. V. MEIGS and H. W. SULKOWITCH: Clinical, psychiatric and psycho-analytic study of a case of male pseudohermaphrositism. Amer. J. Obstet. Gynec. 44, 310 (1942). — GASPAR, M. R., J. H. KIMBER and K. A. BERKAW: Children with hernias testes, and female external genitalia. Amer. J. Dis. Child. 91, 542 (1956). — HEALEY, C. E., and C. C. GUY: Pseudohermaphroditismus masculinus externus associated with suprarenal hyperplasia and vascular hypertension. Arch. Path. (Chicago) 12, 543 (1931). — KEEN, J. A., and D. P. DE VILLIERS: Intersex in man: report of 3 cases. S. Afr. med. J. 23, 172 (1949). — KOLLER, T.: Eine seltene Beobachtung von Pseudohermaphroditismus masculinus. Schweiz. med. Wschr. 1943, 191. — KOZOLL, D. D.: Pseudohermaphroditsm. Arch. Surg.(Chicago) 45, 578 (1942). — KRÜCKMANN, I.: Intersexualität bei beiderseitigen tubulären Hodenadenomen. Virchows Arch. path. Anat. 298, 619 (1937). — MILLER, J. R.: Testicular tubular adenoma (Pick). Amer. J. Obstet. Gynec. 34, 680 (1937). — MISHELL, D. R.: Familial intersexuality. Amer. J. Obstet. Gynec. 35, 960 (1938). — MORRIS, J. M. L.: The syndrome of testicular feminization in the male pseudohermaphrodite. Amer. J. Obstet. Gynec. 65, 1192 (1953). — NILSON, O.: Hernia uteri masculinus. Acta chir. scand. Stkh. 83, 231 (1939/40). — NOVAK, J.: Testicular tubular adenoma in 2 sisters. Amer. J. Obstet. Gynec. 45, 856 (1943). — PRADER, A., u. H. P. GURTNER: Das Syndrom des Pseudohermaphroditismus masculinus bei kongenitaler Nebennierenrinden-Hyperplasie ohne Androgenüberproduktion (adrenaler Pseudohermaphroditismus masculinus). Helv. paediat. Acta **10**, 397 (1955). — RUBOVITZ, W. H., and W. SAPLIN: Intersexuality. J. Amer. med. Ass. **110**, 1823 (1938). — SCHAUMKELL, K. W., u. H. H. STANGE: Klinische, konstitutionsbiologische und histologische Untersuchungen beim Pseudohermaphroditismus masculinus internus mit totaler Verweiblichung. Z. Gynäk. **78**, 1449 (1956). — SCHOEN, E. J., A. L. KING and W. F. KNIGGE: Pseudohermaphroditism with multiple congenital anomalies. Pediatrics **16**, 363 (1955). — SEGAL, S. J., and W. D. NELSON: Developmental aspects of human hermaphroditism: the significance of sex chromatin patterns. J. clin. Endocr. **17**, 676 (1957). — STERN, O. N., and W. J. VANDERVORT: Testicular feminization in a male pseudohermaphrodite. New Engl. J. Med. **254**, 787 (1956). — VAAL, O. M. DE: Genital intersexuality in three brothers, connected with consanguineous marriages in the three previous generations. Acta paediatr. (Uppsala) **44**, 35 (1955).

IV. True hermaphroditism

ARNEAUD, J. D., H. ANNAMUNTHODO and J. H. M. PINKERTON: A case of true hermaphroditism. Brit. med. J. **1956**, ii, 792. — BARR, M. L.: An interim note on the application of the skin biopsy test of chromosomal sex to hermaphrodites. Surg. Gynec. Obstet. **99**, 184 (1954). — In: Modern trends in obstetrics and gynaecology, Editor K. BOWES, 2. Ser. London: Butterworth & Co. 1955. — BROMWICH, A. F.: True hermaphroditism. Brit. med. J. **1955**, i, 395. — GREENE, R., D. MATTHEWS, P. E. HUGHESDON and A. HOWARD: A case of true hermaphroditism. Brit. J. Surg. **40**, 263 (1953); **41**, 548 (1954) and personal communication. — PRADER, A., R. E. SIEBENMANN u. M. BETTEX: Ein Fall von echtem Hermaphroditismus bei einem Kleinkind. Helv. paediat. Acta **11**, 423 (1956). — SEVERINGHAUS, A. E.: Sex chromosomes in a human intersex. Amer. J. Anat. **70**, 73 (1942). — WILLIAMS, D. I.: The diagnosis of intersex. Brit. med. J. **1952**, i, 1264. — YOUNG, H. H.: Genital abnormalities, hermaphroditism and related adrenal diseases. Baltimore: Williams & Wilkins Company 1957.

VI. Gonadal agenesis

EHRENGUT, W.: Über ovarielle Agenesie. Z. Kinderheilk. **75**, 224 (1954/55). — GRUMBACH, M. M., J. J. VAN WYK and L. WILKINS: Chromosomal sex in gonadal agenesis. J. clin. Endocr. **15**, 1161 (1955). — HORTLING, H.: Congenital kidney anomalies in "Turner's syndrome". Acta endocr. (Kbh.) **18**, 548 (1955). — JOST, A.: Recherches sur le controlle hormonal de l'organogenèse sexuelle du lapin et remarques sur certaines malformations de l'appareil génital humain. Gynéc. et Obstétr. **49**, 44 (1950). — POLANI, P. E., W. F. HUNTER and B. LENNOX: Chromosomal sex in Turner's syndrome with co-arctation of the aorta. Lancet **1954**, ii, 120. — RUSSELL, A., B. LEVIN and N. E. FRANCE: The webbing syndrome (ULLRICH-TURNER) with and without gonadal agenesis. Proc. roy. Soc. Med. **47**, 318 (1954). — SEGAL, S. J., and W. D. NELSON: Developmental aspects of human hermaphroditism: The significance of sex chromatin patterns. J. clin. Endocr. **17**, 676 (1957). — TURNER, H. H.: A syndrome of infantilism, congenital webbed neck and cubitus valgus. Endocrinology **23**, 566 (1938).

VII. Hypogonadism

ALBERT, A., L. O. UNDERDAHL, L. F. GREENE and N. LORENZ: Male hypogonadism: classification. Proc. Mayo Clin. **28**, 557 (1953). — Male hypogonadism: normal testis. Proc. Mayo Clin. **28**, 409 (1953). — The testis in prepubertal or pubertal gonadotropic failure. Proc. Mayo Clin. **29**, 131 (1954). — BAUER, H. G.: Endocrine and other clinical manifestations of hypothalamic disease. J. clin. Endocr. **14**, 13 (1954). — BRUCH, H.: The Froehlich syndrome; report of the original case. Amer. J. Dis. Child. **58**, 1282 (1939). — GILBERT-DREYFUS, J. C., ŠAVOIE et J. SEBAOUN: L'impubérisme hypogonadotrophique masculin. I. Étude clinique biologique et thérapeutique. Sem. Hôp. Paris **32**, 3127/SP, 267/SP, 282 (1956). — GRUMBACH, M. M., W. A. BLANC and E. T. ENGLE: Sex chromatin pattern in seminiferous tubule dysgenesis and other testicular disorder. J. clin. Endocr. **17**, 703 (1957). — HELLER, C. G., and W. O. NELSON: Classification of male hypogonadism and a discussion of the pathologic physiology, diagnosis and treatment. J. clin. Endocr. **8**, 345 (1948). — HOWARD, R. P., R. C. SNIFFEN, F. A. SIMMONS and F. ALBRIGHT: Testicular deficiency: a clinical and pathological study. J. clin. Endocr. **10**, 121 (1950). — JACKSON, W. P. U., B. G. SHAPIRO, C. J. UYS and R. HOFFENBERG: Primary male hypogonadism with female nuclear sex. Lancet **1956**, ii, 857. — KLINEFELTER, H. F., E. C. RIEFENSTEIN and F. ALBRIGHT: Syndrome characterized by gynecomastia, aspermatogenesis with A-leydigism and increased excretion of follicle stimulating hormone. J. clin. Endocr. **2**, 615 (1942). — McCULLAGH, E. P., J. C. BECK and C. A. SHAFFENBURG: A syndrome of eunuchoidism with spermatogenesis: normal urinary F. S. H. and low or normal I. C. S. H. (fertile eunuchs). J. clin. Endocr. **13**, 489 (1953). — PLUNKETT, E. R., and

M. L. BARR: Testicular dysgenesis. Lancet **1956**, ii, 853. — PRADER, A.: Hypogonadismus beim Knaben. Schweiz. med. Wschr. **1955**, 737. — RIIS, P., S. G. JOHNSEN and J. MOSBECH: Nuclear sex in different types of severe male hypogonadism. Lancet **1957**, ii, 167. — ROTH, A. A.: Familial eunuchoidism: the Lawrence-Moon-Biedl syndrome. J. Urol. (Baltimore) **57**, 427 (1947). — SEGALOFF, A., and W. PARSON: Hypogonadotropic eunuchoidism: a report of a case of failure to respond to chronic gonadotropic hormones due to antihormones. J. clin. Endocr. **7**, 130 (1947). — SNIFFEN, R. C., R. P. HOWARD and F. A. SIMMONS: Testis. IV. Idiopathic eunuchoidism with low FSH; testicular changes secondary to lesions in or near the pituitary and secondary to estrogentherapy. Arch. Path. (Chicago) **57**, 464 (1954). — SOHVAL, A. R., and L. J. SOFFER: Congenital testicular deficiency; defective Sertoli cell differentiation in hypogonadism of so-called "obscure origin". J. clin. Endocr. **13**, 408 (1953). — Congenital familial testicular deficiency. Amer. J. Med. **14**, 328 (1953).

VIII. Sexual precocity

ALBRIGHT, F., W. B. SCOVILLE and H. W. SULKOWITCH: Syndrome characterized by osteitis fibrosa disseminata, areas of pigmentation and gonadal dysfunction; further observations including report of 2 more cases. Endocrinology **22**, 411 (1938). — ARLIEN-SØBORG, U., u. T. IVERSEN: Albright's syndrome. Acta paediat. (Uppsala) **45**, 558 (1956). — BOSSELMAN, H.: Intersexuality and suprarenal virilism. Development of the medulla in hyperplastic adrenals. Endocrinologie **19**, 292 (1937). — CHANNICK, B. J., and D. SOKHOS: Androgenic precocity and congenital crebral cortical atrophy. J. Paediat. **49**, 80 (1956). — COHEN, H.: Hyperplasia of the adrenal cortex associated with bilateral testicular tumours. Amer. J. Path **22**, 157 (1946). — CRAVEN, J. D.: Precocious menstruation. Amer. J. Dis. Child. **43**, 936 (1932). ESCOMEL, E.: La plus jeune mère du monde. Presse méd. **1939**, 875. — FALCONER, M. A., and C. L. COPE: Fibrous dysplasia of bone with endocrine disorders and cutaneous pigmentation. Quart. J. Med. **11**, 121 (1942). — FLANNERY, W. E.: Arrhenoblastoma before puberty. Amer. J. Obstet. **60**, 923 (1950). — GARDNER, L. I., R. C. SNIFFEN, A. S. ZYGMUNTOWICZ and N. B. TALBOT: Follow-up studies in a boy with mixed adrenal cortical disease. Pediatrics **5**, 808 (1950). — HAIN, A. M.: Constitutional precocious puberty. J. clin. Endocr. **7**, 171 (1947). — HAMPSON, J. G., and J. MONEY: Idiopathic sexual precocity in the female. Psychosom. Med. **17**, 16 (1955). — JOLLY, H.: Sexual precocity. Springfield, Ill.: Ch. C. Thomas 1955. — KIMMEL, G. C.: Sexual precocity and accelerated growth in a child with follicular cysts of the ovary. J. Pediat. **30**, 686 (1947). — MONEY, J., and J. G. HAMPSON: Idiopathic sexual precocity in the male. Psychosom.Med. **17**, 1 (1955). — NOVAK, E.: The constitutional type of female precocious puberty with a report of 9 cases. Amer. J. Obstet. Gynec. **47**, 20 (1944). — PERLOFF, W. H., and J. H. NODINE: The association of congenital spastic quadriplegia and androgenic precocity in four patients. J. clin. Endocr. **10**, 721 (1950). — RHODEN, A. E.: Precocious sexual and somatic development in a male infant with presacral teratoma containing androgen-producing tissue. J. clin. Endocr. **4**, 185 (1944). — SCHLESINGER, B. E.: Hydrocephalus with precocious puberty following post-basic meningitis. Proc. roy. Soc. Med. **28**, 149 (1934). — SILAGY, J. M.: Precocious puberty. J. Urol. (Baltimore) **70**, 296 (1953). — WEINBERGER, L. M., and F. C. GRANT: Precocious puberty and tumours of the hypothalamus. Arch. intern. Med. **67**, 762 (1941). — WHITTLE, C. H., and A. LYELL: Precocity in a girl aged 5: due to Stilboestrol inunction. Proc. roy. Soc. Med. **41**, 760 (1948). — WILKINS, L.: Diagnosis and treatment of endocrine disorders in childhood and adolescence. Springfield, Ill.: Ch. C. Thomas 1950. — Feminizing and virilizing adrenal tumours. Classification of adrenal disorders. J. clin. Endocr. **8**, 111 (1948).

Author Index

Subject Index